Advances in Animal Disease Diagnosis

Advances in Animal Disease Diagnosis

Edited by
Suresh Kumar Gahlawat, Ph.D.
Sushila Maan, Ph.D.

CRC Press
Taylor & Francis Group
Boca Raton London New York

CRC Press is an imprint of the
Taylor & Francis Group, an **informa** business

First edition published 2021
by CRC Press
6000 Broken Sound Parkway NW, Suite 300, Boca Raton, FL 33487-2742

and by CRC Press
2 Park Square, Milton Park, Abingdon, Oxon OX14 4RN

Library of Congress Cataloging-in-Publication Data
Names: Gahlawat, Suresh Kumar, editor.
Title: Advances in animal disease diagnosis / edited by Suresh Kumar Gahlawat, Ph.D., Sushila Maan, Ph.D.
Description: First edition. | Boca Raton: CRC Press, 2021. | Includes bibliographical references and index.
Identifiers: LCCN 2020057642 | ISBN 9780367530518 (hardback) | ISBN 9781003080282 (ebook)
Subjects: LCSH: Veterinary medicine–Diagnosis.
Classification: LCC SF771 .A38 2021 | DDC 636.089/6075–dc23
LC record available at https://lccn.loc.gov/2020057642

ISBN: 978-0-367-53051-8 (hbk)
ISBN: 978-0-367-53054-9 (pbk)
ISBN: 978-1-003-08028-2 (ebk)

Typeset in Times
by Newgen Publishing UK

Contents

Figures

Preface

Animal health is under constant threat from various dreaded infectious diseases, which result in significant economic losses to livestock owners. Maintenance of good health status of animals relies on early, precise and rapid diagnosis of a range of animal diseases, which largely consist of infectious diseases. Pathogen detection is an important step for diagnostics, the successful treatment of animal diseases and control management in farm and field conditions. The classical and conventional techniques employed to diagnose pathogens in livestock species are time-consuming, labour-intensive and sometimes give inconclusive results.

Recent advances in molecular biology and biotechnology have opened new avenues in disease diagnosis. These advanced molecular techniques of disease diagnosis have the potential to quickly, reliably and unequivocally diagnose known pathogens/conditions as well as having the potential for novel pathogen detection.

Innovative diagnostic methods play an important role in the detection of new and emerging infectious diseases at the interface between animals, humans and their environment, and may facilitate the discovery of new vaccines that bridge human and animal vaccine development (the One Health Concept). The development and delivery of new veterinary vaccines and diagnostic tests is of primary importance in developing technological strategies for the future, and will provide both opportunities and challenges for animal health.

New advances in diagnostics and vaccine design using genomics have provided powerful new methods that have also set the stage for enhanced diagnosis, surveillance and control of infectious diseases. High-throughput sequencing (HTS), for example, uses the latest DNA sequencing platforms in the detection, identification and detailed analysis of both pathogen and host genomes.

The objective of this book is to instil a broad-based knowledge of the modern advanced diagnostic tools of emerging or re-emerging animal diseases, the movement of pathogens of livestock importance and other clinical conditions affecting livestock industry into its users. This knowledge is a necessary prerequisite for the development of accurate diagnosis, therapy and prevention of infectious diseases.

This book primarily addresses students of biotechnology and related fields. Beyond this academic purpose, its usefulness extends to all veterinary professions and most particularly to diagnosticians working in both clinical and private-practice settings.

This book makes the vast and complex field of animal biotechnology more accessible by the use of graphics and illustrations with detailed explanatory legends. The relevant tables present knowledge in a cogent and useful form. Most chapters begin with an abstract followed by in-depth knowledge given in the main body of text. The book is comprised of chapters covering details of molecular diagnostic methods, biosensors, viral pseudotyping, metagenomics and its applications, toll-like receptors (TLRs), the RPA technique, the role of proteomics and metabolomics in different disease diagnosis, imaging techniques in veterinary diagnostics and programmed cell death, as well as focusing on the specific diagnosis of some important infectious diseases (e.g., enteric viruses, foot-and-mouth disease, listeriosis, rotavirus infections, bovine tuberculosis and the SARS-CoV-2 pandemic). One chapter also focuses on the need for uniform guidelines on the patenting of diagnostic methods, and present global rules, regulations and IPR on diagnostic methods.

The authors would like to thank all colleagues whose contributions and advice have been a great help. The authors are also grateful to the editorial assistant, Ms. Jyotsna Jangra, and other staff at Taylor & Francis Books India Pvt. Ltd for their cooperation.

Editors

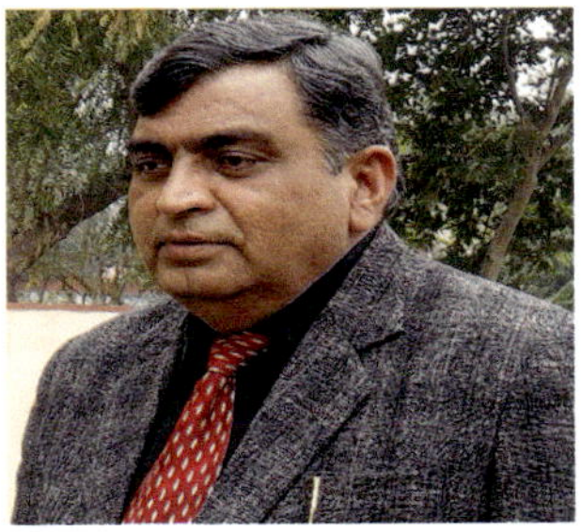

Suresh Kumar Gahlawat

Suresh Kumar Gahlawat is a dedicated teacher with over 26 years of experience, working as Professor of Biotechnology and Dean of Academic Affairs at Chaudhary Devi Lal University, Sirsa, and is the recipient of prestigious fellowships, namely BOYSCASTS and the Biotechnology Overseas Associateship, funded by the Ministry of Science and Technology, Government of India, availed at the FRS Marine Laboratory, Aberdeen, Scotland, in the laboratory of A.E. Ellis and Bertrand Collet. He was appointed as Research Fellow (Honorary) for a period of three months in the School of Biological Sciences by the University of Aberdeen, UK, and has published more than 80 research papers in journals of national and international repute, as well as review articles and book chapters. He has edited seven books, completed four major research projects and supervised 14 M.Phil. and Ph.D. research scholars, as well as having delivered more than 45 invited talks at various academic staff colleges and conferences/seminars in his field of specialisation. During his post-doctoral fellowship he visited several United Kingdom laboratories, including the Centre for Environment, Fisheries and Aquaculture Science (Cefas), Weymouth, the University of Stirling, the Biotechnology and Biologic Sciences Research Council, the Pirbright Institute. During his career he has developed easy and inexpensive methods for the isolation of macrophages; a sensitive, non-destructive method for the detection of IPNV carriers in Atlantic salmon; and a loop-mediated isothermal amplification method for the detection of *Renibacterium salmoninarum*, *Aeromonas hydrophila* and *Pseudomonas florescens*. He has carried out major research work on IPNV carriers; Type-I interferon signaling; expression of interferon and interferon-induced genes; disease diagnosis; probiotics; and nanotechnology on marine/freshwater fish and shellfish species. As an academic administrator, he has served as Dean of Colleges, Dean of Student Welfare, Dean of Research, Dean of the Faculty of Life Sciences, Chairperson of the Department of Biotechnology etc., and has attended several trainings, including the Leadership for Academicians Programme (LeAP-2019) at Aligarh and Monash University, Melbourne, Australia under the MHRD initiative.

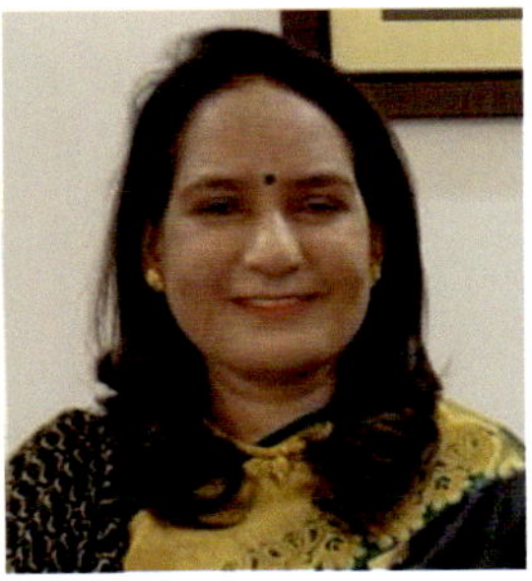

Sushila Maan

Sushila Maan obtained her B.V.Sc. and A.H. (Hons.) and M.V.Sc. (Veterinary Microbiology) degrees with distinction from the College of Veterinary Sciences, Hisar, India. She completed her Ph.D. in Molecular Virology from the Royal Veterinary College, University of London, UK in 2004, under the Commonwealth Scholarship Programme. She was a Post-Doctoral Fellow within the Arbovirus Molecular Research Group at the Institute for Animal Health (IAH), Pirbright, UK from 2006 to 2011.

Sushila Maan led and coordinated an international project funded by BBSRC(UK)-DBT(GOI) under the title "Farmed Animal Disease and Health". She was awarded the prestigious Bio-CARe Fellowship for Women Scientists by the Department of Biotechnology, Government of India, and has been conferred with several awards for her outstanding professional excellence, including becoming a Fellow of the National Academy of Agricultural Sciences (FNAAS) and receiving the ISVIB Scientist Award in 2017, and the LUVAS Best Researcher Award in 2015. During her 25-year research career since 1995, she has published 140 peer-reviewed research articles, of which 81 are in various international journals of repute and 59 in national journals. She has also presented her research findings at several international conferences in the UK, France, Portugal, Italy, the Netherlands, Australia, South Africa, China and the USA. Her work on sequence analyses of bluetongue and other related orbiviruses has revolutionised the genetic studies of these viruses globally. These research findings have led to the development of RT-PCR-based diagnostic kits for molecular detection and the typing of economically important orbiviruses. She has completed seven major research projects and supervised five M.V.Sc projects and a Ph.D student.

She is on the scientific panels (as a referee) of various international and national journals, namely *Virus Research*, *PLOS One*, *Virology*, *Vaccine*, the *Journal of Virology*, *Transboundary and Emerging Diseases*, *Frontiers in Veterinary Science*, *The Lancet* and the *Indian Journal of Virology*, and is also listed as an editorial board member of *The World Scientific Journal*, *Animal and Veterinary Sciences*, *The Haryana Veterinarian* and the *Journal of Veterinary Science and Animal Medicine*.

Contributors

Praveen P. Balgir
Department of Biotechnology
Punjabi University
Patiala-147002, Punjab, India

Meenakshi Balhara
Centre for Biotechnology
Maharshi Dayanand University
Rohtak-124001, Haryana, India

Kanisht Batra
College of Veterinary Sciences
Lala Lajpat Rai University of Veterinary and Animal Sciences (LUVAS)
Hisar-125004, Haryana, India

Sandeep Bhatia
Diagnostic & Vaccine Group
ICAR, National Institute of High Security Animal Diseases
Bhopal-462022, Madhya Pradesh, India

Basanti Brar
Department of Animal Biotechnology
Lala Lajpat Rai University of Veterinary and Animal Sciences (LUVAS)
Hisar-125004, Haryana, India

Barbara Brito Rodriguez
The ithree institute
University of Technology Sydney
Sydney, New South Wales, Australia

Lukumoni Buragohain
Department of Animal Biotechnology
College of Veterinary Science
Assam Agricultural University
Khanapara, Guwahati-781022, Assam, India

Niti Chawla
Department of Biotechnology
Chaudhary Bansi Lal University
Bhiwani-127021, Haryana, India

Anil Kumar Chhillar
Centre for Biotechnology
Maharshi Dayanand University
Rohtak-124001, Haryana, India

Pooja Choudhary
Centre for Biotechnology
Maharshi Dayanand University
Rohtak-124001, Haryana, India

Swati Dahiya
Department of Veterinary Microbiology
Lala Lajpat Rai University of Veterinary and Animal Sciences (LUVAS)
Hisar-125004, Haryana, India

Sweety Dahiya
Centre for Biotechnology
Maharshi Dayanand University
Rohtak-124001, Haryana, India

Mehak Dangi
Centre for Bioinformatics
Maharshi Dayanand University
Rohtak-124001, Haryana, India

P.K. Dubey
Temple University
Philadelphia-19140, Pennsylvania, USA

S. Dubey
Temple University
Philadelphia-19140, Pennsylvania, USA

Neer Gahlawat
O.P. Jindal Global University
Sonepat-131001, Haryana, India

Sarvar Gahlawat
O.P. Jindal Global University
Sonepat-131001, Haryana, India

Suresh Kumar Gahlawat
Department of Biotechnology
Chaudhary Devi Lal University
Sirsa-125055, Haryana, India

Anil Ghanghas
Department of Law
Chaudhary Devi Lal University
Sirsa-125055, Haryana, India

Mayukh Ghosh
Department of Veterinary Physiology and Biochemistry
RGSC, Banaras Hindu University
Mirzapur-231001, Uttar Pradesh, India

Parveen Goel
Department of Veterinary Medicine
College of Veterinary Sciences
Lala Lajpat Rai University of Veterinary and Animal Sciences (LUVAS)
Hisar-125004, Haryana, India

R.S. Kataria
Division of Animal Biotechnology
ICAR, National Bureau of Animal Genetic Resources
Karnal-132001, Haryana, India

Tejinder Kaur
Department of Biotechnology
Punjabi University
Patiala-147002, Punjab, India

Samander Kaushik
Centre for Biotechnology
Maharshi Dayanand University
Rohtak-124001, Haryana, India

Sulochana Kaushik
Department of Genetics
Maharshi Dayanand University
Rohtak-124001, Haryana, India

Aman Kumar
Department of Animal Biotechnology
Lala Lajpat Rai University of Veterinary and Animal Sciences (LUVAS)
Hisar-125004, Haryana, India

Naveen Kumar
Diagnostic & Vaccine Group
ICAR, National Institute of High Security Animal Diseases
Bhopal-462022, Madhya Pradesh, India

Rajesh Kumar
Department of Veterinary Physiology and Biochemistry
Lala Lajpat Rai University of Veterinary and Animal Sciences (LUVAS)
Hisar-125004, Haryana, India

Sandeep Kumar
Department of Veterinary Surgery and Radiology
College of Veterinary Sciences
Lala Lajpat Rai University of Veterinary and Animal Sciences (LUVAS)
Hisar-125004, Haryana, India

Karthik Kumaragurubaran
Centre for Animal Health Studies
Tamil Nadu Veterinary and Animal Sciences University
Madhavaram Milk Colony-600051, Chennai, India

Sushila Maan
College of Veterinary Sciences
Lala Lajpat Rai University of Veterinary and Animal Sciences (LUVAS)
Hisar-125004, Haryana, India

Yashpal Singh Malik
Division of Biological Standardization
ICAR, Indian Veterinary Research Institute
Izatnagar, Bareilly-243122, Uttar Pradesh, India

Jyotsana Mehta
Department of Veterinary Microbiology
Lala Lajpat Rai University of Veterinary and Animal Sciences (LUVAS)
Hisar-125004, Haryana, India

Hari Mohan
Centre for Biotechnology
Maharshi Dayanand University
Rohtak-124001, Haryana, India

Monika
Department of Zoology
Government College Bahadurgarh
Bahadurgarh-124507, Jhajjar, Haryana

Bhuvan Nagpal
Manglam Diagnostics
Hisar-125005, Haryana, India

Aravindh Babu R. Parthiban
Centre for Animal Health Studies
Tamil Nadu Veterinary and Animal Sciences University
Madhavaram Milk Colony-600051, Chennai, India

Harshad Sudhir Patki
Department of Veterinary Anatomy and Histology
College of Veterinary and Animal Sciences
Kerala Veterinary and Animal Sciences University
Pookode-673576, Kerala, India

Asha Poonia
Department of Zoology
Chaudhary Bansi Lal University
Bhiwani-127021, Haryana, India

Minakshi Prasad
Department of Animal Biotechnology
Lala Lajpat Rai University of Veterinary and Animal Sciences (LUVAS)
Hisar-125004, Haryana, India

Aruna Punia
Centre for Biotechnology
Maharshi Dayanand University
Rohtak-124001, Haryana, India

Monika Punia
Department of Biotechnology
Chaudhary Devi Lal University
Sirsa-125055, Haryana, India

Dhinakar Raj Gopal
Centre for Animal Health Studies
Tamil Nadu Veterinary and Animal Sciences University
Madhavaram Milk Colony-600051, Chennai, India

Suman Rani
Department of Biotechnology
Punjabi University
Patiala-147002, Punjab, India

Nidhi Saini
Department of Biotechnology
Chaudhary Devi Lal University
Sirsa-125055, Haryana, India

Anubha Sharma
Department of Animal Biotechnology
Lala Lajpat Rai University of Veterinary and Animal Sciences (LUVAS)
Hisar-125004, Haryana, India

Namita Sharma
Centre for Biotechnology
Maharshi Dayanand University
Rohtak-124001, Haryana, India

Parvati Sharma
Department of Zoology
Chaudhary Bansi Lal University
Bhiwani-127021, Haryana, India

Yashika Sharma
Centre for Biotechnology
Maharshi Dayanand University
Rohtak-124001, Haryana, India

Neelesh Sindhu
Department of Veterinary Medicine
College of Veterinary Sciences
Lala Lajpat Rai University of Veterinary and Animal Sciences (LUVAS)
Hisar-125004, Haryana, India

Renu Singh
College of Veterinary Sciences
Lala Lajpat Rai University of Veterinary and Animal Sciences (LUVAS)
Hisar-125004, Haryana, India

Jaya Parkash Yadav
Department of Genetics
Maharshi Dayanand University
Rohtak-124001, Haryana, India

Abbreviations

ASFV	African swine fever virus
BCoV	bovine coronavirus
BEV	bovine enteric virus
BRD	bovine respiratory disease
CSFV	classical swine fever virus
ELISA	enzyme-linked immunosorbent assay
FAM	carboxyfluorescein
Fpg probe	formamidopyrimidine DNA glycosylase
GNP	gold nanoparticle
HS	haemorrhagic septicaemia
IFN	interferon
LAMP	loop-mediated isothermal amplification
LFD	lateral flow detection
LRR	leucine-rich repeats
MS	mass spectrometry
MSI	mass spectrometry imaging
NA-NOSE	nano artificial NOSE
NMR	nuclear magnetic resonance
PCR	polymerase chain reaction
PCV2	porcine circovirus 2
PRRS	porcine reproductive and respiratory syndrome
PPV	porcine parvovirus
PRRs	pattern recognition receptors
qPCR	(quantitative) real-time polymerase chain reaction
RPA	recombinase polymerase amplification
RT-PCR	reverse-transcription polymerase chain reaction
RT-RAA	reverse-transcription recombinase-aided amplification
RV	rota virus
SARS-CoV-2	severe acute respiratory syndrome coronavirus 2
SDA	strand displacement amplification
SIV	swine influenza A
SSB	single-stranded DNA binding protein
THF	tetrahydrofuran
TLR	toll-like receptors

1

Biosensors: An Advanced System for Infectious Disease Diagnosis

Niti Chawla[1] **and Parvati Sharma**[2]
[1] *Department of Biotechnology, Chaudhary Bansi Lal University, Bhiwani-127021, Haryana, India*
[2] *Department of Zoology, Chaudhary Bansi Lal University, Bhiwani-127021, Haryana, India*
Corresponding author: Parvati Sharma, *parvati.hsr@gmail.com*

1.1 Introduction

A biosensor is defined as a device which can convert signals originating from biological material into detectable electrical signals. "Biosensor" can be divided into two words, "bio" (meaning life) and "sensor" (arising from the Latin *sentire*, which means "to recognize"). The word "sensor" also refers to the concept of the five basic human senses of ophthalmoception (sight), audioception (hearing), gustaoception (taste), olfaction (smell) and tactioception (touch). The senses work on a few basic points: a) sensory cells collect the input signal that comes from external stimuli; b) they send the collected information from external stimuli towards the brain to interpret these signals; c) receptors present in brain respond to these stimuli as per instructions gained from the interoperating center. Thus, the function of the senses can be related to biosensors as they are devices that obtain and give response to stimuli originating from the environment. The senses present in our body respond to external physical stimuli in different ways, such as the sense of hearing responding to acoustic waves, touch to pressure and sight to electromagnetic radiation. In this context, a physical sensor is a gadget which gives a response to a physical property. In the same way, the senses of taste and smell give a response to external chemical stimuli such as the odor, fragrance and particular flavor of certain molecules. In relation to this, a chemical sensor is defined as a gadget that can transform chemical information of a biological system into analytically detectable signals. A sensor contains a specific reacting site that might show a response to a specific sort of analyte that stimulates a chemical reaction at the site of the biological component, at which point these signals are converted into an electrical signal. The electrical signal is further transferred to the processing center to give a detectable response (Yogeswaran and Chen, 2008). The development of biosensors is based on two main components, i.e., synthetic biological agents and cell surface receptors such as enzymes, antibodies, nucleic acids etc. Biosensors have many applications in medical sciences, from the diagnosis of various diseases, such as AIDS, cancer, influenza, hepatitis etc., to food bioanalysis, to the detection of invading sites of microbes in living organisms, heavy metals, harmful chemicals, pesticides or air-borne microorganisms in soil and water. This chapter is dedicated to providing a brief introduction to biosensors and how they help to diagnose infectious diseases in the present scenario.

1.2 Principles of Biosensors

A biosensor is a scientific device which is formed by the combination of biological, physical and chemical components to obtain a powerful signal in the detection of an analyte in order to measure its importance from a biological point of view. Here, biological components act as biosensing components and physicochemical components act as biotransducer components.

The recognition element and the transducing device are the two main components of any kind of sensing platform. In the consideration of biosensors, the recognition element—such as an enzyme, antibody, phage or single-stranded DNA—is a biological component having the capacity of response towards a stimuli, and the transducing device is capable of transforming the response of a biological component or any kind of physicochemical change into a detectable electrical signal (Boeneman *et al.*, 2011; Kazemi-Darsanaki *et al.*, 2013; Dey and Goswami, 2011). The recognition element of a biosensor acts in two ways: a) an affinity biosensor partially or permanently binds with the desired analyte; b) a catalytic biosensor temporarily interacts through a chemical reaction or electron transfer (Boeneman *et al.*, 2011). Cells, tissues, organelles, microbes and enzymes are categories of catalytic sensor, and antibodies, receptors and nucleic acids fall under the category of affinity-type sensors (Hasan *et al.*, 2014).

Biosensors basically have three components:

(i) a recognition element or a detector involving biological structures to recognize the biomolecule and produce a stimulus
(ii) a physical transducer which translates the input signal or stimulus to an output signal or response
(iii) an electronic signal which functions as a processing system to convert an output signal in a presentable form for data representation (Kazemi-Darsanaki *et al.*, 2013)

A *recognition*, *detector* or *bioreceptor* element is the main component of any kind of biosensor because through its use a sensor can produce a selective response towards a specific analyte. Various biomolecular structures, such as enzymes, nucleic acids, antibodies, receptors, bio membranes and living cells, can be used as a detector molecule or bioreceptor in a biosensor.

A *transducer* converts the stimulus that is generated by the detector molecule through the particular biological layer and the analyte into an output signal.

This *output signal* is further measured by using a device such as a light-sensitive and/or electronic mechanism.

Biosensors have great potential in the field of pharmaceuticals and medical diagnostics, with their perfect precision in monitoring disease-specific markers in various experiments held in vivo and in vitro, with the help of the first oxygen biosensor having been developed by Clark and Lyons in 1962. Biosensors are also used in other industries, such as biotechnology, agriculture and food and beverage production, as well as environmental, agricultural and many other biotechnological industries (Nurunnabi *et al.*, 2010). Due to their achievements, there is high demand in the market specifically in the detection of real-time signals of various enzymes, proteins and hormones like glucose, peroxides, lactates, cytokines and antibodies released in different diseases or at the time of tumor formation (Malima *et al.*, 2012). Such biosensors have the ability to measure the desired target molecules in minute quantities and, hence, act as a powerful apparatus to diagnose a disease at its initial level, which is very helpful in the earliest possible initiation of treatment for a particular disease (Giepmans *et al.*, 2006).

1.3 Composition of Biosensors

Biosensing elements are composed of a different biological entity, capable of carrying out specific reactions in which the biological entity combines with a specific group of compounds to create a measurable signal, which is converted by the transducer into a presentable form.

1.3.1 Enzymes

Enzymes, which are widely used in many biosensor studies, are catalysts of various chemical reactions, and as a byproduct of these reactions various compounds are released or generated. These compounds, like hydrogen ions (H^+), hydrogen peroxide (H_2O_2), oxygen (O_2) and carbon dioxide (CO_2), can be easily detected by transducers. The most widely used enzymes in biosensors are glucose oxidase, horseradish peroxidase and alkaline phosphatase, among others.

1.3.2 Microbes

Microbes used as a biosensing mold in the creation of biosensors proved a milestone in the development process. Microbes have various advantages, like their ubiquitous nature, their adaptability to different environmental conditions, their ability to process new molecules either aerobically or anaerobically with the release of different molecules such as NH_4, CO_2, H^+ etc. and the fact that they are more economic than other components as no purification step is required and they are generally less time-consuming to use. With these qualities, microbes are used to find pollutants or pathogens in ecosystems, to exploit hormones, pathogens, toxins and other analytes generated in various disease and to assess biological oxygen demand (BOD) in polluted water.

1.3.3 Cells and Tissues

As a biosensing element cells have various properties, such as the potential to adapt according to their surrounding environmental conditions—like microbes—and their adhesiveness, through which they can immobilize over a matrix surface and adhere to the receptors present on a cell membrane. Cells as biosensors are often used for the duration of treatment of a disease to find out the effect of a drug, its toxicity and different organic derivatives.

Tissues, which are groups of cells, have further advantages over cells and organelles due to their high content of enzymes and their cofactors, and the high reactivity and speed of enzymes working within them. Cells and tissues are useful in the detection of proliferations of cells during tumor formation in cancer, with the help of single-cell resolution using electrochemical impedance biosensors of high density (Kwasny *et al.*, 2011; Arya *et al.*, 2012).

1.3.4 Organelles

A cell has different organelles to carry out specific functions and, thus, organelles can be intended as biosensors of specific analytes. For example, mitochondria, an organelle in a cell with the ability to concentrate calcium, can help to measure calcium in water pollutants (Rizzuto *et al.*, 1999).

1.3.5 Antibodies

The highly selective reaction of antigens and antibodies may enable them to act as immunobiosensors. In immunobiosensors, antibodies are immobilized over the surface of a matrix on the basis of their potential of affinity and covalently combine with transducers with the help of different bonds, like amide (NH_2), esters (-O-) or thiol (-SH-). Antigen–antibody interaction is also dependent upon the orientation of the receptor antibody at the time of immobilization on the surface.

1.3.6 Nucleic Acids

DNA, which is a type of nucleic acid, acts as a suitable candidate for biosensing due to its specificity of base pairing of nucleotides in complementary strands. A nucleic acid biosensor (NAB) is a short single strand of oligo nucleotide that acts as a probe and is immobilized over the platform of the matrix, combining with the transducer to measure the quantity of DNA/RNA in the sample (Palecek, 2002). Such a probe is reusable due to the hybridization property that occurs between probe and sample, which can be regenerated by denaturation (Hong *et al.*, 2013).

1.3.7 Aptamers

Aptamers are derived as a novel frontier to act as a receptor. These are obtained from single-stranded nucleic acid (DNA or RNA) against different biomolecules such as amino acids, proteins and others. Aptamers have the advantage of their stable secondary structure, due to which they can be easily synthesized, and which also helps in their performance. Aptamers bind to particular targets without any discrimination of closely related targets through their selective potency of affinity (Mascini and Tombelli, 2008).

1.4 Classification of Biosensors

Biosensors have been classified on various perspectives; however, they can basically be classified on two aspects: the biorecognition element and signal transduction. Signals are transmuted by transducers, of

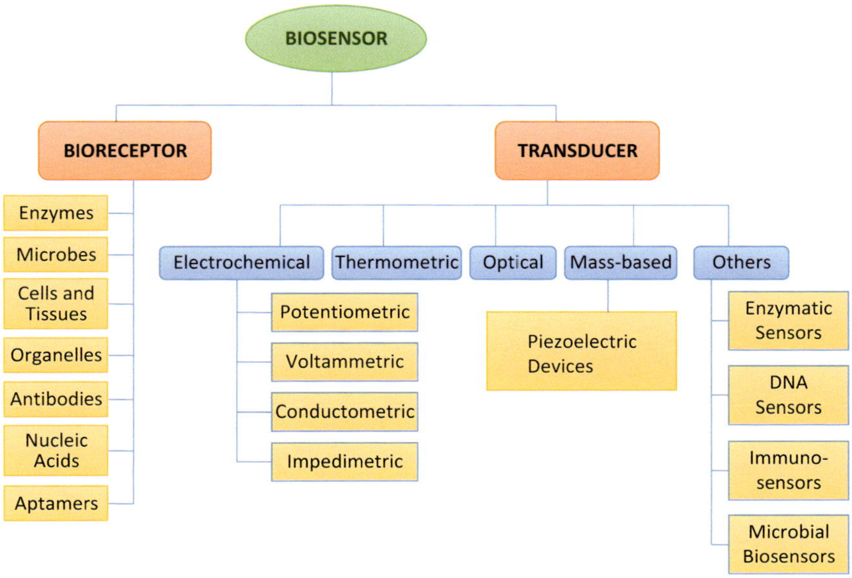

FIGURE 1.1 Biosensors: composition and classification.

which the four basic types are electrochemical transducers, thermometric transducers, optical sensors and mass sensitive sensors (Figure 1.1).

1.4.1 Electrochemical Transducers

Electrochemical transducers are highly sensitive, robust, portable, fast in their detection speed, cost-effective and compatible with modern technologies. These transducers can be distinguished into the various categories given below.

1.4.1.1 Potentiometric Transducers

Potentiometric transducers detect the signals via the potential difference developed between two reference electrodes, or the working electrode and the reference electrode, separated by a semipermeable membrane placed in the electrochemical cell at a zero current. Anion-selective electrodes (ISEs) act as such sensors in order to convert the biological reaction into an electrical signal. A typical example of a potentiometric biosensor is a pH meter. Another example is a urea biosensor, which has been proven to be a valuable tool in detecting urea in milk. There are three types of ion-selective electrode which are used in biosensors, as follows.

(a) A normal pH glass electrode is used for cations in which a very thin hydrated glass membrane acts as a sensing element which generates a transverse electric potential between cations of determined binding sites. The ingredients of glass help to measure the selectivity of this membrane.
(b) A pH electrode of glass is coated with a membrane that is selectively permeable for different gases, such as carbon dioxide (CO_2), ammonia (NH_3) and hydrogen sulphide (H_2S). The pH of the sensing solution changes when gasses pass through the membrane and that change can be measured. The sensing solution lies between the membrane and the electrode, which is then determined.
(c) A thin membrane made up of silver sulphide and allied molecules specific for an ion conductor is used in place of a glass membrane. It is useful in the reaction of peroxidise and cyanide ions.

1.4.1.2 Voltammetric Transducers

Voltammetric transducers measure oxidation or reduction current in electroactive species on the basis of the potential difference between working electrodes, which are referred to as the constant potential electrode and the reference electrode. These sensors responded high current value, low interference and low work potential. The final output of such a transducer is in the form of current that is equivalent to either the concentration of electroactive species, or perhaps to the rate of their disappearance (Hasan *et al.*, 2014). A stripping voltammetry measurement of Pb(II), Clark-type oxygen electrode and oxygen sensor based on nanoporous gold are some examples of this type.

1.4.1.3 Conductometric Transducers

Conductometric transducers are based on the measurement of the electrical conductivity of a solution that occurs during a biochemical reaction, because most enzymatic reactions involve either consumption or release of actively charged species. These enzymatic reactions create a global change in the ionic composition of the desired samples. They are not very common as biosensors, especially in cases when enzyme is used as recognition element (Hasan *et al.*, 2014). These transducers have various advantages, as follows.

(a) No reference electrode is required.
(b) They are not light-sensitive.
(c) Power consumption is low.
(d) A thin film of electrode is sufficient for minute measurements.
(e) They are not expensive.
(f) A large spectrum of various compounds can be obtained on the basis of different reaction and mechanisms.

1.4.1.4 Impedimetric Transducers

Impedimetric transducers are based on the measurement of the variation of impedance with AC frequency in an electrochemical cell (Lang *et al.*, 2007). The high sensitivity and rapid response of this technique makes it useful in the detection of biological interaction with biosensor platforms. Bacteria detection can be measured in two ways: first, by the detection of metabolites produced by bacterial growth which are responsible for the media conductivity changes. Second, selective bacterial response can be measured by the immobilization of bacteria on a sensor platform using various bioreceptors such as antibodies, aptamers and the recorded changes produced in charge transfer resistance or interfacial impedance (Hasan *et al.*, 2014). This system helps in the detection of pathogens and gives an indication of microorganisms in food and water samples, which plays a vital role in public as well as environment health.

1.4.2 Thermometric Transducers

Thermometric transducers are related to temperature and convert thermal energy into physical energy such as mechanical energy, electrical signals etc. These transducers are mainly used for the detection of temperature and heat flow. They consist of a sensing element which alters its properties with changes in temperature. An example is a resistance thermometer in which platinum metal acts as a sensing element, measuring the quantity of heat with a highly sensitive thermal resistor to calculate the analyte concentration. A thermocouple is another example of this type of sensing element, which creates electrical potential difference across its terminals. A thermocouple basically consists of two terminals of dissimilar metals such as copper and constantan; with both metals at different temperatures, a difference of voltage that is developed across the terminals is used to measure the temperature. However, such thermal biosensors are not common.

1.4.3 Optical Transducers

Optical transducers convert light rays into electrical signals. They measure the physical quantity of light and translate it into an electrical signal that can read by an integrated measuring device. These are also known as photo electric transducers. They may be based on light-emitting sources like fluorescence, luminescence, light scattering spectroscopy absorption, internal reflection or surface plasmon resonance. Such a technique is used to determine the levels of casein in milk, with the development of localized surface plasmon resonance on gold nanoparticles (Shao *et al.*, 2010). Several optical devices have been developed and applied successfully in the detection of cancer, arthritis, cardiovascular disease, viral infection, neurodegenerative disease and metastasis, and are helpful in monitoring disease progression and therapy response.

1.4.4 Piezoelectric Devices

Piezoelectric devices (mass-based devices) are based on the electric potential that is generated via elastic deformation of crystals due to changes in potential at a specific frequency. Piezoelectric sensors use the piezoelectric effect to explore physical parameters like temperature, force, acceleration or strain by their few measurable modifications. The piezoelectric effect is the ability of the piezoelectric material to convert applied mechanical pressure into a directly proportional electrical change. Alternation of the resonance frequency is an indication of binding between analyte and the crystal. Here, the crystal is covered with a biological element where analyte adsorption takes place. Recently, piezoelectric immunosensors have been used to detect very small amounts of antigens in a pictogram, so this device is among the most sensitive sensors.

1.4.5 Other Biosensors

Other types of biosensors may include enzymatic biosensors, DNA biosensors, immunobiosensors and microbial biosensors.

1.4.5.1 Enzymatic Sensors

Enzyme-based sensors include highly specific and selective enzyme molecules as recognition elements which are immobilized on transducing surfaces known as electrodes (Boeneman *et al.*, 2011; Monteiro and Almeida *et al.*, 2018). These enzymes catalyze electrochemical reactions that involve electroactive products on the transducer and the sample under the presence of a suitable substrate at measurable electric changes (Zhu *et al.*, 2015; Monteiro and Almeida *et al.*, 2018). The concentration of an analyte in a tested sample can be measured through its current, potential and charge by the use of different techniques, such as amperometric, potentiometric and impedimetric techniques, respectively (Pineda *et al.* 2014; Kurbanoglu *et al.*, 2017; Rocchitta *et al.*, 2016). The amperometric technique is the most appropriate method to detect the transduction of the enzymatic response into a quantifiable signal (Pineda *et al.* 2014).

On the basis of their functions, enzymatic sensors can be further divided into two categories.

1.4.5.1.1 Substrate Biosensors

Substrate biosensors are used to determine the specific substrates of enzymatic reactions. For example, a glucose oxidase-based enzymatic sensor is used to determine glucose, and a urease sensor is used for urea determination (Liu *et al.*, 2012; Nejadnik *et al.*, 2011). These two are the most commonly used biosensors.

1.4.5.1.2 Inhibitor Biosensors

Inhibitor biosensors are capable of determining substances which reduce the action of an enzyme. The determination of organophosphorus pesticides by the use of enzyme acetylcholinesterase, which inhibits acetylcholine hydrolysis, is the best example of an inhibitor biosensor (Brondani *et al.*, 2009).

1.4.5.2 Immunosensors

Immunosensors are based on immunoglobins. Immunoglobins are antibodies secreted by the immune system of an organism in response to foreign biological compounds (antigens) and these are employed in the case of immunobiosensors as biochemical receptors.

1.4.5.3 DNA Sensors

DNA sensors include nucleic acids (DNA) and their fragments like DNA probes or DNA primers. DNA sensors can be further revised or improved to increase their stability and they can also be used as biosensors. The sequence of oligonucleotides that is used in DNA biosensors is selective to the interaction with assured biomolecules. These synthetic nucleic receptors are known as aptamers or apta sensors (Liu *et al.*, 2010; Kang *et al.*, 2009). DNA sensors are mostly used to determine the nucleotide sequence in a desired DNA molecule, which has a complementary sequence to the probes, making such sensors helpful in consistently diagnosing pathogenic microorganisms such as bacteria, viruses and fungi causing different diseases as well as in detecting genetic diseases (Kang *et al.*, 2009).

1.4.5.4 Microbial Biosensors

Microbial biosensors are basically dependent upon the response of microorganisms due to alterations in the chemical composition of a microbial growth culture. A microbial biosensor is immersed in a suspension of microbial culture to detect the state of natural communities of microbes. Such a biosensor may be in the form of a column or membrane reactor (Heath, 2007). Microbial biosensors are mostly utilized in toxin determination systems, which are based on the inhibition of luciferase enzyme activity of luminescence at the time of oxidation in some analytes (Strehlitz *et al.*, 1999; Dolatabadi and Manjulakumari *et al.*, 2012; Chen *et al.*, 2012). They are also used to detect the effect of substances on a cell as a part of a multicellular organism and are also useful in observing the action of biological wastewater treatment systems.

1.5 Biosensors in Diagnosis of Infectious Diseases

Infectious diseases are the prominent cause of death of humans and animals worldwide. Their causative agents are bacteria, viruses, fungi, protozoans etc. The principle factor in the management of these diseases is their early and real-time diagnosis, which cannot be achieved with traditional diagnostic approaches. Therefore, researchers have developed innovative diagnostic tools called "biosensors". In the short span of time since their development, they have become very attractive due to their rapidity, efficiency, sensitivity, simplicity and potential ability for real-time analysis. Below, we describe some of the biosensors recently developed for different infectious diseases.

1.5.1 Acquired Immunodeficiency Syndrome (AIDS)

The causative agent of AIDS is a lentivirus named "human immunodeficiency virus" (HIV), which is actually a subtype of retrovirus. It continues to be a major health problem globally. According to World Health Organization statistics (UNAIDS, 2018), 37.9 million people were living and 7.7 million people died with AIDS worldwide in 2018. Although there are several serological tests available to diagnose HIV, one challenge yet unresolved is diagnosis of the disease at all stages of infection, especially at the early stage, so that it can be successfully treated. Besides that, other problems, such as cross-reactivity, high cost, non-discrimination between HIV-1 and HIV-2 etc., are also associated with conventional diagnostic approaches. To overcome these challenges, several researchers have developed various biosensors, which differ in their sensitivity and accuracy. These biosensors are either based on viral markers such as p24, p17, Tat proteins, CD4+ cells, HIV genes, HIV-1 virus-like particles, enzymes related to HIV etc., or immune markers such as antibodies made against HIV in a patient's body. The detection ultimately measures the progress of the disease or its reaction to the antiviral therapy given to the patient. Below, some of the recently developed advanced biosensors for HIV detection are described.

In 2019, Shamsipur and his coworkers designed a nanotechnology-based biosensor, consisting of a specific polymer film of p-aminobenzoic acid (PABA) between two graphene oxide sub-layers which were electrochemically reduced, with gold nanoparticles as the interfacial layers. This design improved the electrical properties of the surface, which ultimately transduced the signal of binding of the HIV-1 gene and thus detected it at sub-femtomolar level. Besides this, the biosensor was able to operate without any amplification step, capable of producing a repetitive signal and also could maintain its stability during the extensive incubation and detection procedures. It could evaluate a DNA target over a wide concentration range, i.e., from 0.1 fM to 10 nM, with the maximum detection limit of 37 aM.

Similarly, Xiao *et al.* (2019) developed a biosensor consisting of fluorescent immune-chromatographic strips that could detect the disease indirectly by measuring those CD4 antibodies which were not attached with CD4 cells. Actually, the fluorescently labelled antibody-CD4 cell conjugates were blocked by the filter pads that reduced the fluorescence of free CD4 antibodies measured. Thus, the biosensor was based on the inverse relationship between CD4 cells and the fluorescence intensity. The advantages of this biosensor were its rapidity, simple design, accuracy and low expense.

A biosensor for HIV detection was also developed earlier in 2018 by Zhang and his coworkers, based on the detection of HIV-1 protease. They prepared a fluorescence biosensing platform of graphene oxide on which fluorescent-labeled HIV-1 protease could link covalently. It was a rapid, sensitive and accurate biosensor in the detection of HIV-1 protease, successfully detecting as little as 1.18 nanogram/ml of HIV-1 protease.

Another nanobased biosensor for HIV-1 gene detection was developed by Babamiri *et al.* (2018), consisting of a molecularly imprinted polymer electrochemiluminescent sensor that used europium sulfide nanocrystals as a signal-producing compound. With this efficient biosensor, a maximum detection limit of 0.3 fM for HIV gene detection was achieved.

Further, Li *et al.* (2018) developed a mobile phone-mediated biosensor for the detection of HIV p24 antigens. A sandwich immunoassay was performed using covalently immobilized antibodies against p24 antigens on the surface of micro-pits. An image was captured using a mobile phone, which was further analyzed using a computer. This biosensor attained maximum detection limits of 190 pg/ml in buffer and 650 pg/ml in human serum, respectively. Its low cost and easy operation were its main advantages.

Diao *et al.* (2018) also developed another surface plasmon resonance-based biosensor capable of detecting HIV DNA. The principle reaction involved the displacement of a DNA strand leading to the development of DNA tetrahedrons. The biosensor attained a detection limit of 48 fM DNA.

Recently, Zou *et al.* (2019) developed a label-free fluorescent platform based on DNA-stabilized silver nanoclusters for simultaneously detecting two HIV DNAs. That platform was based on enhancement of fluorescence and could detect both HIV-1 and HIV-2 genes. The probe silver nanoclusters/guanine-rich sequence utilized for HIV-1 detection generated a fluorescence signal at 500 nm ex/565 nm em, while the probe silver nanoclusters/silver nanoclusters detected HIV-2 gene-generated fluorescence signals at 580 nm ex/630 nm em, respectively. Moreover, this was the first instance of the simultaneous detection of two HIV DNAs which achieved a maximum detection limit of 11 pM.

1.5.2 Ebola Virus Disease

The Ebola virus belongs to the family *Filoviridae* and causes a rare and lethal disease called the Ebola virus disease. The Ebola virus was transmitted to humans from wild animals and is now capable of transmission from human to human. Several outbreaks have occurred all around the world in the last 40 years since the virus was first observed in 1976. For the diagnosis of the Ebola virus disease, the traditional and most common method is the use of a polymerase chain reaction. However, for this method the virus must be present in a great enough quantity in the blood. To overcome this drawback, Baca *et al.* (2015) developed a surface acoustic wave biosensor for the detection of antigens. This biosensor worked in the concentration-dependent manner, with the potential to detect Ebola viremia prior to the onset of symptoms; it could also detect the virus at low numbers, greatly improving infection control and rapid treatment of the disease.

Similar to this, Tsang *et al.* (2016) developed a nanoparticles-based ultrasensitive system for the early detection of the Ebola virus. This system comprised of a combination of up-conversion nanoparticles linked with an oligonucleotide probe and gold nanoparticles on a nanoporous alumina membrane, linked with target Ebola virus oligonucleotide. A detection limit was achieved up to femtomolar level with this biosensor.

1.5.3 Zika Virus Disease

The Zika virus is a mosquito-borne flavivirus. Till now, several outbreaks of this virus have been faced by many countries. To date, about 86 countries have reported cases of infection. The diagnostic tools most commonly used for Zika infection are RT-PCR, ELISA etc. However, these tools are insufficient due to the nonspecific clinical features of infection with Zika. Laboratory diagnosis is also challenging because of low viremia and cross-reactivity of Zika antibodies with other flaviviruses such as dengue virus, which require confirmation by neutralization assays and thus take lot of time. Advanced research has developed biosensors as innovative tools.

Recently, Chompoonuch Tancharoen *et al.* (2019) prepared an electrochemical biosensor based on a combination of surface-imprinted polymers and graphene oxide for Zika virus detection. The biosensor attained a detection limit similar to the detection limit of the RT-PCR method.

1.5.4 Influenza

Le *et al.* (2014) prepared a biosensor comprised of RNA aptamers specific against different strains of human influenza viruses. These aptamers could assemble onto gold nanoparticles and form gold nanoshells around the viral envelope of gold nanoparticle-coated viruses that were observed by transmission electron microscopy. Visual determination could detect 3×10^8 viral particles.

Krishna *et al.* (2016) developed a giant magneto resistance nano-based biosensor for the detection of the influenza A virus. In it, the influenza virus allowed the interaction of magnetic nanoparticles with the biosensor, which was directly proportional to the concentration of the virus. The biosensor detected as low as 1.5×10^2 TCID50/mL virus and the signal intensity increased with increasing concentration of the virus, up to 1.0×10^5 TCID50/ml.

1.5.5 Hepatitis

Different strains of the hepatitis virus (HAV-HGV) are responsible for causing hepatitis. Giamblanco *et al.* (2015) developed a piezoelectric biosensor which could detect the hepatitis B virus. This biosensor worked on the principle of hybridization between the hepatitis B viral genome and ssDNA probes immobilized on the gold surfaces of a quartz crystal microbalance resonator. This method could be used without amplification or a labelling step and could detect fmol cm^{-2} of the HBV target.

1.5.6 Dengue Fever

Dengue fever is a vector-borne infectious disease, caused by the Dengue virus. It is a major disease that is responsible for killing many people in the world every year. During primary infection not many symptoms are displayed, but later on, if not treated properly, the virus can cause damage to the internal organs and death. Thus, a technique enabling the early detection of the dengue virus could reduce the number of deaths. In view of that, Navakul *et al.* (2017) designed a biosensor based on electrochemical impedance spectroscopy for the early detection of the dengue virus. They prepared a graphene oxide-coated gold electrode; when exposed to viruses, the resistance to transfer of charge varied with type and quantity of viruses. A maximum detection limit of 0.12 pfu/ml was attained with it.

1.5.7 Salmonellosis

Liu *et al.* (2019) prepared a microfluidic biosensor based on impedance for the rapid detection of Salmonella serotypes B and D. This biosensor was capable of detecting even a very low number of cells, i.e., 300 per ml of the sample, within a one-hour detection time.

Similarly, Yongkang *et al.* (2019) developed an electrochemical nano-based genosensor to detect the Salmonella invA gene. It comprised of a polyrole-reduced graphene oxide-layered carbon electrode coated with nanocomposite and horseradish peroxidase-streptavidin bio-functionalized gold nanoparticles (AuNPs-HRP-SA) for signal amplification. Amplification was achieved by reduction of hydrogen peroxide in the presence of hydroquinone using AuNPs-HRP-SA as a nanotag. A limit of detection of the invA gene of 4.7×10^{-17} M was achieved.

1.5.8 Shigellosis

Shigellosis, or bacillary dysentery, is an infectious disease caused by *Shigella* spp. It is a health problem of concern because it is responsible for considerable morbidity and mortality globally per year. Polymerase chain reaction-based techniques are normally used in its detection. Wang *et al.* (2016) developed a simple, rapidly detecting instrument-free biosensor technique for the detection of *Shigella*. This biosensor was based on a combination of multiple cross-displacement amplification and lateral flow biosensors that were capable of visual detection of the pathogen. The detection limit of the assay was 10 fg of genomic templates per reaction in pure culture and 5.86 CFU/tube in human fecal samples.

1.5.9 Tuberculosis

Tuberculosis (TB) is a serious infectious disease caused by the bacterium *Mycobacterium tuberculosis*. It has become a major health concern all around the world due to its high morbidity and mortality rates. Its fatality can also be realized from the data estimated by World Health Organization, according to which a total of 1.5 million people died due to it in 2018. A suitable detection procedure can control this fatal disease, and in view of this, Diouani *et al.* (2017) prepared an electrochemical immune biosensor for its detection that was based on the detection of early secreted antigenic target ESAT-6 proteins that interact with anti-ESAT-6 monoclonal antibodies that were used as the bioreceptor. A maximum detection limit of 7 ng/ml was achieved.

1.5.10 Food-borne Diseases Caused by *Enterococcus faecalis* and *Staphylococcus aureus*

Enterococcus faecalis and *Staphylococcus aureus* are common food-borne pathogens. For their efficient detection, Wang *et al.* (2017b) designed a biosensor based on multiple-loop-mediated isothermal amplification that was capable of detecting the pathogen visually. The detection was based on differentiation between two genes, i.e., Ef0027 and the nuc gene specific to *Enterococcus faecalis* and *Staphylococcus aureus*, respectively.

1.5.11 Listerosis

Listerosis is a serious food-borne infection caused by *Listeria monocytogenes* in both humans and animals. It is a rare disease and cases are few in number, i.e., 0.1–10 cases per 1 million people per year. However, its high rate of mortality makes it a matter of concern. A rapid and efficient detection technique enables the control of disease. To that end, Wang *et al.* (2017a) developed a free gold nanoparticles-based lateral flow biosensor for the detection of *L. monocytogenes*. It could detect 10 fg of genomic DNA templates per reaction in pure culture and could also successfully be applied to detecting *L. monocytogenes* in pork samples.

1.5.12 Leishmaniasis

Leishmaniasis is a parasitic disease caused by a protozoan of *Leishmania* sp. which is transmitted by sand flies, and is a matter of concern especially in developing countries. According to the World Health Organization, around 1 million new cases occur annually. The major risk factors that enhance the chances of the disease are poverty, malnutrition, population mobility, climate change etc. Traditionally, rapid diagnostic tests are in use for the diagnosis of the disease. Sometimes, Chagas fever caused by *Trypanosoma cruzi* gives a false-positive result for Leishmaniasis. Thus, a more reliable and faster diagnostic system should be developed for the safe and effective treatment of the disease.

In view of that, Perinote *et al.* (2010) prepared a nanotechnology-based biosensor capable of distinguishing between cutaneous leishmaniasis and Chagas disease by using an impedence spectroscopy method of detection. The biosensor comprised of nanoparticle-coated films containing antigens of *Leishmania amazonensis* and *Trypanosoma cruzi*. Results were obtained by statistically correlating the antigen-antibody interactions with the electrical impedence.

Recently, Diouani *et al.* (2019) designed a biosensor based on the interaction between casein and GP63 (a major surface protease of the *Leishmania*). This biosensor could detect with a limit of less than 1 parasite/ml of the sample.

1.6 Future Perspectives

Biosensors have been designed specifically to detect certain targets, such as genes, proteins, aptamers, antigens etc. These elements are connected with a transducing element that produces a direct signal when the target is sensed. Since the development of biosensors around 50 years ago, several biosensors have been designed by the researchers so far. These are providing excellent response in the diagnosis of infectious diseases but the use of most is confined to the research level. In the near future, we can likely expect the emergence of more biosensors that will assist us in gaining control over deadly infectious diseases by their timely detection. Thus, there is a strong necessity to develop more biosensors to control the diseases. There is also a need for improvement or refinement of the features of the biosensors. Future biosensors should be easy to handle, transportable, small in size, more powerful, more sensitive and also operable against many targets. Besides these features, one more essential area is to develop the biosensors based on advanced and new technologies such as nanotechnology, microfluidics etc. As we are also aware of infectious diseases, most of which have the potential for transmission and the occurrence of outbreaks, lethality etc., so the availability of strong diagnosis methods, especially based on advanced technologies, is crucial for the diagnosis of deadly infectious diseases.

1.7 Conclusion

We described here the basic principles, structures, techniques and types of biosensors. We expect that this chapter will be helpful in acquiring a detailed understanding of the biosensors and that it brings most of the biosensors developed for the control of infectious diseases together. Thereafter, we summarized the applicability of these biosensors in the diagnosis of different infectious diseases, which have become a major global concern, posing a threat to human life and existence on earth. Conventional diagnostic approaches are time-consuming, labor-intensive and demand the use of sophisticated equipment. But biosensors have many useful features when compared to conventional methods. They are sensitive, specific, fast, operable in real time and have made possible the early or timely detection of deadly diseases. They may therefore be considered a boon to the medical field and are expected to solve many of the problems associated with achieving a healthy life.

References

Arya, S.K., Lee, K.C., Bin Dah'alan, D. and Rahman, A.R.A., "Breast tumor cell detection at single cell resolution using an electrochemical impedance technique," *Lab on a Chip*, vol. 12, no. 13, pp. 2362–2368, 2012.

Babamiri, B., Salimi, A. and Hallaj, R.A., "Molecularly imprinted electro chemiluminescence sensor for ultrasensitive HIV-1 gene detection using EuS nanocrystals as luminophore," *Biosensors and Bioelectronics*, vol. 117, pp. 332–339, 2018.

Baca, J.T., Severns, V. and Lovato, D. *et al.*, "Rapid detection of Ebola virus with a reagent-free, point-of-care biosensor," *Sensors*, vol. 15, pp. 8605–8614, 2015.

Boeneman, K., Delehanty, J.B., Susumu, K., Stewart, M.H., Deschamps, J.R. and Medintz, I.L., "Quantum dots and fluorescent protein FRET-based biosensors," *Advances in Experimental Medicine and Biology*, vol. 733, pp. 63–74, 2011.

Brondani, D., Scheeren, C.W., Dupont, J. and Vieira, I.C., "Biosensor based on platinum nanoparticles dispersed in ionic liquid and laccase for determination of adrenaline," *Sensors and Actuators B: Chemical*, vol. 140, pp. 252–259, 2009.

Chen, Z., Lu, M., Zou, D. and Wang, H., "An E. coli SOS-EGFP biosensor for fast and sensitive detection of DNA damaging agents," *Journal of Environmental Sciences*, vol. 24, no. 3, pp. 541–549, 2012.

Chompoonuch, T., Sukjee, W. and Thepparit, C. *et al.*, "Electrochemical biosensor based on surface imprinting for Zika virus detection in serum," *ACS Sensors*, vol. 4, no. 1, pp. 69–75, 2019.

Clark L.C. and Lyons, C., "Electrode system for continuous monitoring cardiovascular surgery," *Annales Academiae Scientiarum Fennicae Mathematica*, vol. 102, pp. 29–45, 1962.

Dey, D. and Goswami, T., "Optical biosensors: a revolution towards quantum nanoscale electronics device fabrication," *Journal of Biomedicine and Biotechnology*, 2011, article ID 348218.

Diao, W., Tang, M. and Ding, S. *et al.*, "Highly sensitive surface plasmon resonance biosensor for the detection of HIV-related DNA based on dynamic and structural DNA nanodevices," *Biosensors and Bioelectronics*, vol. 100, pp. 228–234, 2018.

Diouani, M.F., Ouerghi, O. and Refai, A. *et al.*, "Detection of ESAT-6 by a label free miniature immuno-electrochemical biosensor as a diagnostic tool for tuberculosis," *Materials Science and Engineering C*, vol. 74, pp. 465–470, 2017.

Diouani, M.F., Ouerghi, O. and Belgacem, K. *et al.*, "Casein-conjugated gold nanoparticles for amperometric detection of Leishmania infantum," *Biosensors*, vol. 9, p. 68, 2019.

Dolatabadi, S. and Manjulakumari, D., "Microbial biosensors and bioelectronics," *Research Journal of Biotechnology*, vol. 7, no. 3, pp. 102–108, 2012.

Giamblanco, N., Conoci, S. and Russo, D. *et al.*, "Single-step label-free hepatitis virus detection by a piezoelectric biosensor," *RSC Advances*, vol. 5, pp. 38152–38158, 2015.

Giepmans, B.N.G., Adams, S.R., Ellisman, M.H. and Tsien, R.Y., "The fluorescent toolbox for assessing protein location and function," *Science*, vol. 312, no. 5771, pp. 217–224, 2006.

Hasan, A., Memic, A. and Annabi, N. *et al.*, "Electro spun scaffolds for tissue engineering of vascular grafts," *Acta Biomaterialia*, vol. 10, no. 1, pp. 11–25, 2014.

Hasan, A., Nurunnabi, M. and Morshed, M. *et al.*, "Recent advances in application of biosensors in tissue engineering," *BioMed Research International*, vol. 2014, article ID 307519, 2014.

Heath, J.R., "Label-free nanowire and nanotube biomolecular sensors for in-vitro diagnosis of cancer and other diseases," in C.A. Mirkin and C.M. Niemeyer (eds), *Nanobiotechnology II: More Concepts and Applications*, John Wiley & Sons, Hoboken, NJ, 2007.

Hong, C.Y., Chen, X. and Liu, T. *et al.*, "Ultra-sensitive electrochemical detection of cancer-associated circulating microRNA in serum samples based on DNA concatamers," *Biosensors and Bioelectronics*, vol. 50, pp. 132–136, 2013.

Kang, X., Wang, J., Wu, H., Aksay, I.A., Liu, J. and Lin, Y., "Glucose oxidase-graphene-chitosan modified electrode for direct electrochemistry and glucose sensing," *Biosensors and Bioelectronics*, vol. 25, no. 4, pp. 901–905, 2009.

Kazemi-Darsanaki, R., Azizzadeh, A., Nourbakhsh, M., Raeisi, G. and Azizollahi Aliabadi, M., "Biosensors: functions and applications," *Journal of Biology and Today's World*, vol. 2, no. 1, pp. 20–23, 2013.

Krishna, V.D., Wu, K. and Perez, A.M. *et al.*, "Giant magnetoresistance-based biosensor for detection of influenza A virus," *Frontiers in Microbiology*, vol. 7, pp. 1–8, 2016.

Kurbanoglu, S., Ozkan, S.A. and Merkoçi, A., "Nanomaterials-based enzyme electrochemical biosensors operating through inhibition for biosensing applications," *Biosensors and Bioelectronics*, vol. 89, pp. 886–898, 2017.

Kwasny, D., Kiilerich-Pedersen, K., Moresco, J., Dimaki, M., Rozlosnik, N. and Svendsen, W.E., "Microfluidic device to study cell transmigration under physiological shear stress conditions," *Biomedical Microdevices*, vol. 13, no. 5, pp. 899–907, 2011.

Lang, H.P., Hegner, M. and Gerber, C., "Cantil ever array sensors for bioanalysis and diagnostics," in C.A. Mirkin and C.M. Niemeyer (eds), *Nanobiotechnology II: More Concepts and Applications*, John Wiley & Sons, Hoboken, NJ, 2007.

Le, T.T., Adamiak, B. and Benton, D.J. *et al.*, "Aptamer-based biosensors for the rapid visual detection of flu viruses," *Chemical Communications*, vol. 50, no. 98, pp. 15533–15536, 2014.

Li, F., Li, H. and Wang, Z. *et al.*, "Mobile phone mediated point-of-care testing of HIV p24 antigen through plastic micro-pit array chips," *Sensors and Actuators B: Chemical*, vol. 271, pp. 189–194, 2018.

Liu, J., Jasim, I. and Shen, Z. *et al.*, "A microfluidic-based biosensor for rapid detection of Salmonella in food products," *PLoS One*, vol. 14, no. 5, e0216873, 2019.

Liu, Y., Matharu, Z., Howland, M.C., Revzin, A. and Simonian, A.L., "Affinity and enzyme-based biosensors: recent advances and emerging applications in cell analysis and point-of-care testing," *Analytical and Bioanalytical Chemistry*, vol. 404, no. 4, pp. 1181–1196, 2012.

Liu, Y., Yu, D., Zeng, C., Miao, Z. and Dai, L., "Biocompatible graphene oxide-based glucose biosensors," *Langmuir*, vol. 26, no. 9, pp. 6158–6160, 2010.

Malima, A., Siavoshi, S. and Musacchio, T. *et al.*, "Highly sensitive microscale in vivo sensor enabled by electrophoretic assembly of nanoparticles for multiple biomarker detection," *Lab on a Chip*, vol. 12, no. 22, pp. 4748–4754, 2012.

Mascini, M. and Tombelli, S., "Biosensors for biomarkers in medical diagnostics," *Biomarkers*, vol. 13, no. 7–8, pp. 637–657, 2008.

Monteiro, T. and Almeida, M.G., "Electrochemical enzyme biosensors revisited: old solutions for new problems," *Critical Reviews in Analytical Chemistry*, vol. 49, no. 1, pp. 1–23, 2019.

Navakul, K., Warakulwit, C. and Yenchitsomanus, P.T. *et al.*, "A novel method for dengue virus detection and antibody screening using a graphene-polymer based electrochemical biosensor," *Nanomedicine*, vol. 13, no. 2, pp. 549–557, 2017.

Nejadnik, M.R., Deepak, F.L. and Garcia, C.D., "Adsorption of glucoseoxidase to 3-scaffolds of carbon nanotubes: analytical applications," *Electroanalysis*, vol. 23, no. 6, pp. 1462–1469, 2011.

Nurunnabi, M., Cho, K.J., Choi, J.S., Huh, K.M. and Lee, Y.K., "Targeted near-IRQDs-loaded micelles for cancer therapy and imaging," *Biomaterials*, vol. 31, no. 20, pp. 5436–5444, 2010.

Palecek, E., "Past, present and future of nucleic acids electrochemistry," *Talanta*, vol. 56, no. 5, pp. 809–819, 2002.

Perinote, A.C., Maki, R.M. and Cothone, M.C. *et al.*, "Biosensors for efficient diagnosis of leishmaniasis: innovations in bioanalytics for a neglected disease," *Analytical Chemistry*, vol. 82, no. 23, pp. 9763–9768, 2010.

Pineda, S., Han, Z.J. and Ostrikov, K., "Plasma-enabled carbon nanostructures for early diagnosis of neurodegenerative diseases," *Materials*, vol. 7, no. 7, pp. 4896–4929, 2014.

Rizzuto, R., Pinton, P., Brini, M., Chiesa, A., Filippin, L. and Pozzan, T., "Mitochondria as biosensors of calcium microdomains," *Cell Calcium*, vol. 26, no. 5, pp. 193–199, 1999.

Rocchitta, G., Spanu, A., Babudieri, S., Latte, G., Madeddu, G., Galleri, G., Nuvoli, S., Bagella, P., Demartis, M. and Fiore, V. *et al.*, "Enzyme biosensors for biomedical applications: strategies for safeguarding analytical performances in biological fluids," *Sensors*, vol. 16, no. 6, p. 780, 2016.

Shamsipur, M., Samandari, L. and Taherpour, A. *et al.*, "Sub-femtomolar detection of HIV-1 gene using DNA immobilized on composite platform reinforced by a conductive polymer sandwiched between two nanostructured layers: a solid signal-amplification strategy," *Analytica Chimica Acta*, vol. 1055, pp. 7–16, 2019.

Shao, Y., Wang, J., Wu, H., Liu, J., Aksay, I.A. and Lin, Y., "Graphene based electrochemical sensors and biosensors: a review," *Electroanalysis*, vol. 22, no. 10, pp. 1027–1036, 2010.

Strehlitz, B., *Methods in Biotechnology, Vol. 6. Enzyme and Microbial Biosensors. Techniques and Protocols*. Humana Press, Totowa, NJ, 1999.

Tsang, M.K., Ye, W. and Wang, G. *et al.*, "Ultrasensitive detection of Ebola virus oligonucleotide based on upconversion nanoprobe/nanoporous membrane system," *ACS Nano*, vol. 10, pp. 598–605, 2016.

Wang, Y., Li, H. and Wang, Y. *et al.*, "Development of multiple cross displacement amplification label-based gold nanoparticles lateral flow biosensor for detection of Listeria monocytogenes," *International Journal of Nanomedicine*, vol. 12, pp. 473–486, 2017a.

Wang, Y., Li, H. and Wang, Y. *et al.*, "Loop-mediated isothermal amplification label-based gold nanoparticles lateral flow biosensor for detection of Enterococcus faecalis and Staphylococcus aureus," *Frontiers in Microbiology*, vol. 8, p. 192, 2017b.

Wang, Y., Wang, Y. and Xu, J. *et al.*, "Development of multiple cross displacement amplification label-based gold nanoparticles lateral flow biosensor for detection of Shigella spp.," *Frontiers in Microbiology*, vol. 7, p. 1834, 2016.

UNAIDS, 2018. "UNAIDS Data 2018". www.unaids.org/en/resources/documents/2018/unaids-data-2018.

Xiao, W., Xiao, M. and Yao, S. *et al.*, "A rapid, simple, and low-cost CD4 cell count sensor based on blocking immunochromatographic strip system," *ACS Sensors*, vol. 4, pp. 1508–1514, 2019.

Yogeswaran, U. and Chen, S.M. "A review on the electrochemical sensors and biosensors composed of nanowires as sensing material," *Sensors*, vol. 8, pp. 290–313, 2008.

Yong, K., Wuwen, Y. and Yaqian, Y. *et al.*, "Electrochemical detection of Salmonella using an invA genosensor on polypyrrole-reduced graphene oxide modified glassy carbon electrode and AuNPs-horseradish peroxidase-streptavidin as nanotag," *Analytica Chimica Acta*, vol. 1074, pp. 80–88, 2019.

Zhang, Y., Chen, X. and Roozbahani, G.M. *et al.*, "Graphene oxide-based biosensing platform for rapid and sensitive detection of HIV-1 protease," *Analytical and Bioanalytical Chemistry*, vol. 410, pp. 6177–6185, 2018.

Zhu, C., Yang, G., Li, H., Du, D. and Lin, Y., "Electrochemical sensors and biosensors based on nanomaterials and nanostructures," *Analytical Chemistry*, vol. 87, pp. 230–249, 2015.

Zou, R., Zhang, F. and Chen, C. *et al.*, "DNA-programming multicolor silver nanoclusters for sensitively simultaneous detection of two HIV DNAs," *Sensors and Actuators B: Chemical*, vol. 296, p. 126608, 2019.

2

Viral Pseudotyping: A Novel Tool to Study Emerging and Transboundary Viruses

Aravindh Babu R. Parthiban,[1] Karthik Kumaragurubaran[1] and Dhinakar Raj Gopal[1]
[1] *Centre for Animal Health Studies, Tamil Nadu Veterinary and Animal Sciences University, Madhavaram Milk Colony-600051, Chennai, India*
Corresponding author: Aravindh Babu R. Parthiban, *aravindhbabu.r.p@tanuvas.ac.in*

2.1 Introduction

The concept of pseudotyping viruses stemmed from several observations of viruses with mixed phenotypes seen in the wild. Such phenotypic mixing has been demonstrated for several viruses that can infect cells at the same time (Boettiger, 1979; Weiss *et al.*, 1975; Závada, 1976, 1972). Earlier studies observed that such phenotypic mixing happened in the envelope glycoproteins only. These studies observed such mixing in both RNA viruses (togavirus, retrovirus, bunyavirus, arenavirus, rhabdovirus, paramyxovirus, orthomyxovirus, coronavirus) and DNA viruses (herpesvirus and poxvirus) (Závada, 1972).

Such observations have led researchers to synthesise pseudotyped viruses. Essentially, a virus pseudotype is a virus with genetic material from one virus and envelope proteins from another virus. The genetic material does not code for the enveloped protein, thus pseudotyped viruses (PVs) can enter a host cell and initiate nucleic acid replication but do not synthesise an infective particle. The viral particles generated are termed pseudotypes, pseudo-viruses, pseudo-particles, trans-complemented viruses, gene transfer vectors, and reporter virus particles.

The outer coat of the pseudotype dictates its cell tropism. In other words, the pseudotyped virus uses the receptors on the target cells for entry. Therefore, the pseudotype can be custom-designed to target specific cell types and deliver the transgene. For example, the human immunodeficiency virus type-1 (HIV-1) pseudotypes by the incorporating heterologous GPs enter cells other than those that express the CD4 receptor.

Pseudotypes have several advantages over their live virus counterparts, especially in situations where the counterparts are emerging/exotic viruses that require high containment facilities for handling.

Moreover, the transfer gene (reporter) in the pseudotype allows easy tracking without having to rely on the virus-specific antiserum.

2.2 How to Make Viral Pseudotypes

There are several pseudotype systems available commercially. The components for making a pseudotyped virus involve plasmid clones of the genes that make the core and the envelope. For example, the commonly used pseudotype backbone is described here. Over a period of time, several improvements have been made on the HIV backbone to develop a safer version (King *et al.*, 2016). There are several iterations of plasmid cocktail systems, such as two- and three-plasmid systems. For ease of understanding, a lentiviral-based pseudotyping system is described below (Figure 2.1). The system consists of the following plasmids.

1. Plasmid encoding the envelope gene. This is a construction whereby the envelope glycoproteins of the target virus are cloned for subsequent incorporation onto the pseudotype virus.
2. Plasmid encoding the retroviral GAG-POL genes. The "GAG" genes form the core of the pseudoptype and the enzyme ("POL") processes the structural proteins.
3. Plasmid encoding the rev gene is sometimes added to increase processivity. However, there are versions that work adequately without the rev gene.
4. Plasmid encoding the transfer gene. The transfer gene is incorporated into the pseudotype core. The plasmid encodes a packaging signal upstream of the gene to ensure efficient packaging of RNA copies into the pseudotype.

All the above plasmids are transfected onto a producer cell line such as HEK 293. The plasmids use the cellular transcription system to transcribe and translate the GAG-POL genes, which form the core of the pseudotype. The transfer gene is incorporated into the pseudotype core through its packaging signal. The transfer gene is more often a reporter gene such as green-fluorescent protein, luciferase or beta- galactosidase. The envelope gene is expressed and integrates onto the cell membrane which then is taken up by the pseudotype while it buds out of the cell. It is to be noted that, although the envelope protein on the pseudotype is the same as that of the corresponding live virus, the density of the envelop proteins and in turn the receptor binding regions may vary.

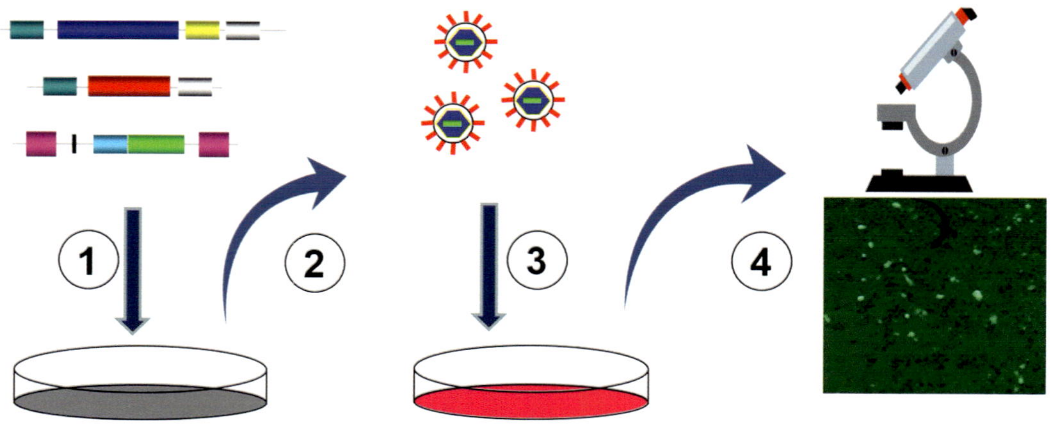

FIGURE 2.1 The schematic of a pseudotype virus production system. 1: The plasmid constructs are transfected into producer cell lines. 2: The pseudotypes produced are harvested by specific purification methods. 3: The pseudotypes are assayed on cell lines expressing suitable receptors. 4: The reporter gene expression is quantified by a suitable assay system.

2.3 Vesicular Stomatitis Virus (VSV)-based Pseudotypes

VSV-based pseudotypes are the most commonly used viral envelopes for the generation of PVs, owing to various positive factors like broad tropism and better physical and thermal stability. PVs with VSV glycoprotein envelopes in the lentivirus vector are considered to be the "gold standard" for gene therapy applications. PVs with vectors bearing an envelope protein from a distant virus can be used for understanding host pathogen interaction, which includes studies on viral entry mechanisms and the blocking of viral entry. Apart from the glycoprotein envelope, the core of VSV can also serve as an excellent vector for PVs (Lawson *et al.*, 1995). Advancement in the field of computational biology has aided in the generation of recombinant VSV through a reverse-genetics approach. When VSV is used as a recombinant vector, the G gene of VSV is replaced with a reporter gene that aids in easy identification of the infectivity of the PVs. Similarly, when the VSV core is used for synthesis of replication-competent PVs, the G gene of VSV is swapped with glycoprotein from a foreign virus.

Though VSV has the potential to be used for the delivery of genes and vaccines, other vectors based on lentivirus are more attractive and used mostly for gene editing and gene therapy. The advantages of the use of lentivirus vectors for gene therapy include their robustness in carrying larger genes, their production of self-inactivating vectors that are thus biologically safe, the compatibility of envelopes with foreign viruses and the prolonged expression of the transgene due to its ability to integrate into the host genome (Naldini *et al.*, 1996). Under these conditions, the VSV G gene is used as the standard envelope glycoprotein on the lentivirus vector. The viral envelope selected for pseudotyping the lentivirus vector (LV) is responsible for the tropism and physical and thermal stability of the PVs.

VSV glycoprotein was used as the envelope for Moloney murine leukemia virus (MoMLV) and avian sarcoma virus-based gene therapy before being used widely for LVs. Though various advantages support the use of the VSV G envelope for LVs, still certain demerits need to be worked upon to improve its efficiency. Transduction in resting lymphocytes is poor and VSV G was found to be hypersensitive in human and mammalian serum studies, thus preventing its wide use under *in vivo* conditions. Cytotoxicity due to VSV G expression has also been reported under *in vitro* conditions, thus making it difficult to produce a self-assembled LV. To alleviate the listed problems, alternatively expressed and purified G protein can be fused into the liposomes to produce virus-like particles. VSV G-based LV pseudotypes produce a strong immune response post-intravenous injection, thereby leading to rapid clearance (Munis *et al.*, 2020).

Despite the various drawbacks related to VSV G-based LV pseudotypes, there are several products (around 150) under clinical trial in the USA for the treatment of ailments. Due to their higher transduction ability, these vectors (VSVGLVs) are used for chimeric antigen receptor-T (CAR-T) cell therapies. Two CD19 specific CAR-T cell therapy-based products—namely, Kymriah and Yescarta—are approved by the Food and Drug Administration (FDA) for the treatment of B-cell malignancies (Sadelain *et al.*, 2017). Currently, HEK 293 or its derivatives are used as cell lines for the production of VSVGLVs.

VSV-based vectors can be used to generate multiple glycoprotein envelopes from different viruses. Simultaneous co-infection of VSV with SV5, MLV, and Sendai viruses can lead to the generation of vectors with heterogeneous envelopes, with glycoproteins from all viruses in various combination. In order to study the nature of foreign envelope proteins it is essential to have a homogeneous protein in the envelope. The use of production-defective or thermosensitive VSV mutants like tlB17 (inactivated at 45°C for 60 minutes) or ts045 can help in the selection of homogeneous pseudotypes, thus enabling studies on envelope proteins (Weiss *et al.*, 1975; Knipe *et al.*, 1977). VSV assembly and budding is dependent to some extent on the nature of the envelope glycoprotein, which was proved by the use of VSV-ΔG to result in the production of more bald particles when compared to native VSV. In the case of retrovirus, the rate of budding of bald particles and viruses with envelope proteins is similar. The PVs with VSV cores have gained popularity in the recent times, where the glycoprotein gene of VSV is swapped with a fluorescent protein, leading to the generation of replication-defective recombinant VSV (rVSV) (Robison and Whitt, 2000). These rVSV PVs were used successfully for studying the entry mechanism of the Ebola virus.

A major advantage of the use of PVs based on rVSV-ΔG is that the work or studies related to high-containment pathogens like Ebola, Nipah, SARS and SARS-CoV-2 can be carried out in lower containment levels (Munis *et al.*, 2020). In an emergency situation or during a pandemic, in order to study the activity of a high-containment pathogen in a host, it can be easily reproduced in lower-containment facilities with the use of PVs if the sequence of envelope glycoprotein of the emerging virus is known.

Major vaccines available on the market are live attenuated vaccines, which generate stronger and longer-lasting immunity but possess various disadvantages, including safety concerns. Recombinant viral vectors like PVs can be a promising alternative for the available live attenuated vaccines. Adenovirus vectors are used successfully as vaccine vectors for prime boost vaccination regimens, but they cannot be dosed repeatedly. Under these circumstances, VSVs possesses certain able qualities, like their inability to integrate into the host, lower toxicity, ability to stably insert transgenes and capacity for production of higher titres, supporting their use as vaccine vectors. Similarly, VSV administration leads to strong activation of both arms of immunity, i.e., humoral and cell-mediated immunity. A report shows that one dose of VSV vector with hemagglutinin of the measles and influenza A viruses could protect laboratory animals against a challenging dose (Schlereth *et al.*, 2000). A VSV vector has been used successfully against various diseases of infectious origin, like hepatitis C and the Ebola virus. Recombinant VSV with glycoprotein of the Zaire Ebola virus (rVSV-ZEBOV) showed promising results in non-human primate studies, and hence this vaccine was used in humans as a phase-III clinical trial during an outbreak (2013–2016) in Africa (Agnandji *et al.*, 2016). The results of the trial showed that the protective efficacy was good and there were no safety issues. Later, in the year 2019, the USA and EU approved this rVSV-ZEBOV vaccine, sold as Erbevo, for human use (FDA, 2019). Thus, there is great potential of VSV PVs as a platform for the production of quality vaccines.

There are safety concerns when replication-competent VSV is used, since VSV is a neurotropic virus. The G protein of VSV is responsible for the neurotropic nature of the virus; hence, a vector or vaccine lacking the G-pseudotyped virus was tested in non-human primates and was found to be safe, without any untoward effect. When rVSV-ZEBOV was tested in immunocompromised NOD-SCID mice and also in rhesus monkeys, the vaccine was safe, without any safety issues (Geisbert *et al.*, 2008). Similarly, since VSV is pathogenic to porcine mammals, studies in pigs showed that rVSV-ZEBOV was safe, without any clinical manifestation. Considering the success obtained in Ebola studies, research is now focused on the generation of a HIV-1 vaccine. In spite of the potential use of VSV as a vaccine vector, re-administration cannot be done due to the development of neutralising antibodies.

2.4 Applications of PVs

2.4.1 Studying Host-Pathogen Interaction

High-risk pathogens (risk group 3 or 4) cannot be handled in every laboratory; hence, PVs can be used safely in lower containment levels. This enables the understanding of virus entry mechanisms inside the host cell, thereby aiding in designing drugs targeting viral entry.

2.4.2 Virus Neutralisation Assays

Virus neutralisation assays are an important component in measuring antibody response against the envelopes of viruses. The first line of assessing the vaccine response against fatal and high-risk viruses such as the Hendra virus, Nipah virus, Ebola virus and, most recently, SARS-CoV-2 is the measurement of the neutralising antibody produced by these vaccines. However, such assays are not widely performed due to the requirement for expensive biocontainment facilities and skilled personnel to work in such facilities. The use of pseudotypes with the envelopes of these high-containment viruses as "surrogate viruses" in neutralisation assays can be performed in less sophisticated laboratories as the pseudotypes are non-infective, replication-competent but transmission defective. Moreover, the pseudotypes encode reporter genes, which help in direct measurement of neutralisation activity without the need for antiserum (antibodies) against the viral envelope.

2.4.3 Gene Transfer

PVs can be directed for delivering genes to the target cells. Previously, retrovirus was mainly used and, in the later stages, heterologous envelope glycoproteins from VSV provide a promising alternative to alleviate the problems associated with the use of retrovirus proteins.

2.4.4 Vaccine

Viral envelope proteins are the primary target for antibodies. Thus, PVs that express different envelope proteins can be a promising tool for designing a vaccine. VSV vector has been widely used as a vaccine against various pathogens, including severe acute respiratory syndrome coronavirus (SARS-CoV), simian immunodeficiency virus (SIV), influenza, Ebola and HPV-16. Due to the problem of genome integration in the case of retrovirus, there is a shift towards the production of virus-like particle vaccines. A list of vaccines based on VSV PVs for emerging diseases is presented in Table 2.1.

References

Agnandji ST, Huttner A, Zinser ME, *et al.* Phase 1 trials of rVSV Ebola vaccine in Africa and Europe. *New Engl. J. Med.* 2016, 374(17): 1647–1660.

TABLE 2.1

Vaccines for emerging diseases under various stages of development based on VSV PVs

S. No.	PV-based Vaccine	Remark	Reference
1	VSV-based H5N1 influenza virus vectors	Single dose in mice provided 100% protection	Furuyama *et al.* (2020)
2	VSV-based Marburg virus vaccine	Single dose provided to nonhuman primates provided uniform protection without viremia	Marzi *et al.* (2019)
3	rVSV expressing the glycoprotein of Zaire-strain Ebola virus	Viremia was noted after single dose in all human participants. Adverse effects were lesser after second dose than the first dose. There was zero conversion after 28 days post-immunisation	Regules *et al.* (2017)
4	VSV-ΔG-spike vaccine for SARS-CoV-2	Single dose in hamster provided safety and reduced viral titres of SARS-CoV-2 post-challenge	Yahalom-Ronen *et al.* (2020)
5	VSV expressing Lassa virus Glycoprotein C	All macaques survived challenge	Stein *et al.* (2019)
6	rVSV expressing glycoprotein precursor (GPC) of Crimean-Congo hemorrhagic fever virus (CCHFV)	All immunocompromised STAT-1 knock-out mice survived challenge	Rodriguez *et al.* (2019)
7	rVSVΔG with Nipah virus glycoprotein or fusion protein	Individual administration of rVSVΔG F/G vaccine in Syrian hamsters led to them not developing disease	Chattopadhyay and Rose (2011)
8	VSV expressing S protein of SARS-CoV	Generation of higher level of neutralising antibodies in mice post-immunisation	Kapadia *et al.* (2005)
9	VSVΔG expressing S protein of MERS	Single dose of immunization resulted in production of neutralizing antibodies and also T cell response	Liu *et al.* (2018)
10	rVSV containing mutated M protein and expressing Zika virus membrane protein (prM)	After vaccine there was no disease in adult mice. Similarly, the offspring of vaccinated mice were also protected against challenge	Emanuel *et al.* (2018)

Boettiger D. Animal virus pseudotypes. *Prog. Med. Virol.* 1979, 25: 37–68.

Chattopadhyay A, Rose JK. Complementing defective viruses that express separate paramyxovirus glycoproteins provide a new vaccine vector approach. *J. Virol.* 2011, 85: 2004–2011.

Emanuel J, Callison J, Dowd KA, Pierson TC, Feldmann H, Marzi A. A VSV-based Zika virus vaccine protects mice from lethal challenge. *Sci. Rep.* 2018, 8: 11043.

First FD. A-approved vaccine for the prevention of Ebola virus disease, marking a critical milestone in public health preparedness and response. [Internet] Silver Spring, MD: US Food and Drug Administration (FDA). 2019, December 19.

Furuyama W, Reynolds P, Haddock E, Meade-White K, Quynh Le M, Kawaoka Y, Feldmann H, Marzi A. A single dose of a vesicular stomatitis virus-based influenza vaccine confers rapid protection against H5 viruses from different clades. *NPJ Vaccines*. 2020, 5: 4.

Geisbert TW, Daddario-Dicaprio KM, Lewis MG, *et al.* Vesicular stomatitis virus-based Ebola vaccine is well-tolerated and protects immunocompromised nonhuman primates. *PLOS Pathog.* 2008, 4(11): e1000225.

Kapadia SU, Rose JK, Lamirande E, Vogel L, Subbarao K, Roberts A. Long-term protection from SARS coronavirus infection conferred by a single immunization with an attenuated VSV-based vaccine. *Virology*. 2005, 340: 174–182.

King B, Temperton NJ, Grehan K, Scott SD, Wright E, Tarr AW, Daly JM. Technical considerations for the generation of novel pseudotyped viruses. *Future Virol.* 2016, 11: 47–59.

Knipe DM, Baltimore D, Lodish HF. Maturation of viral proteins in cells infected with temperature-sensitive mutants of vesicular stomatitis virus. *J. Virol.* 1977, 21(3): 1149–1158.

Lawson ND, Stillman EA, Whitt MA, *et al.* Recombinant vesicular stomatitis viruses from DNA. *Proc. Natl. Acad. Sci. USA*. 1995, 92(10): 4477–4481.

Liu R, Wang J, Shao Y, Wang X, Zhang H, Shuai L, Ge J, Wen Z, Bu Z. A recombinant VSV-vectored MERS-CoV vaccine induces neutralizing antibody and T cell responses in rhesus monkeys after single dose immunization. *Antiviral Res.* 2018, 150: 30–38.

Marzi A, Menicucci AR, Engelmann F, Callison J, Horne EJ, Feldmann F, Jankeel A, Feldmann H, Messaoudi I. Protection against Marburg virus using a recombinant VSV-vaccine depends on T and B cell activation. *Front Immunol.* 2019, 9: 3071.

Munis AM, Bentley EM, Takeuchi Y. A tool with many applications: vesicular stomatitis virus in research and medicine. *Expert Opin. Biol. Ther.* 2020, 20(10): 1187–1201.

Naldini L, Blomer U, Gallay P, *et al.* In vivo gene delivery and stable transduction of nondividing cells by a lentiviral vector. *Science*. 1996, 272(5259): 263–267.

Regules JA, Beigel JH, Paolino KM, Voell J, Castellano AR, Hu Z, Muñoz P, Moon JE, Ruck RC, Bennett JW, Twomey PS, Gutiérrez RL, Remich SA, Hack HR, Wisniewski ML, Josleyn MD, Kwilas SA, Van Deusen N, Mbaya OT, Zhou Y, Stanley DA, Jing W, Smith KS, Shi M, Ledgerwood JE, Graham BS, Sullivan NJ, Jagodzinski LL, Peel SA, Alimonti JB, Hooper JW, Silvera PM, Martin BK, Monath TP, Ramsey WJ, Link CJ, Lane HC, Michael NL, Davey RT Jr, Thomas SJ. rVSVΔG-ZEBOV-GP study group. A recombinant vesicular stomatitis virus Ebola vaccine. *N. Engl. J. Med.* 2017, 376(4): 330–341.

Robison CS, Whitt MA. The membrane-proximal stem region of vesicular stomatitis virus G protein confers efficient virus assembly. *J. Virol.* 2000, 74(5): 2239–2246.

Rodriguez SE, Cross RW, Fenton KA, Bente DA, Mire CE, Geisbert TW. Vesicular stomatitis virus-based vaccine protects mice against Crimean-Congo hemorrhagic fever. *Sci. Rep.* 2019, 9.

Sadelain M, Riviere I, Riddell S. Therapeutic T cell engineering. *Nature*. 2017, 545(7655): 423–431.

Schlereth B, Rose JK, Buonocore L, *et al.* Successful vaccine-induced seroconversion by single-dose immunization in the presence of measles virus-specific maternal antibodies. *J. Virol.* 2000, 74(10): 4652–4657.

Stein DR, Warner BM, Soule G, Tierney K, Frost KL, Booth S, Safronetz D. A recombinant vesicular stomatitis-based Lassa fever vaccine elicits rapid and long-term protection from lethal Lassa virus infection in guinea pigs. *NPJ Vaccines*. 2019, 4.

Weiss RA, Boettiger D, Love DN. Phenotypic mixing between vesicular stomatitis virus and avian RNA tumor viruses. *Cold Spring Harb. Symp. Quant. Biol.* 1975, 39(Pt 2): 913–918.

Yahalom-Ronen Y, Tamir H, Melamed S, Politi B, Shifman O, Achdout H, Vitner EB, Israeli O, Milrot E, Stein D, Cohen-Gihon I, Lazar S, Gutman H, Glinert I, Cherry L, Vagima Y, Lazar S, Weiss S, Ben-Shmuel A, Avraham R, Puni R, Lupu E, Bar David E, Sittner A, Erez N, Zichel R, Mamroud E, Mazor O, Levy H,

Laskar O, Yitzhaki S, Shapira SC, Zvi A, Beth-Din A, Paran N, Israely T. A single dose of recombinant VSV-ΔG-spike vaccine provides protection against SARS-CoV-2 challenge. bioRxiv 2020.06.18.160655; https://doi.org/10.1101/2020.06.18.160655, 2020.

Závada J. Pseudotypes of vesicular stomatitis virus with the coat of murine leukaemia and of avian myeloblastosis viruses. *J. Gen. Virol.* 1972, 15: 183–191.

Závada J. Viral pseudotypes and phenotypic mixing. *Arch. Virol.* 1976, 50(1–2): 1–15.

3

Advanced Sensors for Animal Disease Diagnosis

Swati Dahiya,[1] Jyotsana Mehta[1] and Bhuvan Nagpal[2]
[1] *Department of Veterinary Microbiology, Lala Lajpat Rai University of Veterinary and Animal Sciences, Hisar-125004, Haryana, India*
[2] *Manglam Diagnostics, Hisar-125005, Haryana, India*
Corresponding author: Swati Dahiya, *swatidahiya@luvas.edu.in*

3.1 Introduction to Animal Diseases

Infectious diseases are the primary cause of death of animals worldwide. Animal pathogens are a threat to animal production and subsequently animal product supply. This critically impacts animal well-being and has potential global environmental and biodiversity consequences. The global burden of infectious disease, which accounts for about 42% of the total global burden of disease, indicates the economic costs involved, thus impacting large-scale developmental projects (Pray *et al.*, 2006). In addition, infectious disease-causing agents of animals pose global public health risks due to the emergence of sporadic zoonotic infections and pandemic strains. Animals are the major source of approximately 70% of all human infections. Also, the worldwide population is expected to reach 9.3 billion by 2050 and the subsequent need for food production will have to be doubled to meet the increasing demands. Contrary to this, approximately 20% of animal produce is being lost due to infectious diseases (Tarasov *et al.*, 2016). The essential elements for efficient and effective control of the threat of infectious disease are identification of the causative agents, control of spread and subsequent treatment. Out of these elements, the development of rapid, sensitive and selective assays for pathogen detection has attracted special research orientation worldwide. Early and on-site detection is crucial to control the spread of infectious agents and make improved decisions on treatment procedures. The conventional methods used for the detection of pathogens are culture-based microbiological assays, microscopic examination and biochemical assays (Figure 3.1). Culture-based microbiological assays are the gold standard in most of

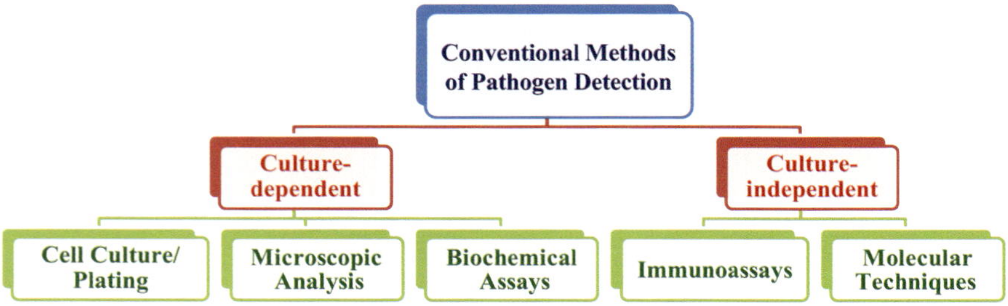

FIGURE 3.1 Conventional methods for the detection of animal pathogens.

the cases and include the isolation of a microbe from a clinical specimen/culture followed by its propagation. Although the method is sensitive and effective, it is costly, time-consuming and labor-intensive. Further, the improvements in pathogen diagnosis include immunological and molecular methods based on enzyme-linked immunosorbent assay (ELISA) techniques, blotting techniques and various forms of polymerase chain reaction (PCR) (Figure 3.1). These techniques are highly specific, sensitive and consume less time. However, the above-mentioned techniques cannot be applied for on-site detection of pathogens. Therefore, the development of highly sensitive, specific, rapid, portable and cost-effective diagnostic platforms for the detection of animal pathogens is the need of the hour.

Sensors—analytical devices comprised of a biological recognition molecule attached to a physiochemical transducer—are an attractive alternative to conventional microbiological and molecular methods, as shown in Figure 3.2. The most common biological components include whole cells, nucleic acids, antibodies, aptamers and enzymes, whereas optical and electrochemical transducers are the major transduction techniques employed. The sensors offer simplicity, miniaturization and on-site applicability along with high specificity and sensitivity. The last three decades have witnessed a number of innovations in the field of biotechnology and nanotechnology for the fabrication of detection platforms for bacterial and viral animal pathogen monitoring. Some of these emerging systems have resulted in various commercialized sensing products for animal pathogens which require a smaller sample and no pretreatment, while being cost-effective and enabling on-site detection.

In this chapter, the focus is on the various sensors explored to date for species-wise animal pathogen diagnostics. Briefly, the conventional and molecular methods are described, along with the associated limitations. Further, the sensors are classified on the basis of target animals. Examples of sensors being used for the detection of pathogens responsible for major economic losses in bovine, caprine, ovine, equine, swine, canine, avian and aquatic animals are elaborated. The different bioprobes, nanomaterials as substrate for bioprobes and transduction platforms are discussed in detail, taking into account the advantages and limitations of each method.

3.2 Common Animal Diseases

An animal disease is an impairment of the normal state of an animal that affects its normal functioning. The economically important emerging and re-emerging diseases of livestock, poultry and aquatic animals needing urgent diagnosis include bovine respiratory disease, infectious bovine rhinotracheitis (IBR), tuberculosis, foot-and-mouth disease (FMD), hemorrhagic septicemia (HS), brucellosis, black quarter (BQ), leptospirosis, trypanosomiasis, theileriosis etc. in cattle and buffaloes; bluetongue (BT), *peste des petites ruminants* (PPR), enterotoxemia, sheeppox and goatpox in sheep and goats; swine fever, swine influenza, colibacillosis, salomonellosis, campylobacteriosis, clostridial infections, swine erysipelas, pasteurellosis, listeriosis, leptospirosis, tuberculosis, brucellosis, *Streptococcus suis* infection in pigs; glanders, corona, equine influenza in equines; canine distemper, canine parvovirus infection and leishmaniasis in dogs; avian influenza, Newcastle disease, fowl pox, picobirnaviral and *Clostridial* infections in poultry; viral haemorrhagic septicemia in fish and some common bacterial infections reported in almost

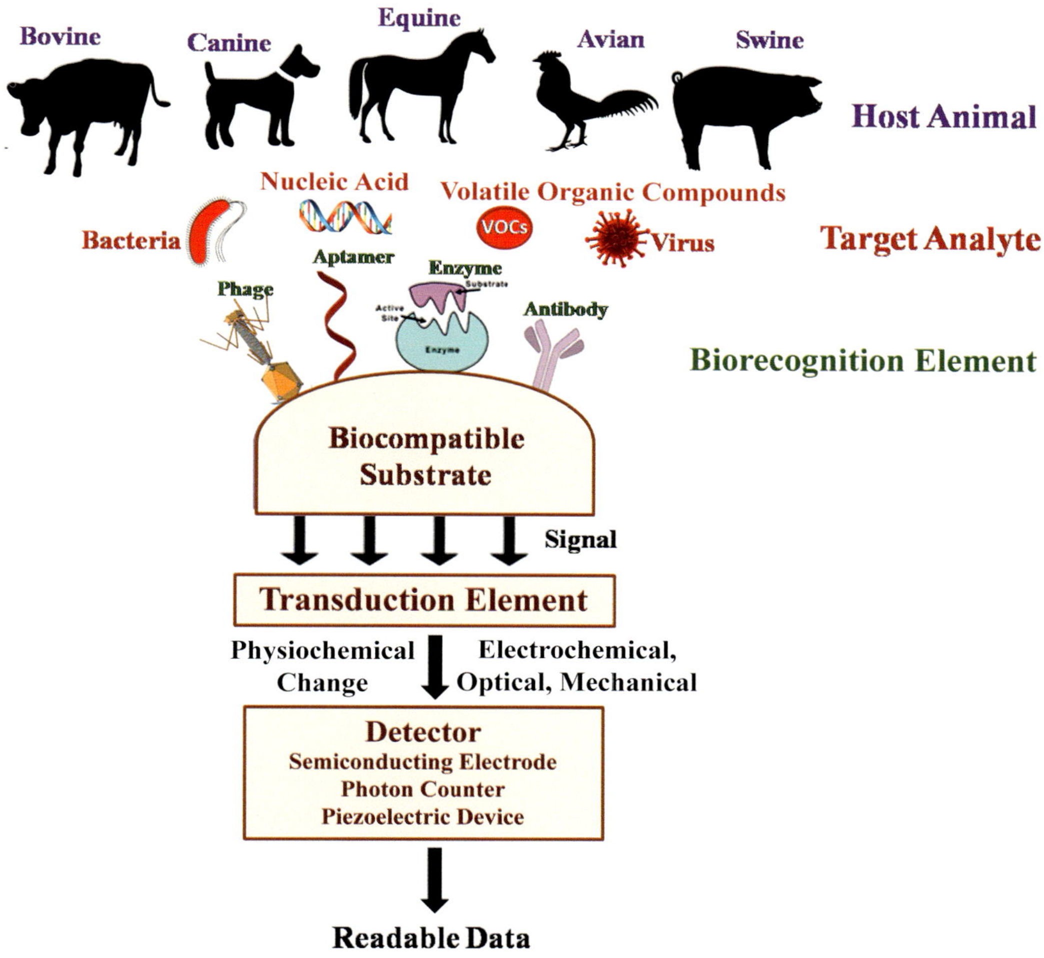

FIGURE 3.2 Schematic of sensors for disease diagnosis of various groups of animals.

all species, like antimicrobial-resistant (AMR) pathogens including methicillin-resistant *Staphylococcus aureus* (MRSA) infection.

3.3 Sensors as New-Generation Diagnostic Platforms for Animal Disease Diagnosis

Traditionally, culture-based microbiological, biochemical and molecular assays have been used for the detection of pathogens. In culture-based assays, either the growth of the pathogen on specific media or the production of biochemical compounds during the growth of a microorganism is monitored and co-related to the initial concentration of the pathogen. The biochemical assays allow pathogen detection through the specific interaction of chemicals with cell components of the pathogen, resulting in a colorimetric signal. On the other hand, molecular assays make use of probes such as antibodies, nucleic acid or other molecules against the complementary component of a pathogen for its highly sensitive and specific detection. The mentioned assays are specific but time-consuming, labor-intensive and costly, and require trained personnel and bulky instrumentation. Further, the conventional methods cannot be applied for on-site detection of pathogens and, thus, cannot facilitate point-of-care (POC) diagnosis.

Sensors, as emerging alternatives to conventional detection methods for animal disease diagnosis, are attracting research and commercial orientation worldwide. Globally, a vast number and variety of sensors are being explored and commercialized for animal health monitoring at various stages. The major advantages facilitating the fast growth of sensors are the low cost of mass production, ease of operation, high sensitivity and specificity, along with POC diagnosis. Sensors are analytical devices that detect a target biomarker which is specific for a particular pathogen, via a bioreceptor (e.g., enzyme, nucleic acid, antibody, whole cells or cell components), a sensing element immobilized onto a physiochemical transducer. The bioreceptor is a key component of a sensing platform as its biochemical properties incorporate high specificity and sensitivity for a target biomarker and circumvent cross-interference from other microorganisms and components present in the sample to be tested. The specific interaction between the bioreceptor and the target analyte produces a physiochemical change which is converted into the readable form of a qualitative and quantitative signal using a transducer. Vidic *et al.* (2017) have reviewed the innovative biosensing systems that can be used for pathogen detection in livestock and poultry. Some of the devices have been validated according to standards of the World Organization for Animal Health. These devices, including the paper-based platforms, are available commercially and are said to be rapid, affordable and easy-to-perform sensing systems for field use.

Researchers worldwide are focusing on improving different aspects of sensors; however, in order to address the main challenges the two major requirements are: (i) improvements in the sensitivity and early detection of pathogens so as to detect them prior to the appearance of clinical signs; (ii) the incorporation of robustness into sensors to make them usable for in-field applications in complex biological samples.

The following sections classify the reported sensors for pathogen detection on the basis of the host animal, i.e., bovine, caprine, ovine, swine, equine, canine, avian and fish. The major focus has been given to electrochemical and optical sensors, attributable to their high sensitivity, ease of readability, portability and diverse functionality. The use of bacteriophages in sensors has been highlighted for the detection of AMR pathogens.

3.3.1 Bovine

Bovine respiratory disease (BRD) has been reported to be the leading cause of \$2 billion of economic loss annually in the USA to the cattle and dairy industry due to concomitant clinical disease, associated therapeutic treatment and decreased animal performance, yield and mortality (Thompson *et al.*, 2006; Snowder *et al.*, 2007). Therefore, exciting and realistic prospects are being explored for developing POC sensing devices facilitating multiplexed and on-site detection and assessment of animal disease prevalence. A novel potentiometric sensor based on extended-gate field-effect transistors in a dual-chip configuration has been presented (Tarasov *et al.*, 2016). The sensor consists of a gold-coated chip incorporated into a microfluidic system for signal production which is electrically connected to the gate terminal of a metal oxide semiconductor field effect transistor (MOSFET) transducer for signal amplification. For the detection of bovine herpesvirus-1 (BHV-1), viral protein gE expressed and immobilized on the gold surface served as a capture antigen for BHV-1-specific antibody (anti-gE). The gE-coated immunosensor exhibited high sensitivity and selectivity to anti-gE in commercially available and real serum samples and the obtained results were found to be in excellent validation with standard surface plasmon resonance (SPR) and ELISA. The explored platform not only achieved performance equivalent to SPR and ELISA, but also offered cost-effectiveness in terms of its inexpensive optical components and faster response.

Infectious bovine rhinotracheitis (IBR), caused by BHV-1, is another highly contagious cattle disease endemic in the UK and other parts of the world (Beer and Dastjerdi, 2018). A commercial, disposable, low-cost electrochemical bioassay for the detection of BHV-1 antibodies has been developed using the Vantix™ biosensor system and well established ELISA reagents (Cork *et al.*, 2013). Vantix™ biosensors consist of a conductive polypyrrole-coated working and reference electrode. The bioassay was based on the formation of an immune-complex on the working electrode resulting in electrochemical changes in the electrical potential (Purvis *et al.*, 2003). The biosensor assay provided quantitative analysis through the measurement of antibody levels in milk samples for routine monitoring in 15 minutes. The results exhibited good correlation with standard ELISA techniques. The results of this study suggested the promising capability of the Vantix™ system for routine immunological testing, with high throughput and rapid results.

Bovine tuberculosis (TB) is another disease of bovines arousing international public health concern. *Mycobacterium bovis* causing bovine tuberculosis has been identified by monitoring changes in the volatile organic compounds (VOCs) profiles of the breath of cattle suffering from the disease (Ellis *et al.*, 2014). A nanotechnology-based sensing array has been fabricated for real-time detection of bovine tuberculosis via breath (Peled *et al.*, 2012). Gas-chromatography/mass-spectrometry (GC-MS) analysis has established the presence of two VOCs linked to disease and the healthy state, each in the exhaled breath yielding distinct VOC patterns for the two study groups. On the basis of the above establishment, a nanotechnology-based sensing array, i.e., nano-artificial nose (NA-NOSE), has been customized for the detection of bovine tuberculosis *via* breath in *M. bovis*-infected cattle. For the development of NA-NOSE, first, an initial pool of an array of 18 chemi-resistive films of gold nanoparticle (GNP) sensors was analyzed using GC-MS for determining the organic functionalities having cross-selective absorption sites for breath VOCs and, thus, six arrays (GNP with either octadecanethiol (2 items), decanethiol, 2-naphthalenethiol, 2-mercaptobenzoazole or 2-nitro-4-trifluoromethylbenzenethiol) were shortlisted. The sensing array was then fabricated by drop-casting modified GNP solutions onto customized titanium/gold (Ti/Au) interdigitated electrodes. The Au particles and organic component in the sensing films provided the electrical conductivity and sorption sites for the guest analyte, respectively. The system was successful in identifying *M. bovis*-infected animals. The NA-NOSE system showed great promise as a detection platform for bovine tuberculosis and offered advantages over the GC-MS technique in terms of cost, portability and response speed. The system could be placed at the barn entrance or beside the milking line for the screening of bovine TB in cattle. This method could also be used for screening other diseases, such as bovine brucellosis and paratuberculosis.

Foot-and-mouth disease (FMD) outbreaks cause major economic losses worldwide and, therefore, early and fast identification of the disease's causative agent, i.e., the FMD virus (FMDV), is of utmost importance. An immunobiosensor using a piezoelectric (PZ) crystal was developed and standardized for FMD diagnosis and virus typing (Gajendragad *et al.*, 2001). The sensor employs an anti-FMDV antibody immobilized onto 6 MHz quartz crystal as the frequency-determining element. In the process, a diluted suspension of clinical samples of tongue and foot epithelium was applied on both sides of the resonating crystal and the change in resonance was observed. A resonance difference of more than 2.5 Hz indicated the presence of FMDV in the tested samples. The sensor was found to be highly sensitive, specific, reproducible and stable up to 18 weeks when stored at room temperature.

Another group of researchers has demonstrated an optical microchip immunosensor, SpectroSens™, for label-free, rapid and robust detection of FMDV based on refractive index changes of high-precision planar Bragg gratings (Bhatta *et al.*, 2012). The sensor is composed of an anti-FMDV antibody immobilized onto a functionalized surface of sensing channels. The specific binding of the target pathogen present in the sample changes the localized refractive index within the sensing channels, which is manifested in the form of increased wavelength from the multi-channel sensor chip. Specific detection of FMDV has been demonstrated within minutes by referenced quantification of reflected wavelength changes in the sensor. Further, simplified "snap-shot" assay data has been displayed in "Turn ON/OFF" format using a hand-held, portable device. The multiplexed SpectroSens™ detection platform exhibits the potential for application in-field for the detection of FMD and template development in the diagnosis of other veterinary diseases.

A rapid and simple chromatographic strip for FMD diagnosis was developed for field application (Reid *et al.*, 2001). This device, which contains a specific monoclonal antibody exhibiting broad reactivity for FMD viruses, has been shown to detect FMDV antigens in the lab as well as in the field. The test has been validated using samples from the nasal passage, epithelial suspensions and probangs from animals infected experimentally, clinical samples and supernatant fluid of their cell culture passage. A similar lateral-flow device for the monitoring of FMDV RNA has been reported (Fowler *et al.*, 2014). The FMDV-specific antibody was immobilized on the test line of the immune-chromatographic strip and the specific interaction of immobilized antibody to the analyte resulting in a highlighted test line. This lateral-flow device can then be used for nucleic acid sequencing, amplification or recovery of the detected virus because of its thermostability, dryness and non-hazardous capillary system.

Another example of a POC lateral-flow device has been validated for FMD diagnosis coupled with reverse transcription loop-mediated isothermal amplification (RT-LAMP) (Waters *et al.*, 2014). The proposed test offered naked-eye diagnosis in less than one hour without the requirement of any instrumentation or a thermocycler for amplification, as the reaction was performed in a standard water bath at a constant temperature. The device has also been able to detect RNA directly from epithelial suspensions without the prior need for RNA extraction. The above-mentioned characteristics advocate the strength of the proposed lateral-flow device as a high-throughput assay format.

3.3.2 Canine

It has been reported in the literature that approximately 17% of households worldwide own dogs as pets (Sudarshan *et al.*, 2006). Despite this, the information available to veterinarians on the prevalence, epidemiology, diagnosis, cure and treatment of canine diseases is scarce (Irwin and Traub, 2006). Rapid and accurate diagnosis is crucial to reduce the incidences and epidemics of canine diseases and their zoonotic counterparts. The quartz crystal microbalance (QCM)-based detection platforms are a new and promising tool for the measurement of frequency changes in antigen-antibody interactions. In a recent study, the QCM biosensor and ProLinker™ B have been combined to enable the rapid diagnosis of canine parvovirus (CPV) (Kim *et al.*, 2015). ProLinker™ B facilitated the attachment of antibodies to a surface of gold-coated quartz crystal in a regular pattern and the proper orientation for binding of the antigen. The binding of the immobilized antibody to the specific target antigen CPV resulted in a change in mass of the quartz crystal and subsequently generated a measurable change in frequency. The QCM biosensor showed sufficiently high sensitivity and specificity of 95.4% and 98.0%, respectively, for the rapid diagnosis of CPV.

Canine distemper (CD), a highly infectious disease, is caused by canine distemper virus (CDV) in canines, Asian elephants, large cats and some primates. An easy and low-cost method for the monitoring of CDV without the need for any instrument has been developed using gold nanoparticle-labeled antibodies (Basso *et al.*, 2015). The attachment of CDV to the specific antibody-conjugated gold nanoparticles resulted in clearly visible colorimetric change. This is attributable to the aggregation of antigen-antibody complex-conjugated gold nanoparticles, exhibiting an extinction peak shift of 30 nm. The proposed method achieved a detection limit of 0.7 mg/L within a linear detection range of 0 to 1.5 mg/L for CDV in real samples of urine in a simple and cost-effective manner. The results correlated well with the conventional standard ELISA technique.

An electrochemical impedance spectroscopy-based sensor for femtomolar detection of *Leishmania* spp. (CL) DNA has been reported using a thiolated carbon nanotube (ThNT) (Frias *et al.*, 2017). The amine-functionalized short single-stranded probes specific to the target DNA were covalently linked to carboxyl-functionalized ThNTs-modified ultrathin Au films. The genosensor exhibited high conductivity on the application of an external magnetic field due to disentangling of ThNTs in oriented covalent immobilization. Under disentangled conditions, the genosensor exhibited a linear detection of the target DNA in the concentration range of 0.1–98.3 fg/μL with a detection limit of 15 fM for CL in genomic samples of infected canine blood. The covalent immobilization of the ThNTs provided incorporated stability by reducing their tendency of being washed out.

Visceral leishmaniasis is a significant cause of mortality and morbidity for both humans and dogs. Researchers worldwide are making attempts to develop improved diagnostic platforms for the detection of associated pathogens even in asymptomatic dogs. Another QCM-based immunosensor using the recombinant antigen of *L. chagasi* (rLci2B-NH6) for the detection of canine visceral leishmaniasis has been developed (Ramos-Jesus *et al.*, 2011). The self-assembled monolayer of rLci2B-NH6 was covalently immobilized in a proper orientation on a quartz crystal gold electrode. Using this strategy, steric hindrance was reduced and major epitopes were exposed by covalently linking the histidine tail of the antigen to glutaraldehyde through the Schiff base reaction. The reported immunosensor showed good productivity, exceptional sensitivity and specificity, along with high reusability.

3.3.3 Equine

A genetically biotinylated single-chain fragment variable antibody (scFv) against Venezuelan equine encephalitis virus (VEE) has been developed (Hu *et al.*, 2004). West Nile virus (WNV) has been detected using biosensors and microfluidic systems using a linear, 15-amino-acid fragment of domain III of WNV as an antigen on an amperometric immunosensor (Ionescu *et al.*, 2007). A surface-enhanced Raman scattering immunoassay has been reported to be highly sensitive for the detection of anti-WNV immunoglobulin. The assay was conducted in solution. The envelope (E) protein of WNV was coated onto the Au nanoparticles for use as the SERS-active substrate. The malachite-green (MG)-conjugated protein A/G (MG-pA/G) was used as a bi-functional Raman tag/antibody binding reporter. The serum collected from rabbits inoculated with E-antigen of WNV was used for incubating these reagents. A SERS signaling response was revealed due to laser interrogation of the sandwiched immunocomplex which is diagnostic for MG. This assay was reported to be >400-fold more sensitive than indirect ELISA conducted using the same concentrations of reagents. Immunocomplex film deposition on solid Au surfaces when subjected to QCM with dissipation monitoring confirmed the formation of antigen-antibody-protein A/G trilayers. The sensitivity and inherent versatility of the sensor suggested that it could be developed as an alternative to ELISA (Neng *et al.*, 2010). The evolution of equine influenza and the origin of canine influenza have been studied with the help of biosensors (Collins *et al.*, 2014).

3.3.4 Swine

Development of a novel diagnostic device for on-site analysis has been reported based on the use of advanced biosensing and photonics technologies to tackle emerging and endemic viruses causing swine epidemics and significant economic damage on pig farms. The device is reported to be under development within the framework of an EU Commission-co-funded project. The technology is able to detect pathogens in different types of biological samples, such as oral fluids, feces, blood or nasal swabs. The SWINOSTICS diagnostics project targets important emerging and endemic swine viruses, namely African swine fever virus (ASFV), classical swine fever virus (CSFV), porcine reproductive and respiratory syndrome virus (PRRSV), porcine parvovirus (PPV), porcine circovirus 2 (PCV2) and swine influenza A virus (SIV). The approach takes advantage of three novel and validated technologies: (i) photonic integrated circuit (PIC) technology; (ii) label-free optical detection, based on refractive index sensing through ring resonators; (iii) a nano-deposition technology used to detect viruses in oral fluid such as saliva. The SWINOSTICS device demonstrated that it could provide results in less than 30 min for five samples simultaneously, making it highly suitable for use in the field by non-technical personnel also (Montagnese *et al.*, 2019).

3.3.5 Avian

Influenza is a highly contagious avian disease caused by the influenza virus. It spreads through saliva, nasal and other secretions as well as excretions from infected organisms (Veerapandian *et al.*, 2016). Real-time PCR (Rt-PCR) is the gold standard for the detection of the influenza virus. Although the technique is very specific, sensitive and accurate, it is labor- and time-intensive. Fluorescence resonance energy transfer (FRET) is a powerful molecular-level method used to detect small changes in response to interaction between biomolecules with high sensitivity. In FRET, non-radioactive energy is transferred from an excited donor to a ground-level acceptor (quencher) placed at distance of 1 to 10 nm. A FRET-based assay for the specific detection of surface antigen haemagglutinins (HAs) of the influenza virus has been developed (Chen and Neethirajan, 2015). The sensor is composed of two nanomaterial-based probes, i.e., luminescent glycan conjugated quantum dots (Gly-QDs) and anti-HA antibody-modified gold nanoparticles (Ab-Au NPs). On exposure to strain-specific HA, the two nanoprobes are brought together due to highly specific binding between HA and both the nanoprobes, forming a sandwich complex. In close proximity, the fluorescence intensity of QDs is quenched due to nonradiative FRET from

QDs to Au NPs. The changes in fluorescence intensity have been correlated to the initial concentration of HA in the tested sample.

Lateral-flow immunoassays are the most convenient method for the commercialized diagnosis of the influenza virus, capable of the detection of a specific analyte in complex media (Sajid *et al.*, 2015). The immunochromatography strips are generally composed of series of pads for spontaneous transporting of samples during analysis. The detection is based on the prior detection of a specific influenza virus onto the antibody-immobilized gold nanoparticles adsorbed on the conjugate pad. The strips consist of two test lines with pre-immobilized antibodies, each specific to either influenza A or B virus. In the presence of the analyte, the formed complex of influenza virus with immune-Au NPs gets transported to reach test lines and binds to specific pre-immobilized antibodies, resulting in a red color appearance due to the accumulation of Au NPs. The unbound immune Au NPs finally arrive at the control line harboring the secondary antibody, which is further shown as a visible red line. If the viral antigen is absent in the sample then the immune-Au NPs move forward and bind to the control line only. Therefore, the presence of two colored lines depicts a positive result, whereas a single red line indicates towards a negative result. Immunosensors are able to differentiate between influenza virus A and B; however, they exhibit inability to distinguish between highly pathogenic avian influenza virus (HPAIV) and low-pathogenic avian influenza virus (LPAIV). More specificity is incorporated in sensors using aptamers as biorecognition elements, which are short nucleic acid sequences that can be generated with high specificity to almost all the antigens. In spite of being simple, efficient, reliable and label-free, the various research groups are exploring ways to improve the sensitivity of lateral-flow devices. In one such report, silver nanoparticles were added to the test line, resulting in 1000-fold amplification of the colorimetric signal (Huang *et al.*, 2016). Quantum dots have also been used to improve sensitivity for avian influenza virus with a detection limit down to 0.09 ng/mL, which is a 100-fold improvement on the standard ELISA technique (Li *et al.*, 2012). Wu *et al.* (2016) reported a QD-based lateral-flow immunoassay which could be used for the quantification of influenza A virus subtype H5 and H9. The attachment of specific antibodies to QDs resulted in significant amplification of the signal and enabled the quantitative read-out of the analyte possible under an ultraviolet lamp.

Campylobacter jejuni is another avian pathogen found on poultry farms, which colonizes the intestine of chickens, waterfowl and turkeys. Poultry is also the main source of campylobacteriosis in humans (Lin, 2009). An optical biosensor has been developed for the detection of *C. jejuni* using a diffraction-based optical strategy and surface plasmon resonance (Gnanaprakasa *et al.*, 2011). The hippuricase gene (hipO) of *C. jejuni* has been used as a target sequence. The thiolated probe complementary to target the hipO gene was immobilized onto a gold-modified surface of a sensing chip. Hybridization of the probe to the target on the chip surface was transduced as the optical signal for *C. jejuni* quantification with a detection limit of 5.0 nM in infected samples.

3.3.6 Fish

Viral haemorrhagic septicaemia (VHS) is one of the most serious viral diseases of both fresh and marine fish species. The detection of the VHS virus is largely dependent on the conventional cell-culture and PCR-based methods, which are time- and labor-consuming. A sensitive and rapid QCM-based DNA biosensor has been demonstrated for the detection of the viral RNS-encoding G-protein in VHS (Hong *et al.*, 2010). The sensitivity of the biosensor was improved using three different DNA probes having 3′ modified ends via amine, biotin or thiol. Further, three different strategies of immobilization on gold-coated quartz surface were compared. First, thiol-labeled probes were immobilized on the naked gold surface. Next, immobilization of amine-functionalized probes on the gold surface fabricated as carxyl chips using methyl propionic acid (MPA) and ethyl (dimethylaminopropyl) carbodiimide/N-hydroxysuccinimide (EDC/NHS) was explored. Last, biotin-labeled DNA probes were attached to an avidin-modified carboxy-functionalized gold surface. All three formats were compared and the avidin-biotin binding was found to be the most effective method for the detection of target DNA. The prepared QCM biosensor exhibited stability of up to 32 repeated regenerations, with a detection limit of 0.0016 μM.

3.4 Bacteriophage-based Sensors for the Detection of Bacterial Pathogens

Bacteriophages, or simply phages, are the most abundant entities on earth, which specifically infect bacterial targets and are harmless to all other organisms, including humans. Due to the huge number of bacteriophages, i.e., 10^{31} particles (Hatfull, 2015) in every type of environment, their low cost of production, high stability in adverse conditions and specificity to targeting bacteria, bacteriophages are being explored as bioprobes for highly sensitive detection of AMR bacterial pathogens. Although significant importance has been given to AMR in humans, the trends in animals are not yet much emphasized. Dairy farming and the poultry industry involve the excessive use of antibiotics as prophylactic and growth-promoting agents (Sharma *et al.*, 2018). Much work is continuing globally on phage therapy (including the effectiveness of phages against MRSA in pigs), but far less information is available on the use of phages for the detection of pathogens in livestock or poultry.

Bacteriophage-based sensors for bacteria detection have been explored through the use of native as well as genetically modified phage particles at varied stages of the phage replication cycle. Several phage-based biosensors have been developed all over the world, involving different mechanical and electronic systems such as QCM, magnetoelastic platforms, SPR and electrochemical methods. Farooq *et al.* (2018) have reported the most recent advancements in whole-phage and phage components-based sensing assays and sensors. The importance of electrochemical biosensors has been emphasized as a simple, cost-effective, reliable and accurate tool for bacterial detection.

Tawil *et al.* (2012) reported the use of SPR for the biodetection of pathogenic bacteria methicillin-resistant *Staphylococcus aureus* (MRSA) and *Escherichia coli* (*E. coli*) O157:H7, using bacteriophages as the recognition elements. The system was found to detect pathogens for concentrations of 10^3 colony-forming units/mL in less than 20 minutes. Hence, the method permits label-free, real-time, rapid, specific and cost-effective detection of pathogens.

An electrochemical sensor for the detection of *C. jejuni* employing a glutathione-S-transferase (GST)-tagged phage receptor binding protein (RPB) Gp48 (GST-Gp48) was immobilized on a gold-modified electrode (Singh *et al.*, 2011). This resulted in oriented immobilization of GST-Gp48 RPB, which improved two- to three-fold bacteria capture efficiency. The sensing platform detected specific bacteria to a detection limit of 100 CFU/mL. Another reproducible, time-efficient and cost-effective bacteriophage assay has been developed to quantify the viable *Mycobacterium avium* subspecies *paratuberculosis* (MAP) in infected samples (Britton *et al.*, 2016). MAP or Johne's disease (paratuberculosis) is a chronic cattle disease posing a danger to economic welfare and health. For analysis, phages infecting MAP were incubated with the sample followed by the addition of a faster-growing bacterium specific to the used phages. In the presence of the target pathogen, the increased number of phages was released, killing neighboring sensor bacteria, resulting in the formation of plaques. A FASTPlaque TB assay was used to quantify the number of plaques, which was correlated to the initial concentration of the target analyte, MAP, with a detection limit of 1-10 CFU/mL. Further, the immunomagnetic separation was incorporated into the assay to achieve a faster response through pre-concentration and enhanced specificity (Britton *et al.*, 2016).

3.5 Conclusion

A profound change has occurred in recent years in veterinary diagnostics with the introduction of new biotechnological assays, which have completely changed the scenario of time-tested, traditional techniques of veterinary disease diagnosis (Prasad *et al.*, 2016). Sensor-based technologies are likely to be widely adopted in the future as they demonstrate the ability to improve diagnostic capabilities while reducing the time and, perhaps, cost associated with more conventional technologies. Biosensors are becoming the choice for mobile and pen-side testing of animal diseases due to their small size and easy handling. Traditionally, pathogens were detected from various biological samples by microscopic examination, biochemical analysis and other conventional methods like animal inoculation. Later on, several molecular and serological assays were employed for diagnostic purposes. Now, the focus is on sensors: wearable biosensors, ingestible biosensors, *in-situ* disease detection devices, online monitoring systems and many other smart nanotechnologies. All these advances are ultimately helping the livestock, poultry and fish industries in the timely detection of diseases so that action can be taken before the situation gets worse. Many such sensors are already on the market and many more are in the pipeline.

References

Basso, C.R., Tozato, C.C., Junior, J.P.A. and Pedrosa, V.A. (2015). A fast and highly sensitive method for the detection of canine distemper virus by the naked eye. *Analytical Methods*, *7*(6), 2264–2267.

Beer, M. and Dastjerdi, A. (2018). Infectious bovine rhinotracheitis/infectious pustular vulvovaginitis. In OIE Biological Standards Commission (ed.), *Manual of Diagnostic Tests and Vaccines for Terrestrial Animals*, pp. 1139–1157. World Organization for Animal Health (OIE), Paris.

Bhatta, D., Villalba, M.M., Johnson, C.L., Emmerson, G.D., Ferris, N.P., King, D.P. and Lowe, C.R. (2012). Rapid detection of foot-and-mouth disease virus with optical microchip sensors. *Procedia Chemistry*, *6*, 2–10.

Britton, L.E., Cassidy, J.P., O'Donovan, J., Gordon, S.V. and Markey, B. (2016). Potential application of emerging diagnostic techniques to the diagnosis of bovine Johne's disease (paratuberculosis). *The Veterinary Journal*, *209*, 32–39.

Chen, L. and Neethirajan, S. (2015). A homogenous fluorescence quenching based assay for specific and sensitive detection of influenza virus A haemagglutinin antigen. *Sensors*, *15*(4), 8852–8865.

Collins, P.J., Vachieri, S.G., Haire, L.F., Ogrodowicz, R.W., Martin, S.R., Walker, P.A. and Skehel, J.J. (2014). Recent evolution of equine influenza and the origin of canine influenza. *Proceedings of the National Academy of Sciences*, *111*(30), 11175–11180.

Cork, J., Jones, R.M. and Sawyer, J. (2013). Low cost, disposable biosensors allow detection of antibodies with results equivalent to ELISA in 15 min. *Journal of Immunological Methods*, *387*(1–2), 140–146.

Ellis, C.K., Stahl, R.S., Nol, P., Waters, W.R., Palmer, M.V., Rhyan, J.C. and Salman, M.D. (2014). A pilot study exploring the use of breath analysis to differentiate healthy cattle from cattle experimentally infected with Mycobacterium bovis. *PloS One*, *9*(2), e89280.

Farooq, U., Yang, Q., Ullah, M.W. and Wang, S. (2018). Bacterial biosensing: recent advances in phage-based bioassays and biosensors. *Biosensors and Bioelectronics*, *118*, 204–216.

Fowler, V., Bashiruddin, J. B., Belsham, G. J., Stenfeldt, C., Bøtner, A., Knowles, N. J. and Barnett, P. (2014). Characteristics of a foot-and-mouth disease virus with a partial VP1 GH loop deletion in experimentally infected cattle. *Veterinary Microbiology*, *169*(1–2), 58–66.

Frias, I.A., Andrade, C.A., Balbino, V.Q. and de Melo, C.P. (2017). Use of magnetically disentangled thiolated carbon nanotubes as a label-free impedimetric genosensor for detecting canine *Leishmaniasis spp*. infection. *Carbon*, *117*, 33–40.

Gajendragad, M.R., Kamath, K.N.Y., Anil, P.Y., Prabhudas, K. and Natarajan, C. (2001). Development and standardization of a piezo electric immunobiosensor for foot and mouth disease virus typing. *Veterinary Microbiology*, *78*(4), 319–330.

Gnanaprakasa, T.J., Oyarzabal, O.A., Olsen, E.V., Pedrosa, V.A. and Simonian, A.L. (2011). Tethered DNA scaffolds on optical sensor platforms for detection of hipO gene from *Campylobacter jejuni*. *Sensors and Actuators B: Chemical*, *156*(1), 304–311.

Hatfull, G.F. (2015). Dark matter of the biosphere: the amazing world of bacteriophage diversity. *Journal of Virology*, *89*, 8107–8110.

Hong, S.R., Jeong, H.D. and Hong, S. (2010). QCM DNA biosensor for the diagnosis of a fish pathogenic virus VHSV. *Talanta*, *82*(3), 899–903.

Hu, W.G., Thompson, H.G., Alvi, A.Z., Nagata, L.P., Suresh, M.R. and Fulton, R.E. (2004). Development of immunofiltration assay by light addressable potentiometric sensor with genetically biotinylated recombinant antibody for rapid identification of Venezuelan equine encephalitis virus. *Journal of Immunological Methods*, *289*(1–2), 27–35.

Huang, X., Aguilar, Z.P., Xu, H., Lai, W. and Xiong, Y. (2016). Membrane-based lateral flow immunochromatographic strip with nanoparticles as reporters for detection: a review. *Biosensors and Bioelectronics*, *75*, 166–180.

Ionescu, R.E., Cosnier, S., Herrmann, S. and Marks, R.S. (2007). Amperometric immunosensor for the detection of anti-West Nile virus IgG. *Analytical Chemistry*, *79*(22), 8662–8668.

Irwin, P. and Traub, R. (2006). Parasitic diseases of cats and dogs in the tropics. *Perspectives in Agriculture Veterinary Science, Nutrition and Natural Resources*, *1*, 21.

Kim, Y.K., Lim, S.I., Choi, S., Cho, I.S., Park, E.H. and An, D.J. (2015). A novel assay for detecting canine parvovirus using a quartz crystal microbalance biosensor. *Journal of Virological Methods*, *219*, 23–27.

Li, X., Lu, D., Sheng, Z., Chen, K., Guo, X., Jin, M. and Han, H. (2012). A fast and sensitive immunoassay of avian influenza virus based on label-free quantum dot probe and lateral flow test strip. *Talanta*, *100*, 1–6.

Lin, J. (2009). Novel approaches for Campylobacter control in poultry. *Foodborne Pathogens and Disease*, *6*(7), 755–765.

Montagnese, C., Barattini, P., Giusti, A., Balka, G., Bruno, U., Bossis, I. and Peransi, S. (2019). A diagnostic device for *in-situ* detection of swine viral diseases: the SWINOSTICS Project. *Sensors*, *19*(2), 407.

Neng, J., Harpster, M.H., Zhang, H., Mecham, J.O., Wilson, W.C. and Johnson, P.A. (2010). A versatile SERS-based immunoassay for immunoglobulin detection using antigen-coated gold nanoparticles and malachite green-conjugated protein A/G. *Biosensors and Bioelectronics*, *26*(3), 1009–1015.

Peled, N., Ionescu, R., Nol, P., Barash, O., McCollum, M., VerCauteren, K. and Haick, H. (2012). Detection of volatile organic compounds in cattle naturally infected with Mycobacterium bovis. *Sensors and Actuators B: Chemical*, *171*, 588–594.

Prasad, M., Brar, B., Ikbal, Ranjan, K., Lambe, U., Manimegalai, J., Vashisht, B., Khurana, S.K. and Prasad, G. (2016) Biotechnological tools for diagnosis of equine infectious diseases. *Journal of Experimental Biology and Agricultural Sciences*, *4* (Spl-4-EHIDZ). http://dx.doi.org/10.18006/2016.4(Spl-4-EHIDZ). S161.S181.

Pray, L., Lemon, S., Mahmoud, A. and Knobler, S. (eds) (2006). *The Impact of Globalization on Infectious Disease Emergence and Control: Exploring the Consequences and Opportunities: Workshop Summary*. National Academies Press, Washington, DC.

Purvis, D., Leonardova, O., Farmakovsky, D. and Cherkasov, V. (2003). An ultrasensitive and stable potentiometric immunosensor. *Biosensors and Bioelectronics*, *18*(11), 1385–1390.

Ramos-Jesus, J., Carvalho, K.A., Fonseca, R.A., Oliveira, G.G., Melo, S.M.B., Alcântara-Neves, N.M. and Dutra, R.F. (2011). A piezoelectric immunosensor for *Leishmania chagasi* antibodies in canine serum. *Analytical and Bioanalytical Chemistry*, *401*(3), 917–925.

Reid, S.M., Ferris, N.P., Brüning, A., Hutchings, G.H., Kowalska, Z. and Åkerblom, L. (2001). Development of a rapid chromatographic strip test for the pen-side detection of foot-and-mouth disease virus antigen. *Journal of Virological Methods*, *96*(2), 189–202.

Sajid, M., Kawde, A.N. and Daud, M. (2015). Designs, formats and applications of lateral flow assay: a literature review. *Journal of Saudi Chemical Society*, *19*(6), 689–705.

Sharma, C., Rokana, N., Chandra, M., Singh, B.P., Gulhane, R.D., Gill, J.P.S., Ray, P., Puniya, A.K. and Panwar, H. (2018). Antimicrobial resistance: its surveillance, impact, and alternative management strategies in dairy animals. *Frontiers in Veterinary Science*, *4*, 237.

Singh, A., Arutyunov, D., McDermott, M.T., Szymanski, C.M. and Evoy, S. (2011). Specific detection of *Campylobacter jejuni* using the bacteriophage NCTC 12673 receptor binding protein as a probe. *Analyst*, *136*(22), 4780–4786.

Snowder, G.D., Van Vleck, L.D., Cundiff, L.V., Bennett, G.L., Koohmaraie, M. and Dikeman, M.E. (2007). Bovine respiratory disease in feedlot cattle: phenotypic, environmental, and genetic correlations with growth, carcass, and longissimus muscle palatability traits. *Journal of Animal Science*, *85*(8), 1885–1892.

Sudarshan, M.K., Mahendra, B.J., Madhusudana, S.N., Narayana, D.A., Rahman, A., Rao, N.S.N. and Ravikumar, K. (2006). An epidemiological study of animal bites in India: results of a WHO sponsored national multi-centric rabies survey. *Journal of Communicable Diseases*, *38*(1), 32.

Tarasov, A., Gray, D.W., Tsai, M.Y., Shields, N., Montrose, A., Creedon, N. and Vogel, E.M. (2016). A potentiometric biosensor for rapid on-site disease diagnostics. *Biosensors and Bioelectronics*, *79*, 669–678.

Tawil, N., Sacher, E., Mandeville, R. and Meunier, M. (2012). Surface plasmon resonance detection of *E. coli* and methicillin-resistant *S. aureus* using bacteriophages. *Biosensors and Bioelectronics*, *37*, 24–29.

Thompson, P.N., Stone, A. and Schultheiss, W.A. (2006). Use of treatment records and lung lesion scoring to estimate the effect of respiratory disease on growth during early and late finishing periods in South African feedlot cattle. *Journal of Animal Science*, *84*(2), 488–498.

Veerapandian, M., Hunter, R. and Neethirajan, S. (2016). Dual immunosensor based on methylene blue-electroadsorbed graphene oxide for rapid detection of the influenza A virus antigen. *Talanta*, *155*, 250–257.

Vidic, J., Manzano, M., Chang, C.M. and Jaffrezic-Renault, N. (2017). Advanced biosensors for detection of pathogens related to livestock and poultry. *Veterinary Research*, *48*(1), 11.

Waters, R.A., Fowler, V.L., Armson, B., Nelson, N., Gloster, J., Paton, D.J. and King, D.P. (2014). Preliminary validation of direct detection of foot-and-mouth disease virus within clinical samples using reverse transcription loop-mediated isothermal amplification coupled with a simple lateral flow device for detection. *PLoS One*, *9*(8), e105630.

Wu, F., Yuan, H., Zhou, C., Mao, M., Liu, Q., Shen, H. and Li, L.S. (2016). Multiplexed detection of influenza A virus subtype H5 and H9 via quantum dot-based immunoassay. *Biosensors and Bioelectronics*, *77*, 464–470.

4

Applications of Metagenomics and Viral Genomics to Investigating Diseases of Livestock

Barbara Brito Rodriguez
The ithree institute, University of Technology Sydney, Sydney, New South Wales, Australia
Corresponding author: Barbara Brito Rodriguez, *barbara.britorodriguez@uts.edu.au*

4.1 Introduction

Sequencing the human genome was a headline-grabbing race that took 13 years from its 1990 start to its 2003 finish (International Human Genome Sequencing Consortium 2004). It was a race that incentivized the development of a number of high-throughput approaches for sequencing nucleic acids, approaches that we now refer to collectively as next-generation sequencing (NGS). By decreasing the cost and increasing the speed of sequencing, NGS ignited the modern genomic era. Release of the human genome sequence was quickly followed by a succession of whole genome sequences for a diversity of animal species, including *Gallus gallus* (completed in 2004), *Bos taurus* (2009), *Ovis aries* (2010), *Sus scrofa* (2012), and *Capra hircus* (2012) (Zimin *et al.* 2009; Groenen *et al.* 2012; International Chicken Genome Sequencing Consortium 2004; Dong *et al.* 2013). But not only we have benefited from completing the whole genome sequences of vertebrates and eukaryotic organisms, the sequencing of microorganisms has also contributed to our knowledge in the genetics and understanding of the genetic determinants of virulence, resistance, evolutionary adaptations and transmission patterns.

Understanding microbial diversity has been enabled by NGS and metagenomics approaches. Metagenomics is a process whereby all the microbial nucleic acids are extracted from a sample or specimen and then simultaneously subjected to sequencing technologies. An important aspect of this technique is that it does not require prior culture or isolation of the virus and it can be performed directly from a clinical or environmental sample or specimen. Using different techniques, we are able to sequence and characterize the "virome", which is the complete collection of viruses present in a sample. The virome can also refer to the complete diversity of viruses found in a specific host or an environment. Viral metagenomic sequencing aims at obtaining the virome in a sample, and it can be performed in either a targeted (using a set of probes or primers to enrich the sequencing of a diversity of viruses) or untargeted (sequencing is obtained without a prior enrichment) manner. NGS targeted to a specific viral species' genome or gene of interest (not metagenomics) is used to study a particular viral specie (not viromes or viral communities) and the sequences are obtained with a higher sensitivity. Both metagenomics and targeted viral species sequencing have important applications to advance our ability to identify and understand livestock diseases.

NGS may have been the spark, but the modern genomic era is fueled by powerful computing capabilities and efficient bioinformatic tools. This is especially true for microbial genomics. The deluge of sequencing data from microbes' metagenomes can be massive. Terabytes of sequence data must be stored and handled, necessitating substantial computing infrastructure and dedicated bioinformatic tools. Data processing and analysis methods and software must be developed or selected to fit the specific task.

This chapter first describes NGS principles and considerations in the context of viral infectious diseases of livestock. It highlights applications in which bioinformatic analysis of sequence data can benefit our ability to discover new viral pathogens, gain insights into their emergence, investigate disease outbreaks, diagnose disease, gain insights into viral ecology in complex diseases, and monitor the ongoing effectiveness of disease-prevention tools such as vaccines.

Metagenomics in the area of virology is challenged by both biological and technical factors. Viruses have a high taxonomic diversity and viral nucleic acid is often present in low amounts in a biological sample compared to the abundance of host and microbial (prokaryotes) nucleic acid. These factors have necessitated the development of approaches tailored to sequencing the communities of DNA and RNA viruses from clinical and environmental samples and in a diversity of vertebrate and invertebrate species. Metagenomics research as it relates to virology has two large demarcations: the study and characterization of prokaryotic viruses (bacteriophages) and the study and characterization of eukaryotic viruses. This chapter discusses the metagenomics of eukaryotic viruses, unless otherwise specified.

4.2 Obtaining Metagenomic Next-generation Sequencing Data for Viruses

The fundamental principle of NGS involves fragmenting the nucleic acid of different samples, adding short "barcode" sequences unique to each sample, and then sequencing the barcoded fragments in parallel during one run. Millions of small fragments from different samples can be sequenced together. Computational approaches subsequently assemble the sequences of fragments into complete or partial collections of viral genomes.

Beyond this fundamental principle, different NGS approaches to obtaining metagenomic sequencing data can be selected to meet a desired sequencing objective. For example, targeted metagenomics can consist of using amplicon sequencing (using PCR primers to amplify sequences of interest) or hybridization capture (using designed oligonucleotides to capture complementary sequences). These approaches are designed to identify a wide range of viruses. They can also be designed to identify conserved regions of viral families and genus. These techniques help overcome sequencing sensitivity due to the low amount of initial viral nucleic acid present in a sample. As a disadvantage, they introduce bias due to the targeted enrichment.

Shotgun viral metagenomics is an untargeted approach in which sequencing is performed without a previous molecular enrichment. The lack of enrichment means that shotgun metagenomics has lower sensitivity than some other NGS approaches, which can be a disadvantage. However, it can be optimized either during sample preparation (i.e., by filtering the sample) or by using a high depth of sequencing. Shotgun viral metagenomics protocols can be designed to obtain DNA and RNA viruses by using DNA and RNA extraction, random amplification and reverse transcription steps. If the focus of the metagenomic sequencing is RNA viruses, "metatranscriptomic" RNA sequencing can be used. The name metatranscriptomic derives from its primary use in sequencing the microbial communities' gene expression (messenger RNA); however, this technique is also useful in obtaining the RNA genome of the viruses. Deep sequencing of all the RNA (excluding ribosomal RNA) in a sample can capture the complete spectrum of the RNA viruses, as well as DNA virus gene expression (Shi *et al.* 2018; Zhang *et al.* 2019). This approach can be especially useful for studying disease complexes, because the gene expression of the bacterial communities and the host can be captured and analyzed in an integrated manner. Advantageously, this method lacks the propensity for bias that sample sequencing involving complex enrichment can have (the sequencing of some viral species may be favored while others are disfavored). However, a disadvantage is that it will not obtain high coverage of DNA viruses.

For the purpose of obtaining metagenomic sequencing data for livestock viruses, some special aspects need to be considered.

4.2.1 Sample Collection

Sampling livestock in the field can be logistically challenging because of the transportation needed from the field to the laboratory. This becomes an issue because the integrity of the viral DNA and RNA in the sample is critical for obtaining good-quality viromes. If possible, samples should be frozen and transported in dry ice or liquid nitrogen. In-house-prepared or commercially available transport media can also be considered to avoid nucleic acid degradation. Several commercial solutions offer formulations that preserve DNA and/or RNA at room temperature for convenient transport. Performance of these methods in molecular assays has been compared by Druce *et al.* (2012). The specific protocol should also balance differences between specimen or sample type (feces, nasal swabs, skin, etc.) and the anatomical site of the animal against the research objective. For example, one study that characterized the bovine respiratory virome found differences in viral species detection and abundance when sampling the upper and lower respiratory tract using nasal swabs or tracheal washes (Zhang *et al.* 2019).

4.2.2 Sample Preparation and Viral Enrichment

The nucleic acid present in a biological specimen will mostly comprise host DNA and RNA, followed by prokaryote nucleic acid. Viral nucleic acid is only a minuscule fraction of the total. Some approaches have been developed to address this issue, for example, different DNA/RNA extraction and purification protocols including centrifugation, filtration (0.22 or 0.45 um pore sizes), nuclease treatments steps (Zhang *et al.* 2018; Kohl *et al.* 2015; Liu *et al.* 2020; Lewandowska *et al.* 2017; Conceicao-Neto *et al.* 2015). As mentioned before, there are commercially available capture probes that hybridize with thousands of known vertebrate viruses, which enrich the amount of viral RNA sequenced (Wylie *et al.* 2015). If the objective is virus detection rather than sequencing, microarrays or pan-virus PCR primers can be employed. These target small conserved genetic regions of a wide arrange of viruses and viral families (Chen *et al.* 2011; Rose 2005).

4.2.3 Library Preparation and Sequencing

In general terms, library preparation consists of fragmenting the nucleic acid of the sample before adding adaptors and barcodes that will allow amplification, sample identification and binding to a surface where the sequencing will take place. The particular library preparation method used will depend on the sequencing platform. Some methods are designed to allow lower input of initial material; others allow for relatively degraded nucleic acid. The final part of library preparation is quality control—checking that the concentration and integrity of the library are compatible with the platform.

4.3 Bioinformatic Analysis of NGS Data

Running parallel sequencing on NGS platforms in the laboratory generates enormous amounts of raw data, which is then processed, analysed and interpreted via bioinformatics. A variety of bioinformatic workflows, each using different software and approaches, can be constructed for obtaining a final taxonomic profile for a sample and the consensus sequences for the viruses it contains (Nooij *et al.* 2018). However, regardless of the choice of workflow, the bioinformatic analysis of the raw data involves three main steps, described below.

4.3.1 Step 1: Quality Assessment of the Data Produced

The sequence of each of the millions of nucleic acid fragments is called a "read". Reads produced by most short-read sequencing platforms are between 50 and 400 base pairs in length. The reads are outputted as a text file, which contains information regarding the quality of each base called. Most sequence analysis algorithms begin by assessing the quality of the reads and then discarding bases that have been called with low quality. This process is known as "trimming" the reads.

4.3.2 Step 2: Assembly of Reads (Fragments)

Once low-quality bases have been removed, the reads are assembled. One of two approaches can be taken to assembly: *De novo* assembly or reference assembly (Figure 4.1). *De novo* assembly works based on algorithms that join reads, based on overlapping patterns of high similarity, into longer sequences called contigs. Contigs can be a few hundred or thousands of bases long. *De novo* assembly only relies on the sequence information contained in the reads and does not use any prior viral genome reference to guide the assembly of reads into contigs. In contrast, reference assembly uses known viral sequences as references, which are used to map the reads to any part of the reference viral genome. Many fragments may overlap in each of the nucleotide positions of the reference genome. The overlapping reads may be highly similar but not completely identical, either because of sequencing errors or because of the existence of minority haplotype variants typical of RNA viruses (a swarm of related viruses as a result of the fast replication rate and the lack of polymerase proof-reading ability) (Domingo and Perales 2019). The consensus sequence corresponds to one linear sequence of the viral genome that, in each of the nucleotide positions, contains the specific nucleotide base that was most frequently observed when assembling overlapping fragments (Figure 4.1).

4.3.3 Step 3: Taxonomic Classification

Contigs generated by *de novo* assembly or short sequenced reads are taxonomically classified by querying their similarity to a database containing thousands of viral genome sequence references that represent all known viral species. The largest and most widely used repository for nucleic acid sharing is NCBI GenBank. More specifically for viral genomes, there is a dedicated platform called NCBI Virus (www.ncbi.nlm.nih.gov/labs/virus/). For metagenomics projects, the raw read data has to be deposited in the NCBI Sequence Read Archive (SRA; www.ncbi.nlm.nih.gov/sra).The extent to which contigs obtained by *de novo* assembly can be taxonomically classified depends on the divergence from the reference database used to query the sequenced nucleic acid. Distant viruses from the same family may be identified as a new viral species if a relatively homologous region of the virus aligns with one existing viral species in the reference database. Completely new viruses that are extremely divergent from those in the reference databases (i.e., new viral families) may be missed. Indeed, when analyzing metagenomic data from different specimens and samples, a large number of reads and contigs cannot be classified (neither as viral, prokaryote nor eukaryote). Such sequences have been referred to as "dark matter" (Krishnamurthy and Wang 2017) and exploring these unknown contigs is a biological and bioinformatic challenge. Overcoming the challenges can deliver rewards. For example, the identification of a sequence common to

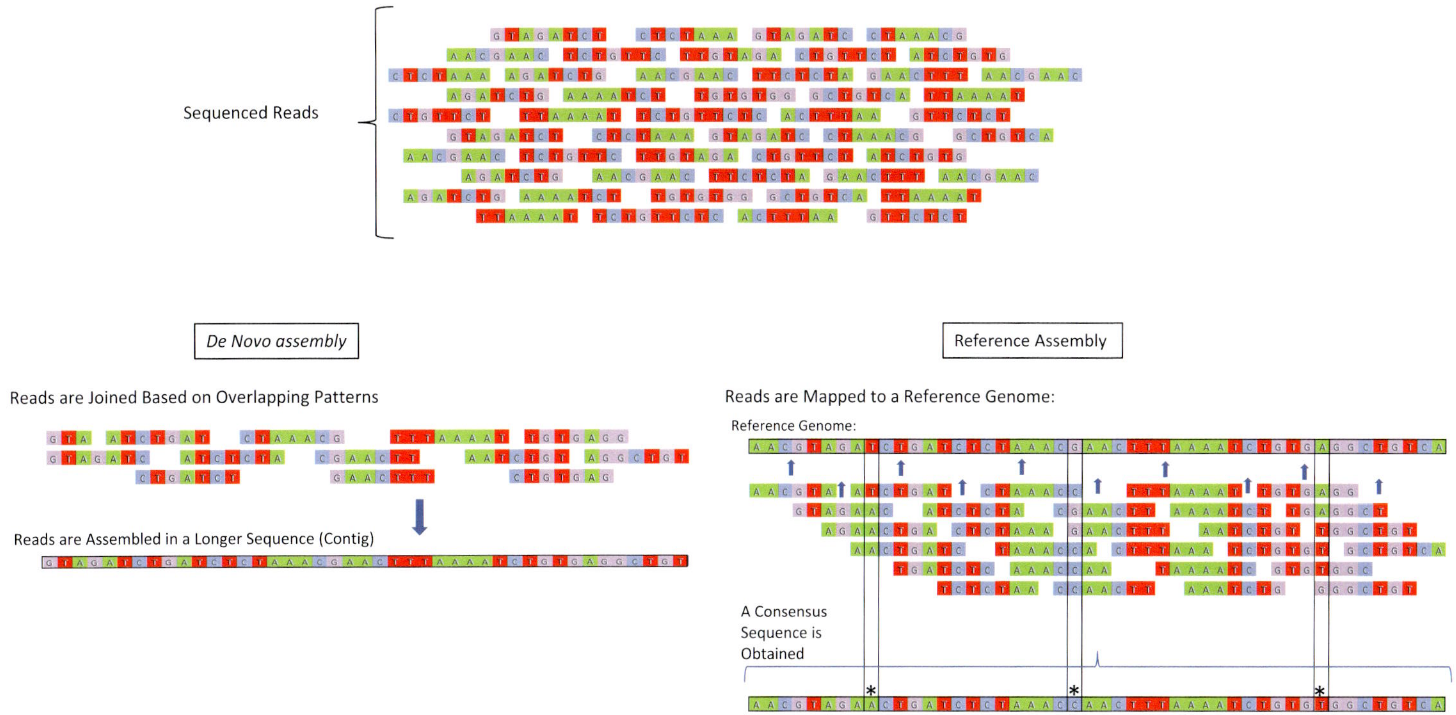

FIGURE 4.1 Simplified representation of *de novo* and reference-guided assembly.

During *de novo* assembly, sequenced reads are joined into a larger contig based on overlapping patterns. In contrast, reference-based assembly is guided by a reference genome. The reads are mapped to a specific part of the genome based on sequence similarity. After the read mapping, a consensus sequence is obtained by calling the most frequent base of the overlapping reads in each position. In the figure, positions indicated by * show different overlapped bases and how consensus sequence is constructed with the most abundant.

most fecal samples in humans led to the discovery of the CrAssphage, the most abundant bacteriophage in the human gut (Dutilh *et al.* 2014).

4.4 Metagenomics and Viral Genomics Can Identify New Viruses and Foster Understanding of Emerging Viruses

By developing different approaches to sequencing the communities of DNA and RNA viruses in environmental samples and a diversity of vertebrate and invertebrate species, we have extended our knowledge of the "virosphere" from 2285 known viral species in 2009 to >6500 as accepted by the International Committee of Taxonomy of Viruses (ICTV 2020). In livestock, viral metagenomic studies have discovered 14 new viruses in pigs, 9 in cattle, 3 in poultry and 1 in small ruminants, in addition to characterizing new genotypes of known viruses. A recent systematic review by Kwok *et al.* (2020) describes the data available from different viral metagenomics studies in livestock.

Whole-genome sequencing creates opportunities to understand routes by which new viruses emerge. When sequencing costs were relatively high, viral sequencing was limited to specific regions of the viral genome, which limited the insights that could be gained. For example, for genotyping assessment most of the attention was typically given to highly variable protein coding genes. Thus, most influenza viruses early studies tended to sequence only the hemagglutinin (HA) segment of the virus (HA is a surface protein subject to antigenic changes due to interaction with the host immune system), or sometimes HA in combination with the neuraminidase (NA) viral segment. Since the introduction of the more affordable NGS has enabled the complete genome of influenza viruses to be efficiently obtained, we now better understand the complex dynamics of influenza A reassortments or rearrangement of all gene segments during co-infection with different influenza A viruses (Chastagner *et al.* 2019). Understanding these dynamics (the emergence of new reassorted viruses) is particularly relevant in species known to harbor influenza viruses that have a zoonotic potential: swine and avian influenza. In a second example, the early focus on sequencing partial viral regions has led to public sequence repositories containing much higher numbers of sequences of the VP1 region of foot-and-mouth disease virus (FMDV) and the ORF5 sequences of porcine reproductive and respiratory syndrome (PRRS) viruses, in comparison to the whole genome sequence of their respective viruses. The availability of complete viral genomes enables proper recombination analysis between different areas within the viral genomes. Sequencing of only one viral "gene" does not allow us to detect and understand recombination between different coding regions of the genome. With more whole genomes of viruses published and available to study, we are understanding frequent patterns of recombination in PRRS and FMDV and their role in genotype emergence (Brito *et al.* 2018; Wang *et al.* 2019; Zhao *et al.* 2015).

4.5 Viral Genomics and Phylogenetics Can Identify Disease Transmission Chains

Knowing the genomic sequences of pathogens is useful for identifying and investigating viral disease outbreaks (disease source and disease spread). Virus detection traditionally relies on molecular and serologic methods that provide information about presence or absence of a pathogen. These methods may provide relatively quantitative information (i.e., Ct values of qPCR) or may differentiate between virus subtypes. For example, there are molecular assays that can detect if an influenza virus is type A, B or C, the type of HA (H1-H18) or can even differentiate within the hemagglutinin H1 subtype at a genotype level (i.e., H1N1pdm09 virus versus other seasonal H1 viruses) (WHO 2017; Chidlow *et al.* 2010). However, knowing the sequence of a pathogen genome takes investigatory powers up a step, offering finer resolution with an ability to differentiate organisms at an individual level. The ability to differentiate means that mutations that inevitably arise in the fast generation of viral progeny can be identified and used as markers to track links between cases. The resolution of the genetic changes is especially relevant for RNA viruses that lack a proofreading mechanism in their polymerase, resulting in high mutation rates. The genetic changes they incur can be tracked in individual transmission events with high resolution. Thus, for example, we now better understand the dynamics of human seasonal influenza virus and how some of these viruses can be transmitted and become endemic in swine populations globally (Rajao *et al.* 2018).

To visualize the genomic differences and evolutionary relationships between organisms, phylogenetic trees are used. Phylogenetic trees were originally used in evolutionary biology to understand the genetic relationship between a wide range of eukaryotic species (for example, the relationship between different mammals, or mammals and other vertebrates). The tree's pattern of branching reflects how species or other groups evolved from a series of common ancestors. The horizontal branch lengths often represent the genetic distance. The genetic relationship between samples obtained from different animals, inferred in a phylogenetic tree, can provide relevant information of the transmission chain. We can also understand the distribution or spread of different viral genotypes within regional and global contexts (Figure 4.2).

Phylogenetic trees can be constructed using different mathematical approaches. The choice of method depends on the objective of the analysis. The simplest methods, such as the neighbor-joining approach, can group sequences based on their total nucleotide similarity, and are useful for a quick general overview of a genetic relationship. More complex approaches, such as maximum likelihood and Bayesian phylogenetic analysis, are more appropriate for detailed analysis.

Phylogenetic analysis can be further combined with time and geographic information of disease occurrence, known now as phylogeographic analysis (Volz *et al.* 2013). The use of phylogeography to study the spread of pathogens (Lemey *et al.* 2009; 2010) increased following the development of Bayesian phylogeographic approaches.

Tailored information systems are important for disseminating viral genetic and spatiotemporal information in near-real time. Typically, they feature graphic interfaces with dynamic genetic and geographic data visualization, making them intuitive systems for interpreting disease occurrence. Information systems have been developed by organized groups to tackle specific health issues, including animal and plant health issues. For instance, Nexstrain (https://nextstrain.org/) is a publicly available platform that

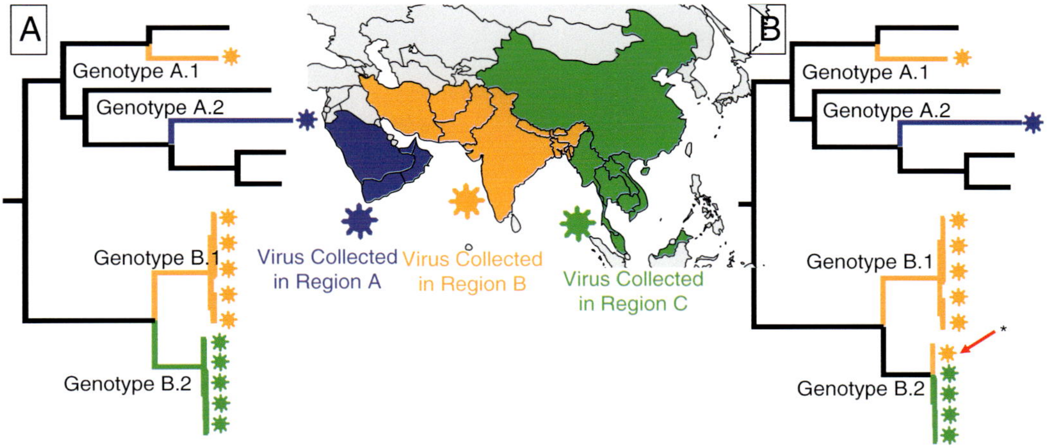

FIGURE 4.2 An example of how a phylogenetic tree and geographic information can provide important insights into virus distribution and spread.

In this example, viruses sequenced from samples collected in regions A, B, and C are depicted. Panel A shows a demarcated difference between the viruses present in the different regions, which may suggest presence of local genotypes without inter-region spread. It also shows that in region B, two different genotypes of the virus circulate. Panel B has a small difference where one sample from region B is grouped with viruses from region C. Depending on the genetic distance and additional epidemiological data, it may be hypothesized that there was an introduction of genotype B2 to region B from region C. All hypothesis and interpretation should be carefully assessed in combination with epidemiological data of the different regions, for example, animal movement, potential route of introduction, and bias in sampling strategies (sampling locations and sampling time).

allows for data sharing and visualization. In the field of animal health, for example, the Disease Bioportal (https://bioportal.ucdavis.edu/), developed by the Center for Animal Disease Modeling and Surveillance at the University of California, Davis, can be used to monitor the distribution of livestock viral diseases.

Pathogen genomic analyses can be applied to surveillance and control of viral animal diseases. Monitoring and controlling PRRS locally and FMDV globally are examples of how this approach can be used in animal health. For PRRS control in the United States, viral sequence data analyses have facilitated the tracking of viral spread (Alkhamis *et al.* 2017). The movement of live pigs between farms is a common practice, and understanding the disease status of each farm is vital to plan animal movement. Because several genotypes of PRRS circulate in the farms, sequencing and characterization enable the monitoring of disease spread. A regional approach that was adopted over a decade ago proposed a framework to share information of disease occurrence (Corzo et al. 2010). This effort has had an important impact in PRRS control by monitoring new PRRS outbreaks in farms using epidemiological and virus sequence data to understand transmission sources. Foot-and-mouth disease is one of the most widely studied livestock diseases, because of its impact in developing countries and the constant threat it presents to disease-free countries. Surveillance of FMD globally has been achieved by coordinating the efforts of a network of diagnostic laboratories across the world. Samples collected in several endemic countries are sequenced and the information is disseminated through quarterly and annual reports to understand the spread of specific viral lineages (www.wrlfmd.org). Based on the reports and spread in different regions, recommendations are made for vaccine formulations. These analyses further help preparation against new introductions of FMD into FMD-free countries by closely monitoring the dynamic distribution of the evolving FMDV lineages.

4.6 Viral Genomics in Monitoring Vaccine Matching

Another useful application of viral sequencing and molecular surveillance is monitoring the effectiveness of vaccination in livestock by identifying the similarity between circulating viruses and vaccine viruses. Divergent vaccine viruses may not correctly match local field strains for specific viruses. Different viruses have different antigenic matching genetic correlations (for example, for influenza A virus, a technique called antigenic cartography can be used to correlate genetic distance data with *in vitro* antigenic data of any two heterologous (different) viruses (Smith *et al.* 2004)). Antigenic cartography makes it possible to detect unexpected changes in antigenicity driven by small genetic changes. Although, there is no unmistakably direct correlation between the genetic distance of a vaccine and a field virus and the level of cross-protection. A proper evaluation of vaccine protection may be conducted when detecting divergent strains through molecular surveillance. One example is the commercial vaccine produced for H1N1pdm09 virus in swine. Failures in protection were observed when using more generic strains of the virus, so the assessment and use of a match vaccine candidate has been recommended (Tapia *et al.* 2020; Everett *et al.* 2019). As mentioned above, FMDV viruses and sequences are continuously monitored by the world reference laboratory, which makes recommendations of antigens to include in vaccines based on quarterly outputs of FMDV sequencing in different geographic regions (WRLFMD *et al.* 2020).

4.7 Viral Genomics and Metagenomics for Improving Molecular Diagnostics

Viral sequences, whether obtained from viral isolates or from metagenomic sequencing of clinical samples, can help improve veterinary molecular diagnostics in two main ways: first, by providing a test for the relevancy of diagnostic PCR primers; and second, by widening the scope of diagnostic assays. Veterinary diagnostic laboratories routinely use sensitive diagnostic assays such as RT-PCR assays that detect RNA viruses using a set of appropriate specific primers. Primer design is based on the genetic information available for the virus being screened for, and targets conserved areas of the virus. Diagnostic assays can fail when the local virus diverges in the region of the genome to which the primer has been designed to bind. This is particularly relevant for some RNA viruses that diverge quickly. The performance of the PCR can be assessed by monitoring viral sequences using the unbiased approaches of NGS.

Metagenomic studies in livestock that have discovered new viruses and characterized new genotypes of known viruses, while valuable, have taken place in limited locations. It is likely that as more metagenomics studies in livestock are carried out across the world, more viral species will be discovered. Including all new viruses in the design of new molecular assays to have available in veterinary diagnostic laboratories can be a critical tool in confirming the diagnosis of clinical diseases.

4.8 Viruses as Communities and Disease Causality

Viral diseases in livestock can be more complex than allowed for by Koch's postulates. Metagenomics and metatranscriptomics offer a handle on this complexity. Traditionally, Koch's postulates were the criteria to establish causality of infectious diseases. The postulates established that to prove causality, an organism must be found in diseased individuals but not in healthy ones. In addition, the disease should be replicated when a microorganism is isolated from a diseased animal, grown, and then used to inoculate a healthy animal. The causal relationship of some bacterial infections satisfies Koch's postulates. However, some infectious diseases depend on additional factors individual to the host, such as immunological conditions, and additional factors such as environmental stressors. A generic causal relationship of diseases caused by a complex of viral and/or bacterial pathogens can't be established by Koch's postulates. Similarly, it is difficult to establish the pathogenesis of the under-studied viruses that are present in healthy and diseased individuals, which have been recently identified by metagenomics studies. Metagenomics and metatranscriptomics can provide a means to understand the interactions of the virome, bacterial pathogens, and the individual host response that result in clinical disease. After establishing associations of pathogen combination, abundance, and host responses, further understanding of the detailed cellular and molecular mechanisms is required to understand the disease process. Assessment of disease causality through the study of metagenomics and viral genomics is still challenging due to the lack of culture systems to isolate and study some of the viruses found using metagenomics.

One example of a disease caused by multiple factors is bovine respiratory complex. Respiratory disease is the costliest disease in beef cattle. Transportation from breeding farms to the feedlot, changed diet, and the mixing of animals from different sources results in a combination of infectious agents and stressor factors that enable respiratory disease. Traditionally, respiratory disease has been attributed to viruses such as bovine respiratory syncytial virus (bovine orthopneumovius), bovine parainfluenza 3 (bovine respirovirus 3), bovine adenovirus, bovine viral diarrhea virus (BVDV or pestivirus), bovine coronavirus and infectious bovine rhinotracheitis virus (bovine alphaherpesvirus 1), and bacteria such as *Pasteurella multocida*, *Mannheimia haemolytica*, *Histophilus somni*, and *Mycoplasma bovis*. Diagnostics for respiratory disease in cattle are generally restricted to detecting these pathogens. More recent metagenomics studies have revealed the existence of a range of other viruses associated with respiratory disease such as influenza D, bovine nidovirus, and bovine rhinovirus A and B (Zhang *et al.* 2019; Ng *et al.* 2015; Mitra *et al.* 2016). Many of these viruses are present both in diseased and apparently healthy cattle, making the causation mechanism difficult to elucidate. Different statistical associations of the presence and abundance of specific viral species and the occurrence of clinical disease can provide initial insights into causation. These insights can help establish appropriate protocols for prevention, control and treatment.

4.9 Challenges and Future Directions

Metagenomics has thus far been applied by only a few groups around the world to study the virome in livestock. Their findings have revealed the existence of more viruses than the ones traditionally included in the detection assays of veterinary diagnostic laboratories. Future research efforts should focus on the role of newly discovered viruses as pathogens, and the development of new systems to effectively culture and study these viruses. Advanced laboratory and data analysis skills are currently required to conduct metagenomics. The development of biotechnologies that make laboratory processes simpler together with the automation of bioinformatics can expand the use of and insights from metagenomics. Training in

NGS and bioinformatics for technicians, veterinarians, and molecular biologists involved in field practice and laboratory diagnostics of livestock diseases may become common practice. This will advance our knowledge of infectious diseases and allow for better control and treatment strategies to improve animal health.

References

Alkhamis, M.A., A.G. Arruda, R.B. Morrison, and A.M. Perez. 2017. "Novel approaches for spatial and molecular surveillance of porcine reproductive and respiratory syndrome virus (PRRSv) in the United States." *Sci Rep* 7: 4343.

Brito, B., S.J. Pauszek, E.J. Hartwig, G.R. Smoliga, L.T. Vu, P.V. Dong, C. Stenfeldt, L.L. Rodriguez, D.P. King, N.J. Knowles, K. Bachanek-Bankowska, N.T. Long, D.H. Dung, and J. Arzt. 2018. "A traditional evolutionary history of foot-and-mouth disease viruses in Southeast Asia challenged by analyses of non-structural protein coding sequences." *Sci Rep* 8 (1): 6472.

Chastagner, A., E. Bonin, C. Fablet, S. Queguiner, E. Hirchaud, P. Lucas, S. Gorin, N. Barbier, V. Beven, E. Garin, Y. Blanchard, N. Rose, S. Herve, and G. Simon. 2019. "Virus persistence in pig herds led to successive reassortment events between swine and human influenza A viruses, resulting in the emergence of a novel triple-reassortant swine influenza virus." *Vet Res* 50 (1): 77.

Chen, E.C., S.A. Miller, J.L. DeRisi, and C.Y. Chiu. 2011. "Using a pan-viral microarray assay (Virochip) to screen clinical samples for viral pathogens." *J Vis Exp* 50: 2536.

Chidlow, G., G. Harnett, S. Williams, A. Levy, D. Speers, and D.W. Smith. 2010. "Duplex real-time reverse transcriptase PCR assays for rapid detection and identification of pandemic (H1N1) 2009 and seasonal influenza A/H1, A/H3, and B viruses." *J Clin Microbiol* 48 (3): 862–866.

Conceicao-Neto, N., M. Zeller, H. Lefrere, P. De Bruyn, L. Beller, W. Deboutte, C.K. Yinda, R. Lavigne, P. Maes, M. Van Ranst, E. Heylen, and J. Matthijnssens. 2015. "Modular approach to customise sample preparation procedures for viral metagenomics: a reproducible protocol for virome analysis." *Sci Rep* 5: 16532.

Corzo, C.A., E. Mondaca, S. Wayne, M. Torremorell, S. Dee, P. Davies, and R.B. Morrison. 2020. "Control and elimination of porcine reproductive and respiratory syndrome virus." *Review Virus Res* 154(1–2): 185–192.

Domingo, E. and C. Perales. 2019. "Viral quasispecies." *PLoS Genet* 15 (10): e1008271.

Dong, Y., M. Xie, Y. Jiang, N. Xiao, X. Du, W. Zhang, G. Tosser-Klopp, J. Wang, S. Yang, J. Liang, W. Chen, J. Chen, P. Zeng, Y. Hou, C. Bian, S. Pan, Y. Li, X. Liu, W. Wang, B. Servin, B. Sayre, B. Zhu, D. Sweeney, R. Moore, W. Nie, Y. Shen, R. Zhao, G. Zhang, J. Li, T. Faraut, J. Womack, Y. Zhang, J. Kijas, N. Cockett, X. Xu, S. Zhao, J. Wang, and W. Wang. 2013. "Sequencing and automated whole-genome optical mapping of the genome of a domestic goat (Capra hircus)." *Nat Biotechnol* 31 (2): 135–141.

Druce, J., K. Garcia, T. Tran, G. Papadakis, and C. Birch. 2012. "Evaluation of swabs, transport media, and specimen transport conditions for optimal detection of viruses by PCR." *J Clin Microbiol* 50 (3): 1064–1065.

Dutilh, B.E., N. Cassman, K. McNair, S.E. Sanchez, G.G. Silva, L. Boling, J.J. Barr, D.R. Speth, V. Seguritan, R.K. Aziz, B. Felts, E.A. Dinsdale, J.L. Mokili, and R.A. Edwards. 2014. "A highly abundant bacteriophage discovered in the unknown sequences of human faecal metagenomes." *Nat Commun* 5: 4498.

Everett, H.E., M. Aramouni, V. Coward, A. Ramsay, M. Kelly, S. Morgan, E. Tchilian, L. Canini, M.E.J. Woolhouse, S. Gilbert, B. Charleston, I.H. Brown, and S.M. Brookes. 2019. "Vaccine-mediated protection of pigs against infection with pandemic H1N1 2009 swine influenza A virus requires a close antigenic match between the vaccine antigen and challenge virus." *Vaccine* 37 (17): 2288–2293.

Groenen, M.A., A.L. Archibald, H. Uenishi, C.K. Tuggle, Y. Takeuchi, M.F. Rothschild, C. Rogel-Gaillard, C. Park, D. Milan, H.J. Megens, S. Li, D.M. Larkin, H. Kim, L.A. Frantz, M. Caccamo, H. Ahn, B.L. Aken, A. Anselmo, C. Anthon, L. Auvil, B. Badaoui, C.W. Beattie, C. Bendixen, D. Berman, F. Blecha, J. Blomberg, L. Bolund, M. Bosse, S. Botti, Z. Bujie, M. Bystrom, B. Capitanu, D. Carvalho-Silva, P. Chardon, C. Chen, R. Cheng, S.H. Choi, W. Chow, R.C. Clark, C. Clee, R.P. Crooijmans, H.D. Dawson, P. Dehais, F. De Sapio, B. Dibbits, N. Drou, Z.Q. Du, K. Eversole, J. Fadista, S. Fairley, T. Faraut, G.J. Faulkner, K.E. Fowler, M. Fredholm, E. Fritz, J.G. Gilbert, E. Giuffra, J. Gorodkin, D.K. Griffin, J.L. Harrow, A. Hayward, K. Howe, Z.L. Hu, S.J. Humphray, T. Hunt, H. Hornshoj, J.T. Jeon, P. Jern, M. Jones, J. Jurka, H. Kanamori, R. Kapetanovic, J. Kim, J.H. Kim, K.W. Kim, T.H. Kim, G. Larson, K. Lee, K.T. Lee, R. Leggett, H.A. Lewin, Y. Li, W. Liu, J.E. Loveland, Y. Lu, J.K. Lunney, J. Ma, O. Madsen, K. Mann, L. Matthews, S. McLaren, T. Morozumi, M.P. Murtaugh, J. Narayan, D.T. Nguyen, P. Ni, S.J. Oh, S. Onteru, F. Panitz, E.W. Park, H.S.

Park, G. Pascal, Y. Paudel, M. Perez-Enciso, R. Ramirez-Gonzalez, J.M. Reecy, S. Rodriguez-Zas, G.A. Rohrer, L. Rund, Y. Sang, K. Schachtschneider, J.G. Schraiber, J. Schwartz, L. Scobie, C. Scott, S. Searle, B. Servin, B.R. Southey, G. Sperber, P. Stadler, J.V. Sweedler, H. Tafer, B. Thomsen, R. Wali, J. Wang, J. Wang, S. White, X. Xu, M. Yerle, G. Zhang, J. Zhang, J. Zhang, S. Zhao, J. Rogers, C. Churcher, and L.B. Schook. 2012. "Analyses of pig genomes provide insight into porcine demography and evolution." *Nature* 491 (7424): 393–398.

International Committee on Taxonomy of Viruses (ICTV). 2020. "Virus taxonomy, the ICTV report on virus classification and taxon nomenclature." https://talk.ictvonline.org/ictv-reports/ictv_online_report/.

International Chicken Genome Sequencing Consortium. 2004. "Sequence and comparative analysis of the chicken genome provide unique perspectives on vertebrate evolution." *Nature* 432 (7018): 695–716.

International Human Genome Sequencing Consortium. 2004. "Finishing the euchromatic sequence of the human genome." *Nature* 431 (7011): 931–945.

Kohl, C., A. Brinkmann, P.W. Dabrowski, A. Radonic, A. Nitsche, and A. Kurth. 2015. "Protocol for metagenomic virus detection in clinical specimens." *Emerg Infect Dis* 21 (1): 48–57.

Krishnamurthy, S.R. and D. Wang. 2017. "Origins and challenges of viral dark matter." *Virus Res* 239: 136–142.

Kwok, K.T.T., D.F. Nieuwenhuijse, M.V.T. Phan, and M.P.G. Koopmans. 2020. "Virus metagenomics in farm animals: a systematic review." *Viruses* 12 (1): 107.

Lemey, P., A. Rambaut, A.J. Drummond, and M.A. Suchard. 2009. "Bayesian phylogeography finds its roots." *PLoS Comput Biol* 5 (9): e1000520.

Lemey, P., A. Rambaut, J.J. Welch, and M.A. Suchard. 2010. "Phylogeography takes a relaxed random walk in continuous space and time." *Mol Biol Evol* 27 (8): 1877–1885.

Lewandowska, D.W., O. Zagordi, F.D. Geissberger, V. Kufner, S. Schmutz, J. Boni, K.J. Metzner, A. Trkola, and M. Huber. 2017. "Optimization and validation of sample preparation for metagenomic sequencing of viruses in clinical samples." *Microbiome* 5 (1): 94.

Liu, B., N. Shao, J. Wang, S. Zhou, H. Su, J. Dong, L. Sun, L. Li, T. Zhang, and F. Yang. 2020. "An optimized metagenomic approach for virome detection of clinical pharyngeal samples with respiratory infection." *Front Microbiol* 11: 1552.

Mitra, N., N. Cernicchiaro, S. Torres, F. Li, and B.M. Hause. 2016. "Metagenomic characterization of the virome associated with bovine respiratory disease in feedlot cattle identified novel viruses and suggests an etiologic role for influenza D virus." *J Gen Virol* 97 (8): 1771–1784.

Ng, T.F., N.O. Kondov, X. Deng, A. Van Eenennaam, H.L. Neibergs, and E. Delwart. 2015. "A metagenomics and case-control study to identify viruses associated with bovine respiratory disease." *J Virol* 89 (10): 5340–5349.

Nooij, S., D. Schmitz, H. Vennema, A. Kroneman, and M.P.G. Koopmans. 2018. "Overview of virus metagenomic classification methods and their biological applications." *Front Microbiol* 9: 749.

Rajao, D.S., A.L. Vincent, and D.R. Perez. 2018. "Adaptation of human influenza viruses to swine." *Front Vet Sci* 5: 347.

Rose, T.M. 2005. "CODEHOP-mediated PCR – a powerful technique for the identification and characterization of viral genomes." *Virol J* 2: 20.

Shi, M., Y.Z. Zhang, and E.C. Holmes. 2018. "Meta-transcriptomics and the evolutionary biology of RNA viruses." *Virus Res* 243: 83–90.

Smith, D.J., A.S. Lapedes, J.C. de Jong, T.M. Bestebroer, G.F. Rimmelzwaan, A.D. Osterhaus, and R.A. Fouchier. 2004. "Mapping the antigenic and genetic evolution of influenza virus." *Science* 305 (5682): 371–376.

Tapia, R., M. Torremorell, M. Culhane, R.A. Medina, and V. Neira. 2020. "Antigenic characterization of novel H1 influenza A viruses in swine." *Sci Rep* 10 (1): 4510.

Volz, E.M., K. Koelle, and T. Bedford. 2013. "Viral phylodynamics." *PLoS Comput Biol* 9 (3): e1002947.

Wang, A., Q. Chen, L. Wang, D. Madson, K. Harmon, P. Gauger, J. Zhang, and G. Li. 2019. "Recombination between Vaccine and Field Strains of Porcine Reproductive and Respiratory Syndrome Virus." *Emerg Infect Dis* 25 (12): 2335–2337.

World Health Organization (WHO). 2017. *WHO Information for the Molecular Detection of Influenza Viruses.* www.who.int/influenza/gisrs_laboratory/WHO_information_for_the_molecular_detection_of_influenza_viruses_20171023_Final.pdf?ua=1.

World Reference Laboratory for Foot-and-Mouth Disease (WRLFMD), World Organization for Animal Health (OIE), and Food and Agriculture Organization (FAO). 2020. "The World Reference Laboratory for Foot-and-Mouth Disease (WRLFMD) reports." www.wrlfmd.org/.

Wylie, T.N., K.M. Wylie, B.N. Herter, and G.A. Storch. 2015. "Enhanced virome sequencing using targeted sequence capture." *Genome Res* 25 (12): 1910–1920.

Zhang, D., X. Lou, H. Yan, J. Pan, H. Mao, H. Tang, Y. Shu, Y. Zhao, L. Liu, J. Li, J. Chen, Y. Zhang, and X. Ma. 2018. "Metagenomic analysis of viral nucleic acid extraction methods in respiratory clinical samples." *BMC Genomics* 19 (1): 773.

Zhang, M., J.E. Hill, C. Fernando, T.W. Alexander, E. Timsit, F. van der Meer, and Y. Huang. 2019. "Respiratory viruses identified in western Canadian beef cattle by metagenomic sequencing and their association with bovine respiratory disease." *Transbound Emerg Dis* 66 (3): 1379–1386.

Zhang, Y.Z., Y.M. Chen, W. Wang, X.C. Qin, and E.C. Holmes. 2019. "Expanding the RNA virosphere by unbiased metagenomics." *Annu Rev Virol* 6 (1): 119–139.

Zhao, K., C. Ye, X.B. Chang, C.G. Jiang, S.J. Wang, X.H. Cai, G.Z. Tong, Z.J. Tian, M. Shi, and T.Q. An. 2015. "Importation and recombination are responsible for the latest emergence of highly pathogenic porcine reproductive and respiratory syndrome virus in China." *J Virol* 89 (20): 10712–10716.

Zimin, A.V., A.L. Delcher, L. Florea, D.R. Kelley, M.C. Schatz, D. Puiu, F. Hanrahan, G. Pertea, C.P. Van Tassell, T.S. Sonstegard, G. Marcais, M. Roberts, P. Subramanian, J.A. Yorke, and S.L. Salzberg. 2009. "A whole-genome assembly of the domestic cow, Bos taurus." *Genome Biol* 10 (4): R42.

5

Toll-like Receptors in Livestock Species

P.K. Dubey,[1] S. Dubey,[1] Suresh Kumar Gahlawat[2] and R.S. Kataria[3]
[1] *Temple University, Philadelphia-19140, Pennsylvania, USA*
[2] *Department of Biotechnology, Chaudhary Devi Lal University, Sirsa-125055, Haryana, India*
[3] *Division of Animal Biotechnology, ICAR, National Bureau of Animal Genetic Resources, Karnal-132001, Haryana, India*
Corresponding author: R.S. Kataria, *katariaranji@yahoo.co.in*

Ever since their domestication, livestock species have played a pivotal role in meeting human demands of food, transportation, clothing and many more. A few of these species moved from place to place, along with the migration of the human race, to settle in different places globally. During the passage of time, these species went onto adapt themselves to local agro-climatic conditions, both naturally and through management practices. These livestock species are a major source of milk, butter, fat and meat, besides also providing an enormous contribution in terms of draught, hide and manure. Many of these species are known for their unique attributes, including their adaptation to tropical or temperate climates, utilization of often-coarse fodder, unique reproduction features and resistance to diseases. Among these characteristic features, tropically adapted species are known for their ability to resist prevalent infectious diseases, such as those caused by tick-borne protozoa and many viral pathogens, better than species adapted to temperate climatic conditions. It is, therefore, important to understand the mechanism of immune activation in these species, for their selection and sustainable use.

Two fundamentally different types of responses of the immune system have been identified in mammals: innate and acquired (adaptive). The innate defence mechanism primarily reduces pathogen load and further activates selective adaptive immunity for final clearance of pathogens. Innate immunity is an important front line in the defense system of a host against infectious diseases by discriminating between self and non-self. Immune cells express different non-clonal receptors, termed "pattern recognition receptors" (PRRs), against the microbial constituents to activate the host's innate immune system. These PRRs selectively recognize conserved domains of microbial components such as pathogen-associated molecular patterns (PAMPs). These PRRs are also constantly monitoring the host's internal environment and clearing it of any endogenous changes due to accumulation of host ligands, which are produced during viral infection and/or tumour formation, tissue injury, apoptosis etc. (Medzhitov *et al.* 1997). Several family proteins of PRRs have been reported which act as the first line of defense: calcium-dependent lectin, leucine-rich repeat (LRR) and scavenger receptor domains etc., stimulated by binding with different PAMPs for immune cell activation.

5.1 Toll-like Receptors

Toll-like receptors are one of the most important pattern recognition receptor families of PRRs, and can discriminate between diverse classes of microbial products and activate the innate immune system for the development of antigen-specific acquired immunity. Toll-like receptors are evolutionarily conserved from worms to mammals and have been identified in vertebrates due to their homology with *Toll*, a molecule identified in *Drosophila* essential for embryonic development (Anderson *et al.* 1985) and later was found to be important for antifungal responses in flies (Lemaitre *et al.* 1996). After the discovery of the role of Drosophila Toll in host defense against fungal infection, a mammalian homologue, now known as TLR4, was identified (Medzhitov *et al.* 1997), later leading to the discovery of other TLRs.

5.1.1 Structure of TLRs

TLRs consist of an extracellular domain, composed of several leucine-rich repeats (LRR) motifs, sandwiched between the LRRNT and LRRCT modules. The LRR domain of the TLRs forms a horseshoe structure ectodomain for the ligand binding to the concave surface (Choe *et al.* 2005), followed by a short transmembrane and conserved cytoplasmic domain. Cytoplasmic domain is highly homologous among TLRs and contains a Toll/IL-1R (TIR) domain similar to the interleukin-1 receptor (IL-1R) that mediates recruitment of downstream signaling proteins (Akira and Takeda 2004; Figure 5.1).

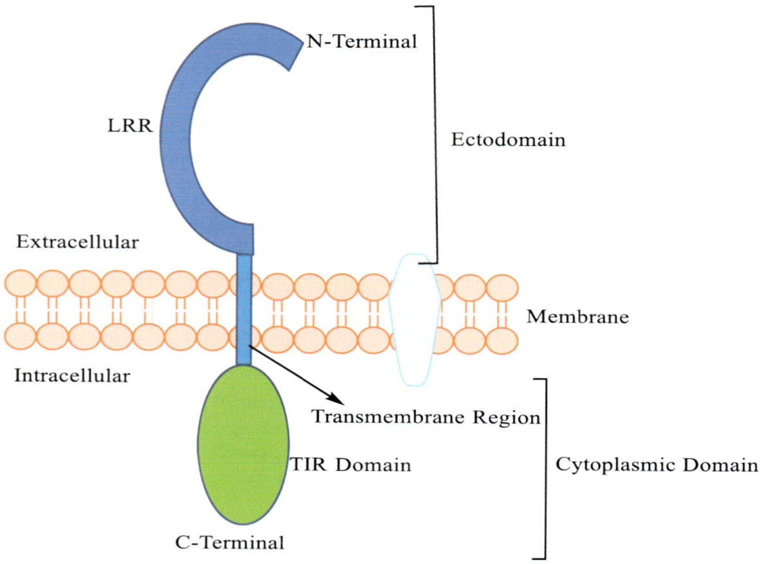

FIGURE 5.1 Structure of typical toll-like receptor.

5.1.2 Ligands of TLRs

Microbial components of bacteria, viruses, fungi and parasites are considered as primary ligands for the TLRs family. These ligands are recognized by different TLRs and elicit a distinct immune response accordingly (Janssens and Beyaert 2003). TLR2 is activated by bacterial cell wall components of Gram-positive bacteria. In response to lipoproteins, lipoteichoic acids, peptidoglycan and zymosan, TLR2 forms heterodimers with TLR1 or TLR6 and, depending upon the heterodimerization of TLR2, it can discriminate between triacyl (TLR2/6) and diacyl (TLR1/2) lipopeptides. TLR2 also forms heterodimers with TLR10 and TLR1, but the specific ligands have not yet been identified. Endosomal expression of TLR3 recognizes double-stranded (ds) RNA viruses, self-mRNA and the synthetic nucleoside moiety (Parker *et al.* 2007). TLR4 mainly recognizes lipopolysaccharides (LPSs) of Gram-negative bacteria and a range of host-derived molecules, such as heat-shock proteins and various extracellular matrix components, including fibronectin, hyaluronic acid and heparan sulfate (Takeda and Akira 2003). TLR5 recognizes flagellin, an essential component of flagella found in both Gram-positive and Gram-negative bacteria (Heine and Lien 2003). Also, TLR5 forms both a homodimer and a heterodimer with TLR4 but they do not alter their function. TLR6 recognizes multiple diacyl lipopeptides of mycoplasma and zymogen, also forming a heterodimer with TLR2. Like TLR1, TLR6 is thought to be specifying or enhancing the PAMP sensitivity of TLR2 and contributes to its signaling capabilities through hetero dimerization. Both TLR7 and TLR8 mediate responses to single-stranded (ss) viral RNA, but they also respond to immunomodulatory drugs such as loxoribine and imidazoquinolines, including imiquimod (R-837) and resiquimod (R-848). TLR9 responds to bacterial and viral DNA containing unmethylated CpG motifs (Takeda and Akira 2003). Much is still unknown about TLR10 associations or ligand recognition, but it is assumed that it may form a heterodimer with TLR2, like TLR1 and TLR6, and thereby be sensitive to similar PAMPs (Table 5.1; Figure 5.2).

TABLE 5.1

Mammalian TLRs cellular locations and their ligands

Receptor	Adapter	Dimerization	Location	Ligand(s)	Ligand Location
TLR1	MyD88	Hetero, TLR2, TLR6, TLR10	Cell surface	Triacyl lipopeptides	Bacteria
TLR2	MyD88	Hetero, TLR1, TLR2, TLR6	Cell surface	Glycolipids, lipopeptides, lipoproteins, lipoteichoic acid, peptidoglycan, HSP70, zymosan	Gram-positive bacteria, host cells, fungi
TLR3	TRIF	Homodimer	Endosome	dsRNA, poly I:C	Viruses
TLR4	MyD88/TRIF	Homo and hetero TLR2	Cell surface	Lipopolysaccharide, heat shock proteins, fibrinogen, hyaluronic acid	Gram-negative bacteria, host cells
TLR5	MyD88	Homo	Cell surface	Flagellin	Bacteria
TLR6	MyD88	Hetero	Cell surface	Diacyl lipopeptides	Mycoplasma
TLR7	MyD88	Homo and hetero	Cell compartment	Imidazoquinoline ssRNA	Small synthetic compounds
TLR8	MyD88	Homo and hetero	Cell compartment	Small synthetic compounds; single-stranded RNA	
TLR9	MyD88	Homo and hetero	Cell compartment	Unmethylated CpG DNA	Bacteria
TLR10	Unknown	Hetero	Cell surface	Unknown	Unknown

(http://en.wikipedia.org/wiki/Toll-like_receptor)

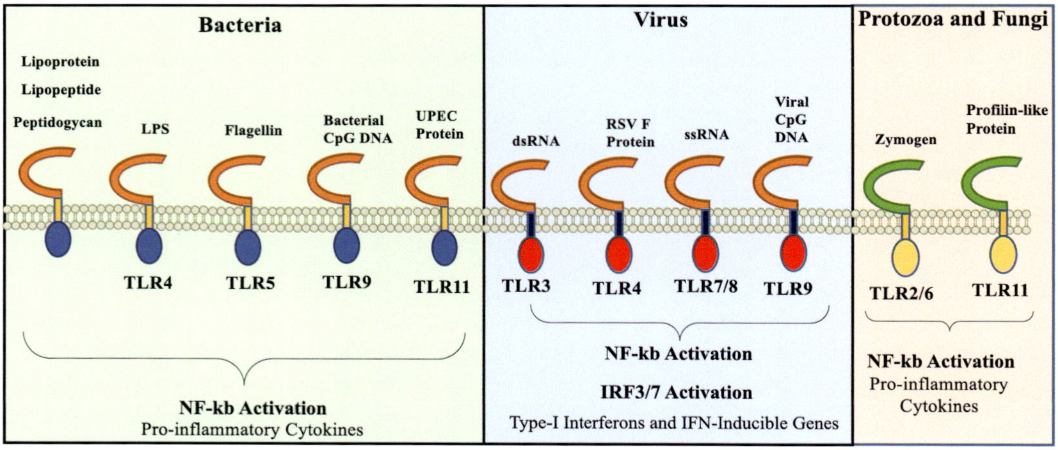

FIGURE 5.2 TLR ligand specificities, recognizing a diverse array of PAMPs from bacteria, viruses, protozoa and fungi.

5.1.3 Cellular Localization of TLRs

In mammals, a total of 13 TLRs (Roach *et al.* 2005) have been identified on the basis of recognition of highly conserved structural motifs of microbial pathogens (Akira and Takeda 2004). Depending on their localization on the cell, they are divided into two groups, the first group (TLRs 1, 2, 4, 5 and 6) being found on the membrane and the second group (TLRs 3, 7, 8 and 9) on the intracellular endosomes. The cellular localization of different TLRs with their respective adapters has been given in Table 5.1.

5.1.4 Tissue Distribution of TLRs

Expression of TLRs is in almost all kinds of cells, but their expression on a few cells is low and upon exposure to pathogen they are upregulated (Dhara *et al.* 2007). TLR expression patterns have been analyzed in different species: humans (Zarember and Godowski 2002), mice (Prueet *et al.* 2004) and chickens (Iqbal and Philbin 2005), but the first study on ruminant TLR expression was given by Menzies and Ingham (2006). TLRs 3, 5 and 6 were maximum expressed in ovine jejunum, while TLRs 6, 7 and 10 were expressed in both ovine Peyer's patch and mesenteric lymph node. In cattle, all TLRs were expressed in bovine skin except TLR6. TLR2 and TLR7 transcripts were most abundant and TLR4 was very low in bovine skin. A similar expression pattern was observed in buffalo and goat (Menzies and Ingham 2006; Raja *et al.* 2011; Goyal *et al.* 2013a). The first report on the expression profiling of different TLRs in buffalo tissues by semi-quantitative PCR was given by Vahanan and coworkers (2008). They reported the expression profile of TLRs 1–10 in buffalo peripheral blood mononuclear cells (PBMNC), neutrophils, spleen, liver, lung, heart, kidney, ovary and uterus using a reverse transcriptase polymerase chain reaction (RT-PCR). Further, the expression profile was confirmed by a real-time PCR quantification method (McGuire *et al.* 2005).

5.1.5 Localization of TLRs on Mammalian Chromosomes

The TLRs identified so far in murine, human, pig, horse and cattle subjects have been successfully mapped to different chromosomes. Bovine TLRs' genomic organization was found to be the same as that of humans and mice (McGuire *et al.* 2005). Bovine TLR1, TLR6 and TLR10 were mapped closely on *Bos taurus* chromosome 6 (BTA6), with results similar to those observed in human chromosome 4, said to result from gene duplication (Beutler and Rehli 2002). Like other species, bovine TLR7 and TLR8 were present on the BTX chromosome. The remaining TLRs (TLRs 2, 3, 4, 5 and 9) were mapped to BTAs 17,

27, 8, 16 and 22, respectively (White *et al.* 2003; Goldammer *et al.* 2004). Amaral and others (2008) have shown whole-genome RH mapping of the riverine buffalo and compared with cattle, BTA6 homologous chromosome map BBU7 (TLRs 1, 6, 10), BTAX homologous chromosome map BBUX (TLRs 7 and 8), BTA17, BTA27, BTA8, BTA16 and BTA22 homologous chromosome map BBU17, BBU1, BBU3, BBU5 and BBU21, respectively.

5.2 TLR Signaling Pathways

Engagement of TLRs with microbial components triggers the activation of signaling cascades, leading to the induction of immune genes involved in antimicrobial host defense (Akira and Takeda 2004). After recognition of ligands, TLRs undergo conformational changes and dimerize for the recruitment of TIR domain-containing adaptor proteins which interact with the TIR domain of TLR. The differential response of TLR mediated by distinct ligands leads to selective usage of adaptor molecules. Two major molecules, MyD88 (myeloid differentiation factor 88) and TRIF (TIR domain-containing adaptor proteins inducing interferon (IFN-β), are responsible for the activation of distinct signaling pathways, leading to the production of pro-inflammatory cytokines and type-I IFN, respectively. MyD88 is critical for the signaling from all TLRs except TLR3. After recognition of pathogens, MyD88 interacts with the TIR domain of TLR and recruits IRAK-4 and IRAK-1 after its phosphorylation, and recruits tumor necrosis factor receptor (TNFR)-associated factor 6 (TRAF6), which acts as ubiquitin ligase. TRAF6, together with an ubiquitination enzyme, itself is ubiquitinated and associates with transforming growth factor (TGF)-β-activated kinase-1 (TAK1) and the TAK1-binding proteins 1 and 2 (TAB1 and TAB2) (Wang *et al.* 2001). TAK1 activates phosphorylation of IκB, which leads to its degradation, translocating NF-κB to the nucleus, and promotes the transcription of multiple pro-inflammatory and chemokines genes. In addition, TAK1 can also activate mitogen-activated protein (MAP) kinases, such as c-Jun N-terminal kinases (JNKs) and p38, leading to the activation of activator protein-1 (AP-1) to regulate the expression of pro-inflammatory cytokine genes (Sato *et al.* 2005).

After activation of TLR3, MyD88-independent pathways are initiated by another TIR domain-containing adaptor, TRIF (Hoebe *et al.* 2003; Yamamoto *et al.* 2003). TRIF interacts with receptor-interacting protein-1 (RIP1), a kinase responsible for the activation of NF-κB (Meylan *et al.* 2004) and TRAF family member-associated NF-κB activator (TANK) binding kinase-1 (TBK1) via TRAF3 (Hacker *et al.* 2006; Oganesyan *et al.* 2006). TBK1 is known to comprise a family of inducible IκB kinases that are able to directly phosphorylate IRF-3 and/or IRF-7 (Fitzgerald *et al.* 2003). Phosphorylated IRF-3 and IRF-7 form homodimers, translocating into the nucleus, binding to the ISRE motifs, resulting in the expression of a set of IFN-inducible genes (Figure 5.3).

5.3 Role of TLRs in Immune Response

The activation of TLRs has wide-ranging effects on both innate and adaptive immunity by releasing pro-inflammatory cytokines and chemokines to clear microbial pathogens. The importance of TLRs in immunity was first demonstrated by MyD88 knockout animals, which exhibited increased susceptibility to *Mycobacterium avium* and *Listerias monocytogenes* infections (Feng *et al.* 2003; Seki *et al.* 2002). TLR2 knockout and MyD88 knockout mice both showed increased susceptibility to infection with *Staphylococcus aureus* (Takeuchi *et al.* 2000). Because of their ability to modulate adaptive immunity, toll-like receptors represent strategic therapeutic targets for diseases that involve inappropriate adaptive immune responses, such as sepsis, autoimmune disorders, cancers and allergies (Lawton and Ghosh 2003). Multiple TLR-ligand interactions are required to induce effective host resistance to pathogens, which has important implications for designing improved strategies for vaccination and immunotherapy against infectious diseases. Individual TLR7, TLR8 and TLR9 agonists have been used successfully as adjuvants to boost $CD4^+$ and $CD8^+$ T-cell response to microbial vaccines (Figure 5.4).

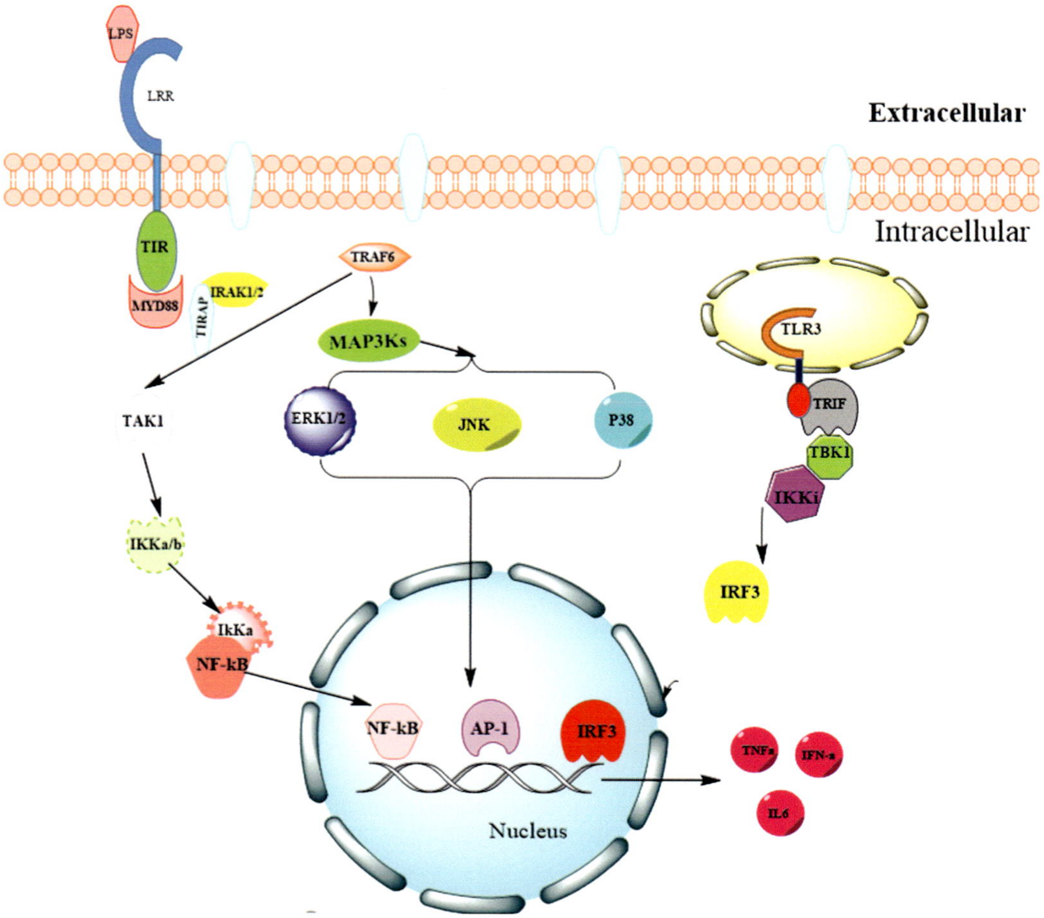

FIGURE 5.3 TLR signaling pathway.

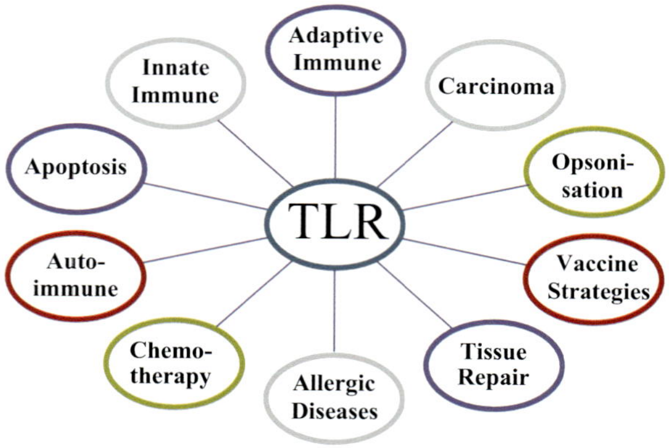

FIGURE 5.4 Role of TLRs in different biological processes.

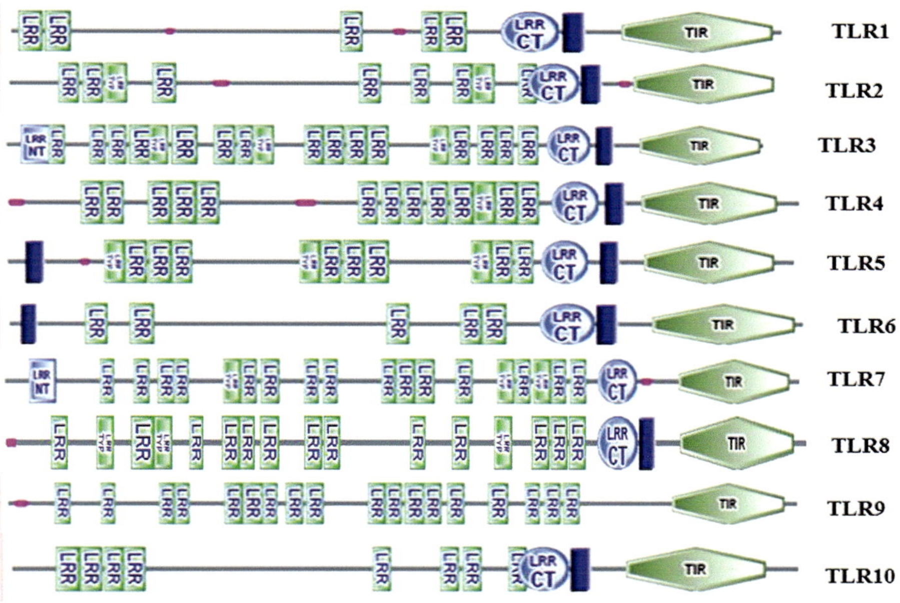

FIGURE 5.5 Predicted functional domains in different TLR proteins (SMART tools).

5.4 Sequence Characterization of Livestock TLRs

Full and partial sequences of TLR genes have been characterized in vertebrates (13 in mice, 11 in humans, 10 in equine, pig, sheep, goat, buffalo and cattle) with their respective functions and ligands (Werling and Coffey 2007; Chang *et al.* 2009; Raja *et al.* 2011; Dubey *et al.* 2012a). Association studies have shown that TLRs act as candidate gene markers for disease resistance and susceptibility. So, additional information on the genomic organization of the TLR genes in different species may help to promote the understanding of TLR evolution. To date, ten TLRs have been reported in livestock species, having respective structures according to the number of exons, introns and the length of UTRs as suggested by different studies.

Different domains of TLRs have been predicted using SMART analysis showing distribution of LRR, LRRNT, LRRCT, TM and TIR domains (Figure 5.5), and further predicted domains were compared with TLRs among livestock species (Table 5.2).

5.5 Polymorphism in TLRs of Livestock Species

Polymorphism in the pattern recognition molecules is associated with alteration of innate and adaptive immunity due to loss of their functional activity. Polymorphism in genetic terms means having multiple alleles of a gene within a population, usually expressing different phenotypes. Due to their central role in triggering innate as well as adaptive immunity, genetic variations within TLR genes are of great significance. Several single-nucleotide polymorphisms within TLR genes have been described and seem to be associated with susceptibility to inflammatory diseases in mammals. Most of the work on the association of SNPs in TLR genes has been carried out in human beings.

Single-nucleotide polymorphism analysis of TLR genes has been used extensively to study their association with susceptibility to various diseases in livestock species. In sheep, allelic variation within TLR4 and TLR9 has been reported (Byun *et al.* 2009) and 12 polymorphic sites were found in TLR4, out of which ten were found to be non-synonymous. In TLR9, four SNPs were reported and two were found to be non-synonymous. The presence of bias SNPs 21, 11, 7, 13 and 11 in porcine TLR1, TLR2, TLR4,

TABLE 5.2

LRRs predicted in TLR genes of different species*

Species	TLR1	TLR2	TLR3	TLR4	TLR5	TLR6	TLR7	TLR8	TLR9	TLR10
Buffalo	18	20	24	21	23	20	26	26	26	19
Cattle	19	20	24	22	21	20	26	25	26	20
Goat	18	18	17	21	22	18	22	20	26	16
Horse	20	20	24	22	-	-	26	26	26	-
Pig	20	20	24	21	22	20	26	26	26	20
Sheep	19	20	24	22	22	20	26	26	26	20

* Domains were analysed using online SMART tools

TLR5 and TLR6 in 96 animals of 11 porcine breeds was reported by Shinkai *et al.* (2006). Polymorphism in the genomic sequences of bovine TLRs 3, 7, 8 and 9 has been analyzed in nine different breeds of *Bos taurus* and *Bos indicus*, but when comparative sequence analysis was done, it revealed a total of 139 polymorphisms, which include single-nucleotide polymorphisms and insertion-deletions. However, Seabury *et al.* (2007) carried out comparative sequence analysis of bovine TLRs 1, 5, and 10 in ten different breeds of *Bos taurus* and *Bos indicus* which revealed a total of 98 polymorphisms, including 92 SNPs and six indels. Out of these SNP sites, 14 were found to be non-synonymous, located within predicted TLR domains and considered to be of functional significance. Through the screening of 11 different breeds of *Bos taurus*, a total of 32 SNPs were identified, 28 of which were found to be in the coding region. Eight SNPs were non-synonymous, potentially altering the specificity of pathogen recognition or efficiency of signaling. Thirty-two SNPs were found to be sharing 20 haplotypes which can be used for assigning the geographic ranges of origin (White *et al.* 2003). In goat TLR5, TLR7 and TLR8, and buffalo TLR2, TLR4 and TLR8, gene polymorphism is reported in their promoter, exon, intron and UTR (Goyal *et al.* 2012; 2013b; 2014; Dubey *et al.* 2013; Dubey, Goyal *et al.* 2010; 2012b; 2013a; 2013b).

5.6 Evolutionary Analysis of Livestock TLR Genes

The phylogenetic analysis of all TLRs has been carried out using Mega4 software following an NJ algorithm (with 1000 bootstrap resampling). The results revealed that dimerizing TLRs 1, 2, 6 and 10 at the same bootstrap have the same pattern of phylogenetic tree, while endosomal expressed TLRs 3, 7, 8 and 9 (viral, bacterial CpG) are grouped at the same clade. Bacterial, Gram-negative-recognizing TLR4 is clustered closer to Gram-positive recognizing TLR2 and flagellin-recognizing TLR5 lying between TLR4 and TLR3, similar to what is reported in other species (Roach *et al.* 2005; Figure 5.6).

5.7 TLRs as Therapeutic Agents

In some diseases like sepsis and several autoimmune disorders, TLR signaling has been found to be an integral component of disease progression. For such diseases, therapeutic approaches aimed at reducing the level of TLR signaling are being explored. In other diseases such as cancer and allergy, where ineffective or inappropriate immune responses are partially to blame for disease progression, therapeutic strategies are being designed to take advantage of the fact that TLR signaling is able to shift the immune system toward an inflammatory TH1 mode, a transition which can, for example, lead to tumor eradication or an amelioration of allergy symptoms (Wooldridge and Weiner 2003; Creticos *et al.* 2006; Klinman 2004; Schetter and Vollmer 2004). Stimulation of TLRs leads to strong protective TH1 immune response, leading to the identification of potential adjuvants such as CpG oligo-deoxy-ribonucleotides, which enhance the effectiveness of vaccination but also enhance overall immune readiness before pathogen

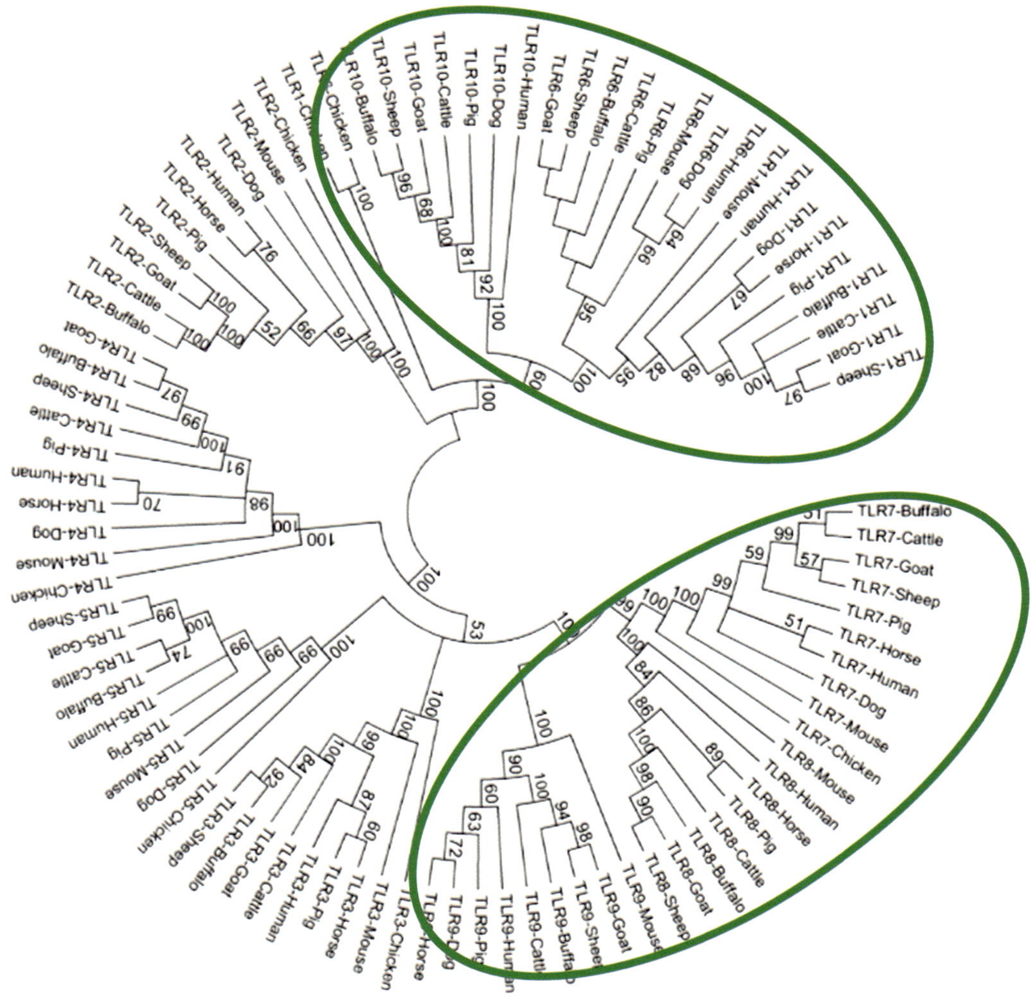

FIGURE 5.6 Phylogenetic analysis of TLR genes.

exposure. The observation that CpG administration leads to a heightened state of innate immune readiness and confers protection against challenge by various deadly bacterial pathogens, suggests that CpG could potentially serve as a universal therapeutic agent in the event of an infectious disease outbreak (Mutwiri *et al.* 2003). Compelling evidence exists for the crucial role of TLRs in inflammation; therefore, targeted inhibition of TLR activation is an attractive therapeutic option in inflammatory conditions. Aldara (Imiquimod) was the first TLR drug to reach the market, having been developed by 3M Pharmaceuticals (Minnesota) and approved for cancer therapy before the TLR mechanism of action was well understood. Many drug candidates have since emerged, of which two are currently in phase-3 clinical trials. Workers (Toshchakov *et al.* 2007) have also identified cell-penetrating peptides as therapeutic, which have the ability to selectively affect different TLRs signaling pathways.

5.8 Conclusion

Investigating disease resistance genes in livestock is gaining importance as improving resistance is perceived as a primary target for genetic improvement along with production traits. For the better understanding of disease resistance traits, it is necessary to investigate the genetic diversity of the immune response genes within and between livestock populations. An approach to detect the polymorphism and diversity in immune response genes specifically encoding for various receptors like TLRs is gaining momentum. Higher polymorphism at these loci increases the probability of recognizing a greater number of pathogens or different antigenic variants, while at the same time reducing the probability for any disease to develop into a catastrophic epidemic. The genomic tools being developed are proving more beneficial in not only understanding the mechanism of disease resistance, but also in identifying functional markers across candidate genes in the globally better-adapted populations within a livestock species.

References

Akira, S. and Takeda, K. 2004. Toll-like receptor signalling. *Nature Reviews Immunology*. 4, 499–511.

Amaral, M.E.J., Grant, J.R., Riggs, P.K., Stafuzza, N.B., Filho, E.A.R., Goldammer, T., Weikard, R., Brunner, R.M., Kochan, K.J., Greco, A.J., Jeong, J., Cai, Z., Lin, G., Prasad, A., Kumar, S., Saradhi, G.P., Mathew, Kumar, M.A., Miziara, M.N., Mariani, P., Caetano, A.R., Galvão, S.R., Tantia, M.S., Vijh, R.K., Mishra, B., Kumar, S.T.B., Pelai, V.A., Santana, A.M., Fornitano, L.C., Jones, B.C., Tonhati, H., Stephen Moore, S., Stothard, P.M. and Womack, J.E. 2008. A first generation whole genome RH map of the river buffalo with comparison to domestic cattle. *BMC Genomics*, 9, 631.

Anderson, K.V., Bokla, L. and Nusslein, V.C. 1985. Establishment of dorsal-ventral polarity in the Drosophila embryo: the induction of polarity by the Toll gene product. *Cell*. 42, 791–798.

Beutler, B. and Rehli, M. 2002. Evolution of the TIR, tolls and TLRs: functional inferences from computational biology. *Current Topics in Microbiology and Immunology*. 270, 1–21.

Byun, S.O., Zhou, O. and Hickford, J.G.H. 2009. Development of a simple typing method for the ovine toll-like receptor 4 gene. *Veterinary Immunology and Immunopathology*. 130, 272–274.

Chang, J.S., Russell, G.C., Jann, O., Glass, E.J., Werling, D. and Haig, D.M. 2009. Molecular cloning and characterization of Toll-like receptors 1–10 in sheep. *Veterinary Immunology and Immunopathology*. 127, 94–105.

Choe, J., Kelker, M.S. and Wilson, I.A. 2005. Crystal structure of human toll-like receptor 3 (TLR3) ectodomain. *Science*. 309, 581–585.

Creticos, P.S., Schroeder, J.T., Hamilton, R.G., Whaley, S.L.B., Khattignavong, A.P., Lindblad, R., Henry Li, Coffman, R., Seyfert, V., Eiden, J.J., Broide, D. and the Immune Tolerance Network Group. 2006. Immunotherapy with a ragweed-toll-like receptor 9 agonist vaccine for allergic rhinitis. *The New England Journal of Medicine*. 355, 1445–1455.

Dhara, A., Saini, M., Das, D.K., Swarup, D., Sharma, B., Kumar, S. and Gupta, P.K. 2007. Molecular characterization of coding sequences and analysis of toll-like receptor 3 mRNA expression in water buffalo (*Bubalus bubalis*) and nilgai (*Boselaphus tragocamelus*). *Immunogenetics*. 59, 69–76.

Dubey, P.K., Aggarwal, J., Goyal, S., Gahlawat, S.K., Kathiravan, P., Mishra, B.P. and Kataria, R.S. 2013a. Sequence and topological characterization of Toll-like receptor 8 gene of Indian riverine buffalo (*Bubalus bubalis*). *Tropical Animal Health and Production*. 45, 91–99.

Dubey, P.K., Goyal, S., Aggarwal, J., Gahlawat, S.K., Kathiravan, P., Mishra, B.P. and Kataria, R.S. 2012b. Development of tetra primers ARMS-PCR assay for the detection of A1551G polymorphism in TLR8 gene of riverine buffalo. *Journal of Applied Animal Research* 40, 17–19.

Dubey, P.K., Goyal, S., Kathiravan, P., Mishra, B.P., Gahlawat, S.K. and Kataria, R.S. 2012a. Sequence characterization of river buffalo Toll-like receptor (TLR) genes 1–10 reveals distinct relationship with cattle and sheep. *International Journal of Immunogenetics*. 40, 140–148.

Dubey, P.K., Goyal, S., Kumari, N., Mishra, S.K., Arora R. and Kataria, R.S. 2013b. Genetic diversity within 5 upstream region of Toll-like receptor 8 gene reveals differentiation of riverine and swamp buffaloes. *Meta Gene*. 1, 24–32.

Dubey, P.K., Selvakumar, M., Kathiravan, P., Yadav, N., Mishra B.P. and Kataria R.S. 2010. Detection of polymorphism in exon 2 of Toll-like receptor 4 gene of Indian buffaloes using PCR –SSCP Technique. *Journal of Applied Animal Research*. 37, 265–268.

Feng, C.G., Scanga, C.A., Collazo, C.C.M., Cheever, A.W., Hieny, S. and Caspar, P. and Sher, A. 2003. Mice lacking myeloid differentiation factor 88 display profound defects in host resistance and immune responses to Mycobacterium avium infection not exhibited by toll like receptor 2 (TLR2)- and TLR4-deficient animals. *The Journal of Immunology*. 171, 4758–4764.

Fitzgerald, K.A., McWhirter, S.M., Faia, K.L., Rowe, D.C., Latz, E., Golenbock, D.T., Coyle, A.J., Liao, S.M. and Maniatis, T. 2003. IKKepsilon and TBK1 are essential components of the IRF3 signaling pathway. *Nature Immunology*. 4, 491–496.

Goldammer, T., Zerbe, H., Molenaar, A. Schuberth, H.J., Brunner, R.M., Kata, S.R. and Seyfert, H.M. 2004. Mastitis increases mammary MRNA abundance of ß-defensin 5, toll-like-receptor 2 (TLR2), and TLR4 but not TLR9 in cattle. *Clinical and Diagnostic Laboratory Immunology*. 11, 174–185.

Goyal, S., Dubey, P.K., Kathiravan, P., Mishra, B.P., Mahajan, R. and Kataria, R.S. 2013a. Expression profiling of Toll-like receptor-7 and 8 genes across caprine tissues using real-time PCR assay. *Indian Journal of Animal Sciences*. 83, 1068–1107.

Goyal, S., Dubey, P.K., Sahoo, B.R., Mishra, S.K., Niranjan, S.K., Singh, S., Mahajan, R. and, Kataria, R.S. 2013b. Sequence based structural characterization and genetic diversity analysis across coding and promoter regions of goat Toll-like receptor 5 gene. *Gene*. 540, 238–245.

Goyal, S., Dubey, P.K., Singh, N., Niranjan, S.K., Kathiravan, P., Mishra, B.P., Mahajan, R. and Kataria, R.S. 2014. Caprine Toll-like receptor 8 gene sequence characterization reveals close relationships among ruminant species. *International Journal of. Immunogenetics*. 41, 81–89.

Goyal, S., Dubey, P.K., Tripathy, K., Mahajan R., Pan, S., Dixit, S.P., Kathiravan, P., Mishra, B.P., Niranjan, S.K. and Kataria, R.S. 2012. Detection of polymorphism and sequence characterization of Toll-like receptor 7 gene of Indian goat revealing close relationship between ruminant species. *Animal Biotechnology*. 23, 194–203.

Hacker, H., Redecke, V., Blagoev, B., Kratchmarova, I., Hsu, L.C., Wang, G.G., Kamps, M.P., Raz, E., Wagner, H., Hacker, G., Mann, M. and Karin, M. 2006. Specificity in toll-like receptor signalling through distinct effector functions of TRAF3 and TRAF6. *Nature*. 439, 204–207.

Heine, H. and Lien, E. 2003. Toll-like receptors and their function in innate and adaptive immunity. *International Archives of Allergy and Immunology*. 130, 180–192.

Hoebe, K., Du, X., Georgel, P., Janssen, E., Tabeta, K., Kim, S.O., Goode, J., Lin, P., Mann, N., Mudd, S., Crozat, K., Sovath, S., Han, J. and Beutler, B. 2003. Identification of Lps2 as a key transducer of MyD88-independent TIR signalling. *Nature*. 424, 743–748.

Iqbal, M. and Philbin, V.J. 2005. Expression pattern of chicken toll-like receptor mRNA in tissues, immune cell subset and cell lines. *Veterinary Immunology and Immunopathology*. 104, 117–127.

Janssens, S. and Beyaert, R. 2003. Role of toll-like receptors in pathogen recognition. *Clinical Microbiology Reviews*. 16, 637–646.

Klinman, D.M. 2004. Immunotherapeutic uses of CpG oligodeoxynucleotides. *Nature Reviews Immunology*. 4, 249–258.

Lawton, J.A. and Ghosh, P. 2003. Novel therapeutic strategies based on toll-like receptor signaling. *Current Opinion in Chemical Biology*. 7, 446–451.

McGuire, K., Jones, M., Werling, D., Williams, J.L., Glass, E.J. and Jann, O. 2005. Radiation hybrid mapping of all 10 characterized bovine toll-like receptors. *Animal Genetics*. 37, 47–50.

Medzhitov, R., Preston, H.P. and Janeway, C.A. Jr. 1997. A human homologue of the Drosophila Toll protein signals activation of adaptive immunity. *Nature*. 388, 394–397.

Menzies, M. and Ingham, A. 2006. Identification and expression of toll like receptors 1–10 in selected bovine and ovine tissues. *Veterinary Immunology and Immunopathology*. 109, 23–30.

Meylan, E., Burns, K., Hofmann, K., Blancheteau, V., Martinon, F., Kelliher, M. and Tschopp, J. 2004. RIP1 is an essential mediator of toll-like receptor 3-induced NF-kappa B activation. *Nature Immunology*. 5, 503–507.

Mutwiri, G., Pontarollo, R., Babiuk, S., Griebel, P., Hvan Drunen Little-van den Hurk, S., Mena, A., Tsang, C., Alcon, V., Nichani, A., Ioannou, X., Gomis, S., Townsend, H., Hecker, R., Potter, A. and Babiuk, L.A. 2003. Biological activity of immunostimulatory CpG DNA motifs in domestic animals. *Veterinary Immunology and Immunopathology*. 91, 89–103.

Oganesyan, G., Saha, S.K., Guo, B., He, J.Q., Shahangian, A., Zarnegar, B., Perry, A. and Cheng, G. 2006. Critical role of TRAF3 in the toll-like receptor-dependent and -independent antiviral response. *Nature*. 439, 208–211.

Parker, L.C., Prince, L.R. and Sabroe, I. 2007. Translational mini-review series on toll-like receptors: networks regulated by toll-like receptors mediate innate and adaptive immunity. *Clinical and Experimental Immunology*. 147, 199–207.

Prueet, S.B., Zheng, Q., Fan, R., Matthews, K. and Schwab, C. 2004. Acute exposure to ethanol affects toll-like receptor signalling and subsequent responses: an overview of recent studies. *Alcohol*. 33, 235–239.

Raja, A., Vignesh, A.R., Mary, B.A., Tirumurugaan, K.G., Raj, G.D., Kataria, R.S., Mishra, B.P. and Kumanan, K. 2011. Sequence analysis of toll-like receptor genes 1—10 of goat (*Capra hircus*). *Veterinary Immunology and Immunopathology*. 140, 252–258.

Roach, J.C., Glusman, G., Rowen, L., Kaur, A., Purcell, M.K., Smith, D.K., Hood, L.E. and Aderem, A. 2005. The evolution of vertebrate Toll-like receptors. *The National Academy of Sciences*. 102, 9577–9582.

Sato, S., Sanjo, H., Takeda, K., Ninomiya, T.J., Yamamoto, M., Kawai, T., Matsumoto, K., Takeuchi, O. and Akira, S. 2005. Essential function for the kinase TAK1 in innate and adaptive immune responses. *Nature Immunology*. 6, 1087–1095.

Schetter, C. and Vollmer, J. 2004. Toll-like receptors involved in the response to microbial pathogens: development of agonists for toll-like receptor 9. *Current Opinion in Drug Discovery and Development*. 7, 204–210.

Seabury, C.M., Cargill, E.J. and Womack J.E. 2007. Sequence variability and protein domain architectures for bovine Toll-like receptors 1, 5, and 10. *Genomics*. 90, 502–515.

Seki, E., Tsutsui, H., Tsuji, N.M., Hayashi, N., Adachi, K., Nakano, H., Yumikura, S.F., Osamu Takeuchi, O., Hoshino, K., Akira, S., Fujimoto, J. and Nakanishi, K. 2002. Critical roles of myeloid differentiation factor 88-dependent proinflammatory cytokine release in early phase clearance of Listeria monocytogenes in mice. *The Journal of Immunology*. 169, 3863–3868.

Shinkai, H., Muneta, Y., Suzuki, K., Eguchi, O.T., Awata, T. and Uenish, H. 2006. Porcine Toll-like receptor 1, 6, and 10 genes: complete sequencing of genomic region and expression analysis. *Molecular Immunology*. 43, 1474–1480.

Takeda, K. and Akira, S. 2003. Toll receptors and pathogen resistance. *Cell Microbiology*. 5, 143–153.

Takeuchi, O., Hoshino, K. and Akira, S. 2000. Cutting edge: TLR2-deficient and MyD88-deficient mice are highly susceptible to *Staphylococcus aureus* infection. *Journal Immunology*. 165, 5392–5396.

Toshchakov, V.Y., Fenton, M.J. and Vogel, S.N. 2007. Cutting edge: differential inhibition of TLR signalling pathways by cell-permeable peptides representing BB loops of TLRs. *The Journal of Immunology*. 178, 2655–2660.

Vahanan, B.M., Raj, G.D., Pawar, R.M.C., Gopinath, V.P., Raja, A. and Thangavelu, A. 2008. Expression profile of toll like receptors in a range of water buffalo tissues (*Bubalus bubalis*). *Veterinary Immunology and Immunopathology*. 126, 149–155.

Wang, C., Deng, L., Hong, M., Akkaraju, G.R., Inoue, J. and Chen, Z.J. 2001. TAK1 is a ubiquitin dependent kinase of MKK and IKK. *Nature*. 412, 346–351.

Werling, D. and Coffey, T.J. 2007. Pattern recognition receptors in companion and farm animals—the key to unlocking the door to animal disease? *The Veterinary Journal*. 174, 240–251.

White, A.N., Kata, S.R. and Womack, J.E. 2003. Comparative fine maps of bovine toll-like receptor 4 and toll-like receptor 2 regions. *Mammalian Genome*. 14, 149–155.

Wooldridge, J.E. and Weiner, G.J. 2003. CpG DNA and cancer immunotherapy: orchestrating the antitumor immune response. *Current Opinion in Oncology*. 15, 440–445.

Yamamoto, M., Sato, S., Hemmi, H., Uematsu, S., Hoshino, K., Kaisho, T., Takeuchi, O., Takeda, K. and Akira, S. 2003. TRAM is specifically involved in the toll-like receptor 4-mediated MyD88-independent signaling pathway. *Nature Immunology*. 4, 1144–1150.

Zarember, K.A. and Godowski, P.J. 2002. Tissue expression of human toll-like receptors and differential regulation of toll-like receptor mRNAs in leukocytes in response to microbes, their products and cytokines. *The Journal of Immunology*. 168, 554–561.

6

COVID-19: An Emerging Pandemic for Mankind

Aman Kumar, Kanisht Batra, Anubha Sharma and Sushila Maan
Department of Animal Biotechnology, Lala Lajpat Rai University of Veterinary and Animal Sciences, Hisar-125004, Haryana, India
Corresponding author: Aman Kumar, *aman.abt@luvas.edu.in*

6.1 Introduction to COVID-19

Despite technological advancement in the area of molecular biology and biotechnology, the entire world is still struggling with the ongoing pandemic of the novel coronavirus (SARS-CoV-2). Once again, viruses have proved themselves smarter than any other species on the earth. On January 8, 2020, a novel coronavirus was officially announced as the causative pathogen of coronavirus infectious disease 2019 (COVID-19) by the Chinese Centre for Disease Control and Prevention (Li *et al.*, 2020). The emergence of the novel coronavirus (SARS-CoV-2) and its subsequent worldwide spread has been challenging to the public health community worldwide. The World Health Organization (WHO) declared the 2019–2020 coronavirus outbreak a Public Health Emergency of International Concern (PHEIC) on January 30, 2020 and a pandemic on March 11, 2020. This coronavirus was initially named the 2019 novel coronavirus (2019-nCoV) on January 12, 2020 by the WHO. On February 11, 2020, the WHO officially named the disease coronavirus infectious disease 2019 (COVID-19) and the Coronaviridae Study Group (CSG) of the International Committee proposed the naming of the new coronavirus as SARS-CoV-2. Before December 2019, six coronaviruses were known to infect humans. Of the six, two were α-CoVs (HCoV-229E, HCoV-NL63) and four were β-CoVs (HCoV-HKU1, HCoV-OC43, SARS-CoV, and MERS-CoV). The β-CoVs, HCoV-HKU1 and HCoV-OC43, were responsible for low pathogenicity and caused mild respiratory symptoms similar to a common cold, respectively. The other two known β-CoVs, SARS-CoV and MERS-CoV, led to severe and potentially fatal respiratory tract infections. Other than the above six, two coronaviruses (HKU2 and beluga whale CoV/SW1) are also important (Burrell *et al.*, 2016; Corman *et al.*, 2020). HKU2 was responsible for the death of 24,000 piglets due to diarrhea in southern China in 2017, which was the first "spillover" from a bat coronavirus to livestock. The other was beluga whale CoV/SW1; although only distantly related to human pathogens, it could reveal how bat viruses get into sea creatures (Chen *et al.*, 2020; Gong *et al.*, 2017).

6.2 Virology

6.2.1 Taxonomy

The Coronaviridae Study Group (CSG) of the International Committee on Taxonomy of Viruses, which is responsible for the classification of viruses and taxon nomenclature of the family *Coronaviridae*, has assessed the placement of the human pathogen, tentatively named 2019-nCoV, within the *Coronaviridae*. Based on phylogeny, taxonomy, and established practice, the CSG recognizes this virus as forming a sister clade to the prototype human and bat severe acute respiratory syndrome coronaviruses (SARS-CoVs) and designated it as SARS-CoV-2, and it has been classified under the order *Nidovirales*, family *Coronaviridae*, subfamily *Coronavirinae*, genus beta-coronavirus and subgenus Sarbecovirus (beta-CoV lineage B) (Gorbalenya *et al.*, 2020) (Figure 6.1).

6.2.2 Virion Structure

SARS-CoV-2 is an enveloped, positive-sense single-stranded RNA (+ssRNA) virus. The viral RNA genome is between 26 and 32 kilobases in length. It is the seventh known human coronavirus which can cause disease in humans after 229E, NL63, OC43, HKU1, MERS-CoV, and the original SARS-CoV (Raoult *et al.*, 2020; Zhu *et al.*, 2020). Each SARS-CoV-2 virion is approximately 50–200 nanometres in diameter (Chen *et al.*, 2020) (Figure 6.2A). Like other coronaviruses, SARS-CoV-2 has four structural proteins, known as the S (spike), E (envelope), M (membrane), and N (nucleocapsid) proteins. The

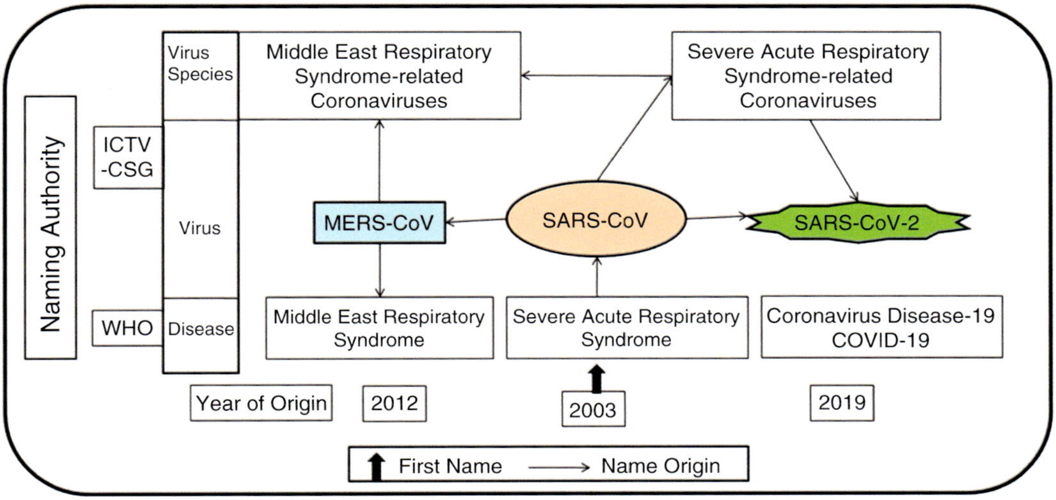

FIGURE 6.1 Flow chart showing chronology of coronavirus naming during the three outbreaks in relation to virus taxonomy and diseases caused by them.

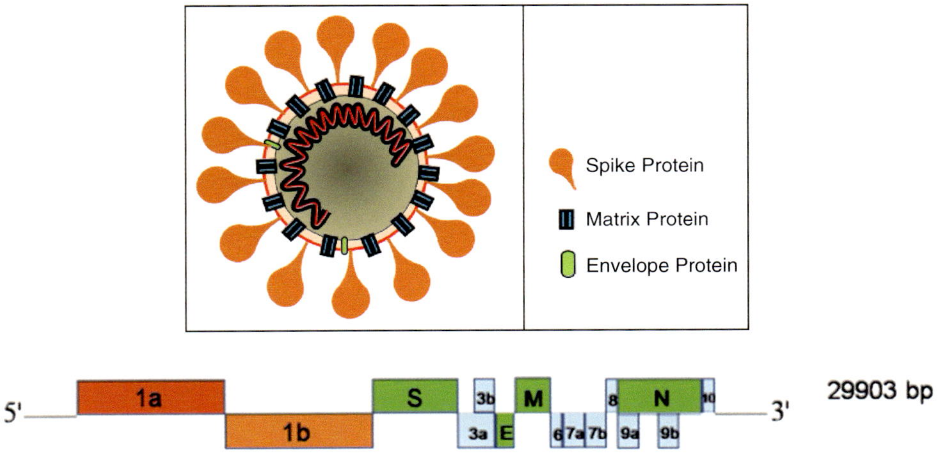

FIGURE 6.2 The β-coronavirus (Lineage B) and its genome.

(A) The β-coronavirus is an enveloped, non-segmented, positive-sense single-stranded RNA virus genome in a size ranging from 26–32 kilobases. (B) 50 and 30 terminal sequences of the SARS-CoV-2 genome. The gene order is 50-replicase ORF1ab-S-envelope (E)-membrane(M)-N-30. ORF3ab, ORF6, ORF7ab, ORF8, ORF9ab, and ORF10 are located at the predicted positions shown in the picture. 1a, 1b, 3a, 3b, 6, 7a, 7b, 8, 9a, 9b, and 10 in the picture represent deferent ORF genes.

N protein codes for the RNA genome while the S, E, and M proteins constitute the viral envelope. The S protein is responsible for the virus' attachment to the membrane of the host cell (Wu *et al.*, 2020).

The first two-thirds of the viral genome encode 16 non-structural proteins which are essential for virus replication. These non-structural proteins are mainly enzymes needed to produce the other encoded proteins, and transcription factors which are required to continually renew the RNA instructions. The remaining third of the viral genome encodes four structural proteins (S, E, M, and N) required for building of the virion. The S protein is synthesized early during infection. The S glycoprotein contains both the receptor-binding domain (RBD) and the domains involved in fusion, rendering it the pivotal protein in the CoV entry process. There are three copies of the S protein and each is responsible for spike formation

(Qian *et al.*, 2015). The membrane (M) glycoprotein lies beneath the spikes, where it shapes mature viral particles and binds the inner layers. Envelope (E) glycoproteins control the assembly, release, and infectivity of mature viruses. The N protein forms a characteristic shell of identical subunits, which binds and packages the RNA genome. It also serves as a cloaking device responsible for hiding viruses from a host's immune system molecules like interferons, siRNA, miRNA, etc. (Chen, Y. *et al.*, 2020).

6.2.3 Genome Characteristics

In general, the members of the family *Coronaviridae* possess a single-strand, positive-sense RNA genome ranging from 26 to 32 kilobases in length. However, the genome of SARS-CoV-2 is in the range of 30 kilobases (Raoult *et al.*, 2020). The SARS-CoV-2 genome has 5' and 3' terminal sequences (265 nt at the 5' terminal and 229 nt at the 3' terminal region), which are present in most CoVs, with a gene order 50-replicase open reading frame (ORF) 1ab-S-envelope(E)-membrane(M)-N-30 (Figure 6.2 B). The predicted S, ORF3a, E, M, and N genes of SARS-CoV-2 are 3822, 828, 228, 669, and 1260 nt in length, respectively. Similar to SARS-CoV, SARS-CoV-2 carries a predicted ORF8 gene (366 nt in length) located between the M and N ORF genes (Wu, F. *et al.*, 2020).

6.2.4 Recent Genome-wide Studies

Genome-wide phylogenetic analysis indicated that SARS-CoV-2 shares 79.5% and 50% sequence identity with SARS-CoV and MERS-CoV, respectively (Lu *et al.*, 2020). However, there is 94.6% sequence identity between the seven conserved replicase domains in ORF1ab of SARS-CoV-2 and SARS-CoV (Zheng *et al.*, 2020), and less than 90% sequence identity with other β-CoVs, implying that SARS-CoV-2 belongs to the lineage B (Sarbecovirus) of β-CoVs (Wu, F. *et al.*, 2020). The genomic sequences of SARS-CoV-2 obtained from the nine initial cases of COVID-19 showed very high sequence identity (>99.98%). A recent study indicated that 120 substitution sites were evenly distributed in eight coding regions, without evident recombination events (Lu *et al.*, 2020). A BLASTn search of the complete genomes of 2019-nCoV revealed that the most closely related viruses available on GenBank were SARS-like betacoronaviruses of bat origin (sequence identity 87.99%; query coverage 99%). In five gene regions (E, M, 7, N, and 14), the sequence identities were greater than 90%, with the highest being 98.7% in the E gene. The S gene of SARS-CoV-2 exhibited the lowest sequence identity (~75%) with bat-derived coronavirus (Acc. Nos. MG772933 and MG772934). Comparison of the predicted coding regions of SARS-CoV-2 showed that they possessed a similar genomic organization to bat-SL-CoVZC45, bat-SL-CoVZXC21, and SARS-CoV. The lengths of most of the proteins encoded by 2019-nCoV, bat-SL-CoVZC45, and bat-SL-CoVZXC21 were similar, with only a few minor insertions or deletions. A notable difference was a longer spike protein encoded by 2019-nCoV compared with the bat SARS-like coronaviruses, SARS-CoV, and MERS-CoV (Lu *et al.*, 2020). However, Tang *et al.* analyzed 103 genomes and found that SARS-CoV-2 had evolved into two types of L and S based on SNP T28,144 (leucine) and C28,144 (serine) and on the basis of prevalence L was the major (~70%) and S the minor (~30%) type. Due to severe selective pressure on the L-type, the L-type might be more aggressive and spread more quickly, while the S-type might remain milder due to relatively weaker selective pressure (Tang *et al.*, 2020).

6.2.5 Specificity of Spike Protein

The SARS-CoV-2 virus is different from other known beta-coronaviruses due to the presence of two specific features of the spike protein. These are:

i) polybasic cleavage site along with O-linked glycans
ii) receptor-binding domain (RBD)

The spike protein has a functional polybasic (furin) cleavage site at the S1–S2 boundary through the insertion of 12 nucleotides, which additionally led to the predicted acquisition of three O-linked glycans around the site (Walls *et al.*, 2020).

6.2.5.1 Polybasic Cleavage Site and O-linked Glycans

The presence of specific polybasic cleavage site RRAR (682–685) in the spike protein at the junction of the S1 and S2 subunit is characteristic of SARS-CoV-2. One proline (P) is also present just proximal to the cleavage site. Hence, the fully inserted sequence is PRRA (681–684). The insertion of proline in the strong turn is predicted to result in the addition of O-linked glycans to S673, T678, and S686, which flank the polybasic cleavage site. Earlier, it was proved in avian influenza virus that acquisition of polybasic cleavage sites converts low-pathogenicity avian influenza viruses into highly pathogenic forms. Similarly, an avirulent isolate of Newcastle disease virus became highly pathogenic during serial passage in chickens by incremental acquisition of a polybasic cleavage site at the junction of its fusion protein subunits. The potential function of the three predicted O-linked glycans is less clear, but they could create a "mucin-like domain" that would shield potential epitopes or key residues on the SARS-CoV-2 spike protein. Further analyses are required to determine whether or not the predicted O-linked glycan sites are utilized toward pathogenicity and/or transmissibility (Andersen *et al.*, 2020).

6.2.5.2 Mutations in the Receptor-binding Domain of SARS-CoV-2

Other than the polybasic cleavage site, the receptor-binding domain (RBD) in the spike protein of SARS-CoV and SARS-related coronaviruses is the most variable part of the virus genome. For critical binding to the ACE2 receptor and for determining the host range of SARS-CoV, six residues (viz. Y442, L472, N479, D480, T487, and Y4911) are present in the RBD of the spike protein. The corresponding residues in SARS-CoV-2 are L455, F486, Q493, S494, N501, and Y505. Five of these six residues are mutated in SARS-CoV-2 compared to its most closely related virus, RaTG13, sampled from a *Rhinolophus affinis* bat, to which it is ~96% identical. SARS-CoV-2 seems to have an RBD that may bind with high affinity to ACE2 from humans, non-human primates, ferrets, pigs, and cats, as well as other species with high receptor homology. In contrast, SARS-CoV-2 may bind less efficiently to ACE2 in other species associated with SARS-like viruses, including rodents and civets. The recent binding studies indicate that SARS-CoV-2 binds with high affinity to human ACE2 (Nguyen *et al.*, 2020).

6.3 Origin and Evolution

Amid the global health emergency, it is important to know the origin and evolution of the virus responsible for COVID-19. The knowledge of the pathway and mechanism by which an animal virus jumped species boundaries to infect humans so efficiently will help in the prevention of future zoonotic probability. Previous outbreaks of beta-coronaviruses in humans involved direct exposure to animals other than bats, particularly in the case of SARS-CoV and MERS-CoV, which were transmitted directly to humans from civet cats and dromedary camels, respectively. Available genome sequence data for known coronavirus strains circulating worldwide depicted that SARS-CoV-2 originated through natural processes (Andersen *et al.*, 2020). The basis of its natural evolution was: i) the binding affinity of its spike protein particularly at the RBD; and ii) the backbone of the virus. Actually, it was observed that the binding of the SARS-CoV-2 spike protein to its ACE2 receptor of the human cell is very effective. Hence, evolution of the virus was the result of natural selection and not the product of genetic engineering. This concept of natural evolution was also supported by its molecular structure, having a distinct backbone which differed substantially from already-known coronaviruses and mostly resembled related viruses found in bats and pangolins. These two features of the virus, the mutations in the RBD portion of the spike protein and its distinct backbone, point toward its natural evolution and rule out laboratory manipulation as a potential origin for SARS-CoV-2 (Andersen *et al.*, 2020).

Another important question concerns from where the virus originated. Genome sequence analysis has shown that SARS-CoV-2 has higher nucleotide sequence identity (96.2%) to the RaTG13 bat virus as compared to pangolin CoV (91.02%). Conversely, it showed higher amino acid (aa) similarity to pangolin CoV (97.5%) than to RaTG13 (95.4%), particularly in the spike (S) protein. The high-S protein amino acid identity implies functional similarity between pangolin CoV and SARS-CoV-2. These findings indicated that pangolin CoV might be the common ancestor of SARS-CoV-2 and RaTG13 (Zhang *et al.*, 2020).

6.4 Pathogenesis

6.4.1 Virus Entry

In general, cell entry of coronaviruses depends on binding of the viral spike (S) proteins to cellular receptors and on S protein priming by host cell proteases. SARS-CoV-2 is transmitted mainly via respiratory droplets and, hence, viral replication is primarily presumed to occur in the mucosal epithelium of the upper respiratory tract (nasal cavity and pharynx), with further multiplication in the lower respiratory tract and gastrointestinal mucosa (Xiao *et al.*, 2020), giving rise to a mild viraemia. The spike protein of SARS-CoV-2 facilitates viral entry into target cells and entry depends on binding of the surface unit, S1, of the S protein to a cellular receptor, which facilitates viral attachment to the surface of target cells (Figure 6.3). Like SARS-CoV, SARS-CoV-2 also engages angiotensin-converting enzyme 2 (ACE2) as the entry receptor (Hoffmann *et al.*, 2020) and employs the cellular serine protease TMPRSS2 for S protein priming. The ACE2-expressing organs, e.g., nasal mucosa, bronchus, lung, heart, esophagus, kidney, stomach, bladder, and ileum, are organs of choice for SARS-CoV-2 (Zou *et al.*, 2020). Recently, potential pathogenicity of SARS-CoV-2 to testicular tissues has also been proposed by clinicians, implying fertility concerns in young patients (Fan *et al.*, 2020). The pathogenesis of SARS-CoV-2 infection is presented in Figure 6.4 as postulated by Jin *et al.* (2020).

6.4.2 Pathological Findings

Xu *et al.* (2020) first reported the pathological findings of severe COVID-19 patients and observed bilateral diffused alveolar damage with cellular fibromyxoid exudates. The right and left lung showed acute respiratory distress syndrome (ARDS) with clear desquamation of pneumocytes and hyaline membrane formation in the right lung and pulmonary edema with hyaline membrane formation in the left lung. Interstitial mononuclear inflammatory infiltrates, dominated by lymphocytes, could be observed in both lungs. Multinucleated syncytial cells with atypical enlarged pneumocytes characterized by large nuclei, amphophilic granular cytoplasm, and prominent nucleoli were identified in the intra-alveolar spaces, indicating viral cytopathic-like changes. These pulmonary pathological findings are very much similar to those reported in SARS and MERS. Moderate microvascular steatosis and mild lobular and portal activity were observed in liver biopsy specimens, which might be caused by either SARS-CoV-2 infection or

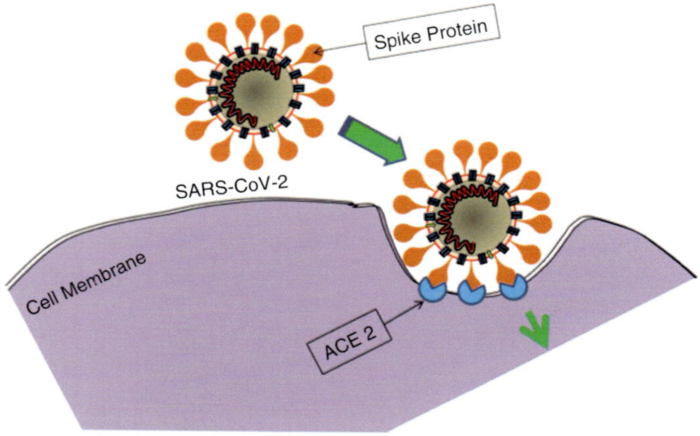

FIGURE 6.3 Cellular entry of SARS-CoV-2 via ACE2.

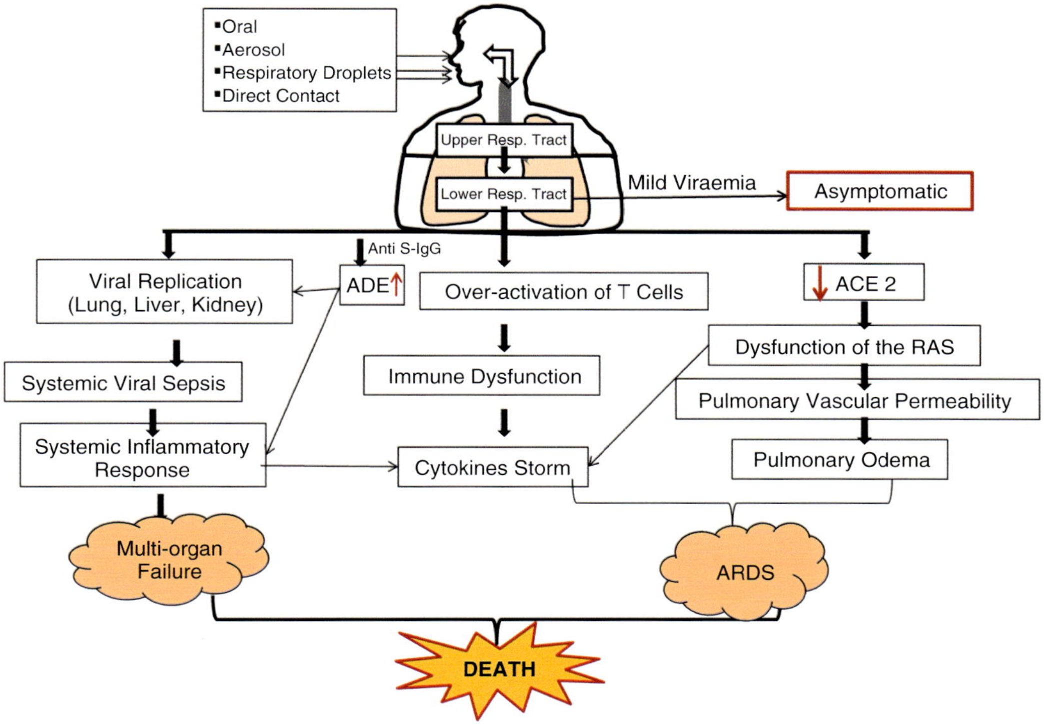

FIGURE 6.4 Pathogenesis of SARS-CoV-2 infection. Antibody-dependent enhancement (ADE).

ACE2: angiotensin-converting enzyme 2; RAS: renin-angiotensin system; ARDS: acute respiratory distress syndrome. Red arrows represent the important turning points in SARS-CoV-2 infection.

drug use. Interestingly, very few interstitial mononuclear inflammatory infiltrates were found in the heart tissue, which means that SARS-CoV-2 might not directly impair the heart (Xu *et al.*, 2020). Massive mucus secretion in both lungs was found in death cases with COVID-19, which was different from SARS and MERS.

6.4.3 Immunopathology

Just like other viral infection, SARS-CoV-2 infection also leads to elicitation of both activate innate and adaptive immune responses. However, uncontrolled inflammatory innate responses and impaired adaptive immune responses may lead to harmful tissue damage, both locally and systemically. Lymphopenia with drastically reduced numbers of CD4+ T-cells, CD8+ T-cells, B-cells, and natural killer (NK) cells is a common feature of severe COVID-19 patients (Huang *et al.*, 2020). The percentage of monocytes, eosinophils, and basophils are also reduced along with lymphopenia in severe cases (Qin *et al.*, 2020). The rise in neutrophil count and the ratio of neutrophil to lymphocyte are also indicative of disease severity and a poor clinical outcome (Zhang *et al.*, 2020). Moreover, immune dysfunction markers (NKG2A) on cytotoxic lymphocytes, NK-cells, and CD8+ T-cells are also upregulated in COVID-19. The numbers of CD4+ T-cells, CD8+ T-cells, B-cells, and NK-cells and the markers of exhaustion on cytotoxic lymphocytes normalize in recovered or convalescent patients (Zheng *et al.*, 2020).

SARS-CoV-2-specific antibodies (IgM and IgG) have also been detected in COVID-19 patients. However, studies of patients with severe disease and worse recovery have also reported an increased IgG response and higher titre of total antibodies. This was suggestive of possible antibody-dependent enhancement (ADE) of SARS-CoV-2 infection (Zhang *et al.*, 2020). ADE can promote viral cellular uptake of infectious virus–antibody complexes following their interaction with Fc receptors (FcR), or other receptors, resulting in enhanced infection of target cells (Takada *et al.*, 2003). The interaction of FcR with the virus-anti-S protein-neutralizing antibodies (anti-S-IgG) complex may facilitate both inflammatory responses and persistent viral replication in the lungs of patients (Fu *et al.*, 2020). The immunopathological effects of ADE have been observed in various viral infections, characterized as antibody-mediated enhancement of viral entry and induction of a severe inflammatory response.

Rapid viral replication and cellular damage, virus-induced ACE2 downregulation and shedding, and antibody-dependent enhancement (ADE) are responsible for aggressive inflammation caused by SARS-CoV-2, as concluded in a recently published review article (Fu *et al.*, 2020). The initial onset of rapid viral replication may cause massive epithelial and endothelial cell death and vascular leakage, triggering the production of exuberant pro-inflammatory cytokines and chemokines (Yang *et al.*, 2020). Substantially elevated serum levels of pro- inflammatory cytokines include IL-6 and IL-1β, as well as IL-2, IL-8, IL-17, G-CSF, GM-CSF, IP10, MCP1, MIP1α (also known as CCL3), and TNF, characterized as cytokine storm (Qin *et al.*, 2020). Also, C-reactive protein and D-dimer are found to be abnormally high. High levels of pro-inflammatory cytokines may lead to shock and tissue damage in the heart, liver, and kidney, as well as respiratory failure. Loss of pulmonary ACE2 function has been proposed to be related to acute lung injury (Imai *et al.*, 2008) because ACE2 downregulation and shedding can lead to dysfunction of the renin-angiotensin system (RAS), and further enhance inflammation and cause vascular permeability. ADE, cytokine storm, and pulmonary oedema leads to a fatal respiratory condition called acute respiratory distress syndrome (ARDS). Elevated levels of IL-6 were found to be a stable indicator of poor outcome in patients with severe COVID-19 with pneumonia and ARDS. Previous studies have found that genetic susceptibility and inflammatory cytokines were closely related to the occurrence of ARDS. More than 40 candidate genes, including ACE2, interleukin-10 (IL-10), tumor necrosis factor (TNF), and vascular endothelial growth factor (VEGF), among others, have been considered to be associated with the development or outcome of ARDS (Meyer *et al.*, 2013). The above biomarkers suggest both a molecular explanation for severe ARDS and a possible treatment for ARDS following SARS-CoV-2 infection.

6.5 Epidemiology

Unfortunately, China has witnessed the emergence of three respiratory virus outbreaks that have turned into epidemics or pandemics: i) avian influenza H5N1 (1997); ii) SARS-CoV (2003); and iii) the ongoing SARS-CoV-2 pandemic (2019–2021).

According to government data seen by the *South China Morning Post*, the first case of COVID-19 is thought to have been found on November 17, 2019. The virus subsequently spread to all provinces of China and at present has spread to more than 200 countries of the world. On January 30, 2020, SARS-CoV-2 was designated a Public Health Emergency of International Concern by the WHO, and on March 11, 2020 the WHO declared it a pandemic (WHO, 2020).

6.5.1 Route of Transmission

To date, the main infection source has been patients with pneumonia due to SARS-CoV-2 and the main route of transmission has been respiratory droplet transmission. However, it can also be transmitted through aerial droplets and contact (Jin *et al.*, 2020). Recently, a new coronavirus was detected in the feces of confirmed patients in Wuhan, Shenzhen, and even the first case in the United States, indicating that the virus can replicate and exist in the digestive tract, suggesting the possibility of fecal-oral transmission (Holshue *et al.*, 2020), but it is not certain that eating virus-contaminated food causes infection and transmission. There have also been views that viruses in feces may be re-transmitted by aerosol formation of virus-containing droplets, requiring further investigation. At present, there is no evidence for aerosol transmission of COVID-19. The WHO also believes that further evidence is needed to assess the possibility of aerosol transmission (WHO, 2020). Moreover, neonatal infection through mother-to-child transmission has also been reported, which needs to be confirmed by further scientific studies (Zhu *et al.*, 2020).

TABLE 6.1

Transmissibility of SARS-CoV-2 in comparison to other viruses involved in previous endemics/pandemics (as described by Azamfirei *et al.*, 2020)

Pathogen	Basic Reproduction Number (R_0)	Severity (CFR %)
SARS	~3.00 (1–2.75)	10
MERS	1.05	37
SARS-CoV-2 (COVID-19)	~3 (2.24–3.58)	~7
HCoVs	1.00	NA
Influenza	1.1–2.3	

6.5.2 Transmissibility

The basic reproduction number (R_0) is the characteristic epidemiological parameter which decides the transmissibility of pathogens. In the case of SARS-COV-2, R_0 is not yet precisely known, but has been estimated to be between 1.4 and 3.9. This indicates that each infection from the virus is expected to result in 1.4 to 3.9 new infections when no members of the community are immune and no preventive measures are taken. However, R_0 may be higher in densely populated regions. Estimates from the SARS outbreak in 2003 reported an R_0 of 3 (Bauch *et al.*, 2005), which means SARS-CoV-2 has a similar ability to infect as SARS or a higher spreading ability than SARS, so that the SARS-CoV-2 outbreak can affect almost the entire world within three to four months (Table 6.1). The slightly higher R_0 for SARS-CoV-2 may be because it has a longer prodromal period, increasing the period during which the infected host is contagious (Rabi *et al.*, 2020).

6.5.3 Viral Shedding

The viral load profile of SARS-CoV-2 is similar to that of influenza, which peaks at around the time of symptom onset, but contrasts with that of SARS, which peaks at around ten days after symptom onset, and that of MERS, which peaks at the second week after symptom onset. It was also observed that older-aged patients have comparatively higher viral loads. The high viral load close to symptom onset suggests that SARS-CoV-2 can be easily transmissible at an early stage of infection (To *et al.*, 2020). In the course of the disease, the virus has been detected one to two days before the onset of symptoms in respiratory tract samples, and can persist up to eight days in mild cases and up to two weeks in severe cases. Viral RNA has also been detected in whole blood, serum, saliva, feces, and urine from day five after symptom onset and up to four to five weeks in moderate cases. Prolonged viral RNA shedding has been reported from nasopharyngeal swabs (up to 37 days among adult patients and in feces—more than one month after infection in pediatric patients). It should be noted that viral RNA shedding does not equate to infectivity. The viral load can be a potentially useful marker for assessing disease severity and prognosis. A recent study indicated that viral loads in severe cases were up to 60 times higher than in mild cases (ECDC, 2020).

6.5.4 Environment Viability

Interestingly, the environmental stability of viable SARS-CoV-2 is up to 3 hours in the air post-aerosolisation, up to 4 hours on copper, up to 24 hours on cardboard, and up to 2 to 3 days on plastic and stainless steel, although with significantly decreased titres (van Doremalen *et al.*, 2020).

6.5.5 Clinical Manifestation

The incubation period for COVID-19 is typically 5 to 6 days, but may range from 2 to 14 days; 97.5% of people who develop symptoms will do so within 11.5 days of infection. Fever has been reported as one

TABLE 6.2

Clinical Symptoms of COVID-19

S.N.	Symptoms	%	S.N.	Symptoms	%
1	Fever	87.9	9	Headache	13.6
2	Dry cough	67.7	10	Chills	11.4
3	Fatigue	38.1	11	Nausea or vomiting	5.0
4	Sputum production	33.4	12	Nasal congestion	4.8
5	Loss of smell and taste	15–30	13	Diarrhoea	4.0
6	Shortness of breath	18.6	14	Haemoptysis	0.9
7	Muscle or joint pain	14.8	15	Conjunctival congestion	0.8
8	Sore throat	13.9	16		

of the most common symptoms of COVID-19 (Table 6.2). Some cases do not develop clinical symptoms at any point in time. These asymptomatic carriers tend not to get tested, and their role in transmission is not yet fully known. However, preliminary evidence suggests that they may contribute to the spread of the disease. The Korea Centres for Disease Control and Prevention (KCDC) reported in March 2020, and the Indian Council of Medical Research (ICMR) reported in April 2020, that ~20% of confirmed cases remained asymptomatic. Infection transmission by asymptomatic individuals can make control of disease spread challenging. Since late January 2020, SARS-CoV-2 transmission from infected but still asymptomatic individuals has been increasingly reported (Mizumoto *et al.*, 2020). Assessment of the viral loads in symptomatic individuals not only showed that the viral loads peak within the first few days of symptoms, but also that asymptomatic patients can have a similarly high viral load without showing symptoms. It was suggested that viral testing should no longer be limited to symptomatic individuals, but also include those who have traveled to affected areas (Lipsitch *et al.*, 2020).

Asymptomatic infection was also documented in Germany; two asymptomatic patients' throat samples were tested positive by reverse transcription (RT)-PCR and by virus isolation, while both patients remained well and afebrile for seven days (Hoehl *et al.*, 2020). Virus infection is not selective in age, having been reported even in a one-month-old infant. Until now, there has been no evidence for intrauterine infection by vertical transmission in women who developed COVID-19 during late pregnancy and no evidence that pregnant women are more susceptible than other adult patients.

6.6 Diagnosis

Laboratory diagnosis should be specific to SARS-CoV-2 and should exclude pneumonia-causing pathogens such as influenza viruses, parainfluenza virus, adenovirus, respiratory syncytial virus, rhinovirus, SARS-CoV, mycoplasma pneumonia, chlamydia pneumonia, and bacterial pneumonia. In addition, the assay should distinguish it from non-infectious diseases, such as vasculitis, dermatomyositis, and organizing pneumonia (Jin *et al.*, 2020).

Identification of SARS-CoV-2 mainly includes virus isolation and viral nucleic acid detection. According to the traditional Koch's postulates, virus isolation is the "gold standard" for virus diagnosis in the laboratory. A variety of biological samples such as swabs, nasal swabs, nasopharynx or trachea extracts, sputum or lung tissue, blood, and feces should be retained for testing in a timely manner, which gives a higher rate of positive detection of lower-respiratory-tract specimens (Wu *et al.*, 2020).

The preliminary identification of the SARS-CoV-2 virus was performed at the viral research institution in China through the classical Koch's postulates, and further characterized in its morphology through electron microscopy (Lu *et al.*, 2020). The gold-standard clinical diagnosis method of SARS-CoV-2 (COVID-19) is nucleic acid detection from nasal and throat swab sampling or blood or other respiratory tract sampling by real-time PCR. The persistence of viral nucleic acid during different stages of COVID-19 favors an RT-qPCR assay as the predominant method to diagnose the disease (Guo *et al.*, 2020). According to WHO guidelines, samples should be taken from both the upper and lower respiratory tracts. This can be achieved through expectorated sputum, bronchoalveolar lavage, or endotracheal aspirate (Cascella *et al.*, 2020). These samples are then assessed for viral RNA using RT-qPCR. If a positive test result is achieved, it is recommended to repeat the test for re-verification purposes. A negative test with a strong clinical suspicion also warrants repeat testing.

6.6.1 Molecular Diagnosis

6.6.1.1 *Real-time Reverse Transcriptase-PCR*

In general, real-time reverse transcriptase PCR (RT-qPCR) is considered to be the gold-standard test for the detection of nucleic acid of pathogen origin (Guo *et al.*, 2020). Particularly, TaqMan chemistry-based real-time PCR is highly specific and sensitive and hence applicable in disease diagnosis. Moreover, RT-qPCR is more sensitive than the conventional RT-PCR assay. Corman *et al.* (2020) developed a dual-labelled RT-qPCR assay for specific and sensitive diagnosis of SARS-CoV-2 (COVID-19). They targeted two structural (E and N) genes and one non-structural (RdRp) gene for confirmatory detection of SARS-CoV-2. The LOD of the assay was 3.9 copies per reaction for the E gene assay and 3.6 copies per reaction for the RdRp assay. The details of the primers and probes used by Corman *et al.* (2020) are mentioned in Table 6.3. The World Health Organization (WHO) also recommended an RT-qPCR assay for the detection of SARS-CoV-2 (COVID-19). The primers and probes selected in the WHO protocol are given in the Table 6.4 (www.who.int/docs/default-source/coronaviruse/protocol-v2-1.pdf?sfvrsn=a9ef618c_2).

6.6.1.2 *SHERLOCK Techniques*

CRISPR/Cas technology has the capability to transfer the nucleic acid sequence information of the gene of interest to detectable signals such as fluorescence and colorimetric values. The RNA-targeting CRISPR-associated enzyme (Cas13) has recently been used for rapid sensing of nucleic acids. Zhang's group demonstrated that Cas13 can be programmed to target and destroy the genomes of diverse mammalian single-stranded RNA viruses (Kellner *et al.*, 2019). Zhang *et al.* developed a platform termed SHERLOCK (Specific High-sensitivity Enzymatic Reporter unLOCKing) that combined isothermal pre-amplification with Cas13 to detect as few as tencopies of RNA of SARS-CoV-2. The SHERLOCK-COVID-19 detection protocol works in three steps and can be completed in one hour, starting from nucleic acid extraction as used for RT-qPCR tests. The first step of 25 minutes of incubation is required for isothermal amplification of the extracted nucleic acid sample using a commercially available recombinase

TABLE 6.3

Oligonucleotide (primers and probes) specific to RT-qPCR for SARS-CoV-2 (COVID-19) detection (Corman *et al.*, 2020)

Targeted Genes	Name of Primers	Oligonucleotide Sequence (5'–3')
RdRpgene	RdRp_SARSr-F	GTGARATGGTCATGTGTGGCGG
	RdRp_SARSr-P2	**FAM**-CAGGTGGAACCTCATCAGGAGATGC-**BBQ**
	RdRp_SARSr-P1	**FAM**-CCAGGTGGWACRTCATCMGGTGATGC-**BBQ**
	RdRp_SARSr-R	CARATGTTAAASACACTATTAGCATA
E gene	E_Sarbeco_F	ACAGGTACGTTAATAGTTAATAGCGT
	E_Sarbeco_P1	**FAM**-ACACTAGCCATCCTTACTGCGCTTCG-**BBQ**
	E_Sarbeco_R	ATATTGCAGCAGTACGCACACA
N gene	N_Sarbeco_F	CACATTGGCACCCGCAATC
	N_Sarbeco_P	**FAM**-ACTTCCTCAAGGAACAACATTGCCA-**BBQ**
	N_Sarbeco_R	GAGGAACGAGAAGAGGCTTG

Note: W is A/T; R is G/A; M is A/C; S is G/C. FAM: 6-carboxyfluorescein; BBQ: blackberry quencher

TABLE 6.4

List of primers and probes recommended by the WHO

Targeted Genes	Name of Primer	Oligonucleotide Sequence (5'–3')	Amlicon Size
RdRP gene	RdRp gene/ nCoV_IP2		108 bp
	nCoV_IP2-12669F	ATGAGCTTAGTCCTGTTG	
	nCoV_IP2-12696b-P1	**Hex**-AGATGTCTTGTGCTGCCGGTA-BHQ-1	
	nCoV_IP2-12759R	CTCCCTTTGTTGTGTTGT	
RdRP gene	RdRp gene/ nCoV_IP4		107 bp
	nCoV_IP4-14059F	GGTAACTGGTATGATTTCG	
	nCoV_IP4- 14084-P2	**FAM**-TCATACAAACCACGCCAGG-**BHQ-1**	
	nCoV_IP4-14146Rv	CTGGTCAAGGTTAATATAGG	
E gene	E_Sarbeco_F	ACAGGTACGTTAATAGTTAATAGCGT	125 bp
	E_Sarbeco_P1	**FAM**-ACACTAGCCATCCTTACTGCGCTTCG-**BBQ**	
	E_Sarbeco_R	ATATTGCAGCAGTACGCACACA	

polymerase amplification (RPA) kit; the second step of 30 minutes of incubation is for the detection of a pre-amplified viral RNA sequence using Cas13; and the third and final step of just 2 minutes of incubation is required for visual detection using a commercially available paper dipstick. The test can be carried out starting with RNA purified from patient samples, as is used for RT-qPCR assays, and can be read out using a dipstick in less than an hour, without requiring sophisticated instrumentation.

6.6.2 Classical Diagnosis

The clinical signs and symptoms are very helpful in diagnosis but not conclusive in SARS-CoV-2 infection. On the basis of clinical symptoms, fever may be considered as the main diagnostic feature. However, various other symptoms, like fatigue, dry cough, dyspnea, etc., with or without nasal congestion, runny nose, or other upper-respiratory symptoms, were also reported (Zhu *et al.*, 2020; Huang *et al.*, 2020). Despite various atypical symptoms, fever is still the typical symptom of SARS-CoV-2 infection (Guan *et al.*, 2020).

6.6.3 Physical Examination

Patients with mild symptoms may not present positive signs. Patients in severe condition may have shortness of breath, moist rales in lungs, weakened breath sounds, dullness in percussion, and increased or decreased tactile speech tremor, etc. (Jin *et al.*, 2020).

6.6.4 Virus Isolation

Virus isolation is one of the oldest gold-standard tests to confirm viral infection. The selection of appropriate samples is very important for the isolation of the virus. SARS-CoV-2 isolation was successfully done from nasopharyngeal and oropharyngeal samples of COVID-19 patients using vero cell lines. Virus replication and isolation were confirmed through cytopathic effects, gene detection, and electron microscopy. Viral culture of SARS-CoV-2 was conducted in a biosafety level-3 facility according to the laboratory biosafety guidelines of the Centers for Disease Control and Prevention (Kim *et al.*, 2020).

6.6.5 Serological Diagnosis

An acute serological response has been reported in patients with SARS-CoV-2 infection. Hence, for the screening of the suspected population, serological tests are very easy and informative. Recently, National

Bio Green Sciences LLC (NBGS) Novel Coronavirus (2019-nCoV) IgM/IgG Antibody Rapid Test Kits have been released. These Rapid Test Kits are for whole blood, serum, and/or plasma, require no special equipment, and are able to deliver results in just 15 minutes (Aurora biomed, 2020). Actually, IgM antibodies provide the first line of defense during viral infections, followed by the generation of adaptive, high-affinity IgG antibody responses for long-term immunity and immunological memory. Therefore, the testing of IgM and IgG antibodies is an effective method for the rapid diagnosis of COVID-19 infection. Moreover, the detection of IgM antibodies tends to indicate a recent exposure to COVID-19, whereas the detection of IgG antibodies indicates a later stage of infection. Thus, this combined antibody test could also provide information on the stage of infection.

6.7 Treatment

To date, no specific antiviral therapy is available against SARS-CoV-2 (COVID-19). In the absence of specific therapy, symptomatic clinical management is the method of choice to control the disease. Several antiviral therapies which were effective against SARS and MERS have also been recommended against SARS-CoV-2 (COVID-19) (Table 6.5).

6.8 Status of Vaccine

It has already been proved that vaccination is the best option for the control of viral diseases and the same is also true for SARS-CoV-2 (COVID-19). However, the CDC has reported that mRNA coronavirus vaccine trials have begun enrolment at Kaiser Permanente Washington Health Research Institute in Seattle, and at Emory Children's Center in Decatur. Other targets like epitopes and S protein-RBD structure-based vaccines have been widely proposed and started. Rapid reconstruction of SARS-CoV-2 using a synthetic genomics platform has been reported, and this technical advance is helpful for vaccine development. Human ACE2 transgenic mouse and rhesus monkey models of SARS-CoV-2 (COVID-19) have been well established for vaccine development (Bao *et al.*, 2020).

6.9 Prevention

Since there is no specific treatment or vaccine against SARS-CoV-2 (COVID-19), the famous proverb "prevention is better than cure" is very much applicable in this pandemic scenario. Preventive measures must focus on optimizing infection control protocols, self-isolation, and patient isolation during the provision of clinical care. The WHO has advised against close contact with patients, farm animals, and wild animals (Cascella *et al.*, 2020). Patients and the general public must cover coughs and sneezes to help prevent aerosol transmission. Frequent handwashing with soap and water is also required. As an alternative measure, hand sanitizers can also be used. Immunocompromised individuals are advised to avoid public gatherings. Emergency medicine departments must apply strict hygiene measures for the control of infections. Healthcare personnel must use personal protective equipment such as N95 masks, FFP3 masks, gowns, eye protection, and gloves. Isolation remains the most effective measure for containment of SARS-CoV-2 (COVID-19) (Cascella *et al.*, 2020).

6.10 Conclusions

On the basis of above-mentioned facts it can be concluded that the SARS-CoV-2 (COVID-19) pandemic is a public health emergency. One of the most worrying things about any outbreak is the spreading of viruses from mild or asymptomatic individuals, which is probably happening in the case of COVID-19. If this trend continues then the virus may establish itself in the population and it will be very difficult to stop the spread of the virus through quarantine. Phylogenetic analysis based on the spike gene nucleotide

TABLE 6.5

List of recommended therapy for clinical management of COVID-19

S.N.	Antiviral Agents	Potential Antiviral Compounds	Reference
1	Ribavirin	It inhibits SARS-associated CoV replication *in vitro*. Due to adverse reactions, the proper dose of ribavirin in clinical application should be given carefully: 500 mg each time, two to three times/day in combination with IFN-α or lopinavir/ritonavir	Dong *et al.*(2020)
2	Lopinavir/ritonavir	The combination of lopinavir/ritonavir is widely used in the treatment of HIV infection. It has been reported that the use of lopinavir/ritonavir with ribavirin has a good therapeutic effect in SARS and MERS and has been recommended for clinical treatment for COVID-19.	Chu *et al.* (2004)
3	Remdesivir (RDV/GS-5734)	It was previously reported to be effective for SARS-CoV*in vivo*, and the antiviral protection of RDV and IFN-_was found to be superior to that of lopinavir/ritonavir-IFN-_ against MERS-CoV *in vitro* and *in vivo*. In addition, remdesivir was used in the treatment of the first COVID-19 patient in the United States and was shown to have antiviral activity against SARS-CoV-2 *in vitro*. However, its effectiveness and safety have not yet been verified in clinical trials.	Holshue*et al.* (2020)
	Favipiravir	Broad-spectrum antiviral with *in vitro* activity against various viruses, including coronaviruses. Early embryonic deaths and teratogenicity observed in animal studies. Favipiravir is contraindicated in women with known or suspected pregnancy and precautions should be taken to avoid pregnancy during treatment with the drug.	www.ashp.org/COVID-19
4	Nelfinavir	It is a selective inhibitor of HIV protease, which has been shown to have a strong inhibition of SARS-CoV, implying a possible therapeutic for COVID-19.	Yamamoto *et al.* (2004)
5	Arbidol	Abroad-spectrum antiviral compound, able to block viral fusion against influenza viruses. In addition, arbidol and its derivative, arbidolmesylate, have been reported to have antiviral activity against SARS-CoV *in vitro*. The antiviral activity of arbidol against SARS-CoV-2 has been confirmed *in vitro* and recommended for clinical treatment.	www.sd.chinanews.com/2/2020/0205/70145.html
6	Chloroquine phosphate	*In vitro* activity against SARS-CoV-2 in infected Vero E6 cells reported. The recommended oral dose is 500 mg twice daily for seven to ten days in adults.	National Health Commission, China
7	Type-I IFNs	Type-I IFNs are antiviral cytokines that induce a large range of proteins that can impair viral replication in targeted cells. Previous studies have reported that IFN-β was superior against SARS-CoV compared to IFN-α. Synergistic effects of leukocytic IFN-α with ribavirin and IFN-β with ribavirin against SARS-CoV were demonstrated *in vitro*.	Jin *et al.* (2020)
8	Convalescent plasma	Recently, convalescent plasma has been widely recommended for use, but the effect of convalescent plasma cannot be discerned from the effects of patient comorbidities, stage of illness, or effect of other treatments.	Li *et al.* (2020)
9	Low-molecular-weight heparin (LMWH)	LMWH anticoagulation therapy is especially recommended in the early stage of the disease, particularly when the D-dimer value is four times higher than the normal upper limit, except for patients with anticoagulant contraindications. The recommended dose is 100U/kg body weight per twelve hours by subcutaneous injection for at least three to five days.	

TABLE 6.5

List of recommended therapy for clinical management of COVID-19 (Cont.)

S.N.	Antiviral Agents	Potential Antiviral Compounds	Reference
10	IVIg	IVIg therapy has already been effective against influenza and SARS. A high dose of IVIg at 0.3–0.5 g per kg weight per day can be given for five days, which can interrupt the storm of inflammatory factors at an early stage, enhancing immune function. A randomized controlled clinical trial of IVIg in patients with severe SARS-CoV-2 infection has been initiated.	
11	Miscellaneous	The binding of S protein to its receptor ACE2 is important for the treatment of COVID-19. ACE2 is an important component of the renin-angiotensin system (RAS). RAS inhibitors (ACEI and AT1R) may be potential therapeutic tools for COVID-19. Moreover, intravenous transplantation of ACE2-mesenchymal stem cells (MSCs), blocking of FcR with immunoglobulin (IVIG), and systemic anti-inflammatory drugs to reduce cytokine storm are also potential therapeutic strategies for severe COVID-19.	Leng *et al.* (2020)

sequence revealed that the SARS-CoV-2 sequences form a single cluster without any branching, indicating SARS-CoV-2 conservation throughout this ongoing outbreak. These findings advocate that the virus that caused the initial outbreak of SARS-CoV-2 is still in circulation, without any significant changes. Moreover, SARS-CoV-2 has lesser CFR as opposed to SARS-CoV and MERS-CoV. To date, most deaths have occurred in the aged population due to novel coronavirus infection, whereas children and young adults exhibit a relatively milder disease. Therefore, SARS-CoV-2 infection will enable the host to develop humoral and cell-mediated immunity and simultaneously the immune-selected viruses may acquire mutations with higher infection potential or altered antigenicity. Since there is no antiviral treatment or vaccine to fight against SARS CoV-2, the development of a vaccine or effective therapeutics is the primary need of the hour.

Acknowledgments

The authors thank the researchers, government agencies, and the WHO, who have generated and shared the experimental data and sequencing data on which this review is based.

References

Andersen, K.G., Rambaut, A., Lipkin, W.I., Holmes, E.C., Garry, R.F. The proximal origin of SARS-CoV-2. *Nature Medicine*, 2020, 26(4), 450–452.

Aurora biomed. Rapid test kit, 2020, www.aurorabiomed.com.

Azamfirei, R. The 2019 novel coronavirus: a crown jewel of pandemics? *Journal of Critical Care Medicien (Targu Mures)*, 2020, 6(1), 3–4.

Bao, L., Deng, W., Huang, B., Gao, H., Liu, J., Ren, L., Wei, Q., Yu, P., Xu, Y., Qi, F., Qu, Y., Li, F., Lv, Q., Wang, W., Xue, J., Gong, S., Liu, M., Wang, G., Wang, S., Song, Z., Qin, C. The pathogenicity of SARS-CoV-2 in hACE2 transgenic mice. *Nature*, 2020, 583(7818), 830–833.

Bauch, C.T., Lloyd-Smith, J.O., Coffee, M.P., Galvani, A.P. Dynamically modeling SARS and other newly emerging respiratory illnesses: past, present, and future. *Epidemiology*, 2005, 16(6), 791–801.

Burrell, C.J., Howard, C.R., Murphy, F.A. Coronaviruses. In Burrell, C.J., Howard, C.R., Murphy, F.A. (eds), *Fenner and White's Medical Virology*, 5th edn, 2016, 437–446. Elsevier.

Cascella, M., Rajnik, M., Cuomo, A., Dulebohn, S.C., Di Napoli, R. Features, evaluation and treatment coronavirus (COVID-19). In StatPearls [Internet], 2020. StatPearls Publishing.

Chen, N., Zhou, M., Dong, X., Qu, J., Gong, F., Han, Y., Qiu, Y., Wang, J., Liu, Y., Wei, Y., Xia, J., Yu, T., Zhang, X., Zhang, L. Epidemiological and clinical characteristics of 99 cases of 2019 novel coronavirus pneumonia in Wuhan, China: a descriptive study. *The Lancet*, 2020, 395(10223), 507–513.

Chen, Y., Liu, Q., Guo, D. Emerging coronaviruses: genome structure, replication, and pathogenesis. *Journal of Medical Virology*, 2020, 92(4), 418–423.

Chu, C.M., Cheng, V.C., Hung, I.F., Wong, M.M., Chan, K.H., Chan, K.S., Kao, R.Y., Poon, L.L., Wong, C.L., Guan, Y., Peiris, J.S., Yuen, K.Y., HKU/UCH SARS Study Group. Role of lopinavir/ritonavir in the treatment of SARS: initial virological and clinical findings. *Thorax*, 2004, 59(3), 252–256.

Corman, V.M., Landt, O., Kaiser, M., Molenkamp, R., Meijer, A., Chu, D.K., Mulders, D.G. Detection of 2019 novel coronavirus (2019-nCoV) by real-time RT-PCR. *Eurosurveillance*, 2020, 25(3), 2000045.

European Centre for Disease Prevention and Control (ECDC). Situation update worldwide [Internet]. Stockholm: ECDC, 2020. Available from: www.ecdc.europa.eu/en/covid-19.

Fan, C., Li, K., Ding, Y., Lu, W., Wang, J. ACE2 Expression in kidney and testis may cause kidney and testis damage after 2019-nCoV infection. medRxiv, 2020. https://doi.org/10.1101/2020.02.12.20022418.

Fu, Y., Cheng, Y., Wu, Y. Understanding SARS-CoV-2-mediated inflammatory responses: from mechanisms to potential therapeutic tools. *Virologica Sinica*, 2020, 35(3), 266–271.

Gheblawi, M., Wang, K., Viveiros, A., Nguyen, Q., Zhong, J.C., Turner, A.J., Oudit, G.Y., *et al.* Angiotensin-converting enzyme 2: SARS-CoV-2 receptor and regulator of the renin-angiotensin system: celebrating the 20th anniversary of the discovery of ACE2. *Circulation Research*, 2020, 126(10), 1456–1474.

Gong, L., Li, J., Zhou, Q., Xu, Z., Chen, L., Zhang, Y., Xue, C., Wen, Z., Cao, Y.A. New bat-HKU2-like coronavirus in swine, China, 2017. *Emerging Infectious Diseases*, 2017, 23(9), 1607.

Gorbalenya, A.E., Baker, S.C., Baric, R.S., Groot, R.J.D., Drosten, C., Gulyaeva, A.A., Haagmans, B.L., Lauber, C., Leontovich, A.M., Neuman, B.W., Penzar, D., Perlman, S., Poon, L.L.M., Samborskiy, D., Sidorov, I.A., Sola, I., Ziebuhr, J. Severe acute respiratory syndrome-related coronavirus: The species and its viruses, a statement of the Coronavirus Study Group. *Nature Microbiology*, 2020. doi: 10.1038/s41564-020-0695.

Guan, W.J., Ni, Z.Y., Hu, Y., Liang, W.H., Ou, C.Q., He, J.X., Liu, L., Shan, H., Lei, C.L., Hui, D., Du, B., Li, L.J., Zeng, G., Yuen, K.Y., Chen, R.C., Tang, C.L., Wang, T., Chen, P.Y., Xiang, J., Li, S.Y. China medical treatment expert group for COVID-19 clinical characteristics of coronavirus disease 2019 in China. *New England Journal of Medicine*, 2020, 382(18), 1708–1720.

Guo, Y.R., Cao, Q.D., Hong, Z.S., Tan, Y.Y., Chen, S.D., Jin, H.J., Tan, K.S., Wang, D.Y., Yan, Y. The origin, transmission and clinical therapies on coronavirus disease 2019 (COVID-19) outbreak: an update on the status. *Military Medical Research*, 2020, 7(1), 11.

Hoehl, S., Rabenau, H., Berger, A., Kortenbusch, M., Cinatl, J., Bojkova, D., Behrens, P., Böddinghaus, B., Götsch, U., Naujoks, F., Neumann, P., Schork, J., Tiarks-Jungk, P., Walczok, A., Eickmann, M., Vehreschild, M.J.G.T, Kann, G., Wolf, T., Gottschalk, R., Ciesek, S. Evidence of SARS-CoV-2 infection in returning travelers from Wuhan, China. *New England Journal of Medicine*, 2020, 382(13), 1278–1280.

Hoffmann, M., Kleine-Weber, H., Schroeder, S., Krüger, N., Herrler, T., Erichsen, S., Schiergens, T.S., Herrler, G., Wu, N.H., Nitsche, A., Müller, M.A., Drosten, C., Pöhlmann, S. SARS-CoV-2 cell entry depends on ACE2 and TMPRSS2 and is blocked by a clinically proven protease inhibitor. *Cell*, 2020, 181(2), 271–280.

Holshue, M.L., DeBolt, C., Lindquist, S., Lofy, K.H., Wiesman, J., Bruce, H., Spitters, C., Ericson, K., Wilkerson, S., Tural, A., Diaz, G., Cohn, A., Fox, L., Patel, A., Gerber, S.I., Kim, L., Tong, S., Lu, X., Lindstrom, S., Pallansch, M.A., Washington State 2019-nCoV Case Investigation Team. First case of 2019 novel coronavirus in the United States. *New England Journal of Medicine*, 2020, 382(10), 929–936.

Huang, C., Wang, Y., Li, X., Ren, L., Zhao, J., Hu, Y., Zhang, L., Fan, G., Xu, J., Gu, X., Cheng, Z., Yu, T., Xia, J., Wei, Y., Wu, W., Xie, X., Yin, W., Li, H., Liu, M., Xiao, Y., Cao, B. Clinical features of patients infected with 2019 novel coronavirus in Wuhan, China. *The Lancet*, 2020, 395(10223), 497–506.

Imai, Y., Kuba, K., Penninger, J.M. The discovery of angiotensin-converting enzyme 2 and its role in acute lung injury in mice. *Experimental Physiology*, 2008, 93(5), 543–548.

Jin, Y.H., Cai, L., Cheng, Z.S., Cheng, H., Deng, T., Fan, Y.P., Fang, C., Huang, D., Huang, L.Q., Huang, Q., Han, Y., Hu, B., Hu, F., Li, B.H., Li, Y.R., Liang, K., Lin, L.K., Luo, L.S., Ma, J., Ma, L.L., Peng, Z.Y., Pan, Y.B., Pan, Z.Y., Ren, X.Q., Sun, H.M., Wang, Y., Wang, Y.Y., Weng, H., Wei, C.J., Wu, D.F., Xia, J., Xiong, Y., Xu, H.B., Yao, X.M., Ye, T.S., Yuan, Y.F., Zhang, X.C., Zhang, Y.W., Zhang, Y.G., Zhang, H.M.,

Zhao, Y., Zhao, M.J., Zi, H., Zeng, X.T., Wang, Y.Y., Wang, X.H. A rapid advice guideline for the diagnosis and treatment of 2019 novel coronavirus (2019-nCoV) infected pneumonia (standard version). Military Medical Research, 2020, 7(4) https://doi.org/10.1186/s40779-020-0233-6

Jin, Y., Yang, H., Ji, W., Wu, W., Chen, S., Zhang, W., Duan, G. Virology, epidemiology, pathogenesis, and control of COVID-19. *Viruses*, 2020, 12(4), 372.

Kellner, M.J., Koob, J.G., Gootenberg, J.S., Abudayyeh, O.O., Zhang, F. SHERLOCK: nucleic acid detection with CRISPR nucleases. *Nature Protocols*, 2019, 14(10), 2986–3012.

Kim, J.M., Chung, Y.S., Jo, H.J., Lee, N.J., Kim, M.S., Woo, S.H., Park, S., Kim, J. W., Kim, H.M., Han, M.G. (2020). Identification of coronavirus isolated from a patient in Korea with COVID-19. *Osong Public Health and Research Perspectives*, 2020, 11(1), 3–7.

Leng, Z., Zhu, R., Hou, W., Feng, Y., Yang, Y., Han, Q., Shan, G., Meng, F., Du, D., Wang, S., Fan, J., Wang, W., Deng, L., Shi, H., Li, H., Hu, Z., Zhang, F., Gao, J., Liu, H., Li, X., Zhao, R.C. Transplantation of ACE2-mesenchymal stem cells improves the outcome of patients with COVID-19 pneumonia. *Aging Disease*, 2020, 11(2), 216–228.

Li, H., Liu, S.M., Yu, X.H., Tang, S.L., Tang, C.K. Coronavirus disease 2019 (COVID-19): current status and future perspective. *International Journal of Antimicrobial Agents*, 2020, 105951.

Lipsitch, M., Swerdlow, D.L., Finelli, L. Defining the epidemiology of Covid-19—studies needed. *New England Journal of Medicine*, 2020, 382(13), 1194–1196.

Lu, R., Zhao, X., Li, J., Niu, P., Yang, B., Wu, H., Wang, W., Song, H., Huang, B., Zhu, N., Bi, Y., Ma, X., Zhan, F., Wang, L., Hu, T., Zhou, H., Hu, Z., Zhou, W., Zhao, L., Chen, J., Meng, Y., Wang, J., Lin, Y., Yuan, J., Xie, Z., Ma, J., Liu, W.J., Wang, D., Xu, W., Holmes, E.C., Gao, G.F., Wu, G., Chen, W., Shi, W., Tan, W. Genomic characterisation and epidemiology of 2019 novel coronavirus: implications for virus origins and receptor binding. *The Lancet*, 2020, 395(10224), 565–574. doi: 10.1016/S0140-6736(20)30251-8. Epub 2020 Jan 30. PMID: 32007145; PMCID: PMC7159086.

Meyer, N.J., Christie, J.D. Genetic heterogeneity and risk of acute respiratory distress syndrome. *Seminars in Respiratory and Critical Care Medicine*, 2013, 34(4), 459–474.

Mizumoto, K., Kagaya, K., Zarebski, A., Chowell, G. Estimating the asymptomatic proportion of coronavirus disease 2019 (COVID-19) cases on board the Diamond Princess cruise ship, Yokohama, Japan, 2020. *Eurosurveillance*, 2020, 25(10), 2000180.

Nguyen, H.L., Lan, P.D., Thai, N.Q., Nissley, D.A., O'Brien, E.P., Li, M.S. Does SARS-CoV-2 bind to human ACE2 more strongly than does SARS-CoV? *Journal of Physical Chemistry B*, 2020, 124(34), 7336–7347.

Qin, C., Zhou, L., Hu, Z., Zhang, S., Yang, S., Tao, Y., Xie, C., Ma, K., Shang, K., Wang, W., Tian, D.S. Dysregulation of immune response in patients with COVID-19 in Wuhan, China. *Clinical Infectious Diseases*, 2020, 71(15), 762–768.

Rabi, F.A., Al Zoubi, M.S., Kasasbeh, G.A., Salameh, D.M., Al-Nasser, A.D. SARS-CoV-2 and coronavirus disease 2019: what we know so far. *Pathogens*, 2020, 9(3), 231.

Raoult, D., Zumla, A., Locatelli, F., Ippolito, G., Kroemer, G. Coronavirus infections: epidemiological, clinical and immunological features and hypotheses. *Cell Stress*, 2020, 4(4), 66–75.

Tang, X., Wu, C., Li, X., Song, Y., Yao, X., Wu, X., Duan, Y., Zhang, H., Wang, Y., Qian, Z., Cui, J., Lu, J. On the origin and continuing evolution of SARS-CoV-2. *National Science Review*, 2020, nwaa036.

To, K.K.W., Tsang, O.T.Y., Leung, W.S., Tam, A.R., Wu, T.C., Lung, D.C., Lau, D.P.L. Temporal profiles of viral load in posterior oropharyngeal saliva samples and serum antibody responses during infection by SARS-CoV-2: an observational cohort study. *The Lancet Infectious Diseases*, 2020, 20(5), 565–574.

van Doremalen, N., Bushmaker, T., Morris, D.H., Holbrook, M.G., Gamble, A., Williamson, B.N., Tamin, A., Harcourt, J.L., Thornburg, N.J., Gerber, S.I., Lloyd-Smith, J.O., de Wit, E., Munster, V.J. Aerosol and surface stability of SARS-CoV-2 as compared with SARS-CoV-1. *New England Journal of Medicine*, 2020, 382(16), 1564–1567.

Walls, A.C., Park, Y.J., Tortorici, M.A., Wall, A., McGuire, A.T., Veesler, D. Structure, function, and antigenicity of the SARS-CoV-2 spike glycoprotein. *Cell*, 2020, 181(2), 281–292.

Wu, D., Wu, T., Liu, Q., Yang, Z. The SARS-CoV-2 outbreak: what we know. *International Journal of Infectious Diseases*, 2020, 94, 44–48.

Wu, F., Zhao, S., Yu, B., Chen, Y.M., Wang, W., Song, Z.G., Hu, Y., Tao, Z.W., Tian, J.H., Pei, Y.Y., Yuan, M.L., Zhang, Y.L., Dai, F.H., Liu, Y., Wang, Q.M., Zheng, J.J., Xu, L., Holmes, E.C., Zhang, Y.Z. A new coronavirus associated with human respiratory disease in China. *Nature*, 2020, 579(7798), 265–269.

Xiao, F., Tang, M., Zheng, X., Liu, Y., Li, X., Shan, H. Evidence for gastrointestinal infection of SARS-CoV-2. *Gastroenterology*, 2020, 158(6), 1831–1833.

Xu, Z., Shi, L., Wang, Y., Zhang, J., Huang, L., Zhang, C., Liu, S., Zhao, P., Liu, H., Zhu, L., Tai, Y., Bai, C., Gao, T., Song, J., Xia, P., Dong, J., Zhao, J., Wang, F.S. Pathological findings of COVID-19 associated with acute respiratory distress syndrome. *The Lancet Respiratory Medicine*, 2020, 8(4), 420–422.

Yamamoto, N., Yang, R., Yoshinaka, Y., Amari, S., Nakano, T., Cinatl, J., Rabenau, H., Doerr, H.W., Hunsmann, G., Otaka, A., Tamamura, H., Fujii, N., Yamamoto, N. HIV protease inhibitor nelfinavir inhibits replication of SARS-associated coronavirus. *Biochemical and Biophysical Research Communications*, 2004, 318(3), 719–725.

Zhang, Z., Wu, Q., Zhang, T. Pangolin homology associated with 2019-nCoV. bioRxiv, 2020. https://doi.org/10.1101/2020.02.19.950253.

Zheng, J. SARS-CoV-2: an emerging coronavirus that causes a global threat. *International Journal of Biological Sciences*, 2020, 16(10), 1678.

Zhou, P., Yang, X.L., Wang, X.G., Hu, B., Zhang, L., Zhang, W., Chen, H.D.A. Pneumonia outbreak associated with a new coronavirus of probable bat origin. *Nature*, 2020, 579(7798), 270–273.

Zhu, H., Wang, L., Fang, C., Peng, S., Zhang, L., Chang, G., Zhou, W. Clinical analysis of 10 neonates born to mothers with 2019-nCoV pneumonia. *Translational Pediatrics*, 2020, 9(1), 51.

Zhu, N., Zhang, D., Wang, W., Li, X., Yang, B., Song, J., Niu, P. China novel coronavirus investigating and research team. A novel coronavirus from patients with pneumonia in China, 2019. *New England Journal of Medicine*, 2020, 382(8), 727–733.

7

Application of Proteomics and Metabolomics in Disease Diagnosis

Lukumoni Buragohain,[1] Mayukh Ghosh,[2] Rajesh Kumar,[3] Swati Dahiya,[4] Yashpal Singh Malik[5] and Minakshi Prasad[6]

[1] *Department of Animal Biotechnology, College of Veterinary Science, Assam Agricultural University, Khanapara, Guwahati-781022, Assam, India*

[2] *Department of Veterinary Physiology and Biochemistry, RGSC, Banaras Hindu University, Mirzapur-231001, Uttar Pradesh, India*

[3] *Department of Veterinary Physiology and Biochemistry, Lala Lajpat Rai University of Veterinary and Animal Sciences, Hisar-125004, Haryana, India*

[4] *Department of Veterinary Microbiology, Lala Lajpat Rai University of Veterinary and Animal Sciences, Hisar-125004, Haryana, India*

[5] *Division of Biological Standardization, Indian Veterinary Research Institute Izatnagar, Bareilly-243122, Uttar Pradesh, India*

[6] *Department of Animal Biotechnology, Lala Lajpat Rai University of Veterinary and Animal Sciences, Hisar-125004, Haryana, India*

Corresponding author: Minakshi Prasad, *minakshi.abt@gmail.com*

7.1 Introduction

Early disease diagnosis is pivotal in customizing an effective treatment regimen for a disease. Identification of disease biomarkers is crucial for early disease diagnosis, disease classification, assessment of disease progression and evaluation of treatment response. The ongoing "omics" era has delivered significant impetus to propel the field of proteomics and metabolomics with marked advancements in analytical platforms such as chromatographic or electrophoretic separation integrated with mass spectrometry (MS), direct analyses through mass spectrometry imaging (MSI), fluorescence-based methods and nuclear magnetic resonance (NMR) spectroscopy in combination with state-of-the-art bioinformatics tools to achieve ample sensitivity along with sufficient precision. The application of proteomics and metabolomics has achieved significant penetration in the arena of clinical medicine by crossing the horizon of basic research and established a strong foot-hold in disease diagnosis of both humans and animals toward securing the "one health" concept. Both of these approaches are predominantly intended to identify the altered proteins or metabolites as indicators of pathophysiological aberrations and establish them as disease-specific diagnostic biomarkers. Proteins are the end products of the central dogma and metabolites are the terminal products of several inter-related metabolic pathways. Thus, proteomics and metabolomics can yield the most nascent information regarding the complex biological networks. Further, both the platforms are equipped with simultaneous identification as well as quantification of multiple key molecules either through a targeted or untargeted approach as promising biomarkers having relevancy in disease diagnosis.

Proteomics refers to the characterization of an absolute complement of proteins, including their identification, localization, function, structure, differential expression and post-translational modifications in a biological system (cell, tissue, biofluid, organ or organism) under certain specified conditions and within a precise temporal framework (Wilkins and Williams, 1995; Shah and Misra, 2011). Mark Wilkins coined the term *proteome*, representing the snapshots of protein composition in a biological system, which was conceptualized by merging the words *genome* and *protein* (Wilkins and Williams, 1995; Wasinger *et al.*, 1995). The classical proteomics approach has evolved from back in the 1970s with the introduction of SDS-PAGE and two-dimensional (2D) gel electrophoresis (Laemmli, 1970; O'Farrell, 1975), followed by persistent developments in high-throughput instrumentation as well as data analysis programs. The proteomics workflow can be broadly classified into the gel-based and gel-free approach. In the gel-based approach, a polyacrylamide gel matrix is used for electrophoretic separation of proteins from a biological cocktail and finally the identification of proteins is performed using mass spectrometry and computational tools. Unlike the gel-based approach, the gel-free approach is independent of using such a gel matrix and alternatively employs other techniques such as chromatography or direct mass spectrometry imaging for protein separation and identification/quantification. Mass spectrometry holds centre stage as the most important analytical platform in proteomics analysis. However, MS was invented much earlier and remained a crucial tool for chemists for a long time. However, in a true sense, the enormous value of this analytical platform has been established through its employment in proteomic and metabolomic introspection (Ahmad *et al.*, 2014). Remarkable sensitivity, considerable precision and an extremely low sample requirement have rendered MS capable of even introspecting single-cell proteomics or metabolomics to unearth valuable information regarding the biomarker dynamics, molecular pathology, therapeutic efficacy etc., thus proving it an indispensable tool not only for diagnosis but also for preventive and therapeutic aspects of several diseases (Minakshi *et al.*, 2019a, 2019b).

Despite significant progress in the field of proteomics, the tempo-spatial dynamics of the proteome is one of the challenges hindering its application in various fields. Occurrence of the disease condition manifests as impairment in cellular processes and pathways leading to variation in the proteome profile of the host (Andersen and Mann, 2006; Di Girolamo *et al.*, 2012) and proteomics assists in identifying those altered proteins, their magnitude and relationship with the disease. Clinical proteomics has emerged as a new domain under the umbrella of proteomics, which has evolved from numerous proteomic interventions in clinical and pre-clinical studies, associated with disease diagnosis and execution of novel therapy by using signature protein(s) involved in the pathological condition of the host (Apweiler *et al.*, 2009). To date, several novel, potentially promising candidate biomarkers pertaining to certain diseases of humans and animals have been identified and validated by proteomics approaches, thus establishing proteomics as a worthy technology in the current "omics era".

Metabolomics is an emerging branch of "omics" that is defined as the global analysis of small molecules (metabolites) which includes identification, characterization and quantification in a biological specimen such as a cell, tissue, biofluid, an organ or an organism at a specific point of time under given genetic and environmental conditions (Oliver *et al.*, 1998; German *et al.*, 2005; Griffin and Vidal-Puig, 2008), and the entire complement of metabolites taken into consideration in a specific biological sample is referred to as the *metabolome* (Querengesser *et al.*, 2007). Although metabolomics in clinical medicine is an emerging field, it was conceptualized by Roger Williams almost 80 years ago based on individual variation and disease-specific "metabolic patterns" in the biological fluids of the diseased subjects (Gates and Sweeley, 1978), while the term "metabolic profile" was coined by Horning and co-workers in 1971 based on quantitative metabolomics of urinary metabolites (Novotny *et al.*, 2008).

Current metabolomic approaches analyze hundreds to thousands of metabolites in biological fluids or tissues to diagnose complex metabolic and other systemic diseases (Clish, 2015). Assessment of metabolites gives a true reflection of the underlying pathophysiological condition of an organism (Tomita and Kami, 2012) because they depict the functional end product of genome, transcriptome and proteome expression (Zhang *et al.*, 2015). Besides endogenous metabolites, there are also exogenous metabolites derived from the metabolism of environmental molecules, xenobiotics, therapeutics agents and metabolites generated due to interaction of host and gut microbiome (Bogdanov *et al.*, 2008). Advancements in science and technology have made metabolomics a robust tool in potential biomarker discovery, investigating metabolic processes, gene-function analysis, systems biology, improvement in treatment regimen and development of diagnostic platforms (Zhang *et al.*, 2015). Moreover, metabolomics has the potential to link environmental and host factors for better understanding the pathogenesis of many diseases (Nicholson *et al.*, 2002), along with identifying the therapeutic checkpoints to develop a broadly specific treatment regimen for multiple infectious agents. It can even assist in drug repurposing by identifying the common host metabolic pathways exploited by similar types of pathogens to combat sudden disease outbreak (Kumar *et al.*, 2020).

The developments in biological sample preparation methodologies and advancements in instrumentation of the analytical modalities—such as nuclear magnetic resonance spectroscopy (NMR), Raman-based methods, chromatography and other separation-based analytical techniques, fluorescence-based methods, microfluidics lab-on-chip platforms and, most importantly, mass spectrometry (MS), along with high-throughput computational tools—have enabled comprehensive and reliable analysis of a broad range of metabolites from a minute amount of diverse biological specimens. These aforementioned qualities and their versatility have rendered metabolomics one of the major platforms in clinical investigations, especially in disease diagnosis (Tsutsui *et al.*, 2011; Zhang *et al.*, 2014). There is probably no novel technology that is devoid of challenges, and metabolomics is not an exception, having some inherent challenges such as the heterogeneous and complex physical properties of a metabolome, rapid metabolite turn-over, the generation of a large volume of data and an immature metabolic database which may create a bottleneck in metabolomic introspection of disease diagnosis (Kuehnbaum and Britz-McKibbin, 2013; Zhang *et al.*, 2015).

Despite the obstacles, state-of-the-art proteomics and metabolomics modalities have not only contributed significantly toward identification and investigation of key proteins and metabolites to monitor the pathophysiological status of the host, but have also assisted in customizing effective individualized therapies to treat several diseases (Zhang *et al.*, 2015). Moreover, proteomic and metabolomic intervention to understand biological systems at the molecular level will usher in the development of advance disease diagnostic tools and effective therapeutics in "personalized medicine" for precise treatment (Nicholson, 2006). The current chapter will highlight various platforms and the significant role of proteomics and metabolomics in the diagnosis of different diseases.

7.2 Basic Strategies and Platforms of Proteomics and Metabolomics

Proteomic and metabolomic introspection approaches function through the identification of a problem, followed by undertaking an effective experimental design to unmask the aberrations at the molecular level, then finding potential solutions toward effective therapeutic intervention. The real task begins after specimen collection and preparation. Collection of an appropriate sample related to the identified problem is a pre-requisite for ultimately achieving fruitful results. Preparation of a pure and uncontaminated sample with adequate analyte concentration is the most crucial and key step for further downstream processing. The quality of data acquired from proteomics and metabolomics analysis is absolutely dependent on proper sample preparation, achieving adequate analyte concentration and maintaining sufficient purity. Methods of sample preparation depend on various factors, such as source, type, location, complexity, abundance and physical properties. Therefore, while there is no gold-standard method of sample preparation, the basic principle is that all the methods are designed to obtain a pure sample with ample concentration along with preventing analyte degradation as much as possible prior to sample analysis.

7.2.1 Biological Specimens for Proteomics and Metabolomics

Any biological system containing protein, such as animal/human tissue, cells, biological fluids (plasma, serum, urine, cerebrospinal fluid, saliva, milk, synovial fluid, seminal plasma, cervical-vaginal fluid, amniotic or allantoic fluid, nasal secretions, bronco-alveolar lavage fluid, tear, vitreous humor, aqueous humor), cancer tissue, stools, bacteriological samples, viral samples etc. can be used for proteomics studies (Catinella *et al.*, 1996; Aldred *et al.*, 2004; Bodzon-Kulakowska *et al.*, 2007; Hanash and Taguchi, 2011; Rodríguez-Suárez *et al.*, 2014; Licier *et al.*, 2016; Castagnola *et al.*, 2017; Camargo *et al.*, 2018; Peffers *et al.*, 2019). Moreover, proteomics analyses are also reported from *in-vitro*-cultured cells, media and cultured embryos (Katz-Jaffe *et al.*, 2006; Geiger *et al.*, 2012; Sinha *et al.*, 2017). However, in clinical proteomics, for biomarker discovery to aid in disease diagnosis, plasma or serum is the choice of sample due to the ease of accessibility (Aldred *et al.*, 2004). Unlike plasma, collection of other samples such as cerebrospinal fluid, synovial fluid, and cancer or other tissues is more invasive in nature and requires special care and skilled personnel (Aldred *et al.*, 2004; Peffers *et al.*, 2019). Depending on disease conditions, saliva and urine specimens are also gaining popularity in clinical proteomics because both can be collected easily, safely and non-invasively (Beeley and Khoo, 1999; Wittke *et al.*, 2003; Bodzon-Kulakowska *et al.*, 2007; Rodríguez-Suárez *et al.*, 2014; Castagnola *et al.*, 2017).

Like proteomics, the most commonly used biofluids for disease diagnosis by metabolomics-based studies are urine and plasma or serum because both can be obtained without or with minimal invasion, respectively, and contain hundreds to thousands of detectable metabolites (Gowda *et al.*, 2008). Moreover, urine contains a low abundance of proteins and high concentrations of low-molecular-weight metabolites which make it easier to produce a pure sample. High-quality metabolomics data can be extrapolated from urine samples through NMR; however, high salt content hinders urinary metabolomic data acquisition through MS, requiring adequate desalting during sample preparation (Gowda *et al.*, 2008). Cerebrospinal fluid, saliva, seminal fluid, amniotic and allantoic fluid, synovial fluid, gut aspirate and bile are other important biological fluids used for metabolomics analysis (Bollard *et al.*, 2005; Bala *et al.*, 2006; Nagana *et al.*, 2006). Specimens such as tissue, cells, lipids and aqueous metabolite extracts are also important for metabolomics-based biomarker discovery (Griffin and Kauppinen, 2007).

Serum or plasma is the most extensively used biological sample, followed by urine, for disease diagnosis and biomarker detection in proteomics and metabolomics platforms. As blood bathes every organ and tissue, thus it contains numerous disease-specific biomarkers released by the tissue. So it has the potential to provide a global view regarding the pathophysiological condition of the host (Aldred *et al.*, 2004; Gowda *et al.*, 2008).

7.2.2 Proteomics Workflow

Currently, the bulk of proteomics introspection broadly follows two approaches: two-dimensional gel electrophoresis coupled with MS (2-DE-MS), and liquid chromatography or capillary electrophoresis coupled with MS (LC-MS or CE-MS) (Figure 7.1). Another approach involves direct sampling and proteomic analysis using mass spectrometry imaging (MSI), which has gained importance in recent times as it facilitates even live single-cell analysis with ultra-low sample requirements and provides enormous

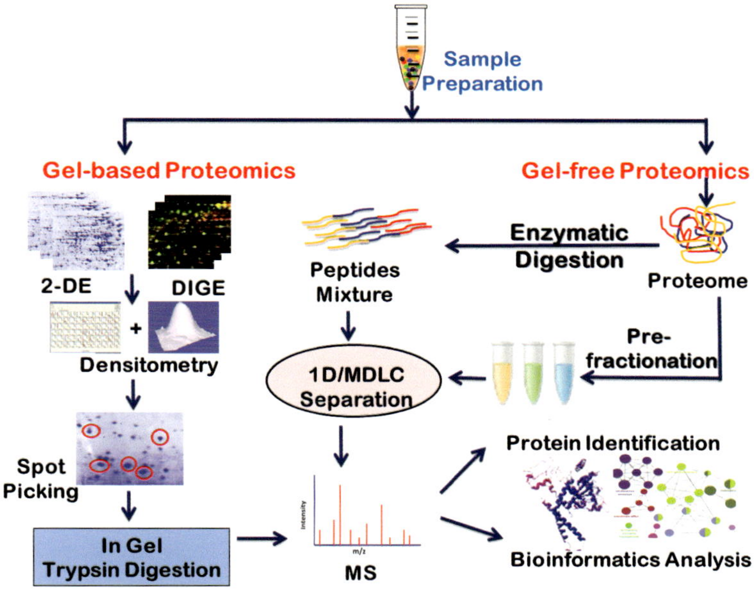

FIGURE 7.1 An overview of a proteomics workflow.

sensitivity (Minakshi *et al.*, 2019b). In the 2-DE-MS approach, complex protein samples are introspected following separation in polyacrylamide gel based on the isoelectric point (pI) and molecular weight of proteins, visualization of protein spots by Coomassie blue or silver staining, densitometry analysis of protein spots followed by enzymatic (trypsin) digestion and finally identification and characterization by MS and other supporting bioinformatics and statistical tools. An initial report of protein identification by 2-DE was published in 1993 (Henzel *et al.*, 1993) and this study actually started the dissemination of proteomics analysis by integrating two-dimension gel electrophoresis and MS, now popularly known as "classical proteomics" (Hixson *et al.*, 2017). The unique characteristic of this method is that thousands of proteins from a complex mixture can be separated with high resolution as individual protein spots. Other advantages are identification of unknown proteins and detection of post-translational modifications (PTMs) of proteins. However, it suffers from low reproducibility and coverage and is a resource-intensive as well as time-consuming method. However, sensitivity was amplified manyfold by introducing fluorescent agents such as CyDye (Cy2, 3 and 5) for labeling samples; this modification is described as differential in-gel electrophoresis (DIGE). Moreover, DIGE reduces gel-to-gel variations and time, and a single gel can be used to resolve control and treated samples by labeling with different fluorescent dyes (Ahmad *et al.*, 2014; Hixson *et al.*, 2017).

The approach of liquid chromatography coupled with MS (LC-MS) is also known as gel-free proteomics, where there is no requirement for polyacrylamide gel electrophoresis. It can further categorize into top-down and bottom-up approaches. Out of these, the bottom-up approach is the most extensively used, and is the method of choice particularly for unknown protein identification; it is also known as "shotgun proteomics". In the bottom-up approach, after sample extraction and preparation, proteins are cleaved to peptides by enzymatic digestion. This is followed by multidimensional LC (MDLC) separation and characterization by tandem MS (MS/MS) along with protein identification using computational and statistical programs (Chait, 2006; Chiou and Wu, 2011; Feist and Hummon, 2015; Hixson *et al.*, 2017). The concept of multidimensional protein separation and identification by LC-MS is also known as multidimensional protein identification technology (MudPIT), which was reported in 1999 (Link *et al.*, 1999). It has revolutionized the execution of high-throughput proteomics to a next level. The top-down approach is devoid of an enzymatic digestion step; instead, whole proteins are ionized directly and subjected to gas-phase fragmentation for MS analysis (Kelleher, 2004; Chait, 2006). This method takes better care of protein isoforms and identifying PTMs than a bottom-up approach, but the top-down method holds good only for small-sized proteins of <100,000 Da with 100% sequence coverage (Sze *et al.*, 2002; Chiou and Wu, 2011; Hixson *et al.*, 2017). To overcome the demerits of top-down and bottom-up approaches, a hybrid approach has been introduced known as middle-down proteomics, which is a combination of bottom-up and top-down proteomics (Zhang *et al.*, 2013). Overall, LC-MS techniques have the ability to identify thousands of known and unknown proteins in one go; moreover, they have improved separation efficiency over 2-DE along with better coverage (Ahmad *et al.*, 2014). The LC-MS approach is robust and regarded as a proteomic workhorse (Jungblut, 2012).

Besides these, there are also many other proteomics techniques used for diagnostic purposes which are either matured or their in nascent stages, such as reverse phase protein array, antibody array, bead-based array and protein microarray. In diagnostic applications these are more specific and some are more sensitive but most of them are dependent on antibodies and have the ability to detect fewer than 100 proteins per run/assay, with the exception of protein microarray (Ahmad *et al.*, 2014).

7.2.3 Quantitative Proteomics

Quantitative proteomics is a relatively new introduction in proteomics that has emerged as a very promising technology. It allows both absolute as well as relative quantification of proteins in given sample(s). Absolute quantitation measures the actual concentration of the protein/peptide in the target sample. It is used for biomarker validation and preference is given when the peptides/proteins of interest are few in number and already known. Relative quantification is applied when the goal of a study is to compare a global proteome between two or more biological samples or to identify differentially expressed proteins on the basis of protein/peptide concentrations. Currently, two approaches are predominantly employed for quantitative proteomics, namely label-based or label-free quantitative proteomics (Chiou and Wu, 2011; Hixson *et al.*, 2017).

In label-based quantitative proteomic techniques, stable isotopes such as isotopic coded affinity tags (ICAT), isobaric tags for relative and absolute quantitation (iTRAQ) and stable isotope labeling amino acids in cell culture (SILAC) are most commonly employed for proteome analysis. ICAT is a thiol-specific reagent that is used to label cysteine residues of proteins for quantitation prior to enzymatic digestion and MS analysis. It is used to determine the relative protein concentration between two samples (Gygi *et al.*, 1999). Amines of lysine residues and the N-terminus of peptides are covalently labeled with the reacting group of iTRAQ. In iTRAQ-based experiments, quantitation can be either absolute or relative and multiplexing can be done up to four-plex or eight-plex. In this method peptides are labeled after digestion of proteins prior to LC-MS analysis (Ross *et al.*, 2004; Zhang *et al.*, 2017). SILAC is an *in-vivo* labeling proteomics technique usually employed for comparative proteome analyses of two cultured cell populations. For quantitation by SILAC, one population of cell is fed with amino acids labeled with stable isotopes, whereas a second cell population is supplied with normal non-labeled amino acids. Therefore, proteins/peptides extracted from a cell population with metabolically incorporated labeled amino acids will be heavier than another (normal) one and this property is utilized for quantitation and analysis by MS (Ong *et al.*, 2002). Although labeling-based proteomic approaches have gained attention in recent times, several inherent challenges, such as limited multiplexing, the expense of chemicals or kits etc., need to be overcome in the near future.

Label-free quantitative proteomics excludes any labeling agents; instead, quantitation is performed based on peptide ion intensity counting and spectral counting. Unlike a labeling-based approach, the chances of sample contamination during the labeling step are limited in label-free proteomics. A simple sample preparation protocol, the detection of a relatively large abundance of changes, greater flexibility for comparative analysis and time savings are some of the advantages of label-free quantitation. Still, intensity-based quantitation is not as precise as stable isotope-labeling approaches and it is heavily dependent on bioinformatics and statistical tools (Chiou and Wu, 2011; Hixson *et al.*, 2017).

7.2.4 Proteomics Analytical Platforms

In 1988, a report of protein identification using MS revolutionized the field of proteomics (Tanaka *et al.*, 1988). Now, MS, either alone or in combination with other separation modalities, has taken the centerstage as the most important analytical platform in the bulk of proteomics investigations. MS is a robust, sensitive and versatile analytical modality which can be employed according to the requirement for targeted as well as untargeted proteomics and qualitative as well as quantitative analysis of proteins present in diverse samples. Protein samples are first ionized, followed by their separation in a mass analyzer based on mass-to-charge ratios (m/z) of the derived ions. Progress in instrumentation has yielded variable types of mass analyzers with diverse specifications and applications in proteomics, such as time-of-flight (TOF) analyzers, ion traps, triple-quadrupoles (QqQ), q-TOF, TOF-TOF and ion traps coupled with Orbitrap mass spectrometers or Fourier transform ion cyclotron resonance mass analyzers. The results are depicted as a mass spectrum with different intensity and identification of proteins is done by using bioinformatics software and a search database like Mascot or Sequest etc. (Chiou and Wu, 2011; Hixson *et al.*, 2017). The most common ionization platforms for MS-based proteomics analyses are matrix-assisted laser desorption/ionization (MALDI) and electrospray ionization (ESI). The application of MALDI with a time-of-flight (TOF) MS for measurement of proteins masses was pioneered by Karas and Hillenkamp (1988). Simultaneously, for soft ionization of proteins, Fenn and co-workers developed another modality known as electrospray ionization (ESI)-MS (Wong *et al.*, 1988). Both MALDI and ESI are tools of choice in the field of proteomics, for which in 2002 John Bennett Fenn and Koichi Tanaka shared the coveted Nobel Prize in Chemistry. Some of the merits and limitations of MALDI and ESI MS in proteomics studies are delineated in Table 7.1.

Surface-enhanced laser desorption/ionization (SELDI) is a modification of MALDI with a protein chip facility enabling high-throughput analysis of multiple protein samples (Hutchens and Yip, 1993). SELDI is optimized for protein expression analysis (protein profiling) and biomarker discovery (Semmes *et al.*, 2005; El Aneed and Banoub, 2006; Bodzon-Kulakowska *et al.*, 2007). Another advantage of SELDI is that crude samples can be analyzed directly as it has the ability to remove salts and other impurities prior to MS analysis (Bodzon-Kulakowska *et al.*, 2007). Desorption electrospray ionization (DESI) is a modified version of ESI, having the capacity to analyze samples in its native form, and can be used for molecular imaging, although resolution is still better in MALDI (Takats *et al.*, 2004; Cooks *et al.*, 2006; Chen, 2008).

7.2.5 Metabolomics Workflow

Metabolomics introspection can be carried out by different approaches, untargeted and targeted metabolomics, depending on the goal of an experiment (Patti *et al.*, 2012). Untargeted metabolomics is a global approach that performs exhaustive metabolite profiling intended to characterize as many metabolites as possible from biological specimens without any partiality. In untargeted metabolomics, metabolomes of two contrasting groups (control and treated) are identified and compared to find the differences between their metabolite profiles which may be relevant to specific biological conditions (disease). Typical workflow of untargeted metabolomics begins with sample preparation, i.e., isolation of metabolites from the biological system. Subsequently, metabolites are detected, identified and

TABLE 7.1

Characteristics of MS platforms used in proteomics studies

Platform	Advantages	Limitations	Reference(s)
ESI-MS	1. Greater accuracy 2. Can be interfaced online	1. More maintenance is required 2. More prone to contamination	Hirsch *et al.* (2004)
MALDI-MS	1. Resilience to salts, buffers and other compounds often used in protein sample preparation 2. MALDI-TOF is highly sensitive with a wide mass range 3. Spectra are relatively easy to interpret	1. Peptides can be less informative 2. Samples must be spotted on metal targets and dried	

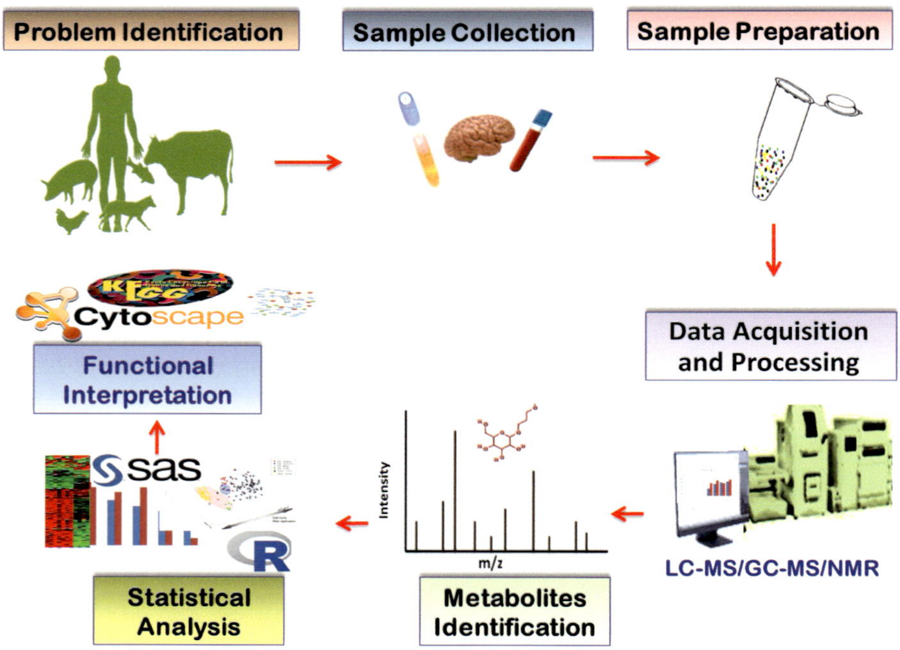

FIGURE 7.2 A simplified outlook of a metabolomics workflow.

characterized through data acquisition, processing and analysis using a suitable analytical platform such as NMR, CE/LC/GC-MS, fluorescence-based methods or MSI using bioinformatics programs and databases such as XCMS (Smith *et al.*, 2006), Pubchem, Metabolights, KEGG, METLIN (Smith *et al.*, 2005), Chemspider, Massbank, MetaboAnalyst, LIPID MAPS, MS-Dial etc. (Minakshi *et al.*, 2019a) (Figure 7.2). Statistical analysis can be performed by principal component analysis (PCA), analysis of variance (ANOVA) etc. for putative biomarker(s) identification and quantitation, which is further validated for its significance to a particular cellular process or metabolic pathway (Gowda *et al.*, 2008; Patti *et al.*, 2012). An untargeted metabolomics approach can also be broadly divided into three steps: metabolite profiling, compound identification and functional interpretation. Profiling includes sample preparation and identifications of differential expressed metabolites, i.e., metabolites with statistically significant variations between samples. Compound identification involves identification and annotation of discovered metabolites in the profiling step by searching against metabolomic databases such as METLIN, mzCloud, HMDB etc. Metabolite identification is followed by interpretation, the final step, which aims to connect the significant metabolites with crucial pathophysiological processes or pathways (Patti *et al.*, 2012). It is important to validate any putative biomarker discovered from metabolomics studies by clinical trials or field studies (Gowda *et al.*, 2008).

A targeted metabolomics approach refers to verification and validation of specified known metabolites, typically focusing their involvement on one or more selected pathways (Dudley *et al.*, 2010). This approach is more effective in pharmacokinetic studies of drug metabolism, determining the influence of therapeutics or genetic modifications induced by a specific enzyme (Nicholson *et al.*, 2002). A high-resolution accurate mass (HRAM) workflow is optimal for large-scale targeted profiling; selected reaction monitoring (SRM) on a triple-quadrupole MS is preferred for routine quantitation. Targeted metabolomics is quantitative and intended to test a hypothesis for known or targeted metabolites information extracted from literature, discovery experiments and/or clinical observations. Typical targeted metabolomics starts with sample preparation for the extraction of specific metabolites followed by metabolite validation and quantitation through data acquisition in analytical platforms like NMR or MS. The acquired data is processed and finally interpretation is done using a specialized program and bioinformatics tools.

Validation of features exhibited by the analyzed metabolite(s) is a pre-requisite to mark their precise role in a complex biological metabolic network (Nalbantoglu, 2019).

7.2.6 Metabolomics Analytical Platforms

The most predominant analytical platforms used in metabolomics are nuclear magnetic resonance (NMR) spectroscopy and mass spectrometry (MS). Of these, different MS modalities, including liquid chromatography-MS (LC-MS) and gas chromatography-MS (GC-MS), are the mainstay of current metabolomics analyses (Shao and Le, 2019). Merits and limitations of metabolomics analytical platforms are highlighted in Table 7.2. Hyphenated LC-MS-NMR is penetrating the field of metabolomics because of its high spectral resolution and great metabolite identification capabilities (Walker *et al.*, 2016).

NMR is a robust tool used in metabolomics studies of various biological samples. Either one-dimensional or two-dimensional NMR methods can be used for metabolomics applications. The most commonly used NMR method for metabolome analysis is a one-dimensional nuclear Overhauser enhancement spectroscopy (NOESY) sequence with water suppression, because of its robustness and its provision of a flatter baseline. Advanced two-dimensional (2D) NMR techniques, including 2D-J spectroscopy, correlation spectroscopy (COSY), total correlation spectroscopy (TOCSY) and heteronuclear single quantum coherence (HSQC) spectroscopy are also gaining in importance in metabolomics studies. The excellent attributes of NMR include, but are not limited to, easy sample preparation and its brief analysis time, robust signal and absolute metabolite quantification. However, low-abundance metabolites can be missed due to the relatively low sensitivity of NMR. Moreover, thousands of metabolite signals are overlapped due to the absence of any prior separation system, which also makes precise structure identification of metabolites a tricky task. Nonetheless, state-of-the-art technological advancements have curtailed these demerits to a great extent, along with upgrades to the sensitivity and resolution of NMR techniques (Gowda *et al.*, 2008; Shao and Le, 2019).

MS is the other platform which is arguably the most widely used modality in metabolomics-based studies because of its better sensitivity, high throughput and its ability to detect a wide array of metabolites from complex biological specimens. MS is usually coupled with prior separation modalities such as LC, GC or capillary electrophoresis (CE). Various mass analyzers commonly used in MS are ion traps, quadrupoles, triple-quads and time-of-flight. In MS, to validate the identity of unknown molecules, tandem MS (MS/

TABLE 7.2

Merits and demerits of metabolomics platforms

Platforms	Merits	Demerits	Reference(s)
NMR	1. Minimum sample preparation 2. Fast sample analysis 3. High reproducibility 4. Rigorous structural analysis of many metabolites 5. Non-destructive and non-invasive	1. Poor sensitivity 2. Signal overlapping 3. Fewer than 100 metabolites can be detected 4. Analysis of organic layer of cell/tissue extract is difficult 5. Expensive and require more space than MS	Gowda *et al.* (2008); Emwas *et al.* (2013); Trushina and Mielke (2014); Shao and Le (2019)
MS	1. More sensitivity than NMR 2. More than 1000 metabolites can be identified in single experiment 3. Potential to analyze any biological sample 4. Less expensive and lower space requirement than NMR	1. Analysis of large molecules and isomers is difficult 2. Lower reproducibility 3. Sample analysis and preparation is time-consuming 4. GC-MS can analyze only volatile metabolites	

MS or even MS^n) methods are employed (Gowda *et al.*, 2008; Shao and Le, 2019; Zhang *et al.*, 2020). By using Fourier-transform ion cyclotron resonance (FT-ICR) and Orbitrap mass analyzers, high resolution and a better mass accuracy can be achieved (Brown *et al.*, 2005; Zhang *et al.*, 2007).

The advantages of GC-MS in metabolomics include, but are not limited to, better separation efficiency, easy operation, relative inexpense, better reproducibility and stability. GC-MS can be employed to analyze volatile metabolites or they can be made volatile by derivatization and thermally stable metabolites. LC-MS is also one of the most popular analytical platforms in metabolomics investigations due to its high sensitivity and the plethora of information provided by the platform regarding diverse metabolites. After achieving adequate concentration, certain biofluids like urine can be directly introduced into the LC system. Separation techniques employed in LC-MS are reverse-phase liquid chromatography (RPLC), high-performance liquid chromatography (HPLC), hydrophilic interaction liquid chromatography (HILIC) etc. Multidimensional LC has emerged as an efficient analytical tool as it can simultaneously analyze metabolome and lipidome in a single run (Gowda *et al.*, 2008; Shao and Le, 2019).

7.3 Proteomics in Animal Disease Diagnosis and Biomarker Discovery

There are numerous proteomics-based documents related to biomarker discovery, disease diagnosis and pathogen identification (Table 7.3). Proteomics not only provides a platform for diagnosis by identifying promising biomarker(s) related to a disease but also aids in identifying targets for drug development and vaccine candidates. Most of the studies are conducted in human diseases, with a special emphasis on cancer for biomarker detection. Laboratory animals, especially rodents, are also in ample use for proteomics-based disease-specific biomarker discovery. Simultaneously, it is also gaining attention in animal science—particularly farm animal health, disease and production—without the exception of pet animals, especially dogs and cats.

7.3.1 Proteomics Biomarkers in Infectious Disease of Farm Animals

Numerous reports of classical proteomic intervention in animals pertaining to infectious diseases are now appearing on a routine basis. One of the most studied animal pathologies through a proteomics approach is mastitis. Apolipoprotein A-I (apo A-I), heat shock 70kD protein, cathelicidin-I and the acute-phase protein serum amyloid A (SAA) were identified in milk samples of cows suffering from mastitis (Smolenski *et al.*, 2007). In a proteomic investigation, another acute-phase protein (APP), α-1-acid-glycoprotein, was identified in mastitis whey samples of cows which were experimentally inoculated with *E. coli* (Boehmer *et al.*, 2008). Similarly, serum proteomics experiments in cows with subclinical mastitis showed differential expression of serpin A3-1, complement factor H proteins and vitronectin-like protein, whereas inter-alpha-trypsin inhibitor heavy chain H4, C4b-binding protein alpha chain, serpin A3-1, apolipoprotein A-I and haptoglobin were differentially expressed in cows with clinical mastitis in comparison to the control animals. But vitronectin was found to be over-expressed in subclinical as well as clinical mastitis (Turk *et al.*, 2012). Over 500 proteins were differentially expressed in the milk of cows with induced mastitis by inoculation with *Streptococcus uberis*. Out of all, the most significantly upregulated proteins were cathelicidins and peptidoglycan recognition protein 1, with other acute-phase proteins being the most over-expressed (Mudaliar *et al.*, 2016). A similar type of introspection was also carried out in other ruminants such as sheep and goats. Core and accessory seroproteome was explored from a serum of mastitis ewes induced by different *S. aureus* strains (Le Maréchal *et al.*, 2009; Le Maréchal *et al.*, 2011). Milk samples collected from ovine clinical mastitis cases showed several differentially expressed proteins (Chiaradia *et al.*, 2013). Twenty-four and 34 differentially expressed proteins in blood and milk, respectively, were identified by Katsafadou *et al.* (2015) in ewes suffering from experimental mastitis caused by *Mannheimia haemolytica*.

Applying 2-DE and LC-MS/MS, Kycko and Reichert (2008, 2012) have detected over-expression of aldolase A, cytokeratin 19 and manganese superoxide dismutase in lung tissue samples of ovine respiratory adenomatosis, caused by Jaagsiekte sheep retrovirus. The molecular pathogenesis of prion diseases of ruminants was investigated using a proteomics approach to identify relevant biomarkers for early diagnosis and customize suitable control strategies (Chich *et al.*, 2007; Batxelli-Molina *et al.*, 2010; Ma and Li, 2012). Proteins such as clusterin, cathelicidin, Ig gamma-2 chain C region, uroguanylin and protease-resistant prion (infectious agent) isoform were depicted as urinary diagnostic biomarkers of bovine spongiform encephalopathy (Shaked *et al.*, 2001; Simon *et al.*, 2008; Ma and Li, 2012). Many unique antimicrobial peptides, acute-phase proteins, complement factors, protease inhibitors and molecules involved in redox reactions were detected by using proteomics tools from bronchoalveolar lavage samples of animals with experimental *Mannheimia haemolytica* infection (Boehmer *et al.*, 2011). By combining chromatographic techniques and MS/MS, transthyretin and α-haemoglobin were identified as two crucial biomarkers from the serum samples of sheep exposed to *M. paratuberculosis* subsp. *avium*. (Zhong *et al.*, 2011). Hughes *et al.* (2013) have proposed that differentially present proteins in the serum of sheep could be used as prospective tools for the precise diagnosis of subclinical paratuberculosis. Shotgun proteomics was used to identify potential footrot-associated proteins present in the plasma of cattle, out of which peptidoglycan recognition protein L and keratansulfate proteoglycan were ascribed to be potential biomarkers (Sun *et al.*, 2013).

Proteomics methodologies were used to understand and identify several viral diseases of swine, such as classical swine fever (CSF), porcine reproductive and respiratory syndrome, foot-and-mouth disease and porcine circovirus infection (Ceciliani *et al.*, 2014). Interaction of *Salmonella typhimurium* and the pig immune system was also investigated by a proteomics approach (Martins *et al.*, 2012). In equine, putative proteomics biomarkers were identified for chronic equine laminitis, and osteoarthritis/osteochondritis in serum and synovial fluid samples, respectively (Chiaradia *et al.*, 2012; Steelman and Chowdhary, 2012). Moreover, to detect doping in game horses, equine plasma proteins were analyzed by multiplexed LC-MS/MS (Barton *et al.*, 2009). A retinal proteome of horses was analyzed to differentiate normal and uvetic conditions. Glial fibrillary acidic protein was found to be up-regulated, whereas pigment epithelium-derived factor and glutamine synthase were reported to be down-regulated in uvetic retina (Deeg *et al.*, 2007). In fowl typhoid, four proteins (fatty acid binding protein, MRP-126, ribosomal protein12 and pyruvate kinase) were found to be altered during proteomic analysis of spleen lymphocytes (So *et al.*, 2009). Proteomics profiling of lung tissue was performed in chickens infected with Newcastle disease virus (Saelao *et al.*, 2018).

7.3.2 Proteomics Biomarkers in Non-infectious Disease of Farm Animals

Proteomic profiling for various skeletal muscle disorders was performed in animal models to discover new reliable biomarkers so that clinical investigation procedures can be optimized for the development of early diagnostics (Doran *et al.*, 2007). Pigs are one of the best models to understand metabolic diseases of humans due to several physiological similarities between pigs and humans; thus, it can be anticipated that disease-specific biomarkers identified in pigs may hold equal potential for diagnosis of human metabolic disorders too. Plasma proteome profiling of pigs leads to the identification of molecular signatures for diet-induced metabolic syndrome, including diabetes biomarkers (te Pas *et al.*, 2013). Different pig models were successfully employed to study highly prevalent human diseases such as diabetes, metabolic syndrome, obesity and cardiovascular diseases for identification of potential biomarkers to be used as diagnostic tool (Bassols *et al.*, 2014). Moreover, pig models are also used to investigate neurodegenerative diseases and brain disorders, including Alzheimer's disease, Parkinson's disease, Huntington's disease and other stress-related disorders (Bassols *et al.*, 2014).

A key cytosolic protein, "ubiquitin C-terminal hydrolase", was revealed when heart muscle proteome was characterized from Simmental Red Holstein crossbred cattle having dilated cardiomyopathy (Weekes *et al.*, 1999). During ketosis, several differentially expressed protein spots were detected in 2-DE analysis of liver between ketotic and normal cows (Xu and Wang, 2008; Xu *et al.*, 2008). In urine samples of cows, differential expression of several proteins such as amyloid precursor protein, serum amyloid A (SAA), VGF (non-acronymic) protein, fibrinogen, C1INH, apolipoprotein C-III, human neutrophil peptides, cystatin C, hepcidin, transthyretin, and osteopontin were elucidated between ketosis and control groups (Xu *et al.*, 2015). Twelve distinctive proteins linked with clinical laminitis in cows were identified and found to be involved in lipid metabolism, carbohydrate metabolism, immune regulation, molecular transport, oxidative stress and inflammatory response (Dong *et al.*, 2015).

7.3.3 Proteomics in Parasitic Disease of Animals

Animals are very much prone to parasitic diseases. Analysis of the bile proteome of sheep infested with fluke indicated six possible protein biomarkers of the cathepsin L protease family (Morphew *et al.*, 2007). *Haemoncus contortus* is a common parasite of sheep. About 150 differentially existing proteins were found in abomasal mucosa between resistant and susceptible sheep. Proteins like galectin-4, trefoil factor-2, DAG and fibrillin-2 were associated with resistant sheep (Nagaraj *et al.*, 2012). Galectin-15 and a few other proteins were observed to be associated with *Teladorsagia circumcincta*-resistant sheep (Athanasiadou *et al.*, 2008; Pemberton *et al.*, 2012).

7.4 Proteomics in Companion Animal Disease Biomarker Discovery

There are many similarities in pathophysiology and clinical responses to therapy between canines and humans. Dogs are of enormous importance in understanding pathophysiological characteristics of human cancer, as they share many common malignancies with humans. Several proteins, such as prolidase, glutathione S-transferase, triosephosphate isomerase and macrophage capping protein, were altered in lymph nodes between dogs with lymphoma and healthy ones (McCaw *et al.*, 2007). Many potential proteins are also identified in sera of dogs with B-cell lymphoma, although further investigation is required for confirmation (Gaines *et al.*, 2007). Proteomic introspection was also carried out to detect protein biomarkers in canine prostate and bladder carcinomas (Leroy *et al.*, 2007). Many proteomics studies were also undertaken to screen biomarkers of canine mammary carcinomas. Mammary tumor stage-specific differential-expressed proteins were also recognized by proteomics intervention (Klopfleisch *et al.*, 2010; Klose *et al.*, 2011).

Proteomics methodologies were also applied to ascertain candidate proteins involved in other diseases, such as Alzheimer's disease, myxomatous mitral valve disease and inherited lethal acrodermatitis (Ceciliani *et al.*, 2014). In canine idiopathic dilated cardiomyopathy (iDCM), signature heart tissue remodeling markers were revealed in the serum proteome of dogs. The identified potential biomarkers of iDCM were inter-alpha-trypsin inhibitor heavy chain H4, apolipoprotein A-IV and microfibril-associated glycoprotein-4 (Bilić*et al.*, 2018). A gel-based proteomics approach was employed for finding signature proteins associated with canine babesiosis (Kuleš *et al.*, 2016). Many altered proteins were also identified in brain spinal tissues of dogs infected with rabies (Thanomsridetchai *et al.*, 2011).

Like canine models, feline models have also been used to study many human diseases, such as type-2 diabetes mellitus, inherited muscular dystrophies and cardiac disorders (Bilić *et al.*, 2018). Urine fibronectin can be used to differentiate cats with idiopathic cystitis (IdC) from healthy ones as fibronectin content increases significantly in urine of cats with IdC (Lemberger *et al.*, 2011). A few proteins such as alpha-1-acid glycoprotein, apolipoprotein-A1 precursor and apolipoprotein-A1 appeared to be differentially expressed in plasma proteomes of cats suffering from pancreatic diseases such as pancreatitis and pancreatic carcinoma (Meachem *et al.*, 2015).

Proteomics not only holds diagnostic importance for pathological status in animals, but also in other physiological diagnosis, such as pregnancy diagnosis in animals. For instance, 2-DE along with MS has been successfully employed for the identification of serum proteomic biomarkers of early pregnancy in buffaloes. Anti-testosterone antibody light chain, serum amyloid A, apolipoprotein A-II precursor, cytokeratin type-II and component-IV isoform-1 are some of the pregnancy-associated up-regulated proteins which in combination can serve in early pregnancy detection (Buragohain *et al.*, 2017).

7.5 Metabolomics in Animal Disease Diagnosis

Metabolomics-based studies for farm animal diseases are still in progressive mode, although significant success has been achieved in recent times (Table 7.3). Moreover, animal models are frequently used for metabolomics studies of several diseases which are also encountered in humans. However, a good number of metabolomics literatures are currently available pertaining to evaluation and biomarker detection in

TABLE 7.3

Application of proteomics and metabolomics in animal disease diagnosis

Disease	Species	Platform Used	Differentially Regulated Proteins/Metabolites	Reference
			Proteomics	
Mastitis	Cattle	2DE, LC-MS/MS	Apolipoprotein A-I (apo A-I), cathelicidin-I, heat shock 70kD etc.	Smolenski *et al.* (2007)
Mastitis	Cattle	2DE + MALDI-TOF-TOF	α-1-acid-glycoprotein, transthyretin, lactadherin, β-2-microglobulin precursor, complement C3, β-fibrinogen, α-2-HS-glycoprotein, and α-1-antiproteinase	Boehmer *et al.* (2008)
Mastitis	Cattle	2DE + MALDI-TOF-TOF	Serpin A3-1, vitronectin-like protein, complement factor H, inter-alpha-trypsin inhibitor heavy chain H4, serpin A3-1, C4b-binding protein alpha chain, haptoglobin and apolipoprotein A-I	Turk *et al.* (2012)
Mastitis	Cattle	LC-MS/MS	Cathelicidins, peptidoglycan recognition protein 1, and other acute phase proteins	Mudaliar *et al.* (2016)
Ovine pulmonary adenocarcinoma	Sheep	2DE, LC-MS/MS	Cytokeratin 19 and aldolase A	Kycko and Reichert (2012)
Bovine spongiform encephalopathy	Cattle	2DE, LC-MS/MS	Clusterin, cathelicidin, Ig gamma-2 chain C region, uroguanylin etc.	Simon *et al.* (2008)
Mannheimia haemolytica infection	Cattle	nanoLC-MS/MS	Antimicrobial peptides, complement factors, acute-phase proteins, protease inhibitors	Boehmer *et al.* (2011)
Johne's disease	Sheep	SELDI TOF-MS	Transthyretin and α-haemoglobin	Zhong *et al.* (2011)
Foot rot	Cattle	LC-MS/MS	Peptidoglycan recognition protein L and keratin sulfate proteoglycan	Sun *et al.* (2013)
Uvetic retina	Horse	2DE + MALDI-TOF-TOF	Glial fibrillary acidic protein, pigment epithelium-derived factor and glutamine synthase	Deeg *et al.* (2007)
Fowl typhoid	Chicken	2DE + MALDI-TOF-TOF	Fatty acid binding protein, MRP-126, ribosomal protein12 and pyruvate kinase	So *et al.* (2009)
Dilated cardiomyopathy	Cattle	2DE, MALDI-MS	Ubiquitin C-terminal hydrolase	Weekes *et al.* (1999)
Ketosis	Cattle	SELDI-TOF-MS	Amyloid precursor protein, serum amyloid A (SAA), VGF (non-acronymic) protein, fibrinogen, C1INH, apolipoprotein C-III, human neutrophil peptides, cystatin C, hepcidin, transthyretin, and osteopontin	Xu *et al.* (2015)
Haemoncus contortus infestation	Sheep	iTRAQ + LC-MS/MS	Galectin-4, trefoil factor 2, DAG and fibrillin-2 were associated with resistance	Nagaraj *et al.* (2012).
Lymphoma	Dog	2DE, MALDI-MS	Prolidase, triosephosphate isomerase, glutathione S-transferase and macrophage capping protein	McCaw *et al.* (2007)

(*continued*)

TABLE 7.3

Application of proteomics and metabolomics in animal disease diagnosis (Cont.)

Disease	Species	Platform Used	Differentially Regulated Proteins/Metabolites	Reference
Idiopathic dilated cardiomyopathy	Dog	TMT, LC-MS/MS	Inter-alpha-trypsin inhibitor heavy chain H4, microfibril-associated glycoprotein 4 and apolipoprotein A-IV	Bilić *et al.* (2018)
Idiopathic cystitis	Cat	SDS-PAGE, MS, western blotting	Urine fibronectin	Lemberger *et al.* (2011)
Pancreatitis and pancreatic carcinoma	Cat	2DE, nano HPLC-MS/MS	Alpha-1-acid glycoprotein, apolipoprotein-A1, and apolipoprotein-A1 precursor	Meachem *et al.* (2015)
			Metabolomics	
Obesity	Dog	NMR	Taurine	Soder *et al.* (2017)
Obesity	Dog	GC +LC-MS	Plasma phospholipid moieties and faecal volatile fatty acids	Forster *et al.* (2018)
Degenerative mitral valve disease	Dog	GC/LC-MS	γ-glutamylmethionine, oxidized glutathione, asymmetric, dimethylarginine, glucose, hexanoyl-carnitine, lactate, deoxycarnitine etc.	Li *et al.* (2015)
Acute diarrhea	Dog	GC/MS, UPLC/MS and HPLC/MS	Kynurenic acid, 2-methyl-1H-indole and 5-methoxy-1H-indole-3-carbaldehyde	Guard *et al.* (2015)
Inflammatory bowel disease	Dog	GC-TOF/MS	3-hydroxybutyrate, hexuronic acid, ribose, and gluconic acid lactone	Minamoto *et al.* (2015)
Bladder cancer	Dog	NMR	Urea, choline, methylguanidine, citrate, acetone and β-hydroxybutyrate	Zhang *et al.* (2012)
Lymphoma	Dog	GC-MS	Palmitoleic acid, oleic acid, palmitic acid, glutamic acid, benzoic acid, inositoletc.	Tamai *et al.* (2014)
Muscular dystrophy	Dog	GC-MS	Stearamide, carnosine, fumaric acid, lactamide, myoinositol-2-phosphate, oleic acid, glutamic acid and proline	Abdullah *et al.* (2017)
Gall bladder mucocele formation	Dog	GC/MS &UPLC-MS/MS	1-stearoyl glycerophosphoserine	Gookin *et al.* (2018)
Bovine respiratory disease	Cattle	NMR	Phenylalanine, lactate, hydroxybutyrate, tyrosine, citrate and leucine	Blakebrough-Hall *et al.* (2020)
Displaced abomasum	Cattle	NMR	Serum hippuric acid and glycine	Basoglu *et al.* (2020)
Ketosis	Cattle	GC-MS & LC-MS	Glycochenodeoxycholate, 1-methylimidazoleacetate, 1-nonadecanoylglycerophosphocholine	Shahzad *et al.* (2019)
Retention of placenta	Cattle	RPLC-MS	Serum Lys, Orn, acetylornithine, lysophophatidylcholine Lyso PC a C28:0, Asp, Leu and Ile	Dervishi *et al.* (2018)
Classical swine fever	Pig	UPLC/ESI-Q-TOF/MS	Bilirubin, L-α-hydroxyisovaleric acid, palmitoyl-l-carnitine, linoleic acid, palmitic acid, etc.	Gong *et al.* (2017)
Mycoplasma hyopneumoniae infection	Pig	LC-MS	α-Aminobutyric acid and long-chain fatty acids	Surendran Nair *et al.* (2019)

TABLE 7.3

Application of proteomics and metabolomics in animal disease diagnosis (Cont.)

Disease	Species	Platform Used	Differentially Regulated Proteins/Metabolites	Reference
Scrapie	Sheep	NMR	Alanine, cytosine, creatine, aspartate + N-acetylaspartate, uracil, gamma-aminobutyric acid etc.	Scano *et al.* (2015)
Newcastle disease	Chicken	LC-MS/MS	305 metabolites involved in amino acid and nucleotide metabolic pathway	Liu *et al.* (2019)

metabolic diseases of canines (Table 7.3). Additionally, dogs share a common ecosystem with humans and, therefore, the prevalence of certain lifestyle and metabolic diseases such as obesity, diabetes and cancer can be inter-related between canine and human populations.

7.5.1 Metabolomics in Canine Diseases

The urinary metabolite profile of Labrador Retriever dogs has been effectively exploited to identify metabolites associated with obesity through NMR-based metabolomics. A significant decrease in the concentration of taurine was detected in the urine samples of overweight dogs as compared to lean dogs. So, taurine can be assumed to be a potential biomarker of obesity in the future, although further validation in larger populations is desirable to substantiate the possibility (Soder *et al.*, 2017). Almost 267 compounds which were differentially present in plasma, feces and urine were identified in GC- or LC-MS analysis among normal-weight, overweight or obese dogs. The metabolites linked to overweight or obese dogs were either plasma phospholipid moieties or fecal volatile fatty acids (Forster *et al.*, 2018). Different heart tissues of dogs were introspected to identify potential metabolites pertaining to heart failure conditions (Carlos *et al.*, 2020). A decreased level of glucose and hexanoyl-carnitine and increased level of lactate and deoxycarnitine have been identified to be associated with canine degenerative mitral valve disease (DMVD) through serum metabolomic introspection (Li *et al.*, 2015). In acute diarrhea of dogs, kynurenic acid was found to be reduced in serum, whereas a decreased level of 2-methyl-1H-indole and 5-methoxy-1H-indole-3-carbaldehyde was encountered in urine (Guard *et al.*, 2015). Like in humans, idiopathic inflammatory bowel disease (IBD) is also a common cause of chronic GI disease in dogs. In GC-TOF/MS analysis, an abundance of metabolites such as 3-hydroxybutyrate, ribose, hexuronic acid and gluconic acid lactone has been identified in IBD-affected dogs (Minamoto *et al.*, 2015). Dogs suffering from bladder cancer (TCC) exhibited six biomarkers (urea, choline, methylguanidine, citrate, acetone and β-hydroxybutyrate) with higher urinary concentration than control dogs (Zhang *et al.*, 2012). Another GC-MS-based serum metabolomics analysis of lymphoma in canines revealed palmitoleic acid, oleic acid, palmitic acid and inositol as potential candidate metabolites for lymphoma diagnosis in dogs (Tamai *et al.*, 2014). Serum metabolic analysis of diabetic (diabetes mellitus) dogs revealed a significantly different metabolite profile from healthy dogs and shares considerable similarity with those reported in human type-1 diabetes. Diabetic dogs exhibited significant up-regulation of glycolysis/gluconeogenesis intermediates, whereas significant down-regulation in bile acids and multiple amino acids was observed (O'Kell *et al.*, 2017). Muscular dystrophy is commonly encountered in certain breeds of dogs. An untargeted metabolomics approach was applied to study the metabolite profile of muscle tissues of dogs. Interestingly, eight significantly altered metabolites (stearamide, fumaric acid, carnosine, myoinositol-2-phosphate, lactamide, oleic acid, glutamic acid and proline) have been reported in relation with muscular dystrophy (Abdullah *et al.*, 2017). The bile metabolome of dogs with gall bladder mucocele formation represented a higher concentration of a compound, 1-stearoyl glycerophosphoserine (Gookin *et al.*, 2018).

7.5.2 Metabolomics in Farm Animal Disease Diagnosis

Metabolomics can be regarded as a next-generation diagnostic tool. Although there has been tremendous advancement in the metabolomics tool in the last decade, its use in diagnosis of livestock diseases is still in its infancy. Blakebrough-Hall *et al.* (2020) used an untargeted NMR metabolomics approach to diagnose bovine respiratory disease (BRD) in cattle. Six altered metabolites, including phenylalanine, tyrosine, lactate, hydroxybutyrate, citrate and leucine, were identified in blood as discriminating features between animals having BRD or not. In another study employing GC-MS, four volatile compounds were identified as differentially present in nasal swab samples between BRD and non-BRD, whereas in serum five volatile compounds were present at significantly different levels. The common marker in both types of samples was phenol (Maurer *et al.*, 2018). About 15 metabolites were depicted to be differentially present in the livers of cows showing clinical ketosis (Shahzad *et al.*, 2019). Plasma profiling by a metabolomics approach has the potential to discriminate normal cows from cows with subclinical or clinical ketosis (Zhang *et al.*, 2013; Li *et al.*, 2014; Sun *et al.*, 2014). Serum metabolite fingerprints were identified to predict retained placenta (RP) in cows prior to parturition (Dervishi *et al.*, 2018). A panel of metabolites were suggested by Hailemariam *et al.* (2014) to predict periparturient diseases in cows. Serum metabolites are also depicted to carry enough potential to be employed as diagnostic biomarkers for the detection of metritis in transition dairy cows (Zhang *et al.*, 2017). In a metabolomics experiment, serum hippuric acid and glycine concentrations were documented to be significantly lower in dairy cows with displaced abomasum compared to normal subjects (Basoglu *et al.*, 2020).

Altered serum metabolites associated with classical swine fever were recognized to differentiate the diseased piglets from the healthy ones (Gong *et al.*, 2017). LC-MS analysis of serum can recognize signature metabolites to discriminate between healthy and *Mycoplasma hyopneumoniae*-infected pigs (Surendran Nair *et al.*, 2019). Sheep with caseous lymphadenitis can also be distinguished from normal ones by evaluating the serum metabolome (De Moraes Pontes *et al.*, 2017). A concentration of several metabolites get remodeled in the brain tissue of sheep exhibiting scrapie with or without clinical signs, and alanine was indicated to be a biomarker of scrapie in sheep (Scano *et al.*, 2015). A targeted LC/MS metabolomics approach was applied to detect Huntington's disease (HD) by using pre-symptomatic HD transgenic sheep. A panel of eight biomarkers were suggested which can identify 80% of pre-symptomatic HD transgenic sheep with 90% confidence (Skene *et al.*, 2017). Significant differences in metabolite concentration were detected between obese and non-obese horses (Coleman *et al.*, 2019). Potential synovial fluid metabolites related to palmar osteochondral disease in horses were identified and quantified by metabolomics platforms (Graham *et al.*, 2020). Lung tissue metabolic profiling of chicks infected with virulent Newcastle disease virus was successfully analyzed by using an MS-based tool (Liu *et al.*, 2019).

7.6 Proteomics and Metabolomics in Human Disease Diagnosis

Numerous human diseases were introspected by using powerful proteomics and metabolomics techniques for potential biomarker discovery toward early and reliable diagnosis. Out of all human diseases, proteomics and metabolomics tools are most extensively applied in the diagnosis of varieties of cancers. Several signature molecules, either proteins or metabolites, are identified, characterized and validated specific to a type of cancer. Among neurological diseases, Huntington's disease, Parkinson's disease and Alzheimer's disease are well studied by proteomics and metabolomics platforms. Inborn errors of metabolic diseases can be diagnosed rapidly by metabolomics methodologies. Promising metabolites are identified for different cancers and cardiovascular diseases such as coronary artery disease, inflammatory diseases, chronic kidney diseases, osteoarthritis, diabetes etc. Other diseases of humans, including fabry disease, hepatitis B virus-infected cirrhosis and alcoholic cirrhosis, non-alcoholic fatty disease, hepatitis C virus infection, HIV-1 and malaria were studied for diagnosis using metabolomics approaches (Gowda *et al.*, 2008; Emwas *et al.*, 2013; Emwas *et al.*, 2015; Zhang *et al.*, 2020). Besides cancer, proteomics techniques are exploited in several other human disease diagnoses such as cardiac diseases, dilated cardiomyopathy, obesity, diabetes, inflammatory bowel disease, autoimmune diseases, kidney diseases etc. (Barbosa *et al.*, 2012; Lippolis and De Angelis, 2016). Proteomics biomarkers are also equally effective for infectious disease diagnosis such as cerebral malaria, acute bacterial meningitis, Human African Trypanosomiasis, severe acute respiratory syndrome (SARS), tuberculosis, Lyme disease, toxoplasmosis, HIV or AIDS (Jungblut *et al.*, 1999; Kavallaris and Marshall, 2005; List *et al.*, 2008; Abdullah Alharbi, 2020).

7.7 Conclusion

Proteomics and metabolomics techniques are providing excellent opportunities in the arena of human and animal health by exploring novel and potential biomarkers for disease diagnosis. In the last decade, significant applications of proteomics and metabolomics platforms have improved the understanding of disease process, diagnosis and treatment. The list of potential disease-specific biomarkers has prospered significantly in recent times, and the trend will obviously be unremitting in the coming years, empowered by state-of-the-art proteomics and metabolomics techniques toward the unearthing of more effective biomarkers for advanced and precise clinical disease diagnosis with widespread execution in personalized medicine. In the near future, it will be a pre-requisite to validate the potential biomarkers in larger populations with thorough investigation of their limitations for the accomplishment of successful lab-to-land transition as stout and reliable early and specific point-of-care disease diagnostic modality.

References

Abdullah, M., Kornegay, J.N., Honcoop, A. *et al.* (2017). Non-targeted metabolomics analysis of Golden Retriever muscular dystrophy-affected muscles reveals alterations in arginine and proline metabolism, and elevations in glutamic and oleic acid in vivo. *Metabolites*, 7(3), 1–19.

Ahmad, Y., Arya, A., Gangwar, A., Paul, S. and Bhargava, K. (2014). Proteomics in diagnosis: past, present and future. *Journal of Proteomics and Genomics*, 1(1), 103.

Aldred, S., Grant, M.M. and Griffiths, H.R. (2004). The use of proteomics for the assessment of clinical samples in research. *Clinical Biochemistry*, 37(11), 943–952.

Alharbi, R.A. (2020). Proteomics approach and techniques in identification of reliable biomarkers for diseases. *Saudi Journal of Biological Sciences*, 27(3), 968–974.

Andersen, J.S. and Mann, M. (2006). Organellar proteomics: turning inventories into insights. *EMBO Reports*, 7, 874–879.

Apweiler, R., Aslanidis, C., Deufel, T. *et al.* (2009). Approaching clinical proteomics: current state and future fields of application in fluid proteomics. *Clinical Chemistry and Laboratory Medicine*, 47(6), 724–744.

Athanasiadou, S., Pemberton, A., Jackson, F. *et al.* (2008). Proteomic approach to identify candidate effector molecules during the in vitro immune exclusion of infective *Teladorsagia circumcincta* in the abomasum of sheep. *Veterinary Research*, 39(6), 58.

Bala, L., Ghoshal, U.C., Ghoshal, U. *et al.* (2006). Malabsorption syndrome with and without small intestinal bacterial overgrowth: a study on upper-gut aspirate using 1H NMR spectroscopy. *Magnetic Resonance in Medicine*, 56, 738–744.

Barbosa, E.B., Vidotto, A., Polachini, G.M. *et al.* (2012). Proteomics: methodologies and applications to the study of human diseases. *Revista da Associação Médica Brasileira*, 58(3), 366–375.

Barton, C., Beck, P., Kay, R. *et al.* (2009). Multiplexed LC-MS/MS analysis of horse plasma proteins to study doping in sport. *Proteomics*, 9(11), 3058–3065.

Basoglu, A., Baspinar, N., Tenori, L. *et al.* (2020). Nuclear magnetic resonance (NMR)-based metabolome profile evaluation in dairy cows with and without displaced abomasum. *Veterinary Quarterly*, 40(1), 1–15.

Bassols, A., Costa, C., Eckersall, P.D. *et al.* (2014). The pig as an animal model for human pathologies: A proteomics perspective. *Proteomics Clinical Application*, 8, 715–731.

Batxelli-Molina, I., Salvetat, N., Andréoletti, O. *et al.* (2010). Ovine serum biomarkers of early and late phase scrapie. *BMC Veterinary Research*, 6, 49.

Beeley, J.A. and Khoo, K.S. (1999). Salivary proteins in rheumatoid arthritis and Sjogren's syndrome: one-dimensional and two-dimensional electrophoretic studies. *Electrophoresis*, 20, 1652–1660.

Bilić, P., Guillemin, N., Kovačević, A. *et al.* (2018). Serum proteome profiling in canine idiopathic dilated cardiomyopathy using TMT-based quantitative proteomics approach. *Journal of Proteomics*, 179, 110–121.

Bilić, P., Kuleš, J., Galan, A. *et al.* (2018). Proteomics in veterinary medicine and animal science: neglected scientific opportunities with immediate impact. *Proteomics*, 18, 1800047.

Blakebrough-Hall, C., Dona, A., D'occhio, M.J. *et al.* (2020). Diagnosis of bovine respiratory disease in feedlot cattle using blood 1H NMR metabolomics. *Scientific Reports*, 10, 115.

Bodzon-Kulakowska, A., Bierczynska-Krzysik, A., Dylag, T. *et al.* (2007). Methods for samples preparation in proteomic research. *Journal of Chromatography B*, 849(1–2), 1–31.

Boehmer, J.L., Bannerman, D.D., Shefcheck, K. *et al.* (2008). Proteomic analysis of differentially expressed proteins in bovine milk during experimentally induced *Escherichia coli* mastitis. *Journal of Dairy Science*, 91(11), 4206–4218.

Boehmer, J.L., Degrasse, J.A., Lancaster, V.A. *et al.* (2011). Evaluation of protein expression in bovine bronchoalveolar fluid following challenge with *Mannheimia haemolytica*. *Proetomics*, 18, 3685–3697.

Bogdanov, M., Matson, W.R., Wang, L. *et al.* (2008). Metabolomic profiling to develop blood biomarkers for Parkinson's disease. *Brain*, 131, 389–396.

Bollard, M.E., Stanley, E.G., Lindon, J.C. *et al.* (2005). NMR-based metabonomic approaches for evaluating physiological influences on biofluid composition. *NMR Biomedicine*, 18, 143–162.

Brown, S.C., Kruppa, G. and Dasseux, J.L. (2005). Metabolomics applications of FT-ICR mass spectrometry. *Mass Spectrometry Reviews*, 24, 223–231.

Buragohain, L., Nanda, T., Ghosh, A. *et al.* (2017). Identification of serum protein markers for early diagnosis of pregnancy in buffalo. *Journal of Animal Science*, 88(8), 1189–1197.

Camargo, M., Intasqui, P. and Bertolla, R.P. (2018). Understanding the seminal plasma proteome and its role in male fertility. *Basic and Clinical Andrology*, 28, 6. https://doi.org/10.1186/s12610-018-0071-5.

Carlos, G., dos Santos, F.P. and Fröehlich, P.E. (2020). Canine metabolomics advances. *Metabolomics*, 16, 16. https://doi.org/10.1007/s11306-020-1638-7.

Castagnola, M., Scarano, E., Passali, G.C. *et al.* (2017). Salivary biomarkers and proteomics: future diagnostic and clinical utilities. *Acta Otorhinolaryngol Italica*, 37(2), 94–101.

Catinella, S., Traldi, P., Pinelli, C. *et al.* (1996). Matrix-assisted laser desorption/ionization mass spectrometry in milk science. *Rapid Communications in Mass Spectrometry*, 10(13), 1629–1637.

Ceciliani, F., Eckersall, D., Burchmore, R. *et al.* (2014). Proteomics in veterinary medicine: applications and trends in disease pathogenesis and diagnostics. *Veterinary Pathology* , 51(2), 351–362.

Chait, B.T. (2006). Chemistry. Mass spectrometry: bottom-up or top-down? *Science*, 314(5796), 65–66.

Chen, C.H.W. (2008). Review of a current role of mass spectrometry for proteome research. *Analytica Chimica Acta*, 624(1), 16–36.

Chiaradia, E., Pepe, M., Tartaglia, M. *et al.* (2012). Gambling on putative biomarkers of osteoarthritis and osteochondrosis by equine synovial fluid proteomics. *Journal of Proteomics*, 75(14), 4478–4493.

Chiaradia, E., Valiani, A., Tartaglia, M. *et al.* (2013). Ovine subclinical mastitis: proteomic analysis of whey and milk fat globules unveils putative diagnostic biomarkers in milk. *Journal of Proteomics*, 83, 144–159.

Chich, J.F., Schaeffer, B., Bouin, A.P. *et al.* (2007). Prion infection-impaired functional blocks identified by proteomics enlighten the targets and the curing pathways of an anti-prion drug. *Biochimica et Biophysica Acta*, 1774(1), 154–167.

Chiou, S.H. and Wu, C.Y. (2011). Clinical proteomics: current status, challenges, and future perspectives. *The Kaohsiung Journal of Medical Sciences*, 27(1), 1–14.

Xu, C., Shu, S., Xia, C., Wang, P., *et al.* (2015). Mass spectral analysis of urine proteomic profiles of dairy cows suffering from clinical ketosis. *Veterinary Quarterly*, 35(3), 133–141.

Clish, C.B. (2015). Metabolomics: an emerging but powerful tool for precision medicine. *Cold Spring Harbor Molecular Case Studies*, 1(1), a000588.

Coleman, M.C., Whitfield-Cargile, C.M., Madrigal, R.G. *et al.* (2019). Comparison of the microbiome, metabolome, and lipidome of obese and non-obese horses. *PloS One*, 14(4), e0215918.

Cooks, R.G., Ouyang, Z., Takats, Z. *et al.* (2006) Detection technologies. Ambient mass spectrometry. *Science*, 311, 1566–1570.

De Moraes Pontes, J.G., De Santana, F.B., Portela, R.W. *et al.* (2017). Biomarkers of the caseous lymphadenitis in sheep by NMR-based metabolomics. *Metabolomics*, 7, 190.

Deeg, C.A., Altmann, F., Hauck, S.M. *et al.* (2007). Down-regulation of pigment epithelium-derived factor in uveitic lesion associates with focal vascular endothelial growth factor expression and breakdown of the blood-brain barrier. *Proteomics*, 7, 1540–1548.

Dervishi, E., Zhang, G., Mandal, R. *et al.* (2018). Targeted metabolomics: new insights into pathobiology of retained placenta in dairy cows and potential risk biomarkers. *Animal*, 12(5), 1050–1059.

Di Girolamo, F., Del Chierico, F., Caenaro, G. *et al.* (2012). Human serum proteome analysis: new source of markers in metabolic disorders. *Biomarkers in Medicine*, 6, 759–773.

Dong, S.W., Zhang, S.D., Wang, D.S. *et al.* (2015). Comparative proteomics analysis provide novel insight into laminitis in Chinese Holstein cows. *BMC Veterinary Research*, 11, 161.

Doran, P., Gannon, J., O'Connell, K. and Ohlendieck, K. (2007). Proteomic profiling of animal models mimicking skeletal muscle disorders. *Proteomics Clinical Applications*, 1, 1169–1184.

Dudley, E., Yousef, M., Wang, Y. *et al.* (2010).Targeted metabolomics and mass spectrometry. *Advances in Protein Chemistry and Structural Biology*, 80, 45–83.

El Aneed, A. and Banoub, J. (2006). Proteomics in the diagnosis of hepatocellular carcinoma: focus on high risk hepatitis B and C patients. *Anticancer Research*, 26(5A), 3293–3300.

Emwas, A.-H.M., Merzaban, J.S. and Serrai, H. (2015). Theory and applications of NMR-based metabolomics in human disease diagnosis. In Rahman, A.-u. and Choudhary, M.I. (eds), *Applications of NMR Spectroscopy*, 93–130. Bentham Science Publishers.

Emwas, A.M., Salek, R.M., Griffin, J.L. *et al.* (2013). NMR-based metabolomics in human disease diagnosis: applications, limitations, and recommendations. *Metabolomics*, 9, 1048–1072.

Feist, P. and Hummon, A.B. (2015). Proteomic challenges: sample preparation techniques for microgram-quantity protein analysis from biological samples. *International Journal of Molecular Sciences*, 16(2), 3537–3563.

Forster, G.M., Stockman, J., Noyes, N. *et al.* (2018). A comparative study of serum biochemistry, metabolome and microbiome parameters of clinically healthy, normal weight, overweight, and obese companion dogs. *Topics in Companion Animal Medicine*, 33(4), 126–135.

Gaines, P.J., Powell, T.D., Walmsley, S.J. *et al.* (2007). Identification of serum biomarkers for canine B-cell lymphoma by use of surface-enhanced laser desorption-ionization time-of-flight mass spectrometry. *American Journal of Veterinary Research*, 68, 405–410.

Gates, S.C. and Sweeley, C.C. (1978). Quantitative metabolic profiling based on gas chromatography. *Clinical Chemistry*, 24(10), 1663–1673.

Geiger, T., Wehner, A., Schaab, C. *et al.* (2012). Comparative proteomic analysis of eleven common cell lines reveals ubiquitous but varying expression of most proteins. *Molecular & Cellular Proteomics*, 11(3), M111.014050.

German, J.B., Hammock, B.D. and Watkins, S.M. (2005). Metabolomics: building on a century of biochemistry to guide human health. *Metabolomics*, 1(1), 3–9.

Gong, W., Jia, J., Zhang, B. *et al.* (2017). Serum metabolomic profiling of piglets infected with virulent classical swine fever virus. *Frontiers in Microbiology*, 8, 731.

Gookin, J.L., Mathews, K.G., Cullen, J. *et al.* (2018). Qualitative metabolomics profiling of serum and bile from dogs with gallbladder mucocele formation. *PLoS One*, 13(1), 1–18.

Gowda, G.A., Zhang, S., Gu, H. *et al.* (2008). Metabolomics-based methods for early disease diagnostics. *Expert Review of Molecular Diagnostics*, 8(5), 617–633.

Graham, R.J.T.Y., Anderson, J.R., Phelan, M.M. *et al.* (2020). Metabolomic analysis of synovial fluid from thoroughbred racehorses diagnosed with palmar osteochondral disease using magnetic resonance imaging. *Equine Veterinary Journal*, 52, 384–390.

Griffin, J.L. and Kauppinen, R.A. (2007). Tumour metabolomics in animal models of human cancer. *Journal of Proteome Research*, 6, 498–505.

Griffin, J.L. and Vidal-Puig, A. (2008). Current challenges in metabolomics for diabetes research: a vital functional genomic tool or just a ploy for gaining funding? *Physiological Genomics*, 34(1), 1–5.

Guard, B.C., Barr, J.W., Reddivari, L. *et al.* (2015). Characterization of microbial dysbiosis and metabolomic changes in dogs with acute diarrhea. *PLoS One*, 10(5), 1–24.

Gutierrez, A.M., Ceron, J.J., Fuentes-Rubio, M. *et al.* (2014). A proteomic approach to porcine saliva. *Current Protein and Peptide Science*, 15, 56–63.

Gygi, S.P., Rist, B., Gerber, S.A., *et al.* (1999). Quantitative analysis of complex protein mixtures using isotope-coded affinity tags. *Nature Biotechnology*, 17(10), 994–999.

Hailemariam, D., Mandal, R., Saleem, F. *et al.* (2014). Identification of predictive biomarkers of disease state in transition dairy cows. *Journal of Dairy Science*, 97(5), 2680–2693.

Hanash, S. and Taguchi, A. (2011). Application of proteomics to cancer early detection. *Cancer Journal (Sudbury, MA)*, 17(6), 423–428.

Henzel, W.J., Billeci, T.M., Stults, J.T. *et al.* (1993). Identifying proteins from two-dimensional gels by molecular mass searching of peptide fragments in protein sequence databases. *Proceedings of the National Academy of Science USA*, 90, 5011e5.

Hirsch, J., Hansen, K.C., Burlingame, A.L. *et al.* (2004). Proteomics: current techniques and potential applications to lung disease. *American Journal of Physiology – Lung Cellular and Molecular Physiology*, 287(1), L1–L23.

Hixson, K.K., Lopez-Ferrer, D., Robinson, E.W. *et al.* (2017). Proteomics. In Lindon, J.C., Tranter, G.E. and Koppenaal, D.W. (eds), *Encyclopedia of Spectroscopy and Spectrometry*, 766–773. The Academic Press.

Hughes, V., Denham, S., Bannantine, J.P. *et al.* (2013). Interferon gamma responses to proteome-determined specific recombinant proteins: potential as diagnostic markers for ovine Johne's disease. *Veterinary Immunology and Immunopathology*, 155(3), 197–204.

Hutchens, T.W. and Yip, T.T. (1993). New desorption strategies for mass spectrometric analysis of macromolecules. *Rapid Communications in Mass Spectrometry*, 7, 576–580.

Jungblut, P.R., Zimny-Arndt, U., Zeindl-Eberhart, E. *et al.* (1999). Proteomics in human disease: cancer, heart and infectious diseases. *Electrophoresis*, 20(10), 2100–2110.

Jungblut, P.R. (2012). *Protein and Peptide Mass Spectrometry in Drug Discovery*. Edited by Michael L. Gross, Guodong Chen and Birendra N. Pramanik. *ChemMedChem*, 7, 2241–2242.

Karas, M. and Hillenkamp, F. (1988). Laser desorption ionization of proteins with molecular masses exceeding 10,000 daltons. *Analytical Chemistry*, 60, 2299–2301.

Katsafadou, A.I., Tsangaris, G.T., Billinis, C. *et al.* (2015). Use of proteomics in the study of microbial diseases of small ruminants. *Veterinary Microbiology*, 181(1–2), 27–33.

Katz-Jaffe, M.G., Schoolcraft, W.B. and Gardner, D.K. (2006). Analysis of protein expression (secretome) by human and mouse preimplantation embryos. *Fertility and Sterility*, 86(3), 678–685.

Kavallaris, M. and Marshall, G.M. (2005). Proteomics and disease: opportunities and challenges. *The Medical Journal of Australia*, 182(11), 575–579.

Kelleher, N.L. (2004).Top-down proteomics. *Analytical Chemistry*, 76(11), 197A–203A.

Klopfleisch, R., Klose, P., Weise, C. *et al.* (2010). Proteome of metastatic canine mammary carcinomas similarities to and differences from human breast cancer. *Journal of Proteome Research*, 9, 6380–6391.

Klose, P., Weise, C., Bondzio A. *et al.* (2011). Is there a malignant progression associated with a linear change in protein expression levels from normal canine mammary gland to metastatic mammary tumors? *Journal of Proteome Research*, 10, 4405–4415.

Kuehnbaum, N.L. and Britz-McKibbin, P. (2013). New advances in separation science for metabolomics: resolving chemical diversity in a post-genomic era. *Chemical Reviews*, 113(4), 2437–2468.

Kuleš, J., de Torre-Minguela, C., Barić Rafaj, R. *et al.* (2016). Plasma biomarkers of SIRS and MODS associated with canine babesiosis. *Research in Veterinary Science*, 105, 222–228.

Kumar, R., Ghosh, M., Kumar, S. *et al.* (2020). Single cell metabolomics: a future tool to unmask cellular heterogeneity and virus-host interaction in context of emerging viral diseases. *Frontiers in Microbiology*, 11, 1152.

Kycko, A. and Reichert, M. (2008). Two-dimensional electrophoretic analysis of polypeptides expressed by normal and ovine pulmonary adenocarcinoma affected lung tissues. *Bulletin of the Veterinary Institute in Pulawy*, 52, 3–8.

Kycko, A. and Reichert, M. (2012). Overexpression of aldolase A and cytokeratin 19 in ovine pulmonary adenocarcinoma. *Polish Journal of Veterinary Science*, 15, 703–709.

Laemmli, U.K. (1970). Cleavage of structural proteins during the assembly of the head of bacteriophage T4. *Nature*, 227(5259), 680–685.

Le Maréchal, C., Jan, G., Even, S. *et al.* (2009). Development of serological proteome analysis of mastitis by Staphylococcus aureus in ewes. *Journal of Microbiological Methods*, 79(1), 131–136.

Le Maréchal, C., Jardin, J., Jan, G. *et al.* (2011). Staphylococcus aureus seroproteomes discriminate ruminant isolates causing mild or severe mastitis. *Veterinary Research*, 42, 35.

Licier, R., Miranda, E. and Serrano, H. (2016). A quantitative proteomics approach to clinical research with non-traditional samples. *Proteomes*, 4(4), 31.

Lemberger, S.I., Deeg, C.A., Hauck, S.M. *et al.* (2011). Comparison of urine protein profiles in cats without urinary tract disease and cats with idiopathic cystitis, bacterial urinary tract infection, or urolithiasis. *American Journal of Veterinary Research*, 72(10), 1407–1415.

Leroy, B., Painter, A., Sheppard, H. *et al.* (2007). Protein expression profiling of normal and neoplastic canine prostate and bladder tissue. *Veterinary and Comparative Oncology*, 5, 119–130.

Li, Y., Xu, C., Xia, C. *et al.* (2014). Plasma metabolic profiling of dairy cows affected with clinical ketosis using LC/MS technology. *Veterinary Quarterly*, 34, 152–158.

Li, Q., Freeman, L.M., Rush, J.E. *et al.* (2015). Veterinary medicine and multi-omics research for future nutrition targets: Metabolomics and transcriptomics of the common degenerative mitral valve disease in dogs. *OMICS: A Journal of Integrative Biology*, 19(8), 461–470.

Link, A.J., Eng, J., Schieltz, D.M. *et al.* (1999). Direct analysis of protein complexes using mass spectrometry. *Nature Biotechnology*, 17, 676–682.

Lippolis, R. and De Angelis, M. (2016). Proteomics and human diseases. *Journal of Proteomics and Bioinformatics*, 9, 63–74.

List, E., Berryman, D., Bower, B. *et al.* (2008). The use of proteomics to study infectious diseases. *Infectious Disorders–Drug Targets*, 8(1), 31–45.

Liu, P., Yin, Y., Gong, Y. *et al.* (2019). In vitro and in vivo metabolomic profiling after infection with virulent Newcastle disease virus. *Viruses*, 11(10), 962.

Luan, H., Wang, X. and Cai, Z. (2019). Mass spectrometry-based metabolomics: Targeting the crosstalk between gut microbiota and brain in neurodegenerative disorders. *Mass Spectrometry Reviews*, 38(1), 22–33.

Ma, D. and Li, L. (2012). Searching for reliable premortem protein biomarkers for prion diseases: progress and challenges to date. *Expert Review of Proteomics*, 9, 267–280.

Peffers, M.J., Smagul, A. and Anderson, J.R. (2019). Proteomic analysis of synovial fluid: current and potential uses to improve clinical outcomes. *Expert Review of Proteomics*, 16(4), 287–302.

Martins, R.P., Collado-Romero, M., Martínez-Gomáriz, M. *et al.* (2012). Proteomic analysis of porcine mesenteric lymph-nodes alter salmonella typhimurium infection. *Journal of Proteomics*, 75, 4457–4470.

Maurer, D., Koziel, J., Engelken, T. *et al.* (2018). Detection of volatile compounds emitted from nasal secretions and serum: towards non-invasive identification of diseased cattle biomarkers. *Separations*, 5(1), 18.

McCaw, D.L., Chan, A.S., Stenger, A.L. *et al.* (2007). Proteomics of canine lymphoma identifies potential cancer specific protein markers. *Clinical Cancer Research*, 13, 2496–2503.

Meachem, M.D., Snead, E.R., Kidney, B.A. *et al.* (2015). A comparative proteomic study of plasma in feline pancreatitis and pancreatic carcinoma using 2-dimensional gel electrophoresis to identify diagnostic biomarkers: A pilot study. *Canadian Journal of Veterinary Research* (*Revue canadienne de recherche vétérinaire*), 79(3), 184–189.

Minakshi, P., Ghosh, M., Kumar, R. *et al.* (2019a). Single-cell metabolomics: technology and applications. In Barh, D. and Azevedo, V. (eds), *Single-Cell Omics*, 319–353. The Academic Press.

Minakshi, P., Kumar, R., Ghosh, M. *et al.* (2019b). Single-cell proteomics: technology and applications. In Barh, D. and Azevedo, V. (eds), *Single-Cell Omics*, 283–318. The Academic Press.

Minamoto, Y., Otoni, C.C., Steelman, S.M. *et al.* (2015). Alteration of the fecal microbiota and serum metabolite profiles in dogs with idiopathic inflammatory bowel disease Alteration of the fecal microbiota and serum metabolite profiles in dogs with idiopathic in flammatory bowel disease. *Gut Microbes*, 6(1), 33–47.

Morphew, R.M., Wright, H.A., Lacourse, E.J. *et al.* (2007). Comparative proteomics of excretory-secretory proteins released by the liver fluke *Fasciola hepatica* in sheep host bile during in vitro culture ex-host. *Molecular and Cellular Proteomics*, 6, 963–972.

Mudaliar, M., Tassi, R., Thomas, F.C. *et al.* (2016). Mastitomics, the integrated omics of bovine milk in an experimental model of *Streptococcus uberis* mastitis: 2. Label-free relative quantitative proteomics. *Molecular Biosystems*, 12(9), 2748–2761.

Nagana Gowda, G.A., Ijare, O.B., Somashekar, B.S. *et al.* (2006). Single-step analysis of individual conjugated bile acids in human bile using 1H NMR spectroscopy. *Lipids*, 41, 591–603.

Nagaraj, S.H., Harsha, H.C., Reverter, A. *et al.* (2012). Proteomic analysis of the abomasal mucosal response following infection by the nematode, *Haemonchus contortus*, in genetically resistant and susceptible sheep. *Journal of Proteomics*, 75, 7, 2141–2152.

Nalbantoglu, S. (2019). Metabolomics: basic principles and strategies. *Molecular Medicine*. https://doi.org/10.5772/intechopen.88563.

Nicholson, J.K., Connelly, J., Lindon, J.C. *et al.* (2002). Metabonomics: a platform for studying drug toxicity and gene function. *Nature Reviews Drug Discovery*, 1, 153–161.

Nicholson, J.K. (2006). Global systems biology, personalized medicine and molecular epidemiology. *Molecular Systems Biology*, 2, 52.

Novotny, M.V., Soini, H.A. and Mechref, Y. (2008). Biochemical individuality reflected in chromatographic, electrophoretic and mass-spectrometric profiles. *Journal of Chromatography B: Analytical Technologies in the Biomedical and Life Sciences*, 866(1–2), 26–47.

O'Farrell, P.H. (1975). High resolution two-dimensional electrophoresis of proteins. *Journal of Biological Chemistry*, 250(10), 4007–4021.

O'Kell, A.L., Garrett, T.J., Wasserfall, C. *et al.* (2017). Untargeted metabolomic analysis in naturally occurring canine diabetes mellitus identifies similarities to human Type 1 Diabetes. *Scientific Reports*, 7(1), 1–7.

Oliver, S.G., Winson, M.K., Kell, D.B. *et al.* (1998). Systematic functional analysis of the yeast genome. *Trends in Biotechnology*, 16(9), 373–378.

Ong, S.E., Blagoev, B., Kratchmarova, I. *et al.* (2002). Stable isotope labeling by amino acids in cell culture, SILAC, as a simple and accurate approach to expression proteomics. *Molecular and Cellular Proteomics*, 1, 376e86.

Patti, G.J., Yanes, O. and Siuzdak, G. (2012). Innovation: metabolomics: the apogee of the omics trilogy. *Nature Reviews Molecular Cell Biology*, 13(4), 263–269.

Pemberton, A.D., Brown, J.K., Craig, N.M. *et al.* (2012). Changes in protein expression in the sheep abomasum following trickle infection with *Teladorsagia circumcincta*. *Parasitology*, 139(3), 375–385.

Querengesser, L., Vogel, H.J., Sykes, B.D. *et al.* (2007). HMDB: the Human Metabolome Database. *Nucleic Acids Research*, 35(suppl. 1), D521–D526.

Rodríguez-Suárez, E., Siwy, J., Zürbig, P. *et al.* (2014). Urine as a source for clinical proteome analysis: From discovery to clinical application. *Biochimica et Biophysica Acta (BBA)–Proteins and Proteomics*, 1844(5), 884–898.

Ross, P.L., Huang, Y.N., Marchese, J.N. *et al.* (2004). Multiplexed protein quantitation in Saccharomyces cerevisiae using amine-reactive isobaric tagging reagents. *Molecular and Cellular Proteomics*, 3, 1154e69.

Saelao, P., Wang, Y., Chanthavixay, G. *et al.* (2018). Integrated proteomic and transcriptomic analysis of differential expression of chicken lung tissue in response to NDV infection during heat stress. *Genes*, 9(12), 579.

Scano, P., Rosa, A., Incani, A. *et al.* (2015). (1)H NMR brain metabonomics of scrapie exposed sheep. *Molecular Biosystems*, 11(7), 2008–2016.

Semmes, O.J., Feng, Z., Adam, B.L. *et al.* (2005). Evaluation of serum protein profiling by surface-enhanced laser desorption/ionization time-of-flight mass spectrometry for the detection of prostate cancer: I. Assessment of platform reproducibility. *Clinical Chemistry*, 51(1), 102–112.

Shah, T.R. and Misra, A. (2011). Proteomics. In Misra, A. (ed.), *Challenges in Delivery of Therapeutic Genomics and Proteomics*, 387–427. Elsevier.

Shahzad, K., Lopreiato, V., Liang, Y. *et al.* (2019). Hepatic metabolomics and transcriptomics to study susceptibility to ketosis in response to prepartal nutritional management. *Journal of Animal Science and Biotechnology*, 10, 96.

Shaked, G.M., Shaked, Y., Kariv-Inbal, Z. *et al.* (2001). A protease-resistant prion protein isoform is present in urine of animals and humans affected with prion diseases. *Journal of Biological Chemistry*, 276, 31479–31482.

Shao, Y. and Le, W. (2019). Recent advances and perspectives of metabolomics-based investigations in Parkinson's disease. *Molecular Neurodegeneration*, 14, 3.

Simon, S.L., Lamoureux, L., Plews, M. *et al.* (2008). The identification of disease-induced biomarkers in the urine of BSE infected cattle. *Proteome Science*, 6, 23.

Sinha, A., Principe, S., Alfaro, J. *et al.* (2017). Proteomic profiling of secreted proteins, exosomes, and microvesicles in cell culture conditioned media. In Boheler, K.R. and Gundry, R.L. (eds), *The Surfaceome: Methods and Protocols*, 91–102. Humana Press.

Skene, D., Middleton, B., Fraser, C. *et al.* (2017). Metabolic profiling of presymptomatic Huntington's disease sheep reveals novel biomarkers. *Scientific Reports*, 7, 43030.

Smith, C.A., O'Maille, G., Want, E.J. *et al.* (2005). METLIN: a metabolite mass spectral database. *Therapeutic Drug Monitoring*, 27(6), 747–751.

Smith, C.A., Want, E.J., O'Maille, G. *et al.* (2006). XCMS: processing mass spectrometry data for metabolite profiling using nonlinear peak alignment, matching, and identification. *Analytical Chemistry*, 78(3), 779–787.

Smolenski, G., Haines, S., Kwan, F.Y. *et al.* (2007). Characterisation of host defence proteins in milk using a proteomic approach. *Journal of Proteome Research*, 6(1), 207–215.

So, H.-K., Mandal, P.K., Baatartsogt, O. *et al.* (2009). Biomarkers identified by proteomic study of spleen lymphocyte from broilers infected with *Salmonella gallinarum* after feeding Korean mistletoe (*Viscum album coloratum*). *Asian Journal of Animal and Veterinary Advances*, 4, 148–159.

Soder, J., Hagman, R., Dicksved, J. *et al.* (2017). The urine metabolome differs between lean and overweight Labrador Retriever dogs during a feed-challenge. *PLoS One*, 12(6), 1–17.

Steelman, S.M. and Chowdhary, B.P. (2012). Plasma proteomics shows an elevation of the anti-inflammatory protein APOA-IV in chronic equine laminitis. *BMC Veterinary Research*, 8, 179.

Sun, D., Zhang, H., Guo, D. *et al.* (2013). Shotgun proteomic analysis of plasma from dairy cattle suffering from footrot: characterization of potential disease-associated factors. *PLoS One*, 8(2), e55973.

Sun, L.W., Zhang, H.Y., Wu, L. *et al.* (2014). 1H-Nuclear magnetic resonance-based plasma metabolic profiling of dairy cows with clinical and subclinical ketosis. *Journal of Dairy Science*, 97, 1552–1562.

Surendran Nair, M., Yao, D., Chen, C. *et al.* (2019). Serum metabolite markers of early Mycoplasma hyopneumoniae infection in pigs. *Veterinary Research*, 50, 98.

Sze, S.K., Ge, Y., Oh, H. *et al.* (2002). Top-down mass spectrometry of a 29-k Da protein for characterization of any post translational modification to within one residue. *Proceedings of the National Academy of Sciences of the United States of America*, 99(4), 1774–1779.

Takats, Z., Wiseman, J.M., Gologan, B. *et al.* (2004). Mass spectrometry sampling under ambient conditions with desorption electrospray ionization. *Science*, 306, 471–473.

Tamai, R., Furuya, M., Hatoya, S. *et al.* (2014). Profiling of serum metabolites in canine lymphoma using gas chromatography mass spectrometry. *Journal of Veterinary Medical Science*, 76, 1513–1518.

Tanaka, K., Waki, H., Ido, Y. *et al.* (1988). Protein and polymer analyses up to m/z 100,000 by laser ionization time-of-flight mass spectrometry. *Rapid Communications in Mass Spectrometry*, 2, 151–153.

te Pas, M.F.W., Koopmans, S.-J., Kruijt, L. *et al.* (2013). Plasma proteome profiles associated with diet-induced metabolic syndrome and the early onset of metabolic syndrome in a pig model. *PLoS One*, 8(9), e73087.

Thanomsridetchai, N., Singhto, N., Tepsumethanon, V. *et al.* (2011). Comprehensive proteome analysis of hippocampus, brainstem, and spinal cord from paralytic and furious dogs naturally infected with rabies. *Journal of Proteome Research*, 10, 4911–4924.

Tomita, M. and Kami, K. (2012). Systems biology, metabolomics, and cancer metabolism. *Science*, 336(6084), 990–991.

Trushina, E.andMielke, M.M. (2014). Recent advances in the application of metabolomics to Alzheimer's disease. *Biochimica et Biophysica Acta*, 1842(8), 1232–1239.

Tsutsui, H., Maeda, T., Min, J.Z. *et al.* (2011). Biomarker discovery in biological specimens (plasma, hair, liver and kidney) of diabetic mice based upon metabolite profiling using ultra-performance liquid chromatography with electrospray ionization time-of flight mass spectrometry. *Clinica Chimica Acta*, 412(11–12), 861–872.

Turk, R., Piras, C., Kovačić, M. *et al.* (2012). Proteomics of inflammatory and oxidative stress response in cows with subclinical and clinical mastitis. *Journal of Proteomics*, 75(14), 4412–4428.

Walker, L.R., Hoyt, D.W., Walker, S.M. II *et al.* (2016). Unambiguous metabolite identification in high-throughput metabolomics by hybrid 1D (1) H NMR/ESI MS(1) approach. *Magnetic Resonance in Chemistry*, 54, 998–1003.

Wasinger, V.C., Cordwell, S.J., Cerpa-Poljak, A. *et al.* (1995). Progress with gene-product mapping of the Mollicutes: Mycoplasma genitalium. *Electrophoresis*, 16(1), 1090–1094.

Weekes, J., Wheeler, C.H., Yan, J.X. *et al.* (1999). Bovine dilated cardiomyopathy: proteomic analysis of an animal model of human dilated cardiomyopathy. *Electrophoresis*, 20, 898–906.

Wilkins, M.R. and Williams, K.L. (1995). The extracellular matrix of the *Dictyostelium discoideum* slug. *Experientia*, 51, 1189–1196.

Wittke, S., Fliser, D., Haubitz, M. *et al.* (2003). Determination of peptides and proteins in human urine with capillary electrophoresis-mass spectrometry, a suitable tool for the establishment of new diagnostic markers. *Journal of Chromatography*, 1013, 173–181.

Xu, C., Shu, S., Xia, C. *et al.* (2015). Mass spectral analysis of urine proteomic profiles of dairy cows suffering from clinical ketosis. *Veterinary Quarterly*, 35, 3, 133–141.

Xu, C. and Wang, Z. (2008). Comparative proteomic analysis of livers from ketotic cows. *Veterinary Research Communications*, 32, 263–273.

Xu, C., Wang, Z., Liu, G.W. *et al.* (2008). Metabolic characteristic of the liver of dairy cows during ketosis based on comparative proteomics. *Asian-Australian Journal of Animal Sciences*, 21(7), 1003–1010.

Wong, S.F., Meng, C.K. and Fenn, J.B. (1988). Multiple charging in electrospray ionization of poly(ethylene glycols). *Journal of Physical Chemistry A*, 92, 546–550.

Zhang, A., Sun, H., Yan, G. *et al.* (2015). Metabolomics for biomarker discovery: moving to the clinic. *Biomedical Research Institute*, 354671. https://doi.org/10.1155/2015/354671.

Zhang, A., Sun, H., Yan, G. *et al.* (2014). Metabolomics in diagnosis and biomarker discovery of colorectal cancer. *Cancer Letters*, 345(1), 17–20.

Zhang, G., Deng, Q., Mandal, R. *et al.* (2017). DI/LC-MS/MS-based metabolic profiling for identification of early predictive serum biomarkers of metritis in transition dairy cows. *Journal of Agricultural and Food Chemistry*, 65, 8510–8521.

Zhang, J., Wei, S., Liu, L. *et al.* (2012). NMR-based metabolomics study of canine bladder cancer. *Biochimica et Biophysica Acta–Molecular Basis of Disease*, 1822(11), 1807–1814.

Zhang, Q., Huang, S., Luo, H. *et al.* (2017). Eight-plex iTRAQ labeling and quantitative proteomic analysis for human bladder cancer. *American Journal of Cancer Research*, 7(4), 935–945.

Zhang, X., Davis, M.E., Moeller, S.J. *et al.* (2013). Effects of selection for blood serum IGF-I concentration on reproductive performance of female Angus beef cattle. *Journal of Animal Science*, 91, 4104–4115.

Zhang, X., Wei, D., Yap, Y. *et al.* (2007). Mass spectrometry-based "omics" technologies in cancer diagnostics. *Mass Spectrometry Reviews*, 26, 403–431.

Zhang, X.W., Li, Q.H., Xu, Z.D. *et al.* (2020). Mass spectrometry-based metabolomics in health and medical science: A systematic review. *RSC Advances*, 10, 3092–3104.

Zhang, Y., Fonslow, B.R., Shan, B. *et al.* (2013). Protein analysis by shotgun/bottom-up proteomics. *Chemical Reviews*, 113(4), 2343–2394.

Zhong, L., Taylor, D., Begg, D.J. *et al.* (2011). Biomarker discovery for ovine paratuberculosis (Johne's disease) by proteomic serum profiling. *Comparative Immunology, Microbiology and Infectious Diseases*, 34, 315–326.

8

Imaging Techniques in Veterinary Disease Diagnosis

Minakshi Prasad,[1] Mayukh Ghosh,[2] Suman,[3] Harshad Sudhir Patki,[4] Sandeep Kumar,[5] Basanti Brar,[1] Neelesh Sindhu,[6] Parveen Goel,[6] Samander Kaushik,[7] Hari Mohan,[7] Shafiq Syed[8] and Rajesh Kumar[9]

[1] *Department of Animal Biotechnology, Lala Lajpat Rai University of Veterinary and Animal Sciences, Hisar-125004, Haryana, India*

[2] *Department of Veterinary Physiology and Biochemistry, RGSC, Banaras Hindu University, Mirzapur-231001, Uttar Pradesh, India*

[3] *ICAR, Central Institute for Research on Buffaloes, Hisar-125004, Haryana, India*

[4] *Department of Veterinary Anatomy and Histology, College of Veterinary and Animal Sciences, Kerala Veterinary and Animal Sciences University, Pookode-673576, Kerala, India*

[5] *Department of Veterinary Surgery and Radiology, College of Veterinary Sciences, Lala Lajpat Rai University of Veterinary and Animal Sciences, Hisar-125004, Haryana, India*

[6] *Department of Veterinary Medicine, College of Veterinary Sciences, Lala Lajpat Rai University of Veterinary and Animal Sciences, Hisar-125004, Haryana, India*

[7] *Centre for Biotechnology, Maharshi Dayanand University, Rohtak-124001, Haryana, India*

[8] *Faculty of Health, School of Biomedical Sciences & Pharmacy, University of Newcastle, Newcastle, New South Wales, Australia*

[9] *Department of Veterinary Physiology and Biochemistry, Lala Lajpat Rai University of Veterinary and Animal Sciences, Hisar-125004, Haryana, India*

Corresponding authors: Minakshi Prasad, *minakshi.abt@gmail.com;* **Mayukh Ghosh,** *ghosh.mayukh87@gmail.com*

8.1 Introduction

Early and precise diagnosis paves the path for effective treatment and sketches the landscape of disease progression, outcome and possible eradication. The basis of disease diagnosis may span from visual symptoms to the extraction of minute details of organs, tissues and sub-cellular machineries through the employment of state-of-the-art diagnostic platforms. Irrespective of the diagnostic tools used, the aberrations in the biological system must be recorded in an interpretable manner to identify the deviation(s). Evidently, diagnostic imaging comes into play to capture the signal(s) generated from the altered homeostasis and display them in a meaningful manner. The authenticity of the information extrapolated from such images can be attested by the words "seeing is believing". Arguably, every investigator tenders undoubted faith over a quality diagnostic image recorded by following standard protocol. The array of valuable information carried by a diagnostic image regarding the underlined etiology, disease progression, therapeutic outcome and the prognosis can be depicted through the phrase "a picture is worth a thousand words". The importance of imaging techniques can be justified by several Nobel Prizes awarded for substantial developments in the mentioned field that include but are not limited to the 2008 Nobel Prize in Chemistry for the development of the green fluorescent protein (GFP), the 2014 Nobel Prize in Chemistry for the introduction of super-resolution fluorescence microscopy and the contribution in cryogenic electron microscopy (cryoEM) that won the coveted award in 2017.

Arguably, the onset of modern imaging technology was pioneered by Robert Hooke with the discovery of cells using a microscope in 1665, followed by elucidation of microbial life from dental plaque in sketches by Antonie Philips van Leeuwenhoek using his own customized microscope (actually a powerful magnifying glass, instead of today's compound microscope) in 1676. Initially, imaging was intended toward amplification of a target to visualize its minute details. Subsequently the potential has been explored further toward diverse applications, including disease diagnosis. In the early era, visible light was used as the sole energy source for imaging an object. However, continuous progress in instrumentation and material science has rendered the other alternate energy sources equally relevant for advanced imaging techniques, such as X-rays for radiography and CT scanning, magnetic field for NMR, infrared light for thermal imaging, ultrasound for ultrasonography, differences in electric potential for ECG, EKG, EEG etc. (Figure 8.1).

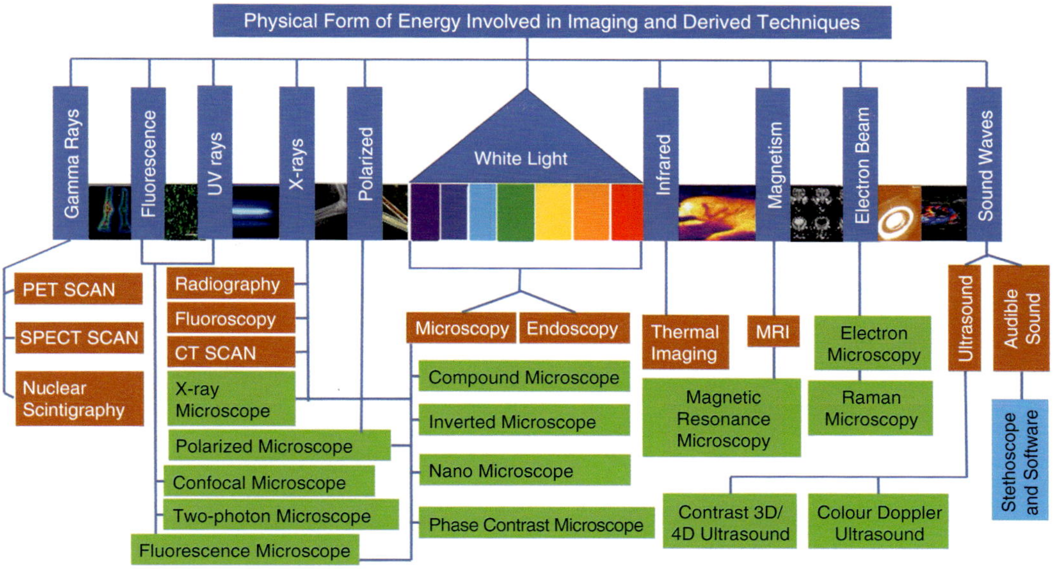

FIGURE 8.1 Different imaging techniques with source of energy at a glance.

Advancements in medical diagnosis have gained concomitant progress along with diagnostic imaging techniques. Currently, the global market for medical imaging systems achieved a valuation of around US$20.13 billion in 2017 and is predicted to inflate at a compound annual growth rate (CAGR) of 4.0% over the future period. The emergence of various infectious and lifestyle diseases accompanied by the urge for their early detection, socio-economic solvency and growing health awareness are some of the crucial factors propelling growth in the upcoming era. Besides the Western world, developing countries such as India, Brazil, China etc. are also contributing immensely in terms of customizing cutting-edge instrumentations, drawing investments and funds, along with providing huge market support for holding the persistent growth in the diagnostic imaging market. The effect of a secured market has been reflected through the continuous development of the existing tools (www.grandviewresearch.com/industry-analysis/medical-imaging-systems-market).

Although the global market for veterinary imaging is lagging behind the human diagnostic imaging market due to some inherent challenges, it still achieved the valuation of US$1.620 billion in 2018. It has been estimated to reach nearly US$2.651 billion by 2026, with a CAGR of 6.3%. The expected growth rate is superior to that of medical diagnostic imaging, which may be due to the enhanced trend of the keeping of companion animals, the spike in expenditure on animal health to maximize the yield from productive animals, the focus toward wildlife disease diagnosis and the rapid emergence of infectious zoonoses, along with technological advancements in veterinary imaging systems (www.alliedmarketresearch.com/veterinary-imaging-market). Veterinary imaging comes under the umbrella of veterinary medicine and deals with obtaining diagnostic images of animals to facilitate the diagnosis of diseases of animal origin. The scope of veterinary diagnostic imaging spans from small laboratory animals like mice to large wild animals like elephants, including pets, livestock animals and even birds. Although the subjects vary widely in veterinary imaging, the imaging systems are very similar to those used in human diagnostic imaging such as radiography, ultrasound imaging, thermal imaging, ECG, EEG, MRI, CT scanning and others. Necessary modification in instrumentation is often required to accommodate the variable size of the veterinary subjects and depending upon the target body parts to be introspected. Prioritizing the integrity of the "one health" concept, as nearly 70% of infectious disease are zoonotic in nature, and considering the growing human interaction with animals due to expansion in global trade and travel, climate change and alteration in biodiversity and changes in food habit due to urbanization, veterinary diagnostic imaging must be strengthened to secure animal health. Development of devoted instrumentations and skilled personnel in a cost-effective manner is the need of the hour for the more commonplace application of imaging techniques in veterinary disease diagnosis. Discussing all these diagnostic imaging techniques at length in one chapter is a daunting task. However, sincere efforts have been extended to accommodate various relevant veterinary imaging techniques and their applicability in animal subjects, as well as their advancements, limitations and future prospects, within the current chapter in a concise manner.

8.2 Microscopy

Microscopy deals with the use of microscopes to visualize an object which is beyond the resolution range of the naked eye. Microscopy is a versatile technique spanning across disciplines with various principles and modifications developed in unison in physics, chemistry, mathematics and engineering; for our purposes, however, it may still be discussed generally. While the underlying principle behind microscopy remains the same—that of illumination of a sample by waves, called primary waves here (electromagnetic, particle, sound), and the detection of waves left after the illumination, called secondary waves here—it may still be useful to categorize them on the basis of the nature of primary waves used as optical microscopy, including X-ray microscopy (electromagnetic), electron microscopy and scanning tunneling microscopy (particles, electrons) (Figure 8.2). The detection of waves resulting from illumination depends on whether the secondary waves are due to reflection, transmission, absorption-emission, scattering or diffraction of the original waves. In most cases, we are usually interested in only one of the many different types of secondary waves produced. In theory, multiple or even all of the aforementioned secondary waves may be generated during illumination; however, due to the rapid progress of instrumentation and material science as well as the development of sophisticated deconvolution approaches, it is possible to disentangle these various secondary waves and use this information to create a holistic picture of the object under study. The field of microscopy has indeed come very far from its humble origins that emerged out of the work of Janssen and his son in optical microscopy by assembling several lenses in a cylinder to achieve significant magnification, which was subsequently developed as a compound microscope. Subsequently, the field prospered through the contributions of two contemporary stalwarts, Robert Hooke and Antonie Philips van Leeuwenhoek. The prime focus until recent times was to increase the magnification and other developments in conventional optical microscopy, following the same path to reach the limit of spatial resolution by magnification. The limit of spatial resolution using light of the visible wavelength in optical microscopy is 0.2 μm, and visualization of objects smaller than this is beyond the limit, urging alternate strategies. Reducing the wavelength of the light source is an option, as is the use of a fast-moving electron beam which releases high-energy waves with shorter wavelengths to replace the conventional light source and increase the spatial resolution. From here, the transmission electron microscope (TEM) was conceptualized by the German scientists Max Knoll and Ernst Ruska in 1938, and the scanning electron microscope (SEM) was introduced by British scientist Charles Oatley in 1952 to usher in the age of electron microscopy. A spatial resolution up to 0.3 nm can be achieved through electron microscopy, expanding the scope to explore tiny objects like viruses. Scanning tunneling microscopy (STM) was introduced by Gerd Binning and Heinrich Rohrer in 1981, which works on an entirely different principle. Devoid of any lens, it exploits a quantum phenomenon called the "tunneling effect" to visualize an object. A probe is used, and a voltage is applied between the probe and the target object. When the probe and the object are nanometers apart, electrons start to jump from the probe to the object, resulting in a weak electronic current. The distance variation between the probe and different parts of the object leads to fluctuation in electronic current. This varying electric current can be mapped to the distance between the probe and object which, in turn, can be used to reproduce the spatial shape of an object with a spatial resolution limit of up to a single atom. Another branch of microscopy is X-ray microscopy, which also follows the principle that a decrease in wavelength increases the spatial resolution. X-ray microscopy employs electromagnetic radiation, typically a soft X-ray having a wavelength of 0.03–10 nm to achieve an optical resolution of nearly 20 nm. The incident wavelength and spatial resolution achieved in X-ray microscopy stands in between the ranges of visible light microscopy and electron microscopy.

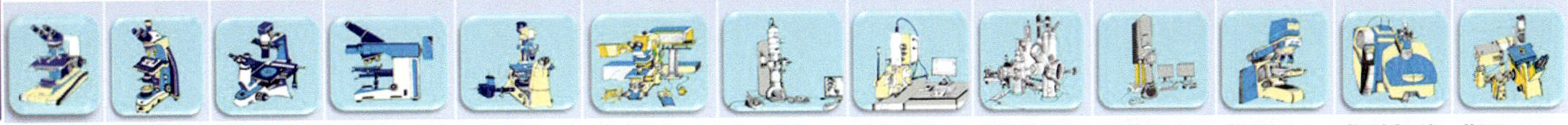

Points of variation / Type of Microscope	Compound	Dark Field	Phase Contrast	Fluorescent	Confocal	Two photon Microscope	TEM	SEM	STEM	Cryo-EM	Atomic force Microscope	Raman Microscope	X-ray Microscope
Energy Source	Visible light (Halogen/ LED/ Natural)	Visible light Halogen/ LED/Natural	Visible light Halogen/LED / Natural	Ultraviolet-Visible wave-length	Ultraviolet-Visible wave-length	Near Infrared (NIR)	Electron Beam of extremely short wavelength	Electron Beam of extremely short wavelength	Electron Beam of extremely short wavelength	Electron Beam of extremely short wavelength	Electron beam	Near Infrared (NIR)	X-ray
System between Source of energy and sample	Achromatic Condenser	Condenser lens to focus on the sample	Special condensers results into small phase shifts	LASER to go via excitation filter allowing light passage with a specific wavelength	LASER scanning precisely focuses the incident light onto a minute area	Pulsed near infrared LASER intensifies focus to specified area only	Electron beam pass through Electro-magnetic fields as lens to reach the section	Electron beam pass through electro-magnetic fields as lens to scan over tissue	Current is produced by tunneling of electrons between probe and the sample	Plunge frozen sample is subjected to electron beam	Scanning tip is made up of etched silicon attached to a cantilever moves over target surface	Energy exchange between incident light and molecular system	Imaging based on difference in absorption of soft X-rays
Sample	Sectioned, stained and mounted on slide	Unstained sample allows scattering of light	Transparent sample allows light to pass based upon varying speed	Specimen previously labeled with fluorescent dyes	Scanning the object at different focal plane by processing 2D Z-stacks/slices to get 3D data	Only excites the fluorophore of the target point to absorb and emit light to form the image	Ultrathin Sections (100 nm) are mounted on metallic grids	Tissue samples coated with metal & held on metallic stubs or metal coated coverslips	A piezoelectric tube attached to probe scans the target surface	Frozen-hydrated grid fixed samples at -173.1°C embedded in amorphous ice/vitreous water	3D Viewing of Non-conducting samples is possible with ease of sample preparation	Transmission, absorption and scattering of near-infrared alters photon frequency	Structures in natural dynamic state, no staining is required
Detector system	Eye lens and Digital display	Only Scattered light passes through objective lens for imaging	Transmitted & scattered light is converted into amplitude (brightness)	Fluorophore tagging allows specific cell type/target molecule identification	Sensitive detection (Photo-multiplier tube) is a must for successful imaging	Fluorophore is excited using two photons with half energy instead of one photon	Specific detectors, Sensors coupled with charge-coupled device (CCD) detector	Secondary electron detectors	Deviation in current flow is deconvoluted to form 3D image of the specimen surface	Specific detectors	Deflection perceived by tip is detected by LASER that is decoded to have AFM image	Raman spectra	Charge-coupled device (CCD) detector
Character istics	Needs staining	Finetunes contrast in unstained live objects	No staining is required	Better intracellular penetration but causes photobleaching & phototoxicity	Deep imaging up to 100 µm but higher illumination may damage live cells	Deep imaging up to 200 µm with reduced photobleaching and phototoxicity	2D Imaging with nano-scale (0.2-0.3nm) resolving power	3D Imaging with resolving power lesser than that of TEM	Depth resolution of 0.01nm can be achieved	Reduces electron beam mediated damage & restores the specimen	Helps in live cell imaging but resolution depends on sharpness of scanning tip	Labelfree, non -destructive but needs careful selection of wavelength	Minimal sample preparation, high spatial resolution & penetration

FIGURE 8.2 Introduction of different microscopes in veterinary imaging.

However, X-ray microscopy carries some advantages over conventional electron microscopy. For one, X-ray microscopy can image an object in its natural form, whereas chemical fixation, dehydration and ultra-thin slicing of a sample is a prerequisite for typical electron microscopy, with the possible exception of cryo-electron microscopy, which allows the imaging of biological samples in their hydrated form. Further insights have been provided regarding the branches and sub-branches of microscopy in the subsequent sections of this chapter (Figure 8.2).

8.2.1 Optical Microscopy

Optical or light microscopy is the most common and the earliest-developed microscopy technique, which employs light of visible wavelength to pass through the object or be reflected and channeled through a lens system for magnification, leading to visualization of the image on a suitable platform. The image can be captured on a photographic film or using a digital camera system. The source of light can be natural or artificial, but the wavelength must be in the visible range. A compound light microscope, working on this basic principle, is the most frequently used microscope in veterinary diagnostics. This has the advantages of low cost, a minimum of instrumentation, ease of operation and maintenance.

Optical microscopy has found application in almost every branch of veterinary science. This platform has been employed routinely for hematological analysis to diagnose anemia, polycythemia or infection by total WBC, RBC or platelet count. It is also used for differential leukocyte count, having diagnostic value in identifying the type of infection. It is indispensible for examination of blood smear and identification of hemoprotozoan diseases such as trypanosomiasis, theileriosis, babesiosis and anaplasmosis etc. Several parameters for semen quality estimation are performed through light microscopy, such as morphological analyses, sperm count, live and dead percentage, sperm motility etc. Microscopical examination is also compulsory for routine urine analyses to identify casts, crystals, bacteria and inflammatory cells in urine. Routine parasitological examinations include fecal egg count and the identification of endoparasite eggs, microscopic ectoparasites and protozoa which require optical microscopy. The utility of this platform in veterinary microbiology is quite predictable, such as for the examination of direct/indirect impression smears with staining for yeast, fungi, bacteria and cells, and smears for inflammatory or neoplastic cells, usually using specific stains. Similarly, light microscopy occupies center stage of histopathological examination for disease diagnosis using specific staining procedures. It can offer magnification from 40 to 1000 times, and is relatively inexpensive and easy to handle. However, in certain cases sample preparation is cumbersome or needs expertise, and a major drawback is the lack of automation to enhance sampling rates. Recent advancement in terms of automatic slide makers and stainers has reduced the uncertainty in sample preparation to some extent. Image acquisition and analysis has also improved recently. Nowadays, digital microscopes fitted with wide screens are used for better imaging, along with several free image analysis software options, which have not only helped in better diagnosis but also in establishing databanks for histopathology. Digitalization and the fast export of figures has also eased the opportunity to obtain expert views from an outstation on a case-by-case basis according to requirements. Software like ImageJ (https://imagej.nih.gov/ij) is useful in rotation, pointing, measurement of length and areas, histogram and profile plot creation; CellProfiler Analyst (https://cellprofiler.org/cp-analyst/) is another interactive program used for exploration, analysis and classification of large biological images and is hence helpful in the annotation of large, high-dimensional image-derived data. Large datasets generated from such software-based analyses can provide the scope to develop artificial intelligence (AI)-based programs in the near future. Neuron Studio (https://biii.eu/neuronstudio) is software for the 3D reconstruction of neurons from 3D confocal images. The program is very helpful in brain tissue imaging and provides morphology study tools for dendrites etc., but its algorithms have not been updated for a long time. L-measure (http://cng.gmu.edu:8080/Lm/help/index.htm) is another free open-access platform which can be used for neuronal reconstruction from brightfield or fluorescence microscopy data and helps in the measurement of volume, asymmetry, angle etc. Similarly, Icy is another open-access platform used to visualize, annotate and quantify images (www.bioimageanalysis.org), which can help in two-dimensional object identification and spot detection. Digimizer (www.digimizer.com/index.php) is freely available software for object detection and measurements. QuPath (https://qupath.github.io/) is a pathology image analysis software which is useful in the analysis of whole-slide images and can rapidly generate ultra-large 2D images. Aperio ImageScope (www.leicabiosystems.com/digital-pathology/manage/aperio-imagescope/) is another example of freely available image analysis software. Several paid programs are also available to digitize, analyze and share larger microscopic images, such as MetaferMetaSystems (https://metasystems-international.com/in/products/solutions/tissue-imaging/), Imaris (https://imaris.oxinst.com/) and Image-Pro (www.mediacy.com/pathology). These programs, with some free accessibility, can be used for analyzing percentage area of staining, color deconvolution, whole-slide analysis, identifying, quantifying and classifying nuclei etc., along with artificial learning platforms for histopathological analysis for better diagnostics. However, the utilization of such software-based advanced imaging platforms is mostly restricted to research purposes only, and their commonplace application in veterinary field diagnosis is still some time away. The development of devoted diagnostic image databases employing such advanced imaging platforms, much like nucleic acid and protein databases, would be very useful for veterinary disease diagnosis.

However, conventional optical microscopy carries some limitations, such as its limitation to facilitating efficient imaging of dark or strongly refracting objects only. For example, a live cell is colorless and transparent, lacking enough contrast to be imaged properly; thus, fixing the cell and staining are usually performed to attain sufficient contrast for effective visualization of the interior details of the cell. Moreover, the spatial resolution limit of 0.2 μm of optical microscopy and the reduction in image clarity arising from off-focus light are certain limitations of this platform. Therefore, improvements in contrast media or precise focusing to certain targeted structures of a sample have urged modification in the existing techniques and now several advanced imaging platforms based on optical microscopy are available; some of them are discussed below.

8.2.2 Dark-field Microscopy

The objective of dark-field microscopy is to enhance the contrast of an unstained translucent object. Here the incident light passes through the condenser lens to focus on the sample. Most of the light that falls on the sample is directly transmitted; only some portion gets scattered by the sample. Only the scattered light passes through the objective lens to form the image, while directly transmitted light is blocked. Hence, the object is seen on a dark background. It is a very simple but efficient technique to image live unstained objects and is used to observe live spirochetes, syphilis-causing organisms and other water-borne, single-celled organisms. In veterinary diagnostics, it is also a very simple method in the diagnosis of leptospirosis. The method is equally applicable in optical as well as electron microscopy. Some modification is also available which employs colored filters to get a stained image of an unstained object against a blue-white background. The low light intensity of a dark-field microscopy image is a major limitation and increasing illumination to get a brighter image can lead to sample damage. Further modifications in dark-field microscopy could provide smartphone-based dark-field microscopes for point-of-care (POC) detection of blood-cell disorders, and visualization of live bacteria, algae, mounted cells and tissues.

8.2.3 Phase-contrast Microscopy

Phase-contrast microscopy is a modified optical microscopy technique developed by Frits Zernike in the 1930s which earned the Nobel Prize in Physics in 1953. Light passing through special condensers results in small phase shifts, leading to light passing through a transparent specimen at different speeds ("out of phase"). These phase shifts in transmitted and scattered light are converted into amplitude (brightness) or contrast changes to construct the image; phase shifts are invisible but can be visualized if converted into brightness changes. Here, no staining is required; hence, live organisms and cells can be imaged, even down to sub-cellular level. It has found its application in the clinical diagnosis of nephrological disorders as a reliable and simple method (Racki *et al.*, 2003). Furthermore, it has been an excellent tool to identify localized sources of bleeding in hematuria cases by identifying dysmorphic and isomorphic red blood cells (Mohammad *et al.*, 1993). It has been successfully employed to diagnose Campylobacterenteritis through visualization of *Campylobacter jejuni* and related species along with red blood cells and neutrophils in fecal samples (Alberer *et al.*, 2017). Easy visualization of endospores is possible by phase-contrast microscopy, with its diagnostic importance for several endospore-forming bacteria, most importantly

Bacillus and Clostridium (Abel-Santos, 2015). Platelet count and tuberculosis identification can also be performed on this platform. The above are a few examples of the wide scope of the diagnostic importance of this imaging platform.

8.2.4 Polarized-light Microscopy

Polarized-light microscopy employs a polarizing plate to convert natural light into polarized light, which is used for illumination of the samples, particularly the birefringent specimens for optical microscopy-based imaging. This contrast-enhancing technique is helpful for the identification of optically anisotropic materials whose reflective index depends on polarized light and its propagation to yield differential imaging (Hershberger *et al.*, 1976). Polarization microscopy has been successfully used for serum analysis to diagnose metabolic disorders where various patterns have been identified with diagnostic importance, such as fan-type dendrites indicative of hyperoxaluria; druses and dendrite-like spherulites indicating hypercreatinemia; oolite spherulites indicative of hypercalcemia; fine-grained particles typical of hyperglycinemia; feather-like rays typical of hyperuricemia; and cross-like spherulites typical of hypercholesterolemia (Savina *et al.*, 2003). Similarly, gout and pseudogout have been successfully diagnosed through this technique (Judkins and Joanne, 1997). Malaria diagnosis using a mobile phone coupled with a polarized microscope has further depicted its application potential in the point-of-care diagnosis of different diseases (Pirnstill and Coté, 2015). Similarly, the technique has also produced better efficiency in the diagnosis of respiratory amyloidosis with respect to the conventional Congo red staining by detecting the contrasting yellow-green birefringence body (Ma *et al.*, 2015). It has also been employed for the diagnosis of silicosis (Goldsmith and Kopeloff, 1961).

8.2.5 Fluorescence Microscopy

White light generated from a light source like a xenon arc lamp, mercury-vapor lamp or high-power LEDs and lasers is passed through an exciter filter which allows the passage of light of a specific wavelength(s) (relevant to the absorption spectra of the fluorophore). A dichroic mirror positioned at an angle reflects the light of the specific wavelength(s) to fall on the specimen previously labeled with fluorescent dyes, such as acriflavine, acridine orange, acridine yellow, thioflavine S etc. The light is absorbed by the fluorophore(s), followed by emission of light of longer wavelength(s) by them. The emitted light reaches an emission filter or barrier filter which allows passage of only the light of specific wavelength(s) (relevant to the emission spectra of the fluorophore) to form the image. This is a powerful specific as well as sensitive technique where a fluorophore tagged with antibodies or DNA or RNA can be used to bind its cognate counterpart in the specimen facilitating identification of specific cell types, autoantigens, microorganisms or target molecules. Besides target identification, it can also be used to trace the intra-cellular localization of any target molecule. It can be applied for both living as well as fixed non-living cells. Immuno-histochemistry using fluorescent labeled antibody, chemical staining where targeted chemicals are labeled with fluorochrome and fluorescent DNA aptamers are the most common techniques employed for disease diagnosis using fluorescence microscopy (Musumeci *et al.*, 2017). The platform has helped immensely in cancer research and diagnosis (Martínez *et al.*, 2014). Modified methods based on this principle, such as conventional and widefield epifluorescence microscopy, florescence resonance energy transfer microscopy, confocal microscopy and total internal reflection fluorescence microscopy, have found wide application in life sciences, including in the visualization of living cell markers and dynamicity, tracking up- or down-regulation of signaling pathway molecules related to disease etc. (Daniel *et al.*, 2011). Nonlinear structured-illumination microscopy is a modified wide-field microscopy technique using a single laser for intensity and requiring no scanning, which can experimentally achieve 2D point resolution of less than 50 nm (Gustafsson *et al.*, 2005). Further, using various fluorescence-based material and software, a number of molecules can be imaged at a time, which is very handy for identifying the physiological status of a target cell or tissue and the detection of multiple antigens simultaneously (Daniel *et al.*, 2011). Theoretically, numerous multiplexing is possible in florescence-based methods, but practically only a limited number of fluorophores are used at a time, which have distinct immunofluorescence wavelength. It is advantageous over phase-contrast and differential interference-contrast microscopy for live cell imaging as it has better penetration inside the cell to explore stained intracellular organelles or microorganisms. However, only fluorescent-labeled structures can be visualized. Fluorescence-induced photobleaching and phototoxicity are certain other limitations of fluorescence-based platforms. Some of the modifications of conventional fluorescence microscopy intended toward better resolution or sensitivity are discussed below.

8.2.5.1 Confocal Microscopy

This technique was first conceptualized by Minsky in 1950 to overcome the drawback of standard epifluorescence microscopy where blurring of the image occurs from out-of-focus light arising from outside the focal plane during imaging at high magnifications or in cases of thick sections. Confocal microscopy using laser scanning precisely focuses the incidence light onto a minute area of the target specimen, and the emitted light passes through a pinhole which allows only the light from the specific focal plane to form the image, blocking the blurring effect of out-of-focus lights. Scanning the object at a different focal plane can assist in forming a 3D-reconstructed image of the specimen. Confocal microscopy can achieve penetration of about 100 μm inside the tissue section. However, as the pinhole allows only a fraction of light to pass through, powerful illumination of the sample is essential for successful imaging on this platform, which poses the threat of damaging the live cells being monitored (Daniel *et al.*, 2011). Spinning-disk microscopy is an advanced confocal microscopy platform for routine as well as high-performance fast imaging of dynamic events in living cells on a timescale basis (http://zeiss-campus.magnet.fsu.edu/articles/spinningdisk/introduction.html).

8.2.5.2 Two-photon Microscopy

Two-photon microscopy is a modified fluorescence microscopy platform whereby instead of using one photon for excitation of fluorophore, two photons with half-energy are used. As the simultaneous absorption of two photons is rare, thus a pulsed infrared laser which is precisely focused on a particular point of the specimen only excites the fluorophore of that target point to absorb and emit light to form the image. Fluorophores outside the focal plane are not excited to emit any light. Thus, the limitations of fluorescence-induced photobleaching and phototoxicity can be restricted, while the problems of blurring effects due to out-of-focus light can also be surmounted. The platform is advantageous in live cell imaging, with deeper penetration into tissue as a result of infrared excitation than the visible or ultraviolet light used for confocal or conventional epifluorescence microscopy, thus facilitating deep-tissue imaging to a depth of about 200 μm into the section, which is even beyond the scope of confocal microscopy, and hence also provides better resolution. Phototherapy for cancer and macular degeneration, *in vivo* imaging of neuronal structure and activity, deep-tissue imaging for immune cell dynamics and *in vivo* fluid transport analyses are the major applications in which it has been employed (Benninger and Piston, 2013; Mostany *et al.*, 2014). However, the high cost of the pulsed laser is still an impediment for commonplace application of the technique.

Wide-field multiphoton microscopy is also an optical non-linear imaging technique employing an optically amplified pulsed laser source to achieve high intensities without requiring scanning. The technique can acquire images of a large area of the specimen at 1000-fold increased frame rates as compared to multiphoton scanning microscopy; however, image quality is drastically reduced with increasing depth of the cross-section.

4Pi microscopy is another modified fluorescence microscopy technique whereby resolution in the Z plane is enhanced by increasing the angular aperture which facilitates 3D imaging of the target specimen. Similarly, spatially modulated illumination microscopy and near-field scanning optical microscopy are other advanced techniques with the potential of disease diagnosis by revealing sub-cellular details along with protein structure, localization and dynamics, tissue-level structural and functional changes to elucidate the structure-function relationships corresponding to disease establishment and progression.

8.2.6 Electron Microscopy

Instead of visible light (wavelength range 400–800 nm), the electron microscopy (EM) technique employs an electron beam with an extremely short wavelength (0.0037–0.0086 nm), thus producing high-resolution images as energy. The resolving power of optical microscopy is 200 nm, whereas it can reach up to 0.3 nm in electron microscopy. Magnification can reach up to 2000x in optical microscopy, whereas the same can reach up to 1,000,000x in electron microscopy (Roane and Pepper, 2015). These properties help to visualize even optically invisible specimens, leading to great application in the diagnosis of viruses and intracellular molecules. Varieties of ancillary techniques like sectioning, immunolabeling and negative staining along with some technical variations have made it yet more versatile, and it has broadly sub-branched into several platforms such as scanning EM (SEM), transmission EM (TEM) and cryogenic EM.

8.2.6.1 Scanning Electron Microscopy

In this platform, a focused electron beam scans the specimen surface and interacts with the sample atoms to produce several signals such as secondary electrons, reflected or back-scattered electrons, X-rays along with electrons and photons of various energies, which are captured by specific detectors. Secondary electron detectors are common in all the SEM instruments along with the other additional detectors. Such signals derived from various depths of the specimen are used to produce the three-dimensional surface image of the specimen. Secondary electrons possess low energies (~50 eV), thus having poor penetration and being restricted to the surface, as well as highly localized, corresponding to the impact of the primary electron beam. Therefore, a surface image with an optical resolution of below 1 nm can be achieved using this platform. The minimum sample preparation required and obtaining a high-resolution, three-dimensional image of the surface of a target specimen are the key advantages of this platform, rendering it a valuable diagnostic tool for routine morphological examination in microbiological samples. Furthermore, application of "wet-SEM" in sample preparation overcomes the limitation of contrast and dehydration-related shrinkage, distortion and collapse of the target sample. Hindrance in high magnification due to the charging of small organic particles (bacteria and viruses) has also been overcome by application of ionic liquid (1-butyl-3-methylimidazolium tetrafluoroborate) and indium-tin oxide, aluminum foil or metal-coated coverslips which act as a conducting surface to prevent charging. These modifications in conventional SEM have helped in the diagnosis of *Leptospira biflexa*, *Salmonella Senftenberg*, vaccinia and the Ebola virus (Golding *et al.*, 2016) in a rapid and reproducible manner. Fungal diseases like onychomycosis caused by dermatophyte, *Candida* or non-dermatophyte mold have been very effectively diagnosed by SEM, even in cases where conventional diagnostics like the use of KOH and fungal culture techniques have given a negative result (Yue *et al.*, 2018). Further, investigation of biofilm chemistry, dental and orthodontic microbiology, changes in cell shape and surface molecules during key biological processes, systematic and taxonomic parasitology, respiratory and gastrointestinal inflammatory disorders and developmental biology are the key areas of potential SEM intervention (Jáuregui *et al.*, 2012). SEM equipped with energy dispersive X-ray spectroscopy (EDS) is useful in forensic diagnosis, particularly suspected electrocution, analyses of mineral bioaccumulation and bioremediation in environmental pollution and heavy-metal toxicity study (Scimeca *et al.*, 2018; Visonà *et al.*, 2018).

8.2.6.2 Transmission Electron Microscopy

Transmission electron microscopy (TEM) projects a beam of electrons through an ultrathin section (usually below 100 nm) of a specimen which interacts with the specimen molecules to produce a two-dimensional image which is subsequently magnified and captured on a fluorescent screen, photographic film or sensor coupled with a charge-coupled device (CCD). It is extremely sensitive, reliable and widely used for imaging microbial samples in viral and bacterial disease diagnosis. The ample magnification power and excellent resolution provide the opportunity to explore the minute structural detail of the moieties even at the sub-cellular level, which may be very helpful in elucidating virus-host interaction and providing insight about pathogenesis and therapeutic opportunities. TEM can be operated in several modes, such as conventional, scanning TEM (STEM), diffraction, spectroscopy and their combinations, depending upon the requirements. The very low requirements concerning samples are a certain advantage inherent to the platform. Several means have been employed to produce satisfactory contrast in TEM imaging. Negative staining using copper or nickel grids having several contrast chemicals such as ammonium molybdate, methylamine tungstate, sodium silicotungstate, phosphotunstic acid (PTA) and uranyl acetate (heavy-metal salts) are being used for diagnostic purposes. Several viruses, including but not limited to coronavirus, rotavirus, adenovirus, astrovirus, parvovirus, herpes virus from infectious bovine rhinotracheitis and Aujeszky's disease, flavivirus from bovine viral diarrhea, bacteriophages, picnorna virus, reovirus, rubella virus, yellow fever virus, influenza virus, Ebola virus and feline calicivirus (Maxie, 2016) have been identified from various samples such as feces, body fluids, secretions, pathological lesions, crusts etc. (Palmer and Martin, 1988). Similarly, several bacterial diseases of veterinary importance like Leptospira, mycoplasma etc. can also be identified on morphological basis by this method (Catroxo and Martins, 2015). Antigen-antibody-based immunoelectron microscopy is another TEM method, first employed by Derrick (1973) in plant virus diagnosis, which produces excellent results in very low sample availability and in identifying contaminating antigens and/or antibodies. However, it has the disadvantage of taking more time, in excess of an hour, against the 10–15 minutes of sample preparation required in negative staining, but sensitivity increases 100-fold. Several viruses, such as flavivirus, rotavirus, poxvirus, paramyxovirus and parvovirus have also been successfully identified using this method. Another extension is an antigen-coated grid technique to coat the virus called the decoration technique, whereby a carbon grid is coated or incubated with a virus-specific antibody to trap the antigen in suspension. This is basically a positive staining technique used to diagnose very small viruses or bacteria like Leptospira. Similarly, specimens embedded in hydrophobic resin and immuno-labeled with colloidal gold particles are also used for the detection of microorganisms and identification of immunolocalization of proteins or antigens in a tissue section employing TEM. Aptamer-based TEM diagnosis is the future of TEM, as it will further enhance the range of diagnosis with high confirmation and can have potential applications in epidemiological studies, as well as diagnosis. Along with rigorous sample processing, the requirement of high concentrations of microbes or virus particles is another drawback of negative staining TEM, as the organisms need to be adsorbed to a thin support film (Golding *et al.*, 2016).

Both SEM and TEM are invaluable EM techniques, but the choice between them depends upon the requirement of the investigator. If the target is to explore information regarding the inner structure of the tissue or cells, such as their crystal structure, morphology, sub-cellular localization etc., then TEM is the choice, whereas SEM provides information regarding the surface of the target sample, like roughness, abundance or contamination etc. In SEM, acceleration voltages up to 30 kV are usually employed; whereas in TEM, they can be in the range of 60–300 kV. The spatial resolution achievable through SEM is limited to ~0.5 nm, whereas TEM can yield spatial resolution of even less than 50 pm. Magnification over 50 million times can be achieved in TEM, whereas it is restricted to 1–2 million times for SEM. SEM generates a 3D image of the specimen surface, whereas TEM produces 2D images of the sample. Due to its larger field of view (FOV), a broader area of sample surface can be scanned by SEM than the very small part of specimen that can be imaged by TEM. Sample preparation for TEM analysis is complex, cumbersome and skill-intensive, with sections having to be very thin, preferably below 150 nm, and below 30 nm for obtaining high-resolution TEM images. In contrast, SEM requires little sample preparation and no such thickness criteria have been ascribed for SEM samples (Ruska, 1980; McMullan, 2006; Antonis, 2019).

8.2.6.3 Cryogenic Electron Microscopy

Cryogenic electron microscopy (cryoEM) is one of the most recent variants of EM, judged the Technology of the Year in 2016 by *Nature Methods* and yielded the Nobel Prize in Chemistry in 2017 to Jacques Dubochet, Joachim Frank and Richard Henderson for developing the platform, with its enormous potential applications. It provides an alternative to X-ray crystallography or NMR spectroscopy for elucidating the macromolecular structure particularly of proteins in solution without requiring crystallization. The method employs imaging of frozen-hydrated samples at cryogenic temperatures (usually 100 kelvin or

-173.1ºC) by electron microscopy, reducing electron-beam-mediated sample damage. In this technique the samples are cooled to cryogenic temperatures and embedded in an environment of amorphous ice/vitreous water. Amorphous ice is a non-crystalline ice which is produced during ultra-fast cooling of liquid water, as rapid cooling does not allow enough time for the formation of the crystalline lattice. Overall, a small droplet of aqueous sample solution is applied to the hydrophilic carbon surface of an EM grid-mesh and plunge-frozen in liquid ethane or a mixture of liquid ethane and propane, followed by EM imaging. Plunge-freezing restores the specimens to their native state, quenching all the motions and metabolic activities without requiring any dyes or fixatives, facilitating the introspection of cellular ultra-structures, cell organelles, viruses and protein complexes at molecular level. Atomic characterization of amyloid filaments have been performed recently for the diagnosis of neurodegenerative disorders such as Alzheimer's and Parkinson's diseases, which has widened the scope of this platform as a future diagnostic technique (Fitzpatrick *et al.*, 2017; Guerrero-Ferreira *et al.*, 2018). Assessment of environmental pollution and characterization of mineral bioaccumulation is another application of this platform (Scimeca *et al.*, 2019). Besides identification of viruses and bacteria, the platform facilitates visualization of the process of virus entry and exit from mammalian cells to explore virus-host interaction and the viral infection cycle (Dillard *et al.*, 2018). The integration of cryoEM with other atomic and molecular interaction data can be more beneficial in terms of reliability and authenticity. Titan Krios™ is a recently introduced platform which integrates fluorescence and cryoEM at the same time in a single, controlled environment. This has been acclaimed as the world's most powerful microscope, which facilitates three-dimensional sample observation at very high resolution under similar-to-natural conditions with unparalleled accuracy (www.pasteur.fr/en/research-journal/news/titan-krios-tm-inauguration-world-s-most-powerful-microscope-institut-pasteur).

Electron microscopy provides rapid morphological identification of an infectious organism along with differential diagnosis, but it is not well suited for the screening of large numbers of samples; future automation may overcome the limitation. Rather, it would be wiser to employ this platform in critical situations such as for the fast detection of a bioterrorism agent or in countering pandemics through early and rapid pathogen detection. But effective application of diagnostic electron microscopy must be quality-controlled and corroborated with parallel diagnostic techniques (Hazelton and Gelderblom, 2003).

8.2.7 Scanning Probe Microscopy

This non-optical electron-based microscopy technique employs a probe tip to scan the specimen surface, producing a three-dimensional picture of the surface and surface-confined structures at Angstrom-level resolution. This branch of microscopy was developed based on the invention of scanning tunneling microscopy (STM), pioneered by Binnig and Rohrer in 1981, which earned them the Nobel Prize in Physics in 1986. A voltage is passed through the probe tip when it is very close (at Angstrom level) to the target surface. An electrical current is produced due to the tunneling of electrons between the probe and the sample. The tip, attached to a piezoelectric tube, scans the target surface and the deviation in current flow is monitored as a function of their relative position, which is deconvoluted to form a 3D image of the specimen surface.

Atomic force microscopy (AFM) is probably the most commonly employed scanning probe microscopy technique in biological applications due to its easy operation and versatility. Here, the scanning tip, usually made of etched silicon, is attached to a cantilever which moves across the target surface, and the deflection due to the attractive and repulsive forces perceived by the tip originating from the surface topology is recorded using a laser beam. The laser movement is decoded to generate an AFM image. The image resolution is highly dependent on the sharpness of the tip, which is undergoing continuous upgradation to improve the image quality.

The platforms confer important advantages as the biological samples can be imaged in solution form and in near-physiological condition. Although the platforms are not in routine use for diagnostic imaging, they have been successfully employed to explore membrane dynamics, for the imaging of cellular systems and even intracellular features, microtubules, along with surface properties, the imaging of DNA and proteins, nanofabrication etc. AFM has been used in the imaging of live cells along with cytoskeletons, ion channels, chromatin and plasmids and diverse membranes. The monitoring of several dynamic processes, such as the growth and polymerization of fibrinogen as well as the alteration of certain physicochemical properties like elasticity and viscosity within live cells, has been performed using this technique (Lal and John, 1994; Bonnell, 2001; Davis, 2005) (https://analyticalscience.wiley.com/do/10.1002/imaging.2696/full).

8.2.8 X-ray Microscopy

The technique employs a soft X-ray band as electromagnetic radiation to magnify the image of a target object, which is captured using photographic film or a charge-coupled device (CCD) detector as it cannot be visualized with the naked eye due to the non-reflecting and non-refracting nature of X-rays. It has excellent penetrative power and thus no special sample preparation is required. It relies upon contrast imaging based on the difference in absorption of soft X-rays at a particular range of the electromagnetic spectrum where water remains transparent to X-rays while carbon and other organic molecules absorb it. This particular region of the electromagnetic spectrum (wavelengths: 2.34–4.4 nm; energies: 280–530 eV) is known as the water window region. Soft X-rays are specifically used for soft-tissue imaging because such a differential absorption pattern is only shown by soft X-rays, with their lower energy and thus longer wavelengths than hard X-rays, which possess higher-energy photons (above 5–10 keV). Hard X-rays thus penetrate all soft tissues and produce no contrast, making them unsuitable for the X-ray microscopy imaging of soft tissues. After the discovery of X-rays by Röntgen in 1895, they found application in microscopy and finally formed the basis of commercial X-ray microscopy with the conceptualization of shadow X-ray microscopy by Sterling Newberry in the 1950s. Subsequently, several chronological advancements have been introduced to conventional X-ray microscopy for the better suitability of this platform in various scientific arenas such as environmental and soil sciences, chemistry, material sciences and magnetism, including biology. Beamline 2.1 (XM-2) is an advanced transmission soft X-ray microscope, probably the first such microscope to be dedicated to biological and biomedical applications, which was developed by the scientists from the National Center for X-ray Tomography, Advanced Light Source (ALS), Berkeley, California. The platform possesses a cryogenic 360° rotation stage for the acquisition of tomographic data from cryo-preserved cells to obtain a 3D-tomographic image on a CCD detector (Le Gros *et al.*, 2014).

The technique is helpful in visualizing the fine structures of the natural dynamic state of living cells, which is beyond the scope of simple staining, PCR or conventional electron microscopy-based methods of diagnosis. Furthermore, the property of X-ray microscopy of imaging both internal and external morphologies with minimal sample preparation, high spatial resolution and high penetration power helps to attain resolution even in thicker samples for hydrated specimens, which provides some extra edge over conventional light- and electron-microscopy-based pathology or morphology study. There are multiple variants of X-ray microscopy based on energy used and the modulation of other properties. In biology, mostly soft energy-based X-rays under 1 keV with an approximate wavelength range of 1–10 nm are applied, with two major aims: to visualize morphology using full-field transmission and to extract physiological information through scanning in 2D or 3D mode. However, integrating the cellular and molecular data from X-ray microscopy with other modalities such as fluorescence microscopy or spectromicroscopy is preferable to obtain the best results (Weinhardt *et al.*, 2019). It can be used for analyzing red blood cells' morphological alteration in different pathological states and based on shape deviation; disease status can be categorized into "none", "mild", "moderate" and "severe" as done for sickle cell anemia. Similarly, cell size and volume, lipid bodies, mitochondria, vacuoles, nucleus and nucleolus can be recognized, with potential value in disease diagnosis, cell proliferation and morphological alterations. Furthermore, the localization of heavy metals is another area of diagnosis which can employ this technique. However, the technique requires radiation shielding to minimize radiation effects, thermal management for the cooling of instrumentation to avoid damage from high-energy photons, slit and shutter management for controlled scattering, monochromators and bandwidth considerations to maximize contrast, and comes with issues concerning vacuums, contamination and the cleaning of surfaces, requiring special care for the avoidance of any hazards.

8.2.9 Raman Microscopy

Raman microscopy is a fast, label-free, non-destructive method whereby energy exchange between the incident light and molecular system generates alterations in photon frequency which can be recorded for Raman-based imaging. It is based on the principle that transmission, absorption and scattering of near-infrared (NIR) laser light on interaction with biomolecules either through elastic or inelastic collision in aqueous environments can generate scattering over a small range of wave numbers, known as Raman shifts, discovered in 1928 by the Indian physicist Sir C.V. Raman. These Raman shifts, characteristic for specific biomolecules, can be imaged to find distribution of the specific biomolecule in cells or a particular area of a specimen in a label-free manner. The distribution of several biomolecules such as proteins, nucleic acids, cholesterol and fatty acids has been observed in cell cultures or tissue specimens. Raman microscopy can be integrated with several other microscopic imaging platforms such as confocal and inverted confocal Raman imaging, fluorescence microscopy, scanning electron microscopy (SEM) and atomic force microscopy (AFM) for the high-resolution imaging of various biological samples. Biological application of confocal Raman microscopy gained momentum from around 1990 onwards, when Puppels *et al.* recorded Raman spectra of single human cells and polytene chromosomes (Puppels *et al.*, 1990). Subsequently, confocal Raman imaging, which amalgamates confocal microscopy with Raman spectroscopy along with other imaging platforms, has been employed for cancer cell imaging, identification of biomolecules having diagnostic values, bacterial characterization, chemical characterization of tissues such as skin melanoma tissue, brain tissue etc. (Da Costa *et al.*, 2018; Morris and Payne, 2019). Confocal Raman microscopy in combination with confocal reflectance, and quantitative phase microscopy have provided insight into hemozoin and hemoglobin distribution for morphological screening in malaria and different blood disorders (Kang *et al.*, 2011). Recently, Raman-based imaging techniques have gained importance in the research and diagnosis of neurodegenerative disorders such as Alzheimer's disease, Huntington's disease, Parkinson's disease, prion diseases, etc. (Devitt *et al.*, 2018). However, limitations such as cost intensity, the standardization of background removal and the generation of Raman spectra in the perspective of several livestock diseases need to be surmounted for widespread application of the technique in veterinary diagnosis.

8.2.10 Magnetic Resonance Microscopy (MRM)

Magnetic resonance microscopy follows the same principle of magnetic resonance imaging (MRI), which is more popular in clinical diagnosis. However, MRI deals with larger subjects like the entire body of an animal with resolution around 1 mm, whereas MRM investigates microscopic specimens with voxel resolution better than 100 μm or even smaller, to 10 μm (Mendonca and Lauterbur, 1987). MRM is a versatile, non-ionizing and non-invasive diagnostic imaging platform, which can offer a better option to visualize the internal structures of target biological objects, where the scope of conventional optical or electron microscopy may be limited by issues of penetration, poor endogenous contrast, opacity of the specimen, radiation and phototoxicity hazards etc., because MRM is not influenced by sample thickness or opacity and only relies upon the magnetic field strength (Fong *et al.*, 2018). The platform provides 3D imaging of internal structures of living cells or tissue specimens with minimal sample preparation. Different endogenous or exogenous tissue contrasts can be exploited through various available MRM modalities for diverse histological imaging. For example, variable tissue compositions containing iron, plaques or fibers can provide endogenous contrast, while iron- and gadolinium-based contrast agents or marking with magnetic dye can offer exogenous contrast for *in-vivo* cellular or tissue imaging to explore several biochemical, physiological and pathological processes (Bulte *et al.*, 2002; Lee *et al.*, 2017). However, MRM encounters some major bottlenecks for routine practical applications, such as how attaining better resolution in MRM images require an ultra-high magnetic field gradient focused on a smaller area, which is difficult to generate using conventional radio frequency (RF) coils. Second, sensitivity has to be increased enormously to improve the resolution from 1 mm of MRI to 10 μm or lower in MRM, otherwise the signal will be very weak (Johnson *et al.*, 1992). Significant progress has been made to overcome those challenges and has opened the arena for the diverse application of this imaging platform, ranging from neurobiology to cancer biology and from histology to toxicology (Cho *et al.*, 1992; Jacobs and Fraser, 1994; Johnson *et al.*, 1992; Zhou and Lauterbur, 1992). Further, the platform facilitates the introspection of embryonic development in mice in a non-invasive manner. The pathological features of human brain tumor tissue have been identified using MRM imaging (Gonzalez *et al.*, 2011). Single mouse myofibers and myonuclei have been successfully imaged using MRM with 6-μm resolution, which can be exploited to differentiate healthy and myopathic cells (Lee *et al.*, 2017).

8.2.11 Super-resolution Microscopy

This is an umbrella term encompassing several advanced optical microscopy techniques developed precisely to resolve the resolution limit of conventional light microscopy arising from the diffraction of light. According to the Abbe diffraction limit, a conventional optical microscope can achieve a resolution limit of up to approximately 200 nm using the visible light spectrum. Employing shorter-wavelength light such as ultraviolet (UV) or X-rays is an option to increase the resolution, but due to their damaging effect on biological samples, the scope for live-cell imaging is restricted. Super-resolution optical microscopy techniques rely upon near-field or far-field microscopy to provide much better resolution and evidently overcome the limitation of damaging effects of shorter-wavelength light. Photon tunneling microscopy (PTM), structured illumination microscopy (SIM), near-field optical random mapping (NORM) microscopy, 4Pi microscopy, stimulated emission depletion microscopy (STED), RESOLFT microscopy and single-molecule localization microscopy (SMLM) are a few examples of techniques which provide super-resolution images of cells, intra-cellular organelles, cell-cycle dynamics, chromatin structure etc. Although these advanced techniques are yet to be used for routine diagnosis and are thus beyond the scope of detailed discussion in the current context, they definitely hold the potential for replacing conventional microscopy techniques. For instance, the application of electron microscopy in the routine diagnosis of kidney disorders, kidney cancer and hematological diseases can be replaced with SIM microscopy. The application of fluorophores is crucial to several such super-resolution imaging techniques. In 2014, the Noble Prize in Chemistry was awarded to Eric Betzig, W.E. Moerner and Stefan Hell for bringing "optical microscopy into the nanodimension" through the advent of super-resolved fluorescence microscopy. Thus, with the introduction of nanoscopy, the limitations of diffraction and resolution restrictions in conventional optical microscopy have come to an end. These techniques have wide biological applications such as in live-cell imaging to analyze microtubular dynamics in different growth conditions, the imaging of intra-golgi apparatus proteins, identifying protein distributions in cytosol and nuclei etc. DNA points accumulation for imaging in nanoscale topography (DNA-PAINT)-based super-resolution microscopy have facilitated considerable multiplexing, accurate molecule counting and ultra-high, sub-5-nm spatial resolution, achieving ~1-nm localization precision. The modality relies upon transient complementary binding of dye-labeled oligonucleotides to their target, producing an imaging signal (Schnitzbauer *et al.*, 2017). Laser-based single-particle tracking photoactivated localization microscopy (sptPALM) and direct stochastic optical reconstruction microscopy (dSTORM) on a modified inverted microscope have revealed nonaxonemal dynamics of intraflagellar transport proteins in live human retinal pigment epithelial cells (Yang *et al.*, 2019). Basically, single particle tracking relies on scatterers, nanoparticles or fluorescent tags to generate signals related to molecular localization. Nanoparticles like quantum dots can be used as alternatives to fluorescent dyes and proteins, and are superior to the currently used resources in terms of brightness and stability but are difficult to integrate into the biological system. Protein labeled with ATTO655 organic fluorophore using a trimethoprim chemical tag has facilitated dSTORM imaging of living HeLa cells to elucidate the dynamics of histone H2B protein at ~20-nm resolution (Wombacher *et al.*, 2010). MINFLUX nanoscopy is another mode of super-resolution fluorescence microscopy which has achieved resolutions in the range of 1 to 3 nm, and can be suitable for the imaging of protein complexes and their distributions in fixed as well as living cells (Gwosch *et al.*, 2020). Routine applications of these advanced imaging techniques may also not be too far off in clinical diagnosis (Thorley *et al.*, 2014; Schermelleh *et al.*, 2019).

8.3 Ultrasonography/Diagnostic Sonography

Ultrasonography/diagnostic sonography is one of the most popular, reliable and convenient diagnostic imaging techniques in veterinary practice, having several advantages over other imaging modalities (Figure 8.3). It facilitates non-invasive real-time imaging of internal organs and soft tissues. Due to its portable instrumentation, sonography can be brought animal-side, which promotes its field-level application. Pulses of sound waves with frequencies beyond the audible range (the audible frequency range is 20 Hz–20 KHz) are directed to the soft tissues through a probe which is reflected to be recorded for sonographic imaging. No ionizing radiation is used and thus the technique is free from such hazards. Although patient cooperation is desirable, it can be performed in animals without sedation. It is also inexpensive in relation to other advanced imaging techniques such as computerized axial tomography scanning and magnetic resonance imaging. Generally, sound wave frequency in the range of 1–18 megahertz (MHz) is used for medical imaging; however, a lower frequency (3–5 MHz) can be used for better penetration for deep-tissue imaging.

The basic components of ultrasonography include a central processing unit (CPU), a transducer probe, a monitor along with keyboard or cursor, disk storage devices and a printer. The CPU is equipped to control the output by manipulating power, gain/reject control, time gain compensation (TGC), persistence sector, angle and depth control for obtaining better resolution in sonographic imaging. The transducer probe is the most important component of the ultrasound assembly, which generates and emits sound waves in a series of pulses and also receives the echoed-off sound after interaction with the tissues through the piezoelectric effect. One or more piezoelectric crystals in the transducer generate vibration due to rapid shape change when an electric current is applied, producing a series of pulsed ultrasound waves. Subsequently, the sound waves are propagated to the target tissues and echo off from the tissues to be reflected back to the transducer. The piezoelectric crystals receive the echoed sound or pressure waves which hit them to emit electrical current, which is recorded as a sonogram for visualization on the display. Transducers may be mechanical with two to four crystals, on the rim of a rotating wheel or an array of crystals as the electronic probe in which the orientation of the firing arrangement determines the shape of view to be generated; a linear array produces a rectangular image, while a curvilinear array generates a trapezoid image and a phased array yields a sector-beam shaped image. Usually, linear-array transducers operate at higher frequencies (5–15 MHz), resulting in a limited field of view (FOV), and are thus generally used for the imaging of superficial structures such as eyes, joints, surface muscles and peripheral blood vessels etc. Curvilinear array transducers generally operate at lower frequencies (2–5 MHz) and are thus used for visualizing deeper structures and organs such as kidney, liver, spleen, urinary bladder etc. Phased array transducers operate at typically low frequencies (1–5 MHz) facilitating sector scan imaging with a wider FOV through a small acoustic window, suitable for intra-thoracic imaging. The software used for image analysis records echo strength, direction and the time required to return after the generation of a pulse, to assist in better interpretation for diagnosis (Bronzino, 2000; Mudry *et al.*, 2003).

Ultrasonography (USG) can be carried out in different display modes. A (amplitude), B (brightness) and M (motion) mode, along with Doppler-mode, are the commonly employed modes for ultrasound imaging. Different types of images are produced through employing specific modes and corresponding programs according to the requirements. A-mode, or amplitude mode, is the oldest and simplest mode, producing a series of peaks on a graph corresponding to the depth of the internal structures from which the sound waves are echoed off; an increase in returning echo leads to a simultaneous increase in peak. This is generally used for non-moving tissues; for instance, subcutaneous fat in animals, more precisely in pigs, can be diagnosed as indicative of obesity. B-mode ultrasonography is the most commonly employed visualization mode as it gives bright pixels or dots on screen which help in the visualization of a two-dimensional (2D) image of the area of target organs for diagnostic purposes. Here, dot intensity corresponds to depth at which the echo was formed and the amplitude of returning echo determines the brightness of the dots. M-mode helps in projecting an echo from a thin slice of tissue over a period of time and gives the impression of video ultrasound imaging. This mode facilitates the detection of organ structure movement and has thus gained importance in cardiac disease diagnosis as it can be useful for monitoring heart valve and wall movement and size of chamber access (Suri *et al.*, 2008).

Technique / Points of variation	Energy used to diagnose	Source of energy	Receiving system	Visualize system	Applicability	Limitations
Ultrasonography	Ultrasound (1-18 megahertz (MHz)	By piezo crystal	By piezo crystal transducer probe	CPU under different mode	Soft tissues imaging, more frequently use in reproductive system, no ionizing radiation	Air and water filled ,hard tissue like bone hinder quality
Digital stethoscope	Audible sound (20-20000Hz)	Stethoscope diaphragm	Bluetooth	Computer or mobile with algorithm software	Identification and documentation of disease-specific signature frequency sound	Still frequency not standardized for different diseases
Endoscopy	Visual light	Bulb at tip	Camera with optical system	Screen or Computer	Gastrointestinal and other bleeding, dysphagia, unusual symptom based pain, cancer	Need larger variation, camera should not be soiled
Thermal imaging	Infrared (Far and near)	The animal body	Camera with IR detector	Screen of camera with algorithm software	Behavior problem, Heat stress	For outer body diagnosis only, water vapor, gases, and carbon dioxide (CO_2) level, aerosols amount and distance from animal influence the imaging quality
X-ray/ Fluoroscopy	X-ray (5 and 150 keV)	Rotating anode x-ray tube	Light-sensitive negative x-ray–sensitive screens/ film	Screen of computer with algorithm software	Hard tissue like bone, teeth, calcification	Need precautionary measures regarding exposer time and dose
Magnetic Resonance Imaging (MRI)	Magnetic force of 0.2 and 1.5 Tesla	Bore of the magnet producing nuclear magnetic moment (radio wave) by odd number of proton or neutron molecule	Radio frequency detector	Screen of computer with algorithm software	Non invasive zero radiation hazard for brain, heart, lungs, spine, knees, wrist etc.	Costly, still limited use in veterinary, restraining using anaesthesia is a must
Computed tomography (CT)	X-rays	X-ray Tube	Attenuated x–rays by x-ray detectors	Screen of computer with algorithm software	Neurological condition, tumour detection and grading near blood vessels, abscesses	Costly, still limited use in veterinary, restraining using anaesthesia is a must
Nuclear Scintigraphy	Radioactivity / Gamma ray	Radionucleotide given i/v to animal emitting Gamma ray	Gamma ray detector	Detector screen identification of hot and cold spot	Detect more metabolically active tissue	Use of radioactive material, hence, an ethical issue in food animals
positron-emission tomography (PET)	Radioactivity	Short-lived positrons emitted from ^{11}C, ^{13}N, ^{15}O, and ^{18}F of 511 keV energy	combination of crystals arranged multilayered in scintillation detectors camera	Photomultiplier tubes and coding scheme with algorithm software	3-dimensional image, metabolic alteration can be diagnosed even in nanomolar range	Use of radioactive material, hence, an ethical issue in food animals
SPECT (Single-Photon Emission Computed Tomography)	Radioactivity	Radiolabeled pharmaceuticals or metabolites producing energy of lower than 511kev energy	single or multiple NaI (Tl) scintillation detectors	Photomultiplier tubes and coding scheme with algorithm software	3-dimensional image, metabolic alteration can be diagnosed even in nanomolar range	Use of radioactive material, hence, an ethical issue in food animals
Electrical Impedance Tomography	Employing alternating current of 10 Khz to 1 Mhz	Numerous electrodes with current	numerous electrodes measure electrical conductivity, permittivity, and impedance due to changes in free ionic flows	Current detector	All hard and soft tissue analysis	Still in nascent stage in veterinary/ animal uses

FIGURE 8.3 Introduction of live animals in veterinary imaging.

Ultrasonography stands as the second-most commonly employed imaging technique in veterinary practices; B-mode grayscale scanning and Doppler ultrasound are the most practiced USG modes relevant to veterinary diagnostics. USG holds the key for the diagnosis of several vital organ-related disorders in animals but is of paramount importance in assessing reproductive patho-physiological status in large as well as small ruminants and companion animals also. It is routinely used for pregnancy diagnosis and fetal age and sex determination in large domestic animals, along with monitoring ovarian status and dynamicity, uterine pathology-associated reproductive disorders such as cystic ovaries, endometritis, pyometra, mucometra, early embryonic mortality, mummified and macerated fetus, anestrum etc. Even male reproductive disorders like pathological conditions of the accessory sex glands can also be diagnosed using ultrasound imaging. Not restricted to imaging, it is also used further to measure the size of ovarian structures like follicles, corpus luteum, follicular and lutenized cysts etc. (Rajamahendran *et al.*, 1994). Similarly, it is also applied in small animals for the detection of different patho-physiological conditions including normal as well as abnormal pregnancy, developmental disorders in a fetus and fetal number, age and sex determination. Gas-filled or bony tissues pose a difficulty in USG imaging as they are non-responsive; hence, the positioning of the ultrasound probe is important in obtaining a proper image of the surrounding soft tissues. At the tissue-bone interface, a shadow is formed due to the absorbance of ultrasound, while it is totally reflected in the tissue-gas phase; this is a major consideration to be followed carefully during quality ultrasound imaging. Even tissue imaging beyond 24-cm depth is noisy and difficult with USG because of the weakness of the returning echo. So, per-rectal insertion of the ultrasound probe is necessary in large animals to obtain images of the reproductive organs, while in small animals like female cats or dogs abdominal examination is sufficient to serve the purpose. Moving forward from the reproductive system, most soft tissues, including muscles, tendons and ligaments, heart, abdominal organs, urinary bladder etc. can also be imaged through USG for diagnostic purposes. Contact with the skin by the clipping of hair and the application of gel on the skin surface is used to avoid thickness and air issues, which is helpful for better imaging. In cases of bowel imaging, fasting is also recommended for the same reason. Further, controlling the depth (in cm), which means the distance between target tissue and transducer, also helps in proper imaging; as a rule of thumb it is controlled in such a way that two-thirds of the target tissue and/or the organ can be visualized on screen. Similarly, brightness and contrast, which range between 16 and 128 shades in grayscale, are also manipulated for better visualization. These considerations are helpful in overcoming two common artifacts, acoustic shadowing and distance enhancement, to acquire quality ultrasound images (Bronzino, 2000; Mudry *et al.*, 2003; Suri *et al.*, 2008; Easton, 2012).

It is generally accepted that greater resolution is obtained by the use of higher frequencies, at the cost of poorer depth imaging. For instance, in small animals, generally 5-MHz probes will image adequately to a depth of 15 cm, while 7.5-MHz probes will be suitable to get an image of tissue at 7-cm depth, and 10-MHz probes can be used for imaging at a depth of 4–5 cm, whereas 2.5–3.5 MHz is usually suitable for echocardiography in larger breeds of dogs. Further, it can be justified that 5.0–10 MHz is suitable for the examination of a bladder from the ventral or ventro-lateral aspect of the caudal abdominal wall in dogs, while 7.5–10 MHz is required for ventral bladder wall examination from the same point in dogs, and a 7.5-MHz transducer is used for uterus, ovary and testis assessment (sometimes needing a 5-MHz probe). Generally, a 7.5-MHz transducer is sufficient for cranial mediastinum imaging, but for deeper lesions a 5-MHz transducer is required. A transducer of 10 MHz is useful for imaging up to approximately 4-cm depth; 7.5 MHz is suitable for about 6 cm depth; and 5 MHz is suitable for up to 15 cm depth, which can be selected depending upon the distance for non-cardiac thoracic ultrasound. For imaging of the cardiac system, 2D (B-mode), M-mode and Doppler-mode are commonly used; among them, Doppler and specially designed electrocardiography ultrasound examination is preferred. 2-D and M-mode examinations usually require 5-MHz transducers for dogs, and for animals weighing around 50 kg, 3–3.5 MHz is preferred, while for smaller animals like cats, a 7.5-MHz transducer is suitable. However, 7.5-MHz probes can also be used for small to average-sized dogs, and 3.5 MHz for echocardiography and deep structure study in very large-sized dogs. Valve anatomy, chamber volumes, wall thickness, myocardial function, pericardial effusion, endocarditis, types of cardiomyopathies, atrial and ventricular septal defects, aortic and pulmonic stenosis, patent ductus arteriosus, congenital heart disease etc. are a few examples of cardiovascular patho-physiological conditions which can be assessed by USG. The above instances can vividly justify that the requirements of ultrasound frequency closely depend upon positioning, angle, distance from target tissue and depth of target tissue for proper imaging. Similarly, for larger animals, 3.5–5.0 MHz, and in calves 5.0 MHz, can be used for trans-abdominal images from the ventral abdominal wall and the right and left flank, while a 6.0–8.0-MHz rectal linear probe is suitable for left-kidney and bladder examination and the assessment of conditions such as omphalitis, extraumbilical abscess, traumatic reticulitis, urolithiasis and bladder rupture, traumatic reticuloperitonitis, umbilical hernia, omphalophlebitis, urachal fistula, abomasum fistula, hernia ventralis or ruminal fistula etc. (Kurt and Cihan, 2013). Bladder stone, pancreatitis, enlarged abdomen, hepatobiliary disorders or abnormalities in other intra-abdominal organs and cancer diagnoses are a few other examples of when USG has been successfully employed. Even ultrasound-guided tissue biopsy is commonly practiced for normal histopathological diagnosis. Ophthalmology-related applications such as the detection of foreign objects, cataracts, stephylomas, retinal detachments, tumors, glaucoma and hypopyon, and GIT-related diagnosis such as detecting the rate of peristalsis, peritonitis, ascites, changes in organ size or shape and the presence of internal masses (cancer), are other common applications of USG in veterinary practices. In equines, a 4–13-MHz linear probe is required for the imaging of tendons and ligaments; a 1–8-MHz convex probe is required for trans-abdominal imaging, scanning of reproductive and musculoskeletal system etc.; a 5–10-MHz endorectal probe is specialized for reproductive imaging; a 1–4-MHz phased array probe for cardiac examination and a 4–9-MHz microconvex transducer for hoof and pastern imaging can be used for diagnostic purposes (www.imotek.com/products/veterinary-ultrasound-/probes/156/equine-ultrasound-probes/). Further, M-mode and Doppler echocardiography have been successfully employed for imaging the heart in equines (Long *et al.*, 1992).

Doppler ultrasonography exploits the Doppler effect for imaging the movement of tissues and body fluids with respect to the probe. The Doppler effect, or Doppler shift, discovered by C. Doppler in 1842, measures the frequency change of sound waves due to the movement of the target with respect to the wave source. The frequency change assists in monitoring the velocity and direction of blood flow or other body fluids. For instance, sound becomes louder when blood moves towards a transducer, and quieter when moving away. As RBCs are the major blood cell and are very small (diameter 7 μm) as compared to the typical ultrasound wavelength (0.2 to 0.5 mm), they can thus produce a scattering effect for imaging. Doppler echocardiography has become a go-to technique for cardiac imaging and the diagnosis of cardiovascular diseases such as vascular stenosis or occlusion, thrombosis, cardiac valve abnormality etc., as well as for monitoring cranial blood circulation. Doppler ultrasonography is also commonly employed for the diagnosis of renal disorders such as renal parenchymal diseases including hydronephrosis, hydroureter, abscess, subcapsular hematomas, renal cyst, neoplasia, calcification and renal calculi etc. (Espada *et al.*, 2006). The technique is also very useful in animal reproduction, particularly for monitoring uterine and ovarian blood flow during different patho-physiological conditions. Various Doppler USG methods are available, such as pulsed-wave and continuous-wave Doppler. Pulsed-wave Doppler generates short pulses of sound waves and identifies the source of reflected sound waves. The same set of piezoelectric crystals are used for pulse generation and reflected echo analysis. Thus, the location of a flow pattern and sample volume can be measured by this method; however, fluid movement velocity beyond 1.5 to 1.7 meters/sec cannot be measured accurately. In continuous-wave Doppler a separate set of piezoelectric crystals are used for pulse generation and reflected echo analysis, thus enabling use of the technique in continuous operation. This method is ideal for high-fluid-velocity measurement but is unable to determine the depth of the returning signal source precisely. Continuous-wave Doppler is mostly used in cardiac applications for the diagnosis of aortic or pulmonic stenosis, ventricular septal defects or mitral and tricuspid insufficiency and other speed-of-flow-related disorders in various organs. Another variant of USG is color Doppler, whereby a color code is used for demarking the mean shift in frequencies due to fluid movement. Usually, blue and green denote the away-flow of the fluid, and red, orange and yellow indicate fluid flow toward the source, hence elucidating details about the direction and velocity of the fluid flow. This helps in the identification and interpretation of flow in a broader area, thus assisting in the diagnosis of normal and abnormal flow. However, consideration regarding the angle of the transducer is very important in color Doppler. The emergence of power Doppler, whereby a color code determines the magnitude of the Doppler shift and not the flow direction, is less angle-dependent, and thus flow perpendicular to the USG beam can also be visualized. It is very useful in the imaging of smaller vessels, where flow is in lesser speed, rendering it advantageous for the monitoring of blood flow within different organs (Bronzino, 2000; Mudry *et al.*, 2003; Easton, 2012; Gugjoo *et al.*, 2014).

Contrast-enhanced ultrasound imaging is a recent upgrade in normal USG which is applied to obtain better contrast and resolution in vascular medicine. Here, air microbubbles encapsulated by a shell of different material smaller than the wavelength of the beam of the USG are used as a contrast agent for image enhancement. The air bubbles are cleared off after use by the lung while the materials of the shell are eliminated by the liver or kidney, hence not inflicting any health hazard. It can be employed in both conventional grayscale as well as Doppler modalities and the contrast agent requires more sound amplitude or energy for better resolution than normal USG due to local deposition of sound energy; however, energy must be below the level of bubble-bursting, which is another major consideration (Dar *et al.*, 2009). The modality is useful in the diagnosis of several blood-flow-related complications such as occlusive diseases, aneurysms, peripheral arterial diseases etc. and liver fibrosis, and the imaging of microvascular size and volumetric flow for detecting tumor-induced angiogenesis. However, the requirement of a specialized technician, the unavailability of 3D dynamic imaging and the poor acoustic window may pose limitations for this modality (Mehta *et al.*, 2017).

3D and 4D ultrasounds, although slightly different modalities from conventional grayscale 2D ultrasound imaging, rely upon the basic B-mode scanning method. Instead of focusing the sound waves in a straight direction like in 2D ultrasound, sound waves are directed at different angles to the target. The echoes returned from the target are computer-processed to produce a three-dimensional image which ultimately depicts a volumetric account of a target such as a fetus. The 3D imaging offers a static view of the target for structural and anatomical exploration, whereas 4D ultrasound facilitates live video streaming of the target object for the duration by gathering a series of 3D scans over time. Clinical use of this technology spans over fetal imaging and diagnosis of developmental disorders, cardio-vascular imaging, altered blood-flow-associated complications etc. (Benoit and Chaoui, 2004; Benacerraf *et al.*, 2005; Pooh *et al.*, 2016).

Tissue harmonic imaging (THI) is a recent nonlinear acoustics-based grayscale sonographic imaging modality that can generate images with improved contrast and resolution as compared to its conventional counterpart (Tranquart *et al.*, 1999). Based on harmonics, sounds of higher frequency, especially second harmonic sounds, are exploited for imaging of the target object. As only harmonic frequencies are used for THI and conventional echoes are excluded, it thus provides better penetration, minimized loss in detail and lesser noise and clutter, resulting in a better image quality (Uppal, 2010). The technique has been used in the clinical diagnosis of lymph node and thyroid abnormalities, pancreatic and hepato-biliary disorders, renal disorders etc. (Anvari *et al.*, 2015).

The development of battery-operated, hand-carried, wireless, portable ultrasound has been a major advancement in USG hardware in recent times, which has helped to reduce instrumentation size. This is very useful not only for application in far-flung areas as point-of-care diagnostics, but has also been employed in extreme cases such as for wild and captive endangered species including elephants and rhinoceros. Nowadays, new USG platforms such as 3D/4D USG for better real-time imaging have also been developed. Further, various changes have taken place for contrast-enhanced imaging by different external material applications for improved sensitivity, which have been used in tumor detection, volume imaging and several diagnostic purposes. Elastography for liver fibrosis, monitoring of thyroid nodules and lymph nodes and tumor detection are recent technological trends in ultrasound imaging. Other recent trends in imaging software-related advancements include software which employs a program for generating one image from different platforms such as computed tomography (CT), magnetic resonance imaging (MRI) and positron emission tomography (PET) in combination with ultrasound data, and automation-related software for increased output and sensitivity.

8.4 Digital Stethoscope

Another advancement in imaging techniques has been the introduction of the digital stethoscope, which converts auscultated acoustic sound to electronic signals. The technique has empowered the conventional stethoscope, the "doctor's best friend", with a wireless detection system combined with imaging facilities and advanced software for disease diagnosis even from remote locations. The emergence of Bluetooth facilities with data connectivity has paved the way to making a tubeless device which can record data and send it far away to obtain an expert opinion. Different software platforms, both online and offline, have already been developed and a few more are to be introduced soon to visualize the recorded sound frequencies relevant to disease as well as healthy conditions. This may facilitate identification and documentation of disease-specific signature frequency sound with digital stethoscopes under different patho-physiological status. Artificial intelligence has even been introduced into the analysis of digital stethoscope-recorded sound frequencies to bring automation to disease diagnosis; the products M™ Littmann® StethAssist™ Heart and Lung Sound Visualization, Thinklabs Stethoscope App, DAYTON iMM-6 etc. are a few examples of digital stethoscope-based imaging systems which have already been introduced for the diagnosis of cardiovascular and pulmonary diseases by introspecting murmurs, atrial fibrillation, different hemodynamic indices etc. Disease identification relies upon change in wave characteristics in terms of amplitude, energy, time, area of graph, repeatability pattern etc. (Swarup and Makaryus, 2018).

8.5 Endoscopy

Endoscopy is another light (optic)-based imaging technique which is used both for diagnostic and therapeutic purposes (Figure 8.3). Recently, it has found application in veterinary practices, particularly in routine small animal practices. It was first introduced in 1911 by Georg Wolf as rigid endoscopy but gained more practical utility after the discovery of optical fiber by Basil Hirschowitz and Larry Curtiss in 1957, paving the way for the development of the first flexible fiberscope by Harold Hopkins. This comprises of an optical fiber-based system with a source of light for the visualization of the target tissue or organ. A camera for live imaging is attached to a fine needle which is generally used for sampling through biopsy of tissue or internal fluid for the diagnosis of specific diseases such as cancer or further evaluation by bacterial culture. Hence, ideally it is made up of three components: the handpiece (for visualization and control), the insertion tube (an arm made with optical fiber for imaging and illumination) which is rotatable at the end, and the umbilical cord (connecting to supporting apparatus for sampling). Flexible endoscopy is currently becoming more popular in practice in medical imaging. The endoscope is generally inserted through the mouth or natural orifices, or through a very small incision to the target organ; it thus requires minimal invasion for both diagnostic as well as surgical procedures, and can even be used for targeted drug delivery to increase the load of a drug to a particular tissue under special condition. Gastrointestinal bleeding, dysphagia-related problems, unusual-symptom-based pain, coughing with blood or passing blood in stool or urine are common indications of where it can be used for differential diagnosis apart from cancer. Wireless-based endoscopy with the application of a capsule is a recent advancement in the area. The conventional wired-endoscopy system requires sedatives, laxatives or local anesthesia for proper imaging with minimum pain to the subject as per requirements. For instance, colonic endoscopy need laxatives to clear content. Sometimes, chances of infection, chest pain, vomition, shortness of breath or changes in the color of urine, over-sedation and perforation of the internal lining of the stomach or esophagus are common complications which must always be considered. However, endoscopy is further indicative in conditions where parallel techniques like blood chemistry, radiography, ultrasound etc. may not be sensitive, specific or effective enough for confirmative diagnosis. Further selection of the correct method of endoscopy is important for successful introspection, as the anatomical environment, position and structures of target organs vary significantly and the choice should be as per the need; for example, otoscopy is desirable for the diagnosis of external ear disorders, and uses different instrumentation than for rhinoscopy, pharyngoscopy or laryngoscopy. Similarly, for nasal endoscopy and gastroscopy, different variants are available. Rigid endoscopy is most commonly employed for thoracoscopy, urethroscopy and cystoscopy, the last being used to visualize the entire urethra and urinary bladder in small and exotic animals.

Skilled personnel are required for endoscopic operations. Currently, virtual reality simulators are available to facilitate better training and skill development in laparoscopic intervention. Disposable endoscope and capsule-based endoscopy are recent advancements in endoscopy available on the market.

Bleeding is a major problem which leads to the clogging of plastic stents in obstructive biliary and pancreatic disorders. It can be countered with the application of nanoparticles and advanced capsule-based endoscopy. Nanoparticles have depicted advantages in endoscopic hemostasis of peptic ulcer bleeding by introducing hemostatic novel nanopowder (TC-325). The introduction of cadmium selenide NP semiconductors or quantum dots in fluorescence endoscopy has provided better imaging and tissue targeting facilities. Similarly, a "smart robotic beetle" for sampling and treatment is another advancement where nanotechnology converges with endoscopy for better diagnosis (Jha *et al.*, 2012). The application of lectin-functionalized fluorescently labeled mesoporous silica nanoparticles as targeted endoscopic contrast agents in exploring colorectal cancer and other colonic lesions is another instance of nano-intervention in endoscopic diagnosis (Chen *et al.*, 2017). In another instance, the application of near-infrared fluorescent silica nanoparticles (FSN), which are biodegradable, have yielded better results in colorectal adenoma detection than conventional white-light endoscopy (Rogalla *et al.*, 2019). Various NPs such as silica and silica/gold hybrid NPs have already been successfully translated to the clinics and clinical fluorescent/white-light endoscopy systems, ushering in further hopes for enhanced nano-applications in endoscopy-based advanced confirmative disease diagnosis (Rogalla *et al.*, 2019). Recently, a Raman endoscope employing surface-enhanced resonance Raman scattering-based NPs (SERRS-NP), like PEGylated SERRS-NP and thiol-functionalized silica-based SERRS-NP, is also being tried for imaging to detect incipient GI tract cancers and premalignant lesions of the intestines, stomach and esophagus with significant reliability (Harmsen *et al.*, 2019).

8.6 Thermal Imaging

Thermal imaging is a recently introduced technique in the arsenal of imaging-based diagnostics in veterinary practices (Figure 8.3). Conventionally it is employed for the tracking of animals in wildlife for their welfare, but recently has gained a hold in the diagnosis of inflammation, sources of lameness, mastitis and behavior-related disorders, even in estrous detection (Telkanranta *et al.*, 2018). It works on the simple principle that infrared (IR) radiation (heat) is converted into visible images which depict the spatial distribution of temperature differences throughout the body in a landscape to be captured by a thermal camera. It is a non-invasive technique whereby an imaging camera fitted with an IR detector, which may be a cooled type (usually operating in the temperature range of -213 to -173°C) or uncooled type (operating in the ambient temperature), captures IR radiation from an animal body and imaging takes place in pixels. Generally, the color-coding for temperature measurement depicts the brightest (warmest) areas usually colored white, intermediate temperatures are indicated by reds and yellows and the coolest parts are black. The thermal imaging camera was initially developed in the 1950s for night operations for military purposes, but has gained entry in social activities for surveillance purposes, including monitoring movements and locating wild animals in the jungle etc. Cooled and uncooled focal plane arrays are the two modes on which IR imaging takes place; both the modes are useful in conclusive imaging along with other variables such as camera sensitivity, minimum resolvable temperature difference (MRTD) or thermal resolution of camera, and the noise equivalent temperature difference (NETD) or thermal sensitivity.

Thermal imagers work in two bands: one covers the 3–5 mm IR range, or mid-wavelength infrared (MWIR), and the second between 8–12 mm, or the long-wavelength infrared (LWIR) region. Generally, the MWIR band is suitable for imaging high-temperature objects and the LWIR band is preferred for near-room-temperature objects. The distance of the object from the imaging source is also an important consideration as only a small portion of the total emitted radiation is represented by the blackbody curves and factors such as water vapor, gases and carbon dioxide (CO_2) levels influence the imaging quality. Thermal imaging systems have been designed to operate in these two spectral bands because they are the two principal transmission windows in the atmosphere appropriate for thermal imaging operation. As a rule of thumb, the MWIR band is useful for imaging from afar, while LWIR imaging is better suited to imaging near objects, but it must be selected on the basis of spatial resolution and sensitivity. The detectors can be broadly classified as thermal detectors and quantum (or photon) detectors. Thermal detectors work on changes in electric conductivity in response to rises in temperature. Certain chemicals with different temperature-dependent physical properties have been exploited in thermal detectors such as pyroelectric detectors made up of ferroelectric crystals (e.g., triglycine sulfate), polymers (e.g., polyvinylidene fluoride, PVF2) and ceramics (e.g., lanthanum doped lead zirconate titanate, PLZT). Microbolometers are another type of improved thermal detector, usually made up of vanadium oxide (VOx) or amorphous silicon (a-Si), having the advantages of low cost, low weight and resilience to vibration and shock. Quantum detectors rely upon detecting the photons from IR radiations and possess more sensitivity but require cooling for proper operation. Indium antimonide (InSb), mercury-cadmium-telluride (HgCdTe) and platinum silicide (PtSi) are the common materials used in photon detectors (Havens and Sharp, 2016).

The IR released from an animal's body is attenuated by the environment, hence local atmospheric factors at the time of imaging are crucial for image quality. However, considering the whole body is in the same environment, scanning of the entire body to yield relative temperature variations in different body parts has diagnostic value for the aforesaid diseases. All objects, including living beings, above absolute zero ($T > 0$ K) radiate heat and the quantity of heat radiated depends on the temperature and surface condition of the object which is captured by thermal imaging. In disease conditions such as inflammation, mastitis or tissue injury and even in general herd health screening, the rate of heat production increases through the affected tissues, which may be due to internal increases in the activity of cells, increased blood flow or due to infection, and can be differentiated from the healthy tissues with cooler temperatures by thermal imaging to help in the diagnosis of the aberrations. Thermal imagers can detect even temperature change of 0.05°C and with scan rates of 30 times per second; even videos can be made and recorded. In dairy animals, mastitis is one problem leading to average increases in udder temperature of 2.4°C, and hence thermal imaging is helpful in the initial diagnosis of sub-clinical mastitis. Similarly, diagnosis of bluetongue virus (BTV), respiratory diseases, the tele-diagnosis of sarcoptic mange in the Spanish ibex (*Capra pyrenaica*) and whole-herd health screening are the other areas where it has found potential applications with high sensitivity and specificity even in initial stages of the ailments (Zaninelli *et al.*, 2018). Thermography can also be exploited to diagnose muscular sports injuries in equines. Since muscle injuries trigger inflammatory processes accompanied by the generation of heat, thus the intensity of inflammation can be enumerated by evaluating the temperature gradient of IR images, with diagnostic importance in game horses.

8.7 Radiographic Imaging

X-rays are electromagnetic waves with an energy level ranging between 1 and several hundred kiloelectronvolts (keV), but generally only 5–150 keV of energy is suitable for X-ray radiography to produce anatomical images. The diagnosis of fractures and other hard-tissue alignments like in teeth etc. are the most frequent bio-medical applications of this imaging platform (Figure 8.3). It is also used in angiography, both for diagnosis and treatment purposes, and in mammography too. Here, a shadowgram is produced by bombarding X-rays from a point source to a targeted anatomical site, where it is absorbed and scattered differentially by the different density of tissues, producing differential brightness-based two-dimensional images visualized on an X-ray film or screen system. Here, dense tissues such as bone or teeth or other highly calcified organs absorb more X-rays, hence yielding a white shadow, while the least-absorbing, sparse tissues give a darker shadow. The effect is due to interaction with tissues which may be photoelectric effect or scattering-based. Various contrast agents are employed to obtain better contrast; for instance, barium is often used in imaging of the gastrointestinal tract (Bronzino, 2000; Mudry *et al.*, 2003).

The basic components of X-ray instrumentation include the X-ray tube, filtration unit, generator and image detection system using screen film combinations.

X-rays are generated by cathode-originated accelerated electron beams passing through a vacuum to the rotating anode in the X-ray tube. A filament integrated with the cathode is heated by passing a current through it to emit the electrons. As thermal energy overcomes the metal binding energy of the electrons, the beam of electron takes off and flows from the cathode to the anode through the vacuum by the applied voltage difference produced by a generator. When the accelerated electrons are stopped within a short distance, the maximum energy content of the electrons is expended to heat the anode, while some portion of the energy is converted into X-rays. The conversion of energy from the accelerated electrons into X-rays basically follows two principles. The first one is Bremsstrahlung radiation, which relies upon producing electromagnetic radiation by sudden deceleration of the charged electron particles. The output yields a continuous spectrum of X-rays with certain characteristic sharp peaks. The second one is characteristic X-ray generation, which is achieved by striking the accelerated electrons on a rotating anode to create a vacant electron orbital which leads to inflow of outer electrons into the vacant inner orbital with a loss of energy, hence producing large numbers of X-rays at a few discrete energies. Both of the methods follow the law of the conservation of energy as the change of electron energy matches with the resultant X-ray energy. So, it is evident that the material of the anode is a determining factor for the production of X-rays with different energy; thus, the choice should be dependent upon the purpose. For instance, molybdenum produces characteristic discrete energy 20 keV X-rays, which is useful for mammography.

Filtration of the X-ray beam is done by the filtration unit to selectively remove low-energy X-rays for getting better contrast and avoiding unnecessary exposure. These low-energy X-rays become almost entirely absorbed and make no contribution to the final image. In conventional radiography, filtration is achieved by using aluminum or copper filters, whereas a 20- to 35-μm-thick molybdenum filter is suitable for mammography that filters both low- and high-energy X-rays from desired ones.

The generator creates voltage differences and currents which help in the generation and acceleration of electrons from the cathode to the anode through the vacuum of the X-ray tube. This is not only helpful in achieving the desired acceleration for penetration, but also in controlling the number of X-rays generated with an amount of energy, which is useful in avoiding blurring effects on edges and small objects. For instance, greater voltage increases penetration power but will give lower contrast; similarly, regulating the time length of current flows through the generator helps in schematizing the amount of X-ray production and exposure time. It requires three-phase transformers for constant voltage supply, which is difficult in single-phase transformers.

X-ray image detection can be achieved either by film or screen or using a film-screen-combination system which constitutes the detector system of the X-ray machine. In an X-ray film-based cassette system, X-rays coming after exposure are detected and imaged on X-ray-sensitive screens using light-sensitive negative film as a medium. Calcium tungstate ($CaWO_4$) or phosphors using rare earth elements like doped gadolinium oxysulfide (Gd_2O_2S) or lanthanum oxybromide (LaOBr) are the usual components of X-ray screens, giving better-contrast images for diagnosis purposes by converting the absorbed X-rays through the screens to visible light in an efficient manner. The visible light exposes the film in the cassette to be developed as a final X-ray image following a dark room-based film development protocol to obtain better resolution.

The aforementioned system is used in projection radiography, which precisely provides a static two-dimensional image of the projected area without any detail regarding motion. Here comes the importance of fluoroscopy, which generates real-time images of the target internal organ by continuously producing X-rays of lower energy, acquiring many images over time on a fluorescent screen. An image intensifier coupled with a TV camera has been employed to convert the usual weak images into better ones, along with recording of the improved images on a continuous basis. The platform is very efficient for diagnosis on occasions such as during angiography and operational events like the insertion of catheters in blood vessels. However, potential radiation hazards are the major limitations of this diagnostic modality.

The digital imaging system provides improved performance, relying upon an advanced X-ray detector and the display device. The detector in general should possess qualities such as proficient absorption of the incident radiation with linear response spanned over a wide range of incident radiation intensity, low intrinsic noise with better spatial resolution, wider field size, suitable imaging time etc. Either area detectors or slot detectors have been used for digital imaging such as digital mammography, depending upon their merits and limitations.

Recent advancements in X-ray imaging have taken place through the introduction of computed radiography (CR). This imaging system is comprised of an image plate (IP), IP reader, an analog-to-digital converter (ADC) and a computer that processes and visualizes the image. The object is exposed in standard X-rays, followed by capture of the attenuated radiations with flexible image plates. Complex crystalline photosensitive phosphors containing halogens and activators are the basic components of the image plate. Barium fluorohalide as halogen doped with europium as an activator has found utility in most of the applications. Following exposure of the image plate with the attenuated X-rays, a latent image is generated, courtesy of the flourohalide and activator-mediated excitation of the electrons in the crystalline phosphor to higher-energy states, followed by their entrapment at various sites in the phosphor. The latent image in computed radiography usually decays very fast, based on the type of phosphor used, with respect to the conventional film screen-based imaging system. Subsequently, the latent image is processed by the IP reader, which is equipped with laser, optical scanner, photomultiplier tube and motorized platform to generate visible light. The weak light signals are converted to electrical emissions by photomultiplier tube. The analog signals are amplified and passed through ADC, where the signals are assigned with binary numbers corresponding to their brightness according to the degree of attenuation. The data is further processed by computer software to yield a digitalized final image, along with enhancement of the image contrast (Bronzino, 2000; Mudry *et al.*, 2003; Easton, 2012).

8.7.1 Contrast Media

Contrast media are additional chemicals often employed to achieve better resolution of images for diagnosis purposes. They enhance the image quality of structures such as soft tissues, which are often difficult to visualize, and a particular organ owing to its lack of contrast with the surrounding tissues or to outline cavities generally invisible on plain radiographs. Positive and negative contrast mediums are two principally distinct categories. Negative contrast mediums mostly employ air, which appears black in radiographs, whereas positive contrast mediums such as barium- and iodine-based compounds appear white.

In negative contrast mediums, air, oxygen, carbon dioxide or nitrous oxide are usually used, which appear as black in radiographic images, and they can be employed in conjunction with positive contrast mediums to generate a double-contrast study. For instance, in hollow-structure radiography such as of the gastro-intestinal tract, a positive contrast medium is used for coating hollow structures, while a negative contrast medium helps in distending the anatomical structure. The advantage of a negative contrast medium which is generally introduced after coating the lining of the internal hollow organ with a positive contrast medium is to yield a double contrast, highlighting the defects in cystography and barium enema studies etc. It can also be used solo for arthrography, fasciography, detecting pneumoperitoneum and for pneumocystography.

In positive contrast mediums, high-atomic-number non-toxic materials which enhance the absorption of X-rays and give more white appearance on radiographs are usually used. The two available conventional types of positive contrast agents are barium sulphate-based mediums and water-soluble iodine compounds.

Barium sulphate is used as a suspension or powder or paste to outline the alimentary tract. This compound is completely insoluble and non-reactive to digestive enzymes, with no possibility of being absorbed through the alimentary canal, and thus can be used for indications in the esophagus, gastrography, reticulography etc. A major drawback is the resultant granulomatous adhesions or aspiration pneumonia on leakage into the peritoneum or accidental inhalation of the compound. Iodinated compounds are water-soluble and used in varied conditions except alimentary examinations because of the bitter taste which renders them difficult to administer in conscious animals; further, they produce poor contrast as compared to barium sulphate. Meglumineiothalamate, sodium iothalamate, megluminediatrizoate, sodium diatrizoate, iohexol and iopamidol metrizamide are used in intravenous pyelography, urethrography, arthrography, myelography, angiography, osteomedullography, sialography etc. Mostly, these compounds are administered into the vascular system and excreted through the kidneys, hence having application in examinations of the kidneys, ureters and bladder. Viscous and oily preparations of iodine compounds such as propylidione, iodized poppy seed oil and iophendylate are used in lymphangiography, dacrocystorhinnography, hysterosalphingography, myelography, bronchography and sialography, while iopanoic acid and meglumineioglycamate are used in cholecystography, as these preparations get excreted through the biliary system (Bronzino, 2000; Mudry *et al.*, 2003; Easton, 2012).

8.7.2 Recent Advancements in Radiographic Imaging

Radiographic imaging from its time of discovery has undergone continuous modifications spanning almost every aspect of instrumentations, including developments in X-Ray tubes, generators, image detection and storage systems and contrast materials in order to make it more compact and effective, with improved image resolution and sensitivity, broadening the scope of radiographic imaging from initial static 2D bone images by projection radiography to mammography, even achieving dynamic continuous imaging of internal organs by fluoroscopy under the current scenario. The development of open-tube technology has outweighed the requirement of rigorous maintenance from the earlier models. Further, microfocus and nanofocus tubes extend additional advantages in terms of automated control over tube output intensity, oblique viewing, rotation of the image chain and a sophisticated GUI (graphical user interface). Similarly, application of an amorphous-silicon flat panel detector (FPD) features a 16-bit format with over 65,000 shades of gray, and some 1 million pixels, which help in the enhancement of resolution (Vaga and Bryant, 2016). These advancements, made as various commercial manufacturers have developed a range of systems or platforms, have further propelled diverse diagnostic applications, such as AlluraClarity with ClarityIQ technology from Philips, which provides high-quality images at low X-ray dose levels with significant noise reduction for patients of variable sizes. This real-time image acquisition and processing platform has reduced the radiation health hazards to be used successfully in interventional neuroradiology, endovascular interventions, neuroangiography, interventional cardiology, for prolonged fluoroscopic visualization of coronaries and cardiac wall movements, bowel and respiratory movements, visualization of neuro vasculature etc. The Artis Q and Q.zen angiography systems from Siemens facilitate interventional imaging in ultra-low-dose X-ray ranges for diagnostic and therapeutic interventions of coronary artery disease, stroke and cancer. The platform pioneers the integration of intravascular ultrasound (IVUS) with angiographic imaging for versatile diagnostic and therapeutic applications. Similarly, GE Healthcare's Image Guided Systems (IGS) provide excellent image quality with exceptional dose efficiency for versatile application in interventional radiology and oncology. Recently, Toshiba introduced the Infinix product line, including the Elite, Select and Essential X-ray systems, and dedicated software equipped with dose management optimizing tools, along with spot fluoroscopy, a dose tracking system (DTS) and advanced image processing (AIP) for enhanced quality and high-resolution imaging in cardiovascular interventions. RaySafe, DoseWise and DoseWatch are other advanced radiographic modalities which have been developed for monitoring radiation dosage to ensure the safety aspect. Rotational angiographies as well as 3D imaging are the other areas where advancements are ongoing and the integration of multiple platforms such as X-rays with CT has been developed (www.itnonline.com/article/interventional-x-ray-advancements). Recently, sub-micronic Hafnia Nanodots-mediated multi-color-based identification of microfractures in bone has been developed through X-ray imaging and spectral computed tomography, which is beyond the scope of conventional imaging methods. The Hafnia nanoparticles used for developing color are small enough to be excreted safely from the body through the reticuloendothelial system (Ostadhossein *et al.*, 2019). In recent times, nanoparticles have proved their worth in X-ray imaging to obtain better resolution. For instance, gold nanoparticles (AuNP) coated with a bilayer of polyelectrolyte have enhanced X-ray scattered imaging in hepatocellular carcinoma to differentiate labeled cells from the unlabeled ones, paving the way for *in-vivo* diagnosis of tumors. These electron-dense nanoparticles show enhanced X-ray scattering in cancer tissues over normal tissues and overcome the issue of similar radiological densities between water and typical liver tissues (Rand *et al.*, 2011). Similarly, AuNPs have also been used in synchrotron-based X-ray imaging techniques as contrast agents in the detection of cancer-related angiogenesis, and the same effect can be achieved by using other high-Z element-based NPs with or without modifications (Chien *et al.*, 2012). Further, the application of K-shell-based NPs of yttrium, zirconium, niobium, ruthenium and rhodium has produced high-spatial-resolution images of tumors in X-ray fluorescence tomography bioimaging. These NPs can give differential spectra from probe and background and also have a higher payload which can work as a better contrast reagent (Li *et al.*, 2018). Magnetic iron oxide NPs have already been approved by the FDA in MRI and may also get access in current imaging platforms for clinical uses in the near future. AuroVist™ is a gold NP already in use for X-ray-based *in-vivo* imaging and diagnosis of indications in blood vessels, kidneys, tumors and other organs. The NPs possess certain advantages such as low viscosity, toxicity and osmolality and stay longer in blood than iodine-based contrast agents. Further, they also provide better contrast as well as being easily cleared out of the body through the kidney (www.nanoprobes.com/pdf/In1102A.pdf, www.universalbiologicals.com/aurovist-1.9-nm-1102-grp). Recently, smart NPs such as iodine-containing liposomes, dendrimers, emulsions, polymeric microspheres and polymeric micelles have been evaluated as novel contrast agents for radiographic imaging applications. They provide certain advantages over the conventional contrast media such as options for ligand binding and surface modifications, increased half-life, prevention of leakage etc. Iodine-free inorganic NP-based contrast agents such as quantum dots, NPs containing high-atomic-number elements and magnetic NPs have made significant progress in the field of radiographic imaging. Although gold is the most common material of interest, NPs of bismuth, lanthanides and tantalum have gained importance in recent times as they are less expensive (De La Vega and Hafeli, 2014). Silver NPs of 5–20-nm size have also found applications in radiotherapy and radiodiagnostics (Mattea *et al.*, 2017). Recently, self-powered X-ray detectors using 2D layered perovskite thin films rich in heavy elements like lead and iodine along with $CsPbBr_3$ microcrystals can boost sensitivity 100-fold as compared to conventional detectors, also employing low-cost fabrication techniques. They are applicable to low-dose dental and medical imaging, paving the way for making X-rays portable in the future as thick 2D perovskite film works better with a small voltage source, which also reduces the chance of irradiation damage (Gou *et al.*, 2019; Tsai *et al.*, 2020) (www.itnonline.com/content/self-powered-x-ray-detector-hopes-revolutionize-imaging). Similarly, the development of X-ray for soft tissue analysis and 3D imaging have been the focus areas of development in radiographic as well as multi-modality imaging in recent times. General exposure charts for X-ray imaging of different animals have been depicted hereunder. However, it should be carefully considered that the exposure technique chart standardized for one X-ray machine may not give satisfactory results with another X-ray machine, even of the same manufacturer. So, a different exposure technique chart should always be standardized for every machine to be employed for radiographic imaging (Tables 8.1, 8.2 and 8.3).

TABLE 8.1

Exposure chart for buffaloes and cattle

	Young Animal		Medium-sized Animal		Heavy Animal	
Body Part	**mAs**	**kV**	**mAs**	**kV**	**mAs**	**kV**
Head	20–0	55–70	20–40	60–80	30–60	70–90
Spine	12–30	60–70	20–60	70–80	30–80	70–100
Thorax	15–20	60–70	20–40	60–85	60–90	80–100
Abdomen (cranial ventral)	25–30	60–70	60–90	90–100	120–160	100–110
Forelimb	10–20	50–60	20–30	60–80	40–160	70–100
Hindlimb	10–20	50–80	20–40	60–90	40–160	90–110

TABLE 8.2

Exposure chart for equines

	Young Animal		Medium-sized Animal		Heavy Animal	
Body Part	**mAs**	**kV**	**mAs**	**kV**	**mAs**	**kV**
Head	25–30	60–75	20–40	60–85	30–60	70–90
Spine	20–30	60–70	30–40	70–90	40–60	80–110
Thorax	10–20	50–60	20–30	60–80	60–80	70–100
Forelimb	10–30	50–70	20–60	60–80	30–120	70–110
Hindlimb	10–30	50–70	20–60	60–90	40–120	70–120

TABLE 8.3

Exposure chart for dogs and cats

	<10 kg Body Weight		10–30 kg Body Weight		>30 kg Body Weight	
Body Part	**mAs**	**kV**	**mAs**	**kV**	**mAs**	**kV**
Head	5–10	50–60	5–15	50–70	20–40	60–80
Spine	5–15	50–70	10–30	50–75	20–40	60–80
Thorax	10–15	50–60	10–20	50–70	20–40	60–80
Abdomen	5–15	50–60	10–20	50–70	10–40	60–90
Forelimb	5–10	40–50	10–20	50–70	10–30	60–70
Hindlimb	5–15	40–60	10–30	50–80	10–30	60–70

8.8 Computed Tomography

The relevance of computed tomography (CT) for biomedical imaging was pioneered by Geofrey N. Hounsfeld with the first CT imaging of the brain in 1971, yielding him the Nobel Prize in Physiology in 1979 along with physicist Allan M. Cormack. Subsequently, the platform has been efficiently used in diverse clinical indications such as neurological conditions, tumor detection and grading, imaging of abscesses, monitoring changes in blood vessels, evaluating bones and joints problems etc. (Figure 8.3). The basic components of the CT scan instrumentation include a gantry, an animal handling unit or patient table, a control console and a computer. The gantry holds the X-ray source, X-ray detectors and the data-acquisition system (DAS). Computed tomography (CT), computed axial tomography (CAT) or body section roentgenography works on the basic principle of radiography whereby a large doughnut-shaped CT scanner bears a hole at the center and employs a rotating gantry with an X-ray tube mounted on one side and a detector mounted on the opposite side. The patient is placed on the motorized table which moves forward through the center hole of the scanner. The X-ray tube and detector rotate around the patient and a series of X-rays are projected to the target object from different angles by the rotating X-ray tube, while the detector senses the attenuated X-rays. Subsequently, a series of 2D radiographic images are acquired which undergo digital geometry processing to constitute cross-sectional and 3D volumetric images of the target object based on CT numbers. It is a computer-enhanced X-ray procedure whereby high-quality cross-sectional images of visceral structures are obtained with the help of contrast media. In the computer imaging, water is considered as the referral point for contrasting and has been assigned the scale of zero. Any tissue or material below the density of water, like air and fat, has been assigned as negative CT. For instance, air has been assigned with CT number -1000, while tissue denser than water gets a positive CT ranging up to +14000 (for dense bone) for computerized contrasting purposes.

Data-acquisition geometries of CT scan systems have progressed from the first to the fifth generation. The first generation, parallel-beam geometry, employs a single highly collimated X-ray pencil beam to act as an X-ray source, applied in linear motion across the targeted area with isocentric rotation of both the source and detector to achieve 180° rotation. It is a single-detector system and scanning is performed at the rate of 1° rotational movement, hence requiring a longer scan time, around 5 minutes. This is currently not in use due to the prolonged time requirement. The second-generation system employs a similar translate-rotate scanning motion to the first-generation system, but requires a reduced scanning time of up to 30 seconds by recruiting a fan beam source and multiple detectors, along with complicated reconstruction algorithms. A wide fan beam with 360° isocentric rotation and rotating detectors form the module of third-generation CT scanning, with no translation motion used and hundreds of detectors acting as curved detector arrays, providing better focusing. The third-generation module, introduced in 1976, is still in use for diagnostic imaging. In the fourth generation the detector array system, with thousands of independent detectors, remains fixed while the X-ray source and fan beam rotate isocentrically. A scanning electron beam as the unique X-ray source and the use of a stationary detector array system are the principal components of the fifth-generation system. Here, a source of X-rays rotates around the patient with other parts remaining static, resulting in the very fast acquisition of projection data—even in 50 milliseconds. Various further modifications, like spiral/helical scanning for quicker scan times, even in three-dimensional imaging, have evolved, whereby projection data for large parts of the body are generated as multiple images in a single breath and final imaging is reconstructed with more advanced algorithms. Most CT scanners employ Bremsstrahlung X-ray tubes as the X-ray source, which require power of typically 120 kV at 200 to 500 mA, to produce X-rays of 30 and 120 keV, thus necessitating generators with high frequency, in the range of 5–50 kHz.

Solid-state and gas ionization detectors are the two detector types commonly used in commercial CT scanners. Photodiodes and an array of scintillating crystals usually made up of ($CdWO_4$) or ceramics of rare earth oxide are the principal components of solid-state detectors. Gas ionization detectors are comprised of an arrangement of chambers holding compressed xenon gas at up to 30 atm pressure. Both of these detectors possess high efficiency to reduce the radiation dose, have a large dynamic range, remain very stable with time and are have low sensitivity to temperature variations. However, solid-state detectors usually possess very high quantum efficiency as compared to gas ionization detectors.

A data-acquisition system (DAS) helps in accurate measurement by minimizing patient variability, such as obese versus lean, through converting and encoding the results into digital values followed by their logarithmic conversion, and transmitting the values to a computer for reconstruction.

A computer system not only controls the functioning of various system components but also performs data acquisition and reconstruction, and displays the tomographic images.

Currently, a different type of CT scanner, termed a cone beam CT, which uses an image plate instead of detectors and is thus more cost-effective, has been employed in veterinary diagnostics. The image quality and resolution are comparable with the existing analogous modalities; however, the significantly sluggish image acquisition rate is a certain limitation of this platform (Bronzino, 2000; Mudry *et al.*, 2003; Easton, 2012; Gugjoo *et al.*, 2014; Wright, 2014).

Despite the valuable information which can be unearthed by CT scanning, it has certain major limitations. The patient must be restrained properly using anesthesia so that they remain immobilized throughout the examination; otherwise, patient movement will lead to blurring of the image. Hazards from ionizing radiation should be dealt with cautiously, following proper protocol. Further, the high expense, extensive instrumentation and necessity for skilled technicians restricts commonplace field application of this imaging modality for veterinary diagnostics.

CT is extremely useful in detecting, precisely locating and grading tumors, as well as the diagnosis of central nervous system disorders. It can also supplement radiological findings where further detail is required. CT scans of visceral organs, cranial structures, small bones, soft tissues and blood vessels can assist in the diagnosis of aberrations of blood vessels, lymphadenopathy, trauma, kidney stones, intracranial lesions, otitis media, dental diseases and musculoskeletal disorders like dysplasia, lameness etc. Spiral CT angiography has been successfully used for the diagnosis of pulmonary thromboembolism. Further, the platform is also useful in wildlife studies such as age, sex and species differentiation. It can be useful for the detection of cysts, abscesses, congenital deformities, cardiovascular diseases, hydrocephalus and coenurosis lesions in animals. Even beyond diagnosis, it can help in targeted drug delivery, guided biopsies and surgical interventions with minimal invasion. Further, integration of CT with other imaging modalities such as fluoroscopy, ultrasound examination or MRI can put in additional value for advanced veterinary diagnosis.

Various advancements have taken place in CT in recent times. The decades-old workhorse of 64-slice computed tomography (CT) has been challenged by 80-, 128-, 256-, 320- and 640-slice systems, which are more beneficial, particularly for children, with advantages in terms of low radiation, low repeat scan, freeze motion and higher coverage area etc. Similarly, the application of microelectronic circuits in detector systems has reduced the noise level related to electronics and provides sharper images. Further development of advanced software to provide iterative image reconstruction which reduces or removes artifacts because of multiple iterations, leading to clearer images in terms of pixels, has proved to be beneficial over the earlier filtered back-projection. Chest computed tomography (CT) is the choice of imaging in various diseases related to the thorax, like emphysema and small and large airway diseases. The recent introduction of dual-energy CT (spectral XT), where two different kV energies are used to visualize the same anatomy, has proved to be efficient for assessing pulmonary, vascular and neoplastic processes and even for lung cancer screening in high-risk individuals. Spectral CT reduces the time of exposure significantly as a single measurement can generate scans of the same anatomy at different energies, nullifying the requirement for multiple scanning. Various types of advance visualization and analysis software have been developed, such as IQon Spectral technology by Philips Healthcare, which has achieved FDA approval. Software has even been introduced with new algorithms to address irregular heart rate issues (Tabari *et al.*, 2017). Portable computed tomography is another advancement which helps in the scanning of terminally ill patients for whom movement can affect their fate (www.neurologica.com/bodytom). This is a battery-operated platform which paves the way for designing handheld point-of-care CT modalities for easy transportation and field-level operation, particularly suitable for animal diagnostics. (Bronzino, 2000; Mudry *et al.*, 2003; Easton, 2012; Gugjoo *et al.*, 2014; Ginat and Gupta, 2014).

8.9 Magnetic Resonance Imaging

Magnetic resonance imaging (MRI) is a non-invasive technique free from any radiation hazard which produces images due to the proton magnetic field of the atomic nuclei of hydrogen and carbon atoms present in the tissue samples intended for imaging. Bloch and Purcell first evidenced the event of nuclear magnetic resonance (NMR) in 1946, earning them the Nobel Prize in Physics in 1952, while the first clinical application of MRI took place in 1980. The atomic nuclei, having an odd number of protons and/or neutrons, bear a net-positive charge. Based on these proton numbers, charged nuclei from certain atoms such as hydrogen nucleus, ^{1}H, or the carbon nucleus, ^{13}C, possess the property of nuclear spin, which produces a magnetic moment eventually leading to generation of a local magnetic field with precise polarity. The application of large external magnetic field aligns the nuclei of such atoms parallel to the external field. Usually in soft tissue imaging, the hydrogen nuclei will be aligned parallel to the externally applied uniform magnetic field, producing a net magnetic moment. When a short radio-frequency (RF) pulse of microseconds is applied perpendicular to the external magnetic field, it tilts the oriented hydrogen nuclei away from the direction of the external magnetic field. Subsequent withdrawal of the RF pulse again reorients the hydrogen nuclei parallel to the external magnetic field, which is termed relaxation. The relaxation leads to loss of energy by emitting an RF signal from the nuclei which induces a voltage that can be detected by applying a conductive field coil around the object to be imaged. The signal is amplified and depicted as the free-induction decay (FID) response signal, which is reconstructed to form three-dimensional grayscale magnetic resonance images. The signal is predominantly generated by the hydrogen as the most abundant atoms of water and lipid molecules present in the biological samples, but carbon (^{13}C), phosphorus (^{31}P), sodium (^{23}Na) and fluorine (^{19}F) atoms, which have an odd number of protons and/or neutrons, also produce weak but recognizable nuclear magnetic moment which can be imaged through MRI (Figure 8.3) (Bronzino, 2000; Mudry *et al.*, 2003; Easton, 2012; Gugjoo *et al.*, 2014).

An MRI machine appears as a large block with a tube running through the middle of the machine, termed the bore of the magnet, where numerous different magnetic fields are applied simultaneously or sequentially to produce the desired NMR signal. It has two units—the analog domain and the digital domain. The analog domain consists of major hardware including the tube-sized bore where the subject to be imaged is rested during the scan. The source of the magnetic field and radiofrequency signal in MRI relies upon: i) a strong static field magnet in conjunction with a sophisticated set of ii) gradient coils and iii) radiofrequency coils. Static field magnets generate a high-intensity and uniform, static magnetic field spanning the whole region to be imaged, as the primary magnet running uniformly below the tube. This helps in achieving the temporal drift of the field strength less than 0.1 ppm/h so that spatial variation is extremely low, stable, uniform in space and constant in time. Primary magnets of four different classes have been employed in MRI scanners: (1) permanent magnets; (2) electromagnets; (3) resistive magnets; and (4) superconducting magnets. Among them, superconducting magnets, which run as coil and take lesser energy to a produce magnetic field, are the most commonly employed currently. Superconducting magnets are cryogenically cooled as the coils are continuously bathed in liquid helium at -452.4ºC. Such a cold temperature facilitates bringing down the resistance of the wire to near zero, thus lowering the electrical requirements of the system. All of these components contribute to maintaining the instrumentation within a convenient size, while still producing high-quality images and operating in a cost-efficient manner. Typically, a magnetic field is focused on the area of scan for 1–20 minutes or longer, with a strength varying from 0.2 to 1.5 tesla (T; 1T = 10000 gauss, G), but a higher field may be required in spectroscopic and functional imaging work. Remember, the magnetic field of the earth is about 0.05 mT (5000 G).

A gradient coil is composed of three gradient fields, in x, y, and z directions of the coordinate system, used to localize the MRI signal spatially to the target of interest and permitting the imaging of even thin anatomical slices. It assists in 3D image reconstruction from spatial information. In an MRI machine, the direction of the static field, along the axis of the scanner, is conventionally taken as the z direction, which produces a significant contribution to the resonant behavior of the nuclei.

Radiofrequency (RF) coils perform the essential function of transmitting and receiving signals at the resonant frequency of the protons within the patient.

The latter two magnetic components can be controlled in terms of precise timing of exposure or pulse sequence by switching on and off.

The control of timing and other information like signal amplitude to the gradient and RF amplifiers/magnet, to process the MRI signal from the receiver, and the construction of an image for display and storage is achieved by the digital domain or digital data processing system operated through computer. It also provides miscellaneous control functions including positioning of patient etc.

MRI is a very good imaging modality for tissues like brain, heart, lungs, spine, knees, wrist etc., which gives differential magnetic spin in disease and normal condition. As MRI scans the radiofrequency signal generated from nuclear spin, so the NMR signal is not obstructed by air-filled regions or bony structures within the body, which provides a marked benefit over ultrasound imaging. Further, being free from the hazard of ionizing radiation, MRI is safer than CT and PET scanning. However, MRI takes longer and requires the patient to be confined within a narrow tube throughout the examination, which are certain demerits of the imaging modality. Further, patients with metal implants can also produce trouble in MRI. In MR imaging, tissues with higher proton density produce a stronger FID response. MR image contrast also depends upon tissue-specific parameters: T1, or spin-lattice relaxation or the longitudinal relaxation time; and T2, or spin-spin relaxation or the transverse relaxation time. T1 indicates the length of time required for the dissipation of energy into the lattice by the surrounding nucleus to regain thermal equilibrium after excitement by a radiofrequency pulse. T2 indicates transverse relaxation occurring by energy exchange between the nuclei producing reduction in field strength toward the static magnet with more random orientation of the nuclei. The image contrast may be adjusted by altering repetition time (TR) and echo delay time (TE) to produce T1-weighted images or T2-weighted images according to the diagnostic purpose. For instance, fat tissues look bright in T1-weighted images due to their short T1 value, while water-rich fluids like cerebrospinal fluid (CSF) appear black due to their long T1 value, thus T1-weighted images suit better the diagnosis of fatty liver or focal hepatic lesions. In contrast, T2-weighted images highlight the water-rich content and are thus suitable for the diagnosis of edema and inflammation (Bronzino, 2000; Mudry *et al.*, 2003; Easton, 2012; Gugjoo *et al.*, 2014; Rinck, 2018).

8.9.1 Contrast Agents

In addition to the intrinsic tissue contrast properties, exogenous artificial MRI contrast agents can also be applied, such as FDA-approved gadolinium-DTPA (diethylenetriamine penta-acetic acid), which can be introduced intravenously or orally in the area of interest to produce contrast-enhanced regions that show as bright relative to the rest of the MR image. Apart from gadolinium chelates, other popular exogenous contrast agents include manganese chelates and superparamagnetic iron oxide particles.

Apart from the basic MRI instrumentation, various advanced platforms have been introduced recently. For instance, magnetic resonance angiography (MRA) has been employed for the evaluation of blood vessels, more commonly the arteries, to obtain information regarding stenosis, occlusions, aneurysms or other blood vessel indications, including locating portosystemic shunts. Similarly, in phase contrast angiography, monitoring of blood-flow velocity is performed, while in magnetic resonance venography (MRV), imaging of veins is achieved through differential excitation of tissue and vein. Further, functional MRI (fMRI) is used for assessing brain activity by monitoring the associated blood-flow changes. Here, a more frequent signal is produced at lower spatial resolution, which produces better spin-spin-based contrast due to the BOLD (blood-oxygen-level-dependent) effect. Interventional MRI is used to guide a minimally invasive procedure such as neurosurgery.

MRI has immense importance in the diagnosis of brain and CNS disorders. It has proved efficient in the diagnosis of intracranial disorders such as congenital brain disorders, hydrocephalus, brain herniation, vasogenic edema, seizure-associated alterations etc. MRI has also been employed for imaging the internal organs of reptiles such as turtles, snakes etc. In rodents like rats, mice and guinea pigs, MRI has been successfully used for the diagnosis of osteoarthritis, osteomyelitis, musculoskeletal and joint disorders, dental disorders, inflammation and fibrosis in vital organs, glaucoma etc. It is also useful to study neurodegenerative disorders like Alzheimer's or Parkinson's diseases in model animals like rodents and lagomorphs. Other MRI intervention in veterinary diagnosis includes but is not limited to nasal neoplasia, eye and orbital diseases, cranial cruciate ligament injuries, osteochondrosis, canine elbow dysplasia, hemorrhage and infarction, spinal cord and vertebral column disorders etc. Soft tissue imaging without the interference of air or liquid has made it an alternative to USG, along with its low radiation hazard, unlike tomographic imaging, which has added further advantages to MRI; however, the size of the necessary instrumentation, its non-compatibility for larger animals and the requirement of specialized accessories and technicians has hindered the commonplace field application of this imaging modality for veterinary diagnosis.

8.9.2 Recent Advancements in MRI

Various MRI scanners have entered the market in recent times to perform imaging of the cardiovascular system, lungs and other organs with improved functioning, such as simplified cardiac imaging workflows with advanced features. Recently, Bruker has introduced the BioSpec series, equipped with MRI CryoProbe™ technology combined with ultra-high field USR magnets that facilitate high-spatial-resolution, multi-purpose preclinical veterinary MR imaging and molecular MRI. Most of the recent advancements have taken place in order to achieve faster contrast scans and on the imaging software front. Recently, the Food and Drug Administration (FDA) has given clearance for multi-contrast MRI based on MAGiC (magnetic resonance image compilation) software developed by GE Healthcare, which can produce eight contrasts in a single acquisition, where the contrast can even be modified after image formation, also saving time for MRI in respect to conventional imaging. Furthermore, the drawback of conventional MRI for the imaging of patients with metal implants has been surmounted successfully in recent times. Medical devices and implants such as in-joint replacements, spine implants, pacemakers and implantable cardioverter defibrillators (ICDs) compatible with MRI have been introduced, with advanced software like ScanWise Implant, which facilitates MRI of patients carrying such implants. Novel implant materials are also appearing which show compatibility with MRI. Similarly, obtaining better resolution in MRI of the lungs was an issue due to the presence of air, with its low density of hydrogen atoms, which has been overcome by ultrashort echo time (UTE) MRI scanning for pulmonary MR imaging. Similarly, cardiac MRI, which was previously under-rated due to its complexity, longer time requirements and cost, has now been simplified by the newly introduced Signa MRI scanners along with ViosWorks cardiac MRI software by GE Healthcare. Significant automation with full 3D chest volume scanning within ten minutes (against almost 70 minutes required for conventional MRI) has been achieved with this platform. Different manufacturers such as GE Healthcare, Phillips, Siemens, Hitachi etc. are working on more compatible MRI platforms and some of them have already come out with advanced MRI platforms for faster imaging to save time and cost with better resolution and contrast (www.itnonline.com/article/software-advances-mri-technology). MRI advancement has been further boosted through the introduction of a micro-NMR smart phone device developed by Haun and co-workers, which has found application in cancer diagnosis. The modality has been successfully employed for quantitative analyses of multiple cancer-associated protein markers from the fine-needle aspirated tumor samples within 60 minutes with 96% accuracy, even better than conventional immunohistochemistry (Haun *et al.*, 2011). Recent progress in terms of better resolution and image quality in MRI has predominantly relied upon the advances in MRI pulse sequences and hardware along with greater field strengths, better multichannel coils, stronger gradients and more homogeneous magnets, in combination with advanced software, which facilitates even single-atom imaging and ultra-high-field anatomical imaging to yield morphology-associated functional information (Corea *et al.*, 2016; Zhu *et al.*, 2018; Harisinghani *et al.*, 2019). Further advancements may take place by allowing provisions for the integration of multi-modality imaging, compatibility with numerous novel implant materials, adjustability for all kind of animals, time and resource efficiency without compromising resolution and allowing automation in image analysis with the intervention of smart technology like artificial intelligence.

8.10 Radiopharmaceuticals and Nuclear Imaging

The discovery of mysterious "rays" emanating from uranium by Henri Becquerel in 1896, and the application of radium in contact with a tuberculous skin lesion for biomedical study in 1901 by Henri Alexandre Danlos and Eugene Bloch, laid the foundation stone of nuclear medicine. The branch further proved its value in imaging techniques with the application of ^{32}P labeling in rats to demonstrate bone mineral dynamicity by O. Chieivitz and Georg de Hevesy in 1935. The application of radionucleotides as such or inserted in any metabolite or pharmaceutical is used in this imaging technique. This radionucleotides generate X-rays, β-rays, positrons or gamma rays (photons), which are measured and used for imaging (Figure 8.3). Mostly positrons and gamma rays are used as sources due to their properties of high penetration and non-ionization. Various advanced techniques such as positron emission tomography (PET) and single-photon emission computerized tomography (SPECT) with their variances have been developed in recent times for nuclear imaging purposes. The basic principle of action is that a radionucleotide or radiopharmaceutical with a short half-life is either administered in animals for biodistribution in the body to generate positrons or gamma rays after decaying, or the animals are exposed to gamma rays from a source and subsequently detected by a detector which may be fixed or rotating to capture images from multiple planes. The emitting energy differs from the initial source, which is sensed by a highly sensitive and advanced detector system depending upon energy source and amount; subsequently, the acquired data is processed through an analogue system for conversion and the generation of a digital image on a computer. Various nucleotide analogues have been employed for this purpose, like F-18 fluorodeoxyglucose (FDG), which is taken up by cancer cells more rapidly than normal cells due to the structural resemblance of this molecule with glucose, as used in cancer imaging. Copper-64 in cancer diagnosis, bromine-82 for estrogen receptor study, gallium-68 for calibrating PET, iodine-131 for thyroid disorder diagnosis, iron-52 for bone marrow imaging, magnesium-52 for heart muscle imaging, osmium-191 for cardiac study, thallium-201 for myocardial perfusion and the diagnosis as well as locating the site of myocardial infarction, oxygen-15 for blood flow study, rhubidium-82 for heart perfusion study and posphorus-32 in different enzymology and genetic study are a few examples of the use of radiopharmaceuticals for nuclear imaging. Thus, radioimaging has gained diverse applications in the diagnosis of various disorders of the brain, heart, lungs, bone, kidney etc. Among all the radioisotopes, Tc-99m, due to its versatility and approval by the US Food and Drug Administration (FDA), is probably the most extensively used imaging agent across the world. Another commonly used material is ^{18}F-FDG for diagnosis and prognosis of early- to late-stage cancers. Similarly, ^{123}I-ioflupane (DaTscan; GE Healthcare) in imaging of the dopaminergic system is another such example. Various platforms using radioisotopes have been developed for imaging purposes, such as nuclear scintigraphy, PET and SPECT, which are discussed below (Bronzino, 2000; Mudry *et al.*, 2003; Easton, 2012; Gugjoo *et al.*, 2014).

8.10.1 Nuclear Scintigraphy or Gamma Scanning

Nuclear scintigraphy, or gamma scanning, is a highly sensitive platform where imaging is performed to identify hot and cold regions by detection of emitted gamma rays from various parts of the object under investigation after internalization of radioisotope-labeled substances by the target tissues. Here, abnormality is detected by analyzing increased or decreased radioactivity from body parts, which indicates the level of uptake of the radio-labeled metabolites by different regions as specific indicators of diseases. The hot spots have more metabolically active tissues indicated by more radioactivities. Various aberrations of kidney, lungs, liver, GI tract and thyroid gland can be diagnosed by this technique. Occult lameness, lung perfusion, tumor detection and ventilation and patency of the ureter in both large as well as small animals are the indications of where it has been employed successfully. It employs a detector system for 2D imaging of the specimen and differs from other modalities like PET and SPECT, where a 3D image is obtained. Scintigraphy also differs from X-ray imaging in the respect that no external ionizing radiation is applied here; only gamma rays emitted from the tissue-internalized radioisotope-labeled pharmacological agents are captured for imaging. However, a major limitation of the modality is the requirement of a relatively large dose of radioisotopes, and thus it is not encouraged in food animals due to residual effects (Bronzino, 2000; Mudry *et al.*, 2003; Easton, 2012; Gugjoo *et al.*, 2014).

8.10.2 Positron-emission Tomography

Positron-emission tomography (PET) employs short-lived positrons emitted from radioactive compounds such as ^{11}C, ^{13}N, ^{15}O and ^{18}F for the generation of images of the target tissues to analyze the dynamics of ongoing metabolic processes. Here, radioisotopes or radio-tracers are tagged with certain key metabolites or ligands like fluorine-18 (^{18}F) fluorodeoxyglucose (FDG) or ^{11}C-labelled metomidate and injected into the body to be taken up in the tissues as per their metabolic requirements. The unstable nuclei of the radio-tracers on decay emits positrons which in combination with neighbor electrons produce two very-high-energy photons (gamma rays) by a process called annihilation, which travel opposite to each other (at 180 degrees) and are detected by an array of detectors. The level of emitted gamma rays determines the rate of uptake of radio-tracers by the target tissue, giving an account of its metabolic flux. More than 100,000 such radioactive decays are detected in the tissue distribution of the positron-emitting tracers for two-dimensional (2D) image formation, and the compilation of several such 2D scanning data from different angles by suitable algorithms leads to three-dimensional (3D) image formation. Gamma rays produced in annihilation are captured by the detector through a series of events. A number of photon tubes are used which run parallel to scintillators in a coupled manner to capture the gamma rays and convert them into visible light by an array of crystals, ultimately producing an amplified electric current pulse in proportion to the intensity of light falling on the photocathode through the photomultiplier tube. The crystal array, which is at the center stage of the entire detection system, is comprised of multiple layers (at the level of 15 to 47) or transaxial layers producing high sensitivity to capture the cross-sectional data. These cross-plane data are further refined and reconstructed through advanced algorithms-based programs. Lead shielding is employed to reduce the radiation hazard as positron annihilation generates 511-keV photons.

Although emission- and transmission-based tomographic imaging was first conceptualized in the late 1950s, it only became popular in medical imaging around the late 1970s, mostly due to its high sensitivity in soft tissue imaging. PET can detect and visualize compounds in nanomolar range which has rendered it a very efficient diagnostic tool for brain imaging, with the scope of reaching even up to receptor level. Thus, it outweighs the advantage of MRI of being able to detect compounds fairly to millimole level. This makes the modality a good choice in the analysis of CNS- and brain-associated disorders such as Alzheimer's disease, Parkinson's disease, epilepsy etc. It is also useful in coronary artery diseases where the study of cardiac muscle metabolism and blood flow is needed, not only for diagnosis but also for understanding of disease mechanism and progression. The importance, accuracy and sensitivity of PET along with the tracer FDG in cancer diagnosis, including determining the stage, grade of cancer and therapeutic effect, is instrumental. It can be used for the imaging of bones, the musculo-skeletal system, thyroid gland, cardiovascular system including blood-vessels and kidney etc., predominantly in small animals, but can also be applied in equine medicine too. Further, it is a valuable non-invasive modality to study metabolic activity of a particular area, and bio-distribution and imaging in infectious diseases

(Lohrke *et al.*, 2017; Gambhir *et al.*, 2018; Chen *et al.*, 2019). Recent advancements in cameras and detector systems hold promise for the wide application of PET in veterinary medicine in the future. For instance, the development of digital detectors and imaging systems employing a semiconductor-based silicon/cadmium telluride (Si/CdTe) Compton camera has improved the efficiency of this imaging technique (Watanabe *et al.*, 2007). Further, there has been the introduction of intelligent software like artificial intelligence (AI)-powered SubtlePET, which employs deep learning algorithms for denoising to acquire clear images up to four times faster from noisy scans, resulting in a significant reduction in scan times. Similarly, next-generation SPECT cameras with cadmium zinc telluride (CZT) detectors have decreased the system footprint, reduced patient radiation doses and shortened the time duration of examination. Further integration of PET-CT and SPECT-CT scanners facilitates CT attenuation correction of the acquired images while adding CT anatomical image overlays for enhanced visualization of the coronary anatomy to precisely identify the points of blockages resulting perfusion defects. Recently introduced amyloid PET imaging has also enhanced the scope of this platform in the exploration of brain and neurodegenerative disorders. Further, the recently introduced FDA-approved EXPLORER PET-CT scanner, which has been acclaimed as the world's first medical imaging system to acquire 3D images of the entire human body, can perform imaging with extremely low radiation doses and at a significantly faster scan time. This can provide additional advantages such as scanning without requiring anesthesia, improved cancer detection, the study of drug pharmacokinetics and biodistribution throughout the body, introspection of metabolic disorders, autoimmune diseases and other chronic diseases, toxicological studies etc. (Bronzino, 2000; Mudry *et al.*, 2003; Easton, 2012; Gugjoo *et al.*, 2014).

8.10.3 Single-photon Emission Computed Tomography

Single-photon emission computed tomography (SPECT) is another advanced modality under nuclear medicine-based imaging systems. This is a hybrid technology where radiolabeled pharmaceuticals or metabolites are used for imaging the internal organs and detecting them on a CT scan system. It differs from conventional CT in terms of using gamma rays instead of X-rays for imaging. Here, detectors capture cross-sectional images from different planes to generate final images from the emitted radiation by the injected radiopharmaceuticals of lower than 511 keV energy. In this way it also differs from PET, which uses C-11, N-13, O-15 and F-18 radiomaterials to generate two coincident 511-keV annihilation photons instead of single-photon emission in SPECT, hence also reducing the cost. Typically, 70- and 140-keV photons are emitted from TI-201 and Tc-99m respectively in SPECT imaging. The detector system, which uses single or multiple NaI(TI) scintillation detectors working on photoelectric effect, detects the photons, scattered in new directions with lower energy than the original photons, with the amount of energy depending upon the scatter angle. It uses an Anger (or scintillation) camera for detection, which receives an image once gamma rays hit and interact with an array of photomultiplier tubes (PMTs) placed at the back of the scintillation crystal for the generation of signal. Using specific algorithms, the signal is encoded to determine the location of interaction and imaging. A collimator made of parallel holes separated by lead septa in front of the NaI (TI) crystal in the scintillation camera is used for imaging purposes. Lead is used to absorb such protons which do not pass through the collimator in the proper way, hence increasing resolution. This is also used for brain imaging and the diagnosis of diseases related to the brain, but has the drawback of poor spatial resolution. The modality is yet to be commonly used in veterinary practices but it can add value in small-animal medicine, with ample applications in the near future (Jaszczak *et al.*, 1980; Rogers and Ackermann, 1992; Tsui *et al.*, 1994).

The functional information acquired through SPECT and PET imaging may require supplementation with the anatomic/morphologic data achieved from computed tomography (CT). So, SPECT and PET are now more often referred to as SPECT-CT and PET-CT. These integration approaches, known as "hybrid imaging", usually offer several advantages in terms of high sensitivity, good spatial resolution, significant reliability and the capacity to precisely identify the origin of functional abnormalities (Bronzino, 2000; Mudry *et al.*, 2003; Easton, 2012; Gugjoo *et al.*, 2014).

8.11 Electrical Impedance Tomography

Electrical impedance tomography (EIT) is another advanced imaging system, first introduced in 1978 by John G. Webster, mostly employing alternating current to measure electrical conductivity, permittivity and impedance of the targeted body parts based on the basic phenomenon that electrical properties of various tissue differ according to their normal or pathological condition due to changes in free ionic flows (Henderson and Webster, 1978). In this non-invasive technique, body parts under observation are imaged to monitor their electrical properties with the help of numerous electrodes (such as ECG, EMG and EEG) to record the resulting equipotentials and generate an image of impedance using specific algorithms. Alternating currents ranging between 10 kHz and 1 MHz are generally used. Various tissues, based on their different physio-chemical properties, have different conductance, ranging between 15.4 mS/cm for cerebrospinal fluid and 0.06 mS/cm for bone in a healthy human subject. In general, tissue like muscle and blood has better conductance than fat, bone or lung tissue (Frerichs *et al.*, 1998; Brown, 2003; Gaggero *et al.*, 2012). Such standardization for different animal subjects is yet to have been achieved precisely, hence the technology is in the nascent stage of development in animal disease diagnosis. However, it has shown significant sensitivity and specificity in different disease study in animals, such as for lung disorders in pigs (Aguiar *et al.*, 2018) and head trauma in pigs (Manwaring *et al.*, 2013); it has also been employed in aquatic animals (Cibis *et al.*, 2017). Thus, in future, the modality, on its own or in combination with other techniques, may serve considerably in animal disease diagnosis due to the advantages of its simple operational setup, non-invasiveness and safer methods even for food animals.

8.12 Nanoparticles in Diagnostic Imaging

Nano-intervention has extended almost four-fold benefits in medical diagnostics and therapy. The application of nanoparticles produces higher contrast through signal amplification, yielding enhanced sensitivity of the imaging modality. Nanoparticles facilitate enormous surface functionalization with different targeting moieties due to their large surface-to-volume ratio, creating the scope for the targeted detection of various diseases. Further, nanoprobes allow compatibility with multi-modality detection, providing an extra edge over the traditional biological moieties. This extends the scope for the integration of several imaging platforms to surmount the limitations of individual techniques through a complementary manner and to customize a combinatorial approach for precise disease diagnosis. Besides radiolabeling used for nuclear imaging, the intrinsic properties of nanoparticles can also be exploited for diverse molecular imaging platforms. For instance, radiolabeled iron oxide nanoparticles (IONPs) can generate imaging signals for MRI as well as PET; the generated data from both of the platforms can supplement the other toward improved diagnosis. Finally, the concept of theranostics, a single moiety possessing both diagnostic and therapeutic values, has been successfully implemented through functionalized nanoparticles and has already started to contribute in critical diseases such as cancer, infectious and communicable diseases, lifestyle diseases, immune-mediated chronic diseases etc. (Prasad *et al.*, 2019; Prasad *et al.*, 2020a; Prasad *et al.*, 2020b). Here, we delineate some recent nanomaterial-propelled advancement in diagnostic imaging modalities within the limited purview of the current discussion.

The introduction of nanoparticles in EMC imaging has cleared the path for the elucidation of intracellular protein localization and protein-protein interactions in sub-cellular compartments, which can be exploited to understand the molecular pathology of diseases. The cathodoluminescence property of small lanthanide-doped nanoparticles (Eu, Er, Ho, Tb, Sm, Dy, Nd, Tm and Yb) has been utilized to develop nanolabels for high-resolution EMC imaging that potentiates the possibility of multicolor electron microscopy in the future, as ions from the different rare earth elements can produce a spectra of distinct colors (Prigozhin *et al.*, 2019). Similarly, labeling by luminescent nanomaterials such as semiconductor quantum dots (QDots), polymer dots (PDots), carbon-based nanodots (CDots), upconversion nanocrystals (UCNPs), fluorescent nanodiamonds (FNDs) and nonfluorescent surface-enhanced Raman scattering (SERS) nanoparticles has opened the avenue of super-resolution microscopy for even up to single-molecule tracking, due to different properties such as unique optical-switching, greater brightness and stability, having distinct advantages over conventional fluorescent dyes. Various nanoparticles have also been commercialized for this purpose, such as ZnS-coated CdSe QDot 705 by Thermo Fisher, and dTeQDot 700 nm and CdTeQDot 720 nm by PlasmaChem GmbH, which have proved their value in high-resolution STED microscopic imaging (Jin *et al.*, 2018). Similarly, upconversion nanocrystals (UCNPs) in single-molecule imaging and PDots in fluorescence microscopy for superior brightness have established their worth in recent times. Nanoparticles coated with active ingredients could be specifically introduced into the cells to enhance the imaging of sub-cellular components in X-ray microscopy. For instance, gold nanoparticles coated with dendritic polyglycerol sulfate having theranostic potential in inflammation have been used for sub-cellular imaging to yield better efficiency than even confocal microscopy (Kepsutlu *et al.*, 2020). The iron oxide nanoparticle-based FDA-approved MRI contrast agents Feridex, Endorem, Cliavist and Resovist are used for cellular labeling and the imaging of hepatocellular carcinoma, while Combidex and Sinerem are used for imaging lymph nodes. Polyglucose sorbitol carboxymethylether-coated iron oxide nanoparticle-based Faraheme is approved for MRI application in iron-deficiency anemia. Gold nanosphere-based Verigene is another FDA-approved nanoformulation used for *in-vitro* diagnostics in genetics. The FDA-approved quantum dots commercially known as Qdots, EviTags and semiconductor nanocrystals have been employed for fluorescent contrast and *in-vitro* diagnostic imaging of tumors, cells and tissues in different aberrations. Albumin colloid nanoparticles containing ^{99m}Tc-based formulation (Senti-Scint) have been clinically approved for lymphoscintigraphy of the breast, while rhenium heptasulfide colloid nanoparticles containing ^{99m}Tc-based formulation (Nanocis) have found application in lymphoscintigraphy of gastrointestinal, melanoma, prostate tumors in SPECT modality. Similarly, Nanocoll and Technecoll are two ^{99m}Tc-based albumin and sulfur colloid nanoformulations, respectively, which have been approved for clinical application in SPECT imaging of inflammation, melanoma, prostate cancer, bone marrow, gastrointestinal tract, liver and spleen carcinoma. Hepatate is a similar type ^{99m}Tc-based stannous fluoride colloid nanoformulation approved for SPECT imaging of gastrointestinal tract, liver and spleen indications (Thakor *et al.*, 2016). Silica-based ultra-small core-shell hybrid nanoparticle Cornell dots (CDots) have been approved by the FDA for imaging metastatic melanoma. ^{124}I-labeled Cy5 dye-loaded CDots functionalized with PEG and cRGDY peptide have been successfully used for PET-imaging elucidation of integrin-expressing lesions. Dye-incorporated dual-modal CDot silica nanoparticles have also depicted encouraging results for sentinel lymph node imaging (Goel *et al.*, 2017). Silica-coated ytterbium nanoparticles coupled to calcium chelators which bind with the affected bone have been used as a nanoparticle-based CT contrast agent. Similarly, bimetallic FeBi nanoparticles visible in both MRI as well as CT imaging have found application in multi-modality imaging. Lutetium PEGylated nanoparticles like PEGylated NaLuF4 provide added benefits for combinatorial fluorescence and X-ray imaging together (Yeh *et al.*, 2017). Zirconium-89-labeled self-assembly supramolecular nanoparticles of tannic acid and Pluronic F-127 have been successfully employed as bimodal contrast agents for *in-vivo* tumor imaging. A self-assembling supramolecular dendrimer nanosystem has depicted greater imaging sensitivity and specificity, with up to 14-fold-enhanced PET signal ratios as compared to ^{18}F-FDG in tumor imaging. (Garrigue *et al.*, 2018). Recently, gold nanoparticles and nanorods have come out as promising nanoformulations in nuclear medicine. The privileges of stability, bio-compatibility and ease of surface functionalization have rendered them efficient and versatile candidates in therapeutic as well as diagnostic imaging applications (Maccora *et al.*, 2019).

8.13 Future Prospects and Conclusion

Early and precise diagnosis stands as the Achilles heel in paving the way for successful therapeutic outcomes. State-of-the-art, reliable and sensitive diagnostic modalities have armed clinical medicine to combat several complicated diseases, even cancer, effectively by timely intervention. This can be well justified by the increase in life expectancy of humans in recent centuries, even though the rate of emergence and re-emergence of several infectious and communicable diseases has significantly elevated recently, along with the introduction of various lifestyle disorders. The same has been achieved in animals too, although to a limited extent. The major bottlenecks for animal diagnostics and their potential solutions can be summarized as follows.

Most of these cutting-edge diagnostics incur significant cost, which often overshadows the commercial value of the livestock, imposing restrictions for farm animal diagnosis. As most of the advanced imaging platforms are in the nascent phase of development, particularly for veterinary diagnostic purposes, hence the cost-involvement is greater under the current scenario. However, in the near future, with proper standardizations in every aspect, the imaging modalities will certainly help to lower the cost factor. Several commercial manufacturers have shown adequate interest in this arena, which will definitely ensure the cost-effectiveness of the imaging platforms for devoted animal diagnosis.

Further, bulky instrumentation often restricts the application of various advanced imaging platforms to laboratory diagnosis, thus ensuring they are mostly useful for research purposes (Figure 8.3). However, the lack of ample well-equipped veterinary diagnostic laboratories is a common phenomenon particularly in under-developed countries. Hand-held, potable point-of-care diagnostics is more suitable for animal diagnosis, particularly at the terminal end of farm animal practice. As necessity drives development, animal diagnostics is heading in this direction, which can be exemplified by the introduction of portable micro-NMR smart phone devices, digital stethoscopes etc. Several innovations will certainly improve lab-to-land transition of these advanced imaging platforms in the future to assist in field-level animal diagnosis.

Animal-specific versions of different imaging modalities are available under the current scenario. The standardization of animal data is also far from being at a satisfactory level to compare between normal and aberrant health conditions. So, the development of image repository systems or devoted animal data banks, much like the NCBI, PDB and KEG databases for genomic, proteomic and metabolomic data, is urgently required to assist in the interpretation of animal imaging data for precise and accurate veterinary disease diagnosis. A benevolent global alliance of multiple stakeholders is necessary to serve the purpose. Similarly, instrumentation necessitates flexibility to accommodate both large as well as small animals in the same imaging platform; hence, customization needs special efforts to modify advanced imaging systems such as MRI, PET, SPECT etc. accordingly to accommodate this.

Another important issue with these advanced imaging modalities is the requirement of adequate skilled and experienced human resources for the proper operation and maintenance of these platforms, along with the generation of accurate data. Even though technological developments of existing platforms have taken place rapidly with the introduction of several newer models, parallel progress in human resource development is mostly lacking, resulting in the misutilization or under-utilization of this advanced equipment in various laboratories. Proper hands-on training and motivation can resolve this issue, which demands special attention.

Moreover, the integration of multiple imaging modalities is a focus area under the current circumstance. Multiplexing of several imaging platforms can overshadow the limitations of each individual modality, which will certainly enhance diagnostic value and increase their accessibility and applicability in precise disease diagnosis. While this is cumbersome and requires intense engineering skill, it is definitely not impossible, as several of these techniques are joined by the same thread, i.e., energy sources. Efforts have already been directed in this direction and PET-CT or SPECT-CT are the evident outcomes. Certainly, many more such examples will be added to the list in the near future.

In conclusion, veterinary diagnostic imaging is an extremely fertile arena of persistent research and development, empowered by a prolific market, with significant impetus from various stakeholders ensuring a prosperous future in coming times.

References

Abel-Santos, E. Endospores, sporulation and germination. *Molecular Medical Microbiology* (2015): 163–178.

Aguiar, S.S., Czaplik, M., Orschulik, J. *et al.* Lung pathologies analyzed with multi-frequency electrical impedance tomography: pilot animal study. *Respiratory Physiology & Neurobiology* 254 (2018): 1–9.

Alberer, M., Schlenker, N., Bauer, M., *et al.* Detection of gastrointestinal pathogens from stool samples on hemoccult cards by multiplex PCR. *The Canadian Journal of Infectious Diseases & Medical Microbiology* (2017): 3472537. doi:10.1155/2017/3472537.

Antonis, N. SEM and TEM: what's the difference? Thermo Fisher Scientific Blog (2019).

Anvari, A., Forsberg, F. and Samir, A.E. A primer on the physical principles of tissue harmonic imaging. *RadioGraphics* 35 no. 7 (2015): 1955–1964.

Benacerraf, B.R., Benson, C.B., Abuhamad, A.Z. *et al.* Three- and 4-dimensional ultrasound in obstetrics and gynecology. *Journal of Ultrasound in Medicine* 24 no. 12 (2005): 1587–1597.

Benninger, R.K.P. and Piston, D.W. Two-photon excitation microscopy for the study of living cells and tissues. *Current Protocols in Cell Biology* 59 no. 1 (2013): 4.11.1–4.11.24.

Benoit, B. and Chaoui, R. Three-dimensional ultrasound with maximal mode rendering: a novel technique for the diagnosis of bilateral or unilateral absence or hypoplasia of nasal bones in second-trimester screening for Down syndrome. *Ultrasound in Obstetrics and Gynecology* 25 (2004): 19–24.

Bonnell, D.A. Scanning tunneling microscopy. *Encyclopedia of Materials: Science and Technology* (2001): 8269–8281.

Bronzino, D.J. *The Biomedical Engineering Handbook* (Boca Raton, FL: CRC Press, 2nd edn, 2000).

Brown, B.H. Electrical impedance tomography (EIT): A review. *Journal of Medical Engineering & Technology* 27 no. 3 (2003): 97–108.

Bulte, J.W., Van Zijl, P.C. and Mori, S. Magnetic resonance microscopy and histology of the CNS. *Trends in Biotechnology* 20 no. 8 (2002): S24–S28.

Catroxo, M.H.B. and Martins, A.M.C.R.P.F. Veterinary diagnostic using transmission electron microscopy. *The Transmission Electron Microscope – Theory and Applications* (2015). doi:10.5772/61125.

Chen, N.T., Souris, J.S., Cheng, S.H. *et al.* Lectin-functionalized mesoporous silica nanoparticles for endoscopic detection of premalignant colonic lesions. *Nanomedicine: Nanotechnology, Biology and Medicine* 13 no. 6 (2017): 1941–1952.

Chen, W., Huang, Z., Nicholas, E.S. *et al.* Direct arene C–H fluorination with 18F– via organic photoredox catalysis. *Science* 364 no. 6446 (2019): 1170–1174.

Chien, C.C., Chen, H.H., Lai, S.F. *et al.* Gold nanoparticles as high-resolution X-ray imaging contrast agents for the analysis of tumor-related micro-vasculature. *Journal of Nanobiotechnology* 10 no. 1 (2012): 10.

Cho, K.O., Hunt, C.A. and Kennedy, M.B. The rat brain postsynaptic density fraction contains a homolog of the Drosophila discs-large tumor suppressor protein. *Neuron* 9 (1992): 929–942.

Cibis, T., Preikschat, S., Minh, D.N. *et al.* Identification of electrical impedance tomography as simulation system emulating the electroreceptive system in aquatic animals. 2017 *IEEE Life Sciences Conference* (LSC). doi:10.1109/lsc.2017.8268171

Corea, J.R., Flynn, A.M., Lechêne, B. *et al.* Screen-printed flexible MRI receive coils. *Nature Communications* 7 (2016): 10839.

Da Costa, S.G., Richter, A.S., Schmidt, U. *et al.* Confocal Raman microscopy in life sciences. *Morphologie* 103 no. 341 (2018): 11–16.

Daniel, B., Schmolze, B.S., Standley, C. *et al.* Advances in microscopy techniques. *Archives of Pathology and Laboratory Medicine* 135 (2011): 255–263.

Dar, M., Patil, D.B., Joy, N. *et al.* Contrast ultrasound imaging and its veterinary clinical applications. *Veterinary World* 2 no. 7 (2009): 284–285.

Davis, J.J. *Biological Applications of Scanning Probe Microscopy* (Weinheim: Wiley Analytical Science, 2005).

De La Vega, J.C. and Hafeli, U.O. Utilization of nanoparticles as X-ray contrast agents for diagnostic imaging applications. *Contrast Media & Molecular Imaging* 10 no. 2 (2014): 81–95.

Derrick, K.S. Quantitative assay for plant viruses using serologically specific electron microscopy. *Virology* 56 (1973): 652–653.

Devitt, G., Howard, K., Mudher, A. *et al.* Raman spectroscopy: an emerging tool in neurodegenerative disease research and diagnosis. *ACS Chemical Neuroscience* 9 no. 3 (2018): 404–420.

Dillard, R.S., Hampton, C.M., Strauss, J.D. *et al.* Biological applications at the cutting edge of cryo-electron microscopy. *Microscopy and Microanalysis* 24 no. 4 (2018): 406–419.

Easton, S. Practical Veterinary Diagnostic Imaging (West Sussex: Wiley-Blackwell, second edition, 2012).

Espada, Y., Novellas, R. and Ruiz de Gopegui, R. Renal ultrasound in dogs and cats. *Veterinary Research Communications* 30 (S1) (2006): 133–137.

Fitzpatrick, A.W.P., Falcon, B., He, S. *et al.* Cryo-EM structures of tau filaments from Alzheimer's disease. *Nature* 547 no. 7662 (2017): 185–190.

Fong, J.F.Y., Ng, Y.H. and Ng, S.M. Carbon dots as a new class of light emitters for biomedical diagnostics and therapeutic applications. *Fullerens, Graphenes and Nanotubes* (2018): 227–295.

Frerichs, I., Hahn, G., Schröder, T. *et al.* Electrical impedance tomography in monitoring experimental lung injury. *Intensive Care Medicine* 24 no. 8 (1998): 829–836.

Gaggero, P.O., Adler, A., Brunner, J. *et al.* Electrical impedance tomography system based on active electrodes. *Physiological Measurement* 33 no. 5 (2012): 831–847.

Gambhir, S.S., Sun, X., Xiao, Z. *et al.* A PET imaging approach for determining EGFR mutation status for improved lung cancer patient management. *Science Translational Medicine* 7 no. 431 (2018): eaan8840. doi:10.1126/scitranslmed.aan8840.

Garrigue, P., Tang, J., Ding, L. *et al.* Self-assembling supramolecular dendrimer nanosystem for PET imaging of tumors. *Proceedings of the National Academy of Sciences* 115 no. 45 (2018): 201812938.

Ginat, D.T. and Gupta, R. Advances in computed tomography imaging technology. *Annual Review of Biomedical Engineering* 16 no. 1(2014): 431–453.

Goel, S., England, C.G., Chen, F. *et al.* Positron emission tomography and nanotechnology: a dynamic duo for cancer theranostics. *Advanced Drug Delivery Reviews* 113 (2017): 157–176.

Golding, C.G., Lamboo, L.L., Beniac, D.R. *et al.* The scanning electron microscope in microbiology and diagnosis of infectious disease. *Scientific Reports* 6 no. 1 (2016). doi:10.1038/srep26516.

Goldsmith, S. and Kopeloff, A. Use of polarized-light microscopy as an aid in the diagnosis of silicosis. *New England Journal of Medicine* 265 no. 5 (1961): 233–235.

Gonzalez, S.A., Morales, J.M., Gonzalez, D.J.M. *et al.* Magnetic resonance microscopy at 14 tesla and correlative histopathology of human brain tumour tissue. *PLOS One* 6 no. 11 (2011): e27442.

Gou, Z., Huanglong, S., Ke, W. *et al.* (2019). Self-powered X-ray detector based on all-inorganic perovskite thick film with high sensitivity under low dose rate. *Physica Status Solidi (RRL) – Rapid Research Letters* (2019): 1900094. doi:10.1002/pssr.201900094.

Guerrero-Ferreira, R., Taylor, N.M., Mona, D. *et al.* Cryo-EM structure of alpha-synuclein fibrils. *Nanomedicine* 14 no. 4 (2018): 7.

Gugjoo, M.B., Amarpal, K.P. *et al.* An update on diagnostic imaging techniques in veterinary practice. *Advances in Animal and Veterinary Sciences* 2 no. 4S (2014): 64–77.

Gustafsson, M.G.L. Nonlinear structured-illumination microscopy: wide-field fluorescence imaging with theoretically unlimited resolution. *Proceedings of the National Academy of Sciences* 102 (2005): 13081–13086.

Gwosch, K.C., Pape, J.K., Balzarotti, F. *et al.* MINFLUX nanoscopy delivers 3D multicolor nanometer resolution in cells. *Nature Methods* 17 (2020): 217–224.

Harisinghani, M.G., O'Shea, A. and Weissleder, R. Advances in clinical MRI technology. *Science Translational Medicine* 11 no. 523 (2019): eaba2591.

Harmsen, S., Rogalla, S., Huang, R. *et al.* Detection of pre-malignant gastrointestinal lesions using surface-enhanced resonance Raman scattering-nanoparticle endoscopy. *ACS Nano* (2019). doi:10.1021/acsnano.8b06808.

Haun, J.B., Castro, C.M., Wang, R. *et al.* Micro-NMR for rapid molecular analysis of human tumor samples. *Science Translational Medicine* 3 no. 71 (2011): 71ra16–71ra16.

Havens, K.J. and Sharp, E.J. *Thermal Imaging Techniques to Survey and Monitor Animals in the Wild: A Methodology* (Amsterdam; Boston, MA: The Academic Press, 2016).

Hazelton, P.R. and Gelderblom, H.R. Electron microscopy for rapid diagnosis of emerging infectious agents. *Emerging Infectious Diseases* 9 no. 3 (2003): 294–303.

Henderson, R.P. and Webster, J.G. An impedance camera for spatially specific measurements of the thorax. *IEEE Transactions of Biomedical Engineering* 25 no. 3 (1978): 250–254.

Hershberger, M.V. and Lumry, R.W. The photophysics of 5-methoxyindole. A non-exciplex forming indole. *Phororhrmistry and Photohiology* 23 (1976): 391–397.

Jacobs, R.E. and Fraser, S.E. Magnetic resonance microscopy of embryonic cell lineages and movements. *Science* 263 no. 5147 (1994): 681–684.

Jaszczak, R.J., Coleman, R.E. and Lim, C.B. SPECT: Single photon emission computed tomography. *IEEE Transactions on Nuclear Science* 27 no. 3 (1980): 1137–1153.

Jáuregui, O., Casals, I. and Fernández, I. *Handbook of Instrumental Techniques from CCiTUB: Biomedical and Biological Applications of Scanning Electron Microscopy* (2012). Corpus ID: 12439309.

Jha, A.K., Goenka, M.K., Nijhawan, S. *et al.* Nanotechnology in gastrointestinal endoscopy: a primer. *Journal of Digestive Endoscopy* 3 no. S05 (2012): 77–80.

Jin, D., Xi, P., Wang, B. *et al.* Nanoparticles for super-resolution microscopy and single-molecule tracking. *Nature Methods* 15 no. 6 (2018): 415–423.

Johnson, J.E. *et al.* Comparison of the lipid regulation of yeast and rat CTP: phosphocholine cytidylyltransferase expressed in COS cells. *Biochemical Journal* 285 Pt 3 (1992): 815–820.

Judkins, S.W. and Joanne, C.P. Synovial fluid crystal analysis. *Laboratory Medicine* 28 (1997): 774–779.

Kang, J.W., Lue, N., Kong, C.R. *et al.* Combined confocal Raman and quantitative phase microscopy system for biomedical diagnosis. *Biomedical Optics Express* 2 no. 9 (2011): 2484.

Kepsutlu, B., Wycisk, V., Achazi, K. *et al.* Cells undergo major changes in the quantity of cytoplasmic organelles after uptake of gold nanoparticles with biologically relevant surface coatings. *ACS Nano* (2020): 1–26.

Kurt, B. and Cihan, M. Evaluation of the clinical and ultrasonographic findings in abdominal disorders in cattle. *Veterinarski Arhiv* 83 no. 1 (2013): 11–21.

Lal, R. and John, S.A. Biological applications of atomic force microscopy. *American Journal of Physiology-Cell Physiology* 266 no. 1 (1994): C1–21.

Le Gros, M.A., McDermott, G., Cinquin, B.P. *et al.* Biological soft X-ray tomography on beamline. *Advanced Light Source* 21 (2014): 1370–1377.

Lee, C.H., Bengtsson, N., Chrzanowski, S.M. *et al.* (2017). Magnetic resonance microscopy (MRM) of single mammalian myofibers and myonuclei. *Scientific Reports* 7 no. 1 (2017). doi:10.1038/srep39496.

Li, Y., Shaker, K., Larsson, J.C. *et al.* A library of potential nanoparticle contrast agents for x-ray fluorescence tomography bioimaging. *Contrast Media and Molecular Imaging* (2018): 1–7.

Lohrke, J., Siebeneicher, H., Berger, M. *et al.* 18 F-GP1, a Novel PET tracer designed for high-sensitivity, low-background detection of thrombi. *Journal of Nuclear Medicine* 58 no. 7 (2017): 1094–1099.

Long, K.J., Bonagura, J.D. and Darke, P.G.G. Standardised imaging technique for guided M-mode and Doppler echocardiography in the horse. *Equine Veterinary Journal* 24 no. 3 (1992): 226–235.

Ma, D., Lu, H., Zhang, C. *et al.* Use of polarized light microscopy is essential in the efficient diagnosis of respiratory amyloidosis and could decrease disease prevalence. *The Clinical Respiratory Journal* 11 no. 6 (2015): 691–695.

Maccora, D., Dini, V., Battocchio, C. *et al.* Gold nanoparticles and nanorods in nuclear medicine: a mini review. *Applied Sciences* 9 no. 16 (2019): 3232.

Manwaring, P.K., Moodie, K.L., Hartov, A. *et al.* Intracranial electrical impedance tomography. *Anesthesia & Analgesia* 117 no. 4 (2013): 866–875.

Martínez, O., Bellard, E., Golzio, M. *et al.* Direct validation of aptamers as powerful tools to image solid tumor. *Nucleic Acid Therapeutics* 24 no. 3 (2014): 217–225.

Mattea, F., Vedelago, J., Malano, F. *et al.* Silver nanoparticles in X-ray biomedical applications. *Radiation Physics and Chemistry* 130 (2017): 442–450.

Maxie, G. *Jubb, Kennedy & Palmer's Pathology of Domestic Animals, Volume 2* (Amsterdam: Elsevier, 6th edn, 2016).

McMullan, D. Scanning electron microscopy 1928–1965. *Scanning* 17 no. 3 (2006): 175–185.

Mehta, K.S., Lee, J.J., Taha, A.A. *et al.* Vascular applications of contrast-enhanced ultrasound imaging. *Journal of Vascular Surgery* 66 no. 1 (2017): 266–274.

Mendonca, D.M.H. and Lauterbur, P.C. Contrast agents for nuclear magnetic resonance imaging. *Biological Trace Element Research* 13 (1987): 229–239.

Mohammad, K.S., Bdesha, A.S., Snell, M.E. *et al.* Phase contrast microscopic examination of urinary erythrocytes to localise source of bleeding: an overlooked technique. *Journal of Clinical Pathology* 46 no. 7 (1993): 642–645.

Morris, J.D. and Payne, C.K. Microscopy and cell biology: new methods and new questions. *Annual Review of Physical Chemistry* 70 no. 1 (2019). doi:10.1146/annurev-physchem-042018-052527.

Mostany, R., Miquelajauregui, A., Shtrahman, M. *et al.* Two-photon excitation microscopy and its applications in neuroscience. *Advanced Fluorescence Microscopy* (2014): 25–42.

Mudry, K.M., Plonsey, R., Bronzino, J.D. *Principles and Applications in Engineering* (Boca Raton, FL: Biomedical Imaging CRC Press, 2003).

Musumeci, D., Platella, C., Riccardi, C. *et al.* Fluorescence sensing using DNA aptamers in cancer research and clinical diagnostics. *Cancers* 9 no. 12 (2017): 174.

Ostadhossein, F., Tripathi, I., Benig, L. *et al.* Multi-"color" delineation of bone microdamages using ligand-directed sub-5 nm hafnia nanodots and photon counting ct imaging. *Advanced Functional Materials* (2019): 1904936.

Pirnstill, C.W. and Coté, G.L. Malaria diagnosis using a mobile phone polarized microscope. *Scientific Reports* 5 no. 1 (2015): 13368.

Pooh, R.K., Maeda, K., Kurjak, A. *et al.* 3D/4D sonography – any safety problem. *Journal of Perinatal Medicine* 44 no. 2 (2016): 125–129.

Prasad, M., Ghosh, M., Brar, B. *et al.* Nano-antimicrobials: a new paradigm for combating mycobacterial resistance – a review article. *Current Pharmaceutical Design* 25 no. 13 (2019): 1554–1579.

Prasad, M., Ghosh, M., Kumar, R. *et al.* An insight into nanomedicinal approaches to combat viral zoonoses. *Current Topics in Medicinal Chemistry* 20 no. 11 (2020a): 915–962.

Prasad, M., Kumar, R., Ghosh, M. *et al.* Application of polymeric nano-materials in management of inflammatory bowel disease. *Current Topics in Medicinal Chemistry* 20 no. 11 (2020b): 982–1008.

Prigozhin, M.B., Maurer, P.C., Courtis, A.M. *et al.* Bright sub-20-nm cathodoluminescent nanoprobes for electron microscopy. *Nature Nanotechnology* 14 (2019): 420–425.

Puppels, G.J., De Mul, F.F.M., Otto, C. *et al.* Studying single living cells and chromosomes by confocal Raman microspectroscopy. *Nature* 347(1990): 301–303.

Racki, S., Grzetić, M., Prodan-Merlak, Z. *et al.* Clinical use of phase-contrast microscopy in the differential diagnosis of microhematuria. *Acta Med Croatica* 57 no. 1 (2003): 11–16.

Rajamahendran, R., Ambrose, D.J. and Burton, B. Clinical and research applications of real-time ultrasonography in bovine reproduction: A review. *Canadian Veterinary Journal* 35 no. 9 (1994): 563–572.

Rand, D., Ortiz, V., Liu, Y. *et al.* Nanomaterials for X-ray imaging: gold nanoparticle enhancement of X-ray scatter imaging of hepatocellular carcinoma. *Nano Letters* 11 no. 7 (2011): 2678–2683.

Rinck, P.A. *Magnetic Resonance in Medicine: A Critical Introduction* (Norderstedt: European Magnetic Resonance Forum, 12th edn, 2018).

Roane, T.M. and Pepper, I.L. Microscopic techniques. In Pepper, I., Gerba, C. and Gentry, T. (eds), *Environmental Microbiology*, pp. 177–193 (Cambridge, MA: The Academic Press, 2015).

Rogalla, S., Flisikowski, K., Gorpas, D. *et al.* Biodegradable fluorescent nanoparticles for endoscopic detection of colorectal carcinogenesis. *Advanced Functional Materials* (2019): 1904992.

Rogers, W.L. and Ackermann, R.J. SPECT instrumentation. *American Journal of Physiologic Imaging* 7 no. 4 (1992): 105–120.

Ruska, E. *The Early Development of Electron Lenses and Electron Microscopy*. Translation by Mulvey, T. (Stuttgart: S. Hirzel Verlag, 1980).

Savina, L.V., Pavlishchuk, S.A., Samsygin, V.I. *et al.* Polarization microscopy in diagnosis of metabolic disorders. *Kliniceskaja Laboratornaja Diagnostika* 3 (2003): 11–14.

Schermelleh, L., Ferrand, A., Huser, T. *et al.* Super-resolution microscopy demystified. *Nature Cell Biology* 21 no. 1 (2019): 72–84.

Schnitzbauer, J., Strauss, M., Schlichthaerle, T. *et al.* Super-resolution microscopy with DNA-PAINT. *Nature Protocols* 12 (2017): 1198–1228.

Scimeca, M., Montanaro, M., Bonfiglio, R. *et al.* Electron microscopy in human diseases: diagnostic and research perspectives. *Nanomedicine* 14 no. 4 (2019). doi:10.2217/nnm-2018-0407.

Scimeca, M., Bischetti, S., Lamsira, H.K. *et al.* Energy dispersive X-ray (EDX) microanalysis: a powerful tool in biomedical research and diagnosis. *European Journal of Histochemistry* 62 no. 1 (2018). doi:10.4081/ejh.2018.2841.

Suri, J.S., Chang, R.F., Kathuria, C., Fenster, A. and Molinari, F. *Advances in Diagnostic and Therapeutic Ultrasound Imaging* (Norwood, MA: Artech House, 2008).

Swarup, S. and Makaryus, A. Digital stethoscope: technology update. *Medical Devices: Evidence and Research* 11 (2018): 29–36.

Tabari, A., Lo Gullo, R., Murugan, V. *et al.* Recent advances in computed tomographic technology. *Journal of Thoracic Imaging* 32 no. 2 (2017): 89–100.

Telkanranta, H., Paul, E. and Mendl, M. Measuring Animal Emotions with Infrared Thermography: How to Realise the Potential and Avoid the Pitfalls. Conference: Recent Advances in Animal Welfare Science VI. Newcastle, United Kingdom, June 28, 2018.

Thakor, A.S., Jokerst, J.V., Ghanouni, P. *et al.* Clinically approved nanoparticle imaging agents. *Journal of Nuclear Medicine* 57 no. 12 (2016): 1833–1837.

Thorley, J.A., Pike, J. and Rappoport, J.Z. Super-resolution microscopy. *Fluorescence Microscopy* (2014): 199–212.

Tranquart, F., Grenier, N., Eder, V. *et al.* Clinical use of ultrasound tissue harmonic imaging. *Ultrasound in Medicine & Biology* 25 no. 6 (1999): 889–894.

Tsai, H., Liu, F., Shrestha, S. *et al.* A sensitive and robust thin-film X-ray detector using 2D layered perovskite diodes. *Science Advances* 6 no. 15 (2020): eaay0815.

Tsui, B.M.W., Zhao, X., Frey, E.C. *et al.* Quantitative single-photon emission computed tomography: Basic and clinical considerations. *Seminars in Nuclear Medicine* 24 no. 1 (1994): 38–65.

Uppal, T. Tissue harmonic imaging. *Australasian Journal of Ultrasound in Medicine* 13 no. 2 (2010): 29–31.

Vaga, R. and Bryant, K. Recent advances in X-ray technology. Pan Pacific Microelectronics Symposium (Pan Pacific), 2016. doi:10.1109/panpacific.2016.7428397.

Visonà, S.D., Chen, Y., Bernardi, P. *et al.* Diagnosis of electrocution: the application of scanning electron microscope and energy-dispersive X-ray spectroscopy in five cases. *Forensic Science International* 284 (2018): 107–116.

Watanabe, S., Takeda, S., Ishikawa, S. *et al.* Development of semiconductor imaging detectors for a Si/CdTe Compton camera. *Nuclear Instruments and Methods in Physics Research Section A: Accelerators, Spectrometers, Detectors and Associated Equipment* 579 no. 2 (2007): 871–877.

Weinhardt, V., Chen, J.H., Ekman, A. *et al.* Imaging cell morphology and physiology using X-rays – a review article. *Biochemical Society Transactions* 47 no. 2 (2019): 489–508.

Wombacher, R., Heidbreder, M., van de Linde, S. *et al.* Live-cell super-resolution imaging with trimethoprim conjugates. *Nature Methods* 7 (2010): 717–719.

Wright, B. Global biofuels: key to the puzzle of grain market behavior. *Journal of Economic Perspectives* 28 no. 1 (2014): 73–98.

Yang, T.T., Tran, M.N.T., Chong, W.M., Huang, C.E. and Liao, J.C. Single-particle tracking localization microscopy reveals nonaxonemal dynamics of intraflagellar transport proteins at the base of mammalian primary cilia. *Molecular Biology of the Cell* 30 no. 7 (2019): 828–837.

Yeh, B.M., FitzGerald, P.F., Edic, P.M. *et al.* Opportunities for new CT contrast agents to maximize the diagnostic potential of emerging spectral CT technologies. *Advanced Drug Delivery Reviews* 113 (2017): 201–222.

Yue, X., Wang, A. and Li, Q. The role of scanning electron microscopy in the direct diagnosis of onychomycosis. *Scanning* (2018): 1–4.

Zaninelli, M., Redaelli, V., Luzi, F. *et al.* First evaluation of infrared thermography as a tool for the monitoring of udder health status in farms of dairy cows. *Sensors* 18 no. 3 (2018): 862.

Zhou, X. and Lauterbur, P.C. NMR microscopy using projection reconstruction. In Blumich, B. and Kuhn, W. (eds), *Magnetic Resonance Microscopy*, pp. 3–27 (Weinheim: VCH, 1992).

Zhu, B., Liu, J.Z., Cauley, S.F. *et al.* Image reconstruction by domain-transform manifold learning. *Nature* 555 no. 7697 (2018): 487–492.

9

Listeriosis in Animals: Prevalence and Detection

Tejinder Kaur and Praveen P. Balgir
Department of Biotechnology, Punjabi University, Patiala-147002, Punjab, India
Corresponding author: Praveen P. Balgir, *balgirbt@live.com*

9.1 Introduction

Listeriosis is an infectious disease of animals that can infect humans too. Its causative bacteria were first isolated by Murray in 1926, in guinea pigs and rabbits in the lab during investigation of an epidemic (Murray *et al.* 1926). It was named *Bacterium monocytogenes* since an increased count of monocytes was observed in blood of infected animals. A year later, morphologically similar bacteria isolated from diseased livers of gerbils was named *Listerella hepatolytica*, in honor of Sir Joseph Lister, a pioneer of antisepsis. Later, the two names were harmonized to *Listeria monocytogenes*.

9.2 Epidemiology, Transmission and Spread

Listeria have been observed to infect different groups of animals, ranging from birds like chicken, quail, partridge and ostrich, to small ruminants like sheep and goat, to larger cattle like cows and buffaloes (OIE 2014). The pathogen has been identified in the meat and milk of animals, and in fish and fishery products (Dhama *et al.*, 2015).

L. monocytogenes, a Gram-positive bacillus, has been observed to live freely in the environment in water, sludge, soil, plants, vegetation and food, and to infect a wide range of both cold- as well as warm-blooded animal species, including humans. Its natural hosts include small animals like arthropods, fish, birds and rodents, to larger animals such as goats, sheep, dogs, pigs, cattle, buffaloes, camels and animals in the wild (Dhama *et al.* 2013).

The bacterium is observed to transgress across the intestinal, foeto-placental and blood-brain barriers, leading to its systemic spread all over the body of the organism (Vazquez-Boland *et al.* 2001). This spread explains the observed characteristics (OIE 2014), viz., gastroenteritis, septicaemia, encephalitis, meningitis, meningoencephalitis and rhombencephalitis, in a variety of infected animals. If pregnant, the infected animal is also prone to abortion and stillbirth (Cossart and Lebreton 2014; Dhama *et al.* 2015).

9.3 Organism Characteristics and Classification

L. monocytogenes is observed to be a Gram-positive, small, motile flagellate, rod-shaped cocco-bacillus. It is a non-spore-forming, non-capsulated pleomorphic, facultative intracellular anaerobe. It exists as a ubiquitous saprophyte living on decaying organic matter. However, once it enters an animal's body, it can colonize it and ultimately lead to its death (Vazquez-Boland *et al.* 2001). Foraging animals are easily exposed to this environmental uptake and become conduits of the faeco-oral cycle (Campero *et al.* 2002; Milillo *et al.* 2012). A number of virulence factors have been identified and characterized from this pathogen (Vera *et al.*, 2013). These factors have been localized to the pathogenicity island designated as LIPI-1 (Listeria Pathogenicity Island 1) and are regulated by PrfA protein, the master regulator. All these proteins carry the bacterium through various stages of its life cycle, including adhesion, invasion of the host cell, intracellular multiplication and propagation.

Presently, more than 20 species have been included in the genus listeria *L. monocytogenes*. These include *L. ivanovii*, *L. grayi*, *L. innocua*, *L. seeligeri*, *L. welshimeri*, *L. marthii* and *L. rocourtiae*, as reported by Graves *et al.* (2010) and Leclercq *et al.* (2010). Halter *et al.* (2013) reported *L. fleischmannii*, as did Bertsch *et al.* (2013). Later, *L. weihenstephanensis*, *L. floridensis*, *L. aquatica*, *L. cornellensis*, *L. riparia* and *L. grandensi* were reported by den Bakker *et al.* (2014), and *L. booriae* and *L. newyorkensis* by Weller *et al.* (2015). Recently, *L. goaensis* was identified by Doijad *et al.* (2018). Of all the species studied, only *L. monocytogenes* and *L. ivanovii* have been observed to cause disease in animals as well as humans (Guillet *et al.* 2010) and *L. ivanovii* has been mainly isolated from ruminants suffering from listeriosis (McLauchlin 1997).

L. monocytogenes has been classified into four evolutionary lineages (I, II, III and IV) based on their distinct ecologic, genetic and phenotypic characteristics. All these lineages have been found to occupy different but overlapping eco-niches. Human clinical samples are the source of Lineages I and II, which further yield serotypes 1/2b and 4b of Lineage I and 1/2a of Lineage II. Lineage-II strains are widespread in nature, including on farms, and consequently have been isolated from food as contaminants and from farm animal listeriosis cases. Lineage-III and -IV strains have been mainly isolated from animals sources and are encountered rarely compared to the other two (Orsi *et al.* 2011). Further studies have found plasmids to be more numerous in Lineage-II than Lineage-I isolates. The plasmids usually carry bacteriocin resistance, metal and other toxin resistance genes which confer a distinct advantage for its survival in varied environments. Some isolates of Lineage I are distinguished from the other three lineages by the presence of pathogenic listerolysin S haemolysin. Many of the Lineage-II isolates display attenuated virulence due to presence of mutations in *prfA* and *inlA* genes, and also a higher rate of recombination that seems to facilitate their adaptation to various environmental niches.

Based on cellular and flagellar antigens of *L. monocytogenes* it has been classified into 13 serotypes, listed as 1/2a, 1/2b, 1/2c, 3a, 3b, 3c, 4a, 4ab, 4b, 4c, 4d, 4e and 7 by Muñoz (2012). Out of these, the commonly reported serotypes from animals are 1/2a and 4b (Datta *et al.* 2013; Mateus *et al.* 2013).

9.4 Life Cycle

Listeriosis, the clinical manifestation of *L. monocytogenes* infection, is mainly reported in ruminants, whereas pigs and birds generally manifest subclinical carrier status. Usually animals harbour the bacteria asymptomatically but sporadic outbreaks on farms have been reported from all over the world. Animals seem to act as reservoirs and disease is spread to humans when contaminated animal products like beef and milk are consumed by them. A number of outbreaks in human populations have sporadically been reported (USDA 2019).

While the organism can thrive in a wide temperature range of from 4 to 45°C, its optimum growth is observed between 30 and 37°C (Janakiraman 2008). Though the bacterium displays motility at 25°C, at extremes of temperature its growth is minimal. The pH optima for growth of listeria has been reported to range from 4.5 to 9.6 (Barbuddhe and Chakraborty 2009; OIE 2014). Listeria is killed by pasteurization at 72°C for 10 seconds. The bacterium has been observed to survive for years outside the host, even in moist soil. The genus Listeria is characterized by low GC DNA content of 38%, like many organisms belonging to the Firmicutes division.

Listeria infects the host by crossing intestinal, placental and blood-brain barrier. On the intestinal barrier the bacteria first get bound to receptors on the epithelial layer of cells, which they cross to enter the blood stream and the lymphatic system, leading to their systemic spread. *L. monocytogenes*, upon reaching the liver and spleen, replicate preferentially inside splenic and hepatic macrophages or epithelial cells (Lecuit 2007). They also target dendritic cells after intestinal delivery, within which the bacteria escape from phagosomes and spread to neighbouring cells (Guzman *et al.* 1995). If the host innate immune response is able to inhibit pathogen replication they do not cause disease; however, if the bacteria escape from first-line immune clearance they keep on multiplying. The organism multiplies intracellularly and passes from one cell to neighbouring cells without lysis of the first cell. *L. monocytogenes* was long presumed to be a model for cytosolic pathogens, but now it has emerged that the bacterium is also capable of surviving in the vacuoles, where it may have a slow or non-growing existence (Bierne *et al.* 2018). It is found in this state in asymptomatic carrier animals. The significance of this observation of persistent vacuolar listeria is that in this state it is less susceptible to antibiotics and more difficult to treat as well as detect by routine clinical techniques. The life cycle is depicted in Figure 9.1. This ability also explains its pathogenesis and clinical manifestation (Janakiraman 2008).

9.4.1 *L. monocytogenes* Virulence Factors

Several virulence determinants (Figure 9.1) have been reported to play a role in host-pathogen interaction and propagation of the pathogen (Camejo *et al.* 2011). Adhesion and internalization are the initial steps in infection.

9.4.2 Factors for Adhesion

Starting with adhesion, which involves several bacterial surface molecules, like Lap, Ami, dltA, FbpA, InlJ, CtaP, LapB, ActA and InlF. Lap is a 104 kDa adhesion protein, an alcohol acetaldehyde dehydrogenase. Lap binds to Hsp60, which is its receptor on the host cell. This receptor binding leads to bacterial adhesion to the intestinal epithelium. The protein's importance in adhesion can be gauged from the fact that it is found in all listerial species, with the exception of *L. grayi*.

Ami is an N-acetyl muramoyl-L alanine amidase, a protein of 99 kDa. It acts on the peptidoglycans, on the amide bond between N-acetyl muramic acid and L-alanine residues, using its N-terminal domain. Using the eight glycine-tryptophan (GW) modules present in its C-terminal that constitute its cell

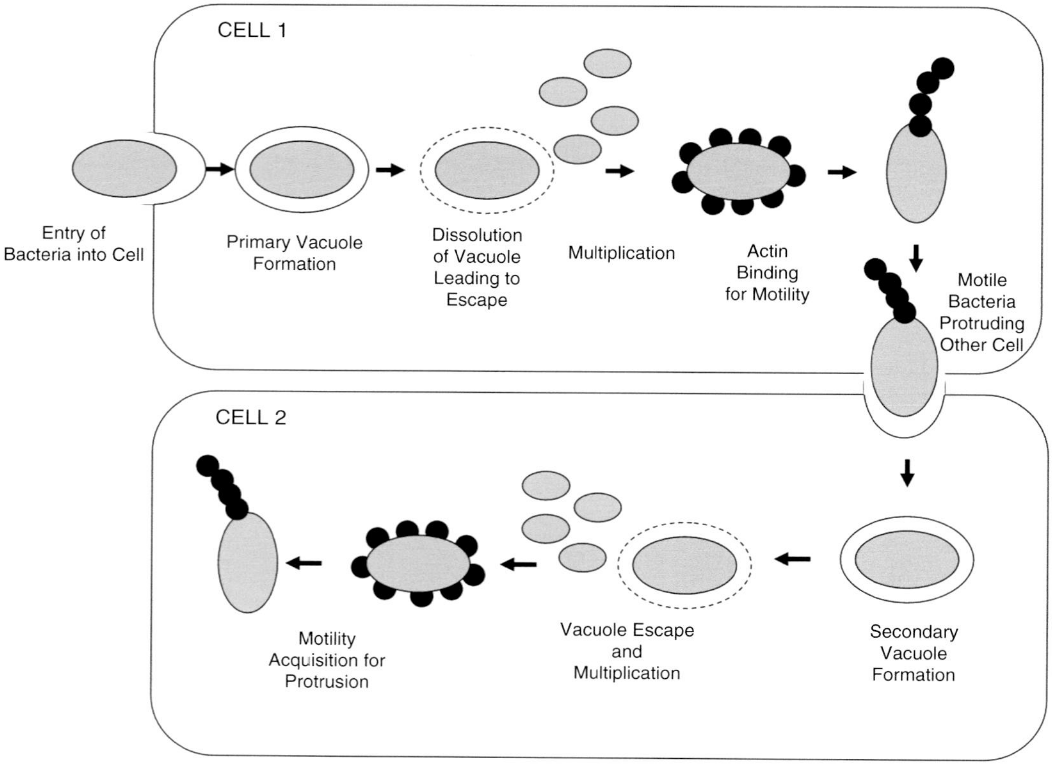

FIGURE 9.1 Life cycle of Listeria.

wall-anchoring (CWA) domain, it anchors to the host cell wall. CWA domain anchors Ami to the bacterial surface, probably by interacting with lipoteichoic acids (LTAs). This CWA domain is also reported to be involved in anchoring the bacteria to the host cells (Camejo *et al.* 2011).

DltA is implicated in D-alanylation of LTAs which leads to bacterial adhesion. FbpA is a strong atypical fibronectin-binding protein. InlJ belongs to the internalin family of proteins present in genome of *L. monocytogenes* strains only, and has leucine-rich repeats (LRRs). Its C-terminus has an LPXTG motif which is covalently bound to the peptidoglycans by the activity of sortase A (SrtA) enzyme. Further *L. monocytogenes* and *L. innocua* strains express inlJ which binds to MUC2, which is the main component of mucosal secretion of the intestine, using its internalin domain (Sabet *et al.* 2008). InlF is an internalin, which is functional only during infection in selected host species.

The CtaP is a cysteine transport-associated protein; as its name suggests, it is functionally associated with cysteine transport. However, it is also involved in acid tolerance, membrane integrity and adhesion to host cells. Its expression is regulated by the master regulator PrfA in Listeria sps.

LapB is a LPXTG domain containing SrtA-anchored protein that is present only in pathogenic Listeria species, under the positive regulation of PrfA. It anchors to the host membrane by its N-terminal binding to a receptor. ActA protein is essential for the intracellular actin-mediated motility of *L. monocytogenes*. By virtue of its recognition of heparin sulfate, it helps host cell attachment and entry. RecA, involved in DNA repair and activation of the SOS response, has a role as an accessory protein in adhesion.

9.4.3 Factors for Host Invasion

L. monocytogenes' entry into macrophages is mainly self-driven by these cells, but phagocyte entry requires bacterial proteins that interact with specific receptors on host cells. Internalins A (InlA) (Gaillard *et al.* 1991) and B (InlB) (Dramsi *et al.* 1995), the two major *L. monocytogenes* invasion proteins, were the first to be identified as assisting entry of Listeria into various non-phagocytic cell types. LPXTG motif present in InlA binds covalently to the host cell wall. InlA binds to E-cadherin, a cell-cell adhesion protein, to facilitate the invasion. Binding of InlA/E-cadherin at the cell surface leads to the activation of host Src kinase, which prompts the recruitment of clathrin and polymerisation of actin at the point of entry, which finally leads to endocytosis of the E-cadherin-enclosed bacterial cell (Bonazzi *et al.* 2008). The InlB protein was observed to have an elongated structure, and thus it was postulated to interact with a number of receptors on the host surface. Its GW (glycine tryptophan) modules mediate non-covalent interactions with the bacterial surface LTAs. The leucine-rich repeats (LRRs) of InlB have been found to bind to various cell surface proteins of the host cell, including gC1qR, c-Met (a tyrosine kinase) and glycosaminoglycans (GAGs). Entry of bacteria into host cells is eased by GAG receptors, which aid in removing bacterial surface InlB, allowing bacterial clustering at the host cell membrane that in turn strongly promotes Met activation. This interaction of InlB with Met induces ubiquitination of Met, which promotes bacterial internalisation in a clathrin-coated vesicle by endocytosis. InlA and InlB interaction is also found to be critical for efficient placental invasion (Disson *et al.* 2008).

Vip is also a LPXTG motif protein, which is attached at the peptidoglycan layer and characterized by ubiquitous presence in all *L. monocytogenes* lineages, except for non-strains. The Vip protein receptor appears to be Gp96 (G protein), which is also known to bind and activate monocytes as well as neutrophils. It is involved in intracellular localisation of Toll-like receptors (TLRs) (Yang *et al.* 2007).

Thus, while promoting invasion of the host cell by bacteria, the binding of Vip with Gp96 interferes with TLR internalisation and influences the host cell innate immune response to *L. monocytogenes.*

The *aut* gene encodes the protein Auto, which is not found in non-pathogenic strains like *L. innocua*; hence, it is also considered a pathogenicity determinant of *L. monocytogenes*. It is autolytic in nature and cleaves its signal peptide, giving rise to its active N-acetyl glucosaminidase domain at the N-terminal, which is functional at acidic pH. Like Ami and InlB, Auto is anchored by its C-terminal domain, made up of GW repeats, to the bacterial cell wall.

The *iap* gene encodes the p60 protein, which is an important bacterial cell surface protein and has hydrolase activity, whose absence disables invasion by bacterial cells. A diacylglyceryl transferase encoded by the *lgt* gene is responsible for lipidation of prolipoproteins to anchoring of lipoproteins, which maintain the net charge of the bacterial surface and hence assist invasion. Another protein, GtcA, which is involved in glycosylation of the cell wall techoic acid, also assists the entry of bacterial cells into host cells.

LpeA is a 35 kD protein especially important for *L. monocytogenes*' entry into mouse hepatocytes and human intestinal epithelial cells (Réglier-Poupet *et al.* 2003). MprF (multiple peptide resistance factor) carries out lysinylation of diphosphatidylglycerol (DPG) within the bacterial membrane, generating lysyl-phosphatidyl-glycerol (L-PG), an important phospholipid of the bacterial membrane, which is crucial for the bacterial invasiveness of both epithelial cells as well as macrophages.

Listeriolysin O (LLO) is the factor mainly responsible for the escape of bacterial cells from the intracellular vacuoles, but has also been shown to facilitate host cell invasion by inducing an influx of calcium ions which results in a transient mitochondrial network fragmentation (Stavru *et al.* 2011), leading to a slowdown in the bio-energetic state of the host cell and promoting invasion by *L. monocytogenes*.

9.4.4 Factors for Escape from Phagocytic Vacuole

The invasion of Listeria into a phagocytic vacuole is a temporary state; it soon escapes into the host cell cytoplasm. This escape is facilitated by various factors.

One of the main proteins involved in the escape of the bacteria from the vacuole is Listeriolysin O (LLO). LLO, encoded by the *hly* gene, is part of the LIPI-1 locus containing the set of virulence genes *prfA*, *plcA*, *hly*, *mpl*, *actA* and *plcB*, respectively. The secreted protein, LLO, belongs to the cholesterol-dependant-cytolysin (CDC) family of toxins. It has optimum activity within the vacuole at acidic pH but is reduced in cytoplasm at neutral pH, thus avoiding damaging effects on the host cell cytoplasm (Beauregard *et al.* 1997). LLO oligomerizes at the membrane of the phagosome, causing perforation and escape of the bacterial cell. It is also reported to influence the host by suppressing protein sumolyation, which results in a decrease in immune response. LLO has been shown to act as a strong signalling molecule that can trigger the apoptotic pathway, upregulate adhesins and cytokines, and activate MAP kinase and protein kinase C pathways. It also plays a role in bacterial invasion by influencing the intracellular Ca^{2+} level.

Two phospholypase C enzymes, a phosphatidylinositol-specific PLC (*plcA*) and a broad-range PC-PLC (*plcB*), have been observed to cooperate with LLO in lysing the phagocytic vacuole, leading to the escape of bacteria into cytoplasm (Goldfine and Knob 1992). A zinc metalloprotease Mpl activates the PC-PLC proenzyme in the acidic environs of the vacuole (Domann *et al.* 1991).

Alonzo *et al.* (2009) reported PrsA2 as another important factor for the vacuolar escape stage of Listeria.

PrsA2 is a chaperone that is functional at the bacterial membrane, interacting with the host cell wall. It is responsible for folding proteins that translocate across the bacterial membrane, e.g., LLO and PC-PLC. PrsA2 is responsible for proper folding, stability and thus activity of LLO and PC-PLC. The factor has been found to be essential for intracellular replication of Listeria.

SvpA, a 64 kDa surface protein, was reported by Borezee *et al.* (2001) to be essential for intracellular survival by promoting escape from the phagocytic vacuole. It is a type-I signal peptidase SipZ that allows processing and secreting of PC-PLC and LLO, helping in vacuolar lysis. Another listerial signal peptidase, Lsp, which converts pre-lipoproteins to mature lipoproteins, has been observed to be highly upregulated within the phagocytic vacuole. Mutation in *lsp* impairs the escape of bacterial cells (Bonnemain *et al.* 2004).

9.4.5 Factors for Intracellular Survival and Multiplication

The escape of listerial cells from the phagocytic vacuole is followed by replication in the host cytoplasm. The energy for this multiplication comes from glucose-1-phosphate of the host cell, which it acquires using its hexose phosphate transporter protein, Hpt. Hence the *hpt* gene product is essential for the survival of Listeria (Chico-Calero *et al.* 2002).

Pyruvate dehydrogenase (PDH) is involved in converting pyruvate to acetyl-coA. This increases the flux of acetyl-coA from the glycolytic pathway into the TCA cycle, for utilisation by the bacteria. Thus, TCA cycle enzymes are essential to the survival and multiplication of the pathogen within the host cell.

Lipoate ligase LplA1 (O'Riordan *et al.* 2003) is an enzyme required by Listeria to perform lipoyl modification in the E2 subunit of host pyruvate dehydrogenase to produce E2-lipoamide, which is utilized by the bacterium for its own growth and metabolism. Lipoic acid (LA) is a cofactor of PDH and other related enzymes; thus, E2 PDH modification targets the meeting point in regulating the metabolism of glucose and fatty acid oxidation pathways. Thus, LplA1 is an essential factor for the intracellular survival and multiplication of Listeria.

Bacterial *pycA*, which encodes a pyruvate carboxylase (Schär *et al.*, 2010), the enzyme of the tricarboxylic acid cycle, is essential for listerial replication. Fri is a unique ferritin involved in iron storage in bacterial cells. Since the host vertebrate cells do not contain free iron, hence all intracellular bacterial pathogens face iron starvation in such host cells. Fri can control the concentration of available iron and hydrogen peroxide, and hence it is an important factor for the growth of Listeria intracellularly (Dussurget *et al.* 2005).

RelA, the main factor responsible for mounting the stringent response in bacterial cells, has been found to be essential for intracellular replication of Listeria. The gene *prsA2* encodes a post-translocation chaperone, and as explained earlier is responsible for the folding of functional proteins which ensure growth and multiplication of *L. monocytogenes* intracellularly in the host cell (Alonzo and Freitag 2010).

The oligopeptide-binding protein OppA, which mediates the transport of oligopeptides, is essential to the intracellular survival and growth of *L. monocytogenes*. About 150 small non-coding RNAs (sRNAs) that are regulatory in nature are also essential (Cossart and Lebreton 2014), as proven by mutation studies by Mraheil *et al.* (2011), for the efficient growth of bacteria in macrophages.

9.4.6 Factors for Intracellular Motility and Intercellular Spread

ActA, a major virulence factor, is a surface protein anchored by its C-terminal transmembrane hydrophobic tail. Once the bacterial cell is released into the host cell cytoplasm, the N-terminal domain of ActA activates polymerisation of actin residues into a tail-like structure at one pole of the bacteria. This tail helps the bacteria in movement within the cell, as well as with inter-cellular escape to neighbouring cells (Campellone and Welch 2010). ActA contains consensus sequences similar to the WASP family of proteins, which are eukaryotic actin nucleator factors. Like other members of this protein family, ActA also contains an actin residue-binding domain and two acidic regions that allow it to bind with the host cell actin nucleator complex Arp2/3 and activate it (Welch *et al.* 1997). The proline-rich repeat region in the middle of ActA recruits the Ena/VASP (vasodilator-stimulated phosphoprotein) family of proteins, which modulate speed and directionality of bacteria. VASP plays two important functions in Listeria actin tail formation. First, it binds the profilin, which is an actin binding protein that helps actin residues to polymerize, and then it ensures the assembly of long parallel filaments by reducing the frequency of actin filament branching.

Tuba and N-WASP in mammals regulate the structure of the apical junction in epithelial cells. The inhibition of these proteins by internalin C (InlC) leads to weakening of the inter-cellular junction, followed by protrusion of the cell membrane. InlC thus increases the capacity of motile bacterial cells to form protrusions on the host plasma membrane and facilitates bacterial spread to neighbouring cells.

PrfA is the protein regulating the expression of more than 150 genes of *L. monocytogenes*, which include all major virulence genes. A homodimer of PrfA binds the promoter, the PrfA box that is made up of a palindromic sequence: tTAACanntGTtAa (the seven conserved nucleotides are depicted in capitals), and activates transcription, regulating the expression of all virulence factors simultaneously (Scortti *et al.* 2007).

As evident from above description of various factors involved in virulence, at various stages of the life cycle of *L. monocytogenes*, it has acted as a model system for the understanding of the mechanisms of other such pathogens. Despite reporting of some polymorphisms in these proteins, the role they play in disease causation and progression has not yet been established (OIE 2018).

This repertoire of factors associated with listerial infection has been exploited in the development of diagnostic tests for the pathogen, as described below.

9.5 Clinical Manifestations

In the case of sheep, goats and cattle, listeriosis presents as rhomboencephalitis, septicaemia and abortion in ruminants. It is observed that when an outbreak is reported in a flock of birds or a herd of animals, only one specific type of pathogen is encountered.

In ruminants the clinical manifestation includes anorexic and depressive symptoms, repeated head-pressing, turning of the head to one side and the appearance of unilateral cranial nerve paralysis. The disease is also known as "circling disease", as one of the signs of suffering in animals is their tendency to circle in one direction. In gravid animals, abortion is reported during the late term, i.e., after 12 weeks in the case of sheep and 7 months in the case of cattle (Hird and Genigeorgis 1990). The neonate, if born, is observed to be septicaemic in many cases, usually marked by inappetence, fever and death. Another symptom observed in ruminants is ophthalmitis. In rare cases, mastitis of ruminants has been associated with *L. monocytogenes*. However, gastroenteritis occurs sometimes in sheep (Clark *et al.* 2004). Meningoencephalitis was reported in ewes by Walker *et al.* (1994). In pigs, the main symptoms are septicaemia, with encephalitis and rarely abortions. As reported by Wesley (2007), birds are mainly carriers and display symptoms as a secondary condition to viral infection and salmonellosis, but disease manifests as septicaemia, and rarely as meningoencephalitis.

Investigation samples of brain tissue from 85 cattle presenting with neurological symptoms were observed for histological changes (Barbuceanu *et al.* 2015); one sample was characterized by microscopic examination of its monocytes, lymphocytes and perivascular sheaths to be a case of listeriosis. The bacteriological tests further confirmed it to be a case of *L. monocytogenes*.

9.6 Disease Diagnosis

The development of diagnostic tests requires evaluation of types of samples that may be easy to obtain and that help in the analysis of *L. monocytogenes*. Next is the need to study sample matrices, along with the determination of appropriate enrichment procedures. This is followed by the choice of appropriate methodology based on test molecule proteins, DNA or a metabolite for the detection of *L. monocytogenes*. This will basically depend on differentiating biochemical characteristics between Listeria monocytogenes and other Listeria spp. Last but not least, the sensitivity (detecting positives) and specificity (detecting negatives) of the test needs to be established.

To begin with, an observation of signs and symptoms along with disease history, pathological lesions, earlier exposure to disease, feed and grazing pasture is helpful in making a preliminary diagnosis. For definitive diagnosis, it is essential to isolate and characterize the bacterium (Kahn 2005).

In general, Listeria can be readily isolated and enriched in culture media designed for the purpose. However, the difficulty lies in establishing the source and spread of the infection amongst animals because of the ubiquitous nature of its occurrence and its ability to survive without a host for a long time (OIE 2014). Some standard methods acceptable for international regulatory purposes for the isolation of *L. monocytogenes* include the official method of the Association of Official Analytical Chemists (AOAC), the United States Food and Drug Administration (FDA) bacteriological and analytical method (BAM) (Hitchins 2001), the ISO 11290 method, the French Standards and the United States Department of Agriculture (USDA) Food Safety and Inspection Service (FSIS) method (OIE 2014).

Most of these methods require enrichment of the sample using a selective broth that incorporates bacteriostatic agents, such as acriflavin and nalidixic acid, which leads to the slowing of growth of competing organisms, followed by plating onto selective agar. Such an enrichment method allows the Listeria to reach detectable levels of 10^4–10^5 cfu/ml, as also for biochemical identification of typical colonies. In the FDA BAM process, first the sample is inoculated into enrichment broth and allowed to grow for 48 hours at 30°C (LEB, FDA, BAM formulation). This contains the selective agents, naladixic acid, acriflavin and cycloheximide, an antifungal agent. The enrichment broth is used for plating onto one of the selective agars: PALCAM, MOX, Oxford or LPM (Hitchins 2001).

In the ISO 11290 method, enrichment is carried out in two steps using Fraser broth, constituted of naladixic acid, acriflavin as a bacteriostatic agent effective against non-listerials and esculin as an indicator glucoside. Esculin hydrolysis by β-D-glucosidase produces aesculetin (6,7-dihydroxycoumarin), which combines with ferric citrate in the broth and creates brown-coloured complexes, where the resultant darkening of media shows the presence of Listeria. In the first step, Fraser broth of half-strength is used for 24 hours of culturing. The aliquots from first step are then added to full-strength Fraser broth in the second step. The samples from both steps are then spread on PALCAM and Oxford agars, for colony isolation.

The broth samples are incubated at 37±1°C for 24 hours on PALCAM agar (polymixin-acriflavine-lithium chloride-ceftazidime-esculin and mannitol). The green -blue colonies representing *L. monocytogenes* as per Ottaviani and Agosti (ISO 2005a) appear to be encircled by an opaque halo. Since the Oxford agar is constituted from acriflavine-lithium chloride-cycloheximide (an antifungal)-colistin (anti-Gram-negative), cefotetan and fosfomycin (antibacterials), it allows the growth of small black listerial colonies encircled by a black halo, which are further incubated in selective media at a specific temperature for a time that allows for luxurious growth.

Sub-culturing the presumptive *L. monocytogenes* needs confirmation by appropriate morphological, physiological and biochemical tests, carried out as per prescribed standards. For the enumeration, the method recommended in EN ISO 11290 Part 2 suggests "agar Listeria according to Ottaviani and Agosti" (ISO 2005b).

The USDA method (2019) involves a two-stage enrichment process using modified University of Vermont Medium (UVM) that is constituted using nalidixic acid and acriflavin in the first step and Fraser broth for the second step. The samples from both steps are then spread on colistin sulphate and moxalactam containing modified Oxford (MOX) agar.

For the isolation and characterisation of listeria sps., tissue samples like brain, liver, heart, spleen, feotus or even aborted placenta can be used. Body fluids like blood, saliva, cerebrospinal fluid meconium from newborns, vomitus or faeces can be the source for culturing and enriching for isolation and diagnostic purposes (Brugere-Picoux 2008; Scott 2013).

To begin with isolation, blood/tryptose agar or brain-heart infusion medium have proven their utility over the years as the best media (Walker *et al.* 1990). Thus, traditionally, the isolation of *L. monocytogenes* sampling from diseased animal tissues has used direct plating of specimens on sheep blood agar or other rich-culture media, simultaneously using cold enrichment with sub-culturing, which takes about 12 weeks.

For selective enrichment various selective media have been designed, including UVM, Fraser's broth, Dominguez Rodriguez isolation agar, PALCAM agar and modified McBride Listeria agar. Commercially, a number of chromogenic agar media for plating and selection are available in place of the conventional media mentioned above, from different sources.

9.7 Pathogen Identification of Cultural Isolates

Listeria spp. can be phenotypically identified using Gram-staining, microscopic morphology and motility observations, biochemical characterization, viz. peroxidase, catalase and sugar fermentation, and in the case of pathogenic strains their haemolytic properties (Dhama *et al.* 2013; OIE 2014). Samples from food are usually tested using the immunofluorescence test (IFT) recommended by the AOAC (2000). These methods are lengthy but they are the gold standard, acceptable the world over (Figure 9.2; Table 9.1).

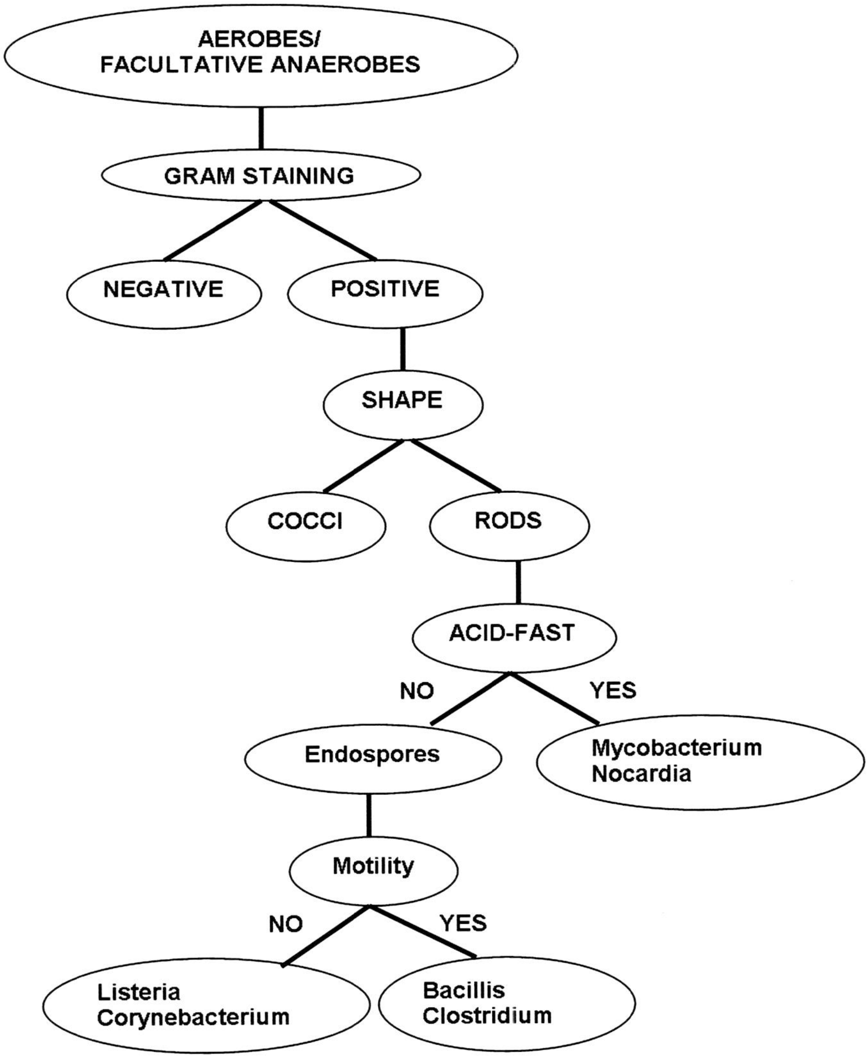

FIGURE 9.2 Biochemical and phenotypic characterization of Listeria.

TABLE 9.1

Biochemical characterization of Listeria spp.

	L. monocytogenes	*L. ivanovii*	*L. seeligeri*
Haemolysin	+	+	+
Catalase	+	+	+
Oxidase	-	-	-
Fermentation			
L-rhamnose	+	-	-
D-mannitol	-	-	-
D-xylose	-	+	+
α-methyl mannoside	+	-	-

Using *in vitro* methods, the pathogenicity testing of Listeria isolates is carried out by culturing on sheep blood agar and chromogenic enzyme assay based on PI-PLC (phosphatidylinositol-specific phospholipase C) activity. Observation of haemolytic activity is usually followed by a CAMP test.

The Christie, Atkins, Munch-Petersen (CAMP) test (Vazquez-Boland *et al.* 1990), is employed to distinguish between *L. monocytogenes*, *L. ivanovii* and *L. seeligeri* species of Listeria.

In this test, two bacterial strains, *Staphylococcus aureus* and *Rhodococcus equi*, which are known producers of β-haemolysin, are streaked on blood agar plates in parallel lines. The listerial isolates are then streaked in between, at right-angles to these lines, without touching them. If haemolysis is observed in the proximity of streaked *R. equi*, the isolate is identified as *L. ivanovii*, whereas haemolysis observed near *S. aureus* is attributed to the presence of *L. monocytogenes* isolates, or to some extent to *L. seeligeri* isolates. Recently, the USDA (2019) recommended use of an rRNA-based test for confirmation at species level.

9.7.1 Enzyme-based Assays

A number of enzyme-based methods using chromogenic substrates have been developed by commercial entities in the form of diagnostic kits. These automated biochemical systems of identification are available around the world; for example, API Listeria and MICRO-ID Listeria, MicroScan (Baxter Healthcare Corporation, West Sacramento), MicroStation (Biolog, Heyward) and Cobas (Becton Dickinson Instrument Systems, Sparks) from the USA and Vitek (bioMerieux, Marcy-l'Etoile) from France are some major systems in use.

Phosphatidylinositol-specific phospholipase C (PIPL-C) is specifically produced by *L. monocytogenes* and *L. ivanovii* species and not any other species of Listeria. Agar media have been developed and commercialized based on chromogenic substrates of PIPL-C. Examples of some commercial chromogenic agar plating methods include Rapid L. mono agar (BioRad), blue colonies producing agar by Marnes de la Coquette (France). Also based on other PIPL-C tests are ALOA of Biolife (Milan, Italy), the BCM chromogenic agar test from Biosynth International (Naperville, USA) and the CHROM agar Listeria test of Mast Diagnostics (Reinfeld, Germany). Alanyl peptidase is another bacterial enzyme that has been found useful for identification of *L. monocytogenes.* It can distinguish all other species which are producers of the enzyme from non-producer *L. monocytogenes*, by a simple colour reaction of the hydrolysis of chromogenic substrates DL-alanine-b-naphthylamide and D-alanine-p-nitroanilide (Clark and McLaughlin 1997). Biolife (Milan, Italy) has also exploited the same enzyme to develop the Monocytogenes ID Disc. However, to complete biochemical identification, *L. ivanovii* can be distinguished from *L. monocytogenes* by its ability to utilize xylose.

In the absence of facilities for the above tests, the Anton test can be used for detecting Listeria. In this test the infected material is applied to the conjunctiva of the eye of a rabbit by simply dropping it over the eye and then observing for development of conjunctivitis or kerato-conjunctivitis within 24–36 hours, confirming the presence of Listeria.

9.7.2 Immunological Assays

Immuno-histochemical testing is usually employed in cases of encephalitic listeriosis, when very few bacteria are suspected to be present. It allows location of antigens in septicaemic tissue lesions in fixed tissues and is useful for the confirmation of listeriosis.

Allen *et al.* (2013), working with goat brain samples, confirmed listeriosis in 33 (89%) out of 37 cases under investigation, using bacterial culturing and immuno-histochemical staining (IHC) or both. IHC was performed on 28 cases, 15 of which were samples from diseased animals and 13 of which were stored samples. IHC successfully detected listeria in 25 out of 28 samples. Out of a total of 50 cases of encephalitic listeriosis, in 15 cases both types of investigative test, viz. IHC and culturing, were performed; 8 out of the 15 yielded bacterial colonies as well as antigen detection by IHC.

Antibody-based tests have mainly been used for analysing environmental and food samples. These tests are simple to perform, with high sensitivity and accuracy (Barbudde *et al.* 2000). The other major advantage is ease of testing by obtaining the sample directly from the enrichment broth without resorting to cumbersome sample preparation procedures. Many commercial kits for performing these immunoassays have been approved by the AOAC (1995). A nanotechnology-based miniaturized immunoassay for the detection of a few Listeria from environmental samples was reported by Jaakohuhta *et al.* (2007).

Enzyme-linked immunosorbent assay (ELISA)-based tests use immobilized antibodies in a microtitre plate for antigen capture along with a second domain of antibody being bound by a secondary antibody which binds an enzyme (or any other label) for detection by a chromogenic substrate. ELISA is a rapid test amenable to miniaturisation. Two examples of commercial tests are TECRA International's Listeria Unique, and BioMerieux's (France) VIDAS Listeria Express.

Mainly LLO and internalin virulent markers have been found to be suitable for the development of ELISA (Amagliani *et al.* 2006). Thus, synthetic peptides of internalins and LLO formed the basis for diagnostic testing of ovine listeriosis caused by *L. monocytogenes* and *L. ivanovii* by Shoukat *et al.* (2013).

9.7.3 Nucleic Acid-based Molecular Assays

Nucleic acid-based assays are helpful in distinguishing *L. monocytogenes* from different listerial species, up to subspecies level, within the same timeframe as ELISA-based assays. The traditional DNA hybridisation assays have now been almost entirely replaced by PCR-based methods. One of the earliest methods (Cocolin *et al.* 1997) combined PCR with DNA hybridisation, using a 96-well high-throughput format using a microtitre plate, to develop a highly specific and sensitive method for diagnosis of Listeria. Later commercial tests like Accuprobe by Gen-Probe Inc. (San Diego, USA) assayed only viable cells, as they were based on DNA probes for detection of virulence factor mRNA, which is produced only in living cells. Similarly, a DNA hybridisation kit named GeneTrak was developed by Neogen Corporation, USA.

PCR is a technique which involves the amplification of a specific fragment of a bacterial gene based on the fragment ends being defined by two primers, the forward and reverse primer. It is the specificity of the oligonucleotide primers that defines the gene segment to be amplified. The fragment thus obtained is analysed on agarose gel as to its size. In comparison to DNA hybridisation methodologies, PCR requires very little sample and takes less time. PCR is thus now a very well established methodology for the identification and characterisation of Listeria spp. For further differentiation of *L. monocytogenes*, separating it from the rest of the listerial species can be carried out based on primers that amplify specific virulence factors or rRNA genes in reverse transcriptase PCR (RT-PCR). PCR can be carried out directly on the test sample, but it gives more reliable results after the samples have been enriched for 24–48 hours. By now, almost all virulence factor genes have been used for developing PCR assays for listeriae (see Table 9.2).

A number of multiplex PCR assays developed by various Labs (Park *et al.* 2006; Kawasaki *et al.* 2009; Lee *et al.* 2014) provide for simultaneous detection of pathogens like *Escherichia coli*, *Salmonella*, *Staphylococcus* and *Listeria*.

A multiplex method for detection of *L. monocytogenes* using *iap*, *hylA* and *actA* virulence genes helped identification of Listeria species of 12 biochemically characterized strains. The samples were examined

TABLE 9.2

Nucleic acid-based assays for Listeria

Gene/ Technique	Forward Primer	Reverse Primer	Reference
16S RNA	L-1 5' CACGTGCTACAATGGATAG 3' L-2 1255 3'GATTAGGGTAITTTGATAAGA 5'	RL-1 3' ATGTTACCTATCATG1TTC 5' RL-2 3' CGATTAGGGTATTWGATA 5' RL-3 5' GTCGCGAAGCCGCGAGGT 3'	Wang *et al.* (1992)
16S-23S RNA intergenic spacer	LA2 5'CTATAGCTCAGCTGGTTAGAG3' L M3F 5'GCAAGGCACTATGC7TGAAGCA3' 5'AGGTAGCCGTATCGGAAGGT 3' 294 – *Listeria*	LB2 5'TTCTCGGTTACTTGTGTCA3' LMIR -5'CCCGATAAAAGG,GATATGATTATT3' 5'GCCCCGTAAAAGGGTATGAT3'	Graham *et al.* (1996, 1997); Suo *et al.* (2010)
23S RNA PCR-RFLP	S1F 5'AGTCGGATAGTATCCTTAC-3'-460 bp digested with *AluI/ CfaI* S2F 5'GCCTACAAGTAGTTAGAGCC3' - 890 bp digested with *XmnI/ CfoI*	S1R5'GGCTCTAACTACTTGTAGGC-3' S2R5'ACTGGTACAGGAATCTCTAC-3'	Paillard *et al.* (2003)
Actin polymerising protein (act A)	F 5' CGCCGCGGAAATTAAAAAAAGA, -839bp	R 5' ACGAAGGAACCGGGCTGCTAG '3	Suarez and Boland (2001)
Aminopeptidase	SK6 5'-GGTCGGTGCATTAATAAG-3' 90bp	AP4-5'CAAGAGTTACAAATTACACC-3'	Winters *et al.* (1999)
Delayed type hypersensitivity factor (dth) Dth18-gene	5'CCGGGAGCTGCTAAAGCGGT3' 326bp 5'GAAGCACCTTTTGACGAAGC3' 122bp	5'GCCAAACCACCGAAAAGACG3' 5'-GCTGGTGCTACAGGTGTTTC-3'	Wernars *et al.* (1991)
Fibrin binding protein (fbp)	G398 -5'TGAAAGAGTTTATCGAGCCATACC-3'	G400 5'CTTATGCTCCTCTAGTACACTTT-3'	Gilot and Content (2002)
Haemolysin (hly) PCR qPCR	5'GCAGTTGCAAGCGCTTGGAGTGAA '3, -456bp HylA-5'ACGCGGATGAAATCGATAAG3' 271bp F: 5'CGGAGGTTCCGCAAAAGATG3' HLYA- 5'ATTGCGAAATTTGGTACAGC3' 234bp	5'GCAACGTATCCTCCAGAGTGATCG '3 5'ACAGGAAGAACATCGGGTTG3' R:5'CCTCCAGAGTGATCGATGTT3' HLYA- 5'ACTTGAGATATATGCAGGAG3'	Liu *et al.* (2003); Suo *et al.* (2010); Swetha *et al.* (2013); Khan *et al.* (2013)

Phospholipase (plcA, plcB)	5'TCCCATTAGGTGGAAAAGCA 3' 193bp 5'CGGCGCACCTAACCAAGTAA3' plcA 5'CTGCTTGAGCGTTCATGTCTCATCCCCC3' 1484bp	5'GTTTGAGCCAGTGGTTTGGT3' 5'CAGTCTGGACAATCTCTTTGAATTTT3' 5'ATGGGTTTCACTCTCCTTCTAC3'	Suo *et al.* (2010); Hage *et al.* (2014) Rawool *et al.* (2007) Kaur *et al.* (2010)
Invasion-associated protein (iap)/ PCR	5'ACAAGCTGCACCTGTTGCAG '3, -131bp 5'GGGTGGTAACGGACCAACTA3' 225bp – *Listeria*	5'TGACAGCGTGTGTAGTAGCA'3 5'TCTTGCGCGTTAATCATTTG3'	Swetha *et al.* (2013); Suo *et al.* (2010)
Metalloprotease (mpl) PCR	*Mpl1* 5' 'TATGACGGTAAAAGCAGATT 3' 1,459bp	MPL2 5'TTCCCAAGCTTCAGCAACTT3'	Vine *et al.* (1992)
L. monocytogenes antigen (lma) PCR	*lma*A-AACAAGGTCTAACTGTAAAC 257bp	*lma*-A-ACTATAGTCAGCTACAATTG	Johnson *et al.* (1992)
Internalin A, B, C and J (inlA, inlB, inlAB)	inlA F 5'ACGAGTAACGGGACAAATGC3' 800bp inlB F 5' TGGGAGAGTAACCCAACCAC 3' 884 inlC F 5' AATTCCCACAGGACACAACC 3' 517 inlJ F 5'TGTAACCCCGCTTACACAGTT 3' 238 5'TGATTCCATGCAATTACTAGAACG3' 545 bp 5'TGTAACCCCGCTTACACAGTT 3'- 611bp	R 5' CCCGACAGTGGTGCTAGATT 3' R 5' GTTGACCTTCGATGGTTGCT 3' R 5' CGGGAATGCAATTTTTCACTA 3' R 5'AGCGGCTTGGCAGTCTAATA 3' 5'AGGATTCTAAACTAGGTAAGTTGGTG3' 5'TTACGGCTGGATTGTCTGTG 3'	Liu *et al.* (2003)
Transcriptional regulator (prfA) PCR, qPCR -	5'GATACAGAAACATCGGTTGGC3' -274 bp PRFI 5'CATGAACGCTCAAGCAGAAG3'- 707bp LIP1: 5'GATACAGAAACATCGGTTGGC3'+ TaqMan™ probes	5'GTGTAACTTGATGCCATCAGG3' PRF2 5'AATTTTCCCAAGTAGGAGGA3' LIP2: 5'GTGTAATCTTGATGCCATCAGG3' 5'-GTGTAATCTTGATGCCATCAGG-3'	Simon *et al.* (1996); Talon *et al.* (2007); Vines *et al.* (1992); Rossmanith *et al.* (2006)

(*continued*)

TABLE 9.2

Nucleic acid-based assays for Listeria (Cont.)

Gene/ Technique	Forward Primer	Reverse Primer	Reference
	FAM-CAGGATTAAAAGTTGACCGCA-MGB-3 FAMCAGGATTAAAAGTTGACCGCA-BHQ1-3- LNA modification 5'-GATACAGAAACATCGGTTGGC-3' 274bp		
Sigma B factor (sigB) SNP analysis	Lineage I Lin IA-F TTA CGT GAT AAA ACA TGG AGT GTG Lin ICA-F[a] CAC ACT CCA TGT TTT ATC ACG TAA 116bp Lineage II ASUA-F GCG AGA ACA GAA GAT TTT GCA ATA ASUCA-F[a] TAT TGC AAA ATC TTC TGT TCT CGC- 151bp Lineage III MPB-F TTA GAA GAT ATG ATG CRA CT MPCB-Fa AGT [b]YGC ATC ATA TCT TCT AA – 223bp [a] denotes SNP specific forward primers	Lin IA-R GCT AAT TTG CGG CGA GCT ASR CAC TTC CTC ATT CTG CAA CG MPB-R CGT GAC ACC [c]RAT GAA ATC AG b Y=C+T. c R=A+G.	Moorhead *et al.* (2003)
lmo0737 multiplex PCR	F AGGGCTTCAAGGACTTACCC 691bp	R ACGATTTCTGCTTGCCATTC	Henerique *et al.* (2017)
lmo1118 multiplex PCR	F AGGGGTCTTAAATCCTGGAA 906bp	R CGGCTTGTTCGGCATACTTA	Henerique *et al.* (2017)
orf2819 multiplex PCR	F AGCAAAATGCCAAAACTCGT 471bp	R CATCACTAAAGCCTCCCATTG	Henerique *et al.* (2017)
orf2110 multiplex PCR	For: AGTGGACAATTGATTGGTGAA 597bp	R CATCCATCCCTTACTTTGGAC	Henerique *et al.* (2017)
flaA multiplex PCR	F TTACTAGATCAAACTGCTCC 538bp	R AAGAAAAGCCCCTCGTCC	Henerique *et al.* (2017)
Fur PCR qPCR	5'-GCCGAGGAAGTTTTCTTGCG-3' 208bpp	5'-TTTCCTCTACAGACCCGCACTC-3'	Author's lab (unpublished data, 2018)

from farm animals and their milk and humans, and reflected the impact of zoonosis on such animals and their milk (El-Gohary *et al.* 2018).

Hu *et al.* (2014) reported the development of a multiplex real-time PCR assay, using molecular beacons that detected eight pathogens simultaneously: *E. coli* O157, *Campylobacter jejuni*, *Enterobacter sakazakii*, *L. monocytogenes*, *Salmonella enterica* subsp. *enterica*, *Shigella* spp., *Vibrio parahaemolyticus* and *V. vulnificus*, claiming 100% sensitive and specific results.

Henriques *et al.* (2017) characterized *L. monocytogenes* using multiplex PCR based on virulence genes *actA*, *hlyA*, *iap*, *inlA*, *inlB*, *inlC*, *inlJ* and *plcA*. They analysed isolates obtained from industrially processed, ready-to-eat meat-based products. The study further carried out PFGE using ApaI and AscI, which grouped these isolates into five clusters based on observation of genetic variability amongst them.

9.7.4 Epidemiological Testing

In times of outbreaks, the identification of Listeria in clinical, environmental or food and feed samples is important to distinguish the pathogenic strain and to delineate the closely related listeriae to establish the source of the outbreak and the pattern of transmission, and to monitor the reservoirs of epidemic strains.

9.7.4.1 Phenotypic Typing Methods

Using phenotypic markers like the H factor of flagella and somatic O factor, antibodies were developed and serological testing carried out which allowed the tests to distinguish Listeria at genus level but not at species level. Such typing methods can assist in tracking the source of environmental contamination (USFDA 2001). Commercial kits for serotyping of Listeria isolates are sold by Denka Seiken (Japan) and antisera are available from Difco (Difco Laboratories/Becton Dickinson and Co., USA).

Multilocus enzyme electrophoresis (MEE) involves the analysis of anywhere between 8 and 23 enzymes in various studies (Gasanov *et al.* 2005). The amino acid variation results in variation in the overall net charge on the protein, which results in differences in the electrophoretic mobility; thus, the isolates can be separated to yield various electrophoretic isotypes. This is also a reflection of the genetic variability of the samples. Gel electrophoresis carried out on starch gel and staining using zymogram methods using enzyme-specific substrates giving colour reactions for detection of enzyme bands were developed during the 1990s and have now been overtaken by molecular methods.

9.7.4.2 Molecular Typing Methods

Molecular typing methods are based on variation in bacteria genomes. Some of these listed by OIE since 2014 include amplified intergenic locus polymorphism (AILP), pulsed-field gel electrophoresis (PFGE), random amplification of polymorphic DNA (RAPD), microarray analysis and, finally, nucleic acid sequencing-based typing. Generally, molecular typing methods are more sensitive and specific when compared with phenotypic typing methods. PFGE involves fragmentation of genomic DNA using restriction enzymes. The World Health Organization has recommended the use of restriction enzymes HaeIII, HhaI and CfoI specifically for serological samples (OIE 2014). Loop-mediated isothermal amplification (LAMP) has been standardized by Tang *et al.* (2011); the technique proved to be 100 times better in terms of sensitivity than traditional PCR and detected up to 2.0 cfu per reaction. Moreover, the assay was found to be 100% accurate as compared to culturing and other antibody-based methods. Direct sequencing of DNA is the gold-standard method that can compare genetic similarities or differences at molecular level. However, it is also the most expensive method of all and requires a lot of time and specialized training to carry out.

A biosensor was developed by Zhao *et al.* (2006) based on secretory LLO for subtyping of *L. monocytogenes*. They developed a uni-lamellar liposome doped with fluorescent dye calcein (50 mM), which was immobilized within porous silica. At such a high concentration the dye, its molecules are self-quenching. They used an alcohol-free sol-gel method for immobilisation of these liposomes, which acted like surrogate cells for attachment and pore-forming activity of LLO secreted by *L. monocytogenes*. LLO activity leads to leaching of the fluorescent dye, which can be detected. The sol-gel system was observed to be stable for five months, and the response time for immobilized the sol-gel biosensor was observed to be 30–100 minutes, below pH 7.4. However, the requirement for a fluorimeter limits the field application of such biosensors.

Dreyer *et al.* (2016) used another molecular technique, that of multilocus sequence typing (MLST), to divide isolates into sequence types (STs) and clonal complexes (CCs, equated to clones). They based their technique on sequencing data from seven housekeeping genes, viz. *abcZ*, *bglA*, *cat*, *dapE*, *dat*, *ldh* and *lhkA2*. The different sequences obtained for each gene were assigned a defining allele number, which were later combined for all the seven loci to define sequence types (STs). Based on their analysis it was reported that the *L. monocytogenes* population can be divided into hypovirulent and hypervirulent clones. These clones were observed to significantly differ in distribution, when comparison was made between non-clinical and clinical samples.

The study reported a specific genotype, ST1, to be isolated dominantly from rhombencephalitis cases, but not from cases displaying other manifestations of the disease. Their observation identified increased neurotropism of ST1 strains in ruminants, being hypervirulent.

Suo *et al.* (2010) designed and prepared a microarray for simultaneous detection of four pathogens: *Escherichia coli* O157:H7, *Salmonella enterica*, *Listeria monocytogenes* and *Campylobacter jejuni*. Prior to detection by microarray, a multiplex PCR amplification step was carried out. For detection of *L. monocytogenes*, four genes, *iap*, *IGS*, *plc* and *hlyA*, were selected for amplification (Table 9.2). After amplification the gene fragments were purified and labeled with Cy3 fluorescent dye. Glass slides were used for preparation of microarrays and each microarray chip was printed with 12 identical arrays for analysis of 12 independent samples. Since microarray assay sensitivity depends on the signal strength after hybridisation of probes, to obtain high fluorescent signal strength 70-mer oligonucleotides were selected as probes, instead of normal 20-mer oligos used in microarrays. Two of the probes, viz. *Hyl* and *Plc*, were species-specific. The assay could detect at a sensitivity of $1x\ 10^{-4}$ ng, i.e., approximately 20 copies of each genomic DNA in the samples analysed. Microarray probes used in the study for detection of *L. monocytogenes* are listed below.

iap-LisM (length 65bp, Tm 80.4°C) ATTGCTCTGGTTACACTAAATATGTATTTGCTAAAGCGGG AATCTCCCTTCCACGTACTTCTGGC

IGS-LisM (length 65bp, Tm 83.9°C) CAGATAAAGTACGCAAGGCAACATGCTTGGAGCATAGC GCCACTACATTTTTGACGGGCCTATAG

plc-LisM (length 65bp, Tm 80.3°C) ACAACGAGCCTAGCAGCACTCTCTATACCAGGTACACAT GATACGATGAGCTATAACGGAGACAT

hlyA-LisM (length 66bp, Tm 80.5°C) AATGTATTAGTATACCACGGAGATGCAGTGACAAATGT GCCGCCAAGAAAAGGTTATAAAGATGGA

9.8 Conclusion

Advancements in micro- and nanotechnologies promise to lead to miniaturisation and availability of diagnostic devices that are accurate and cheap, with high throughput and high sensitivity for a wide range of veterinary applications. Such devices are the need of the hour, especially in field applications to reach remote areas in veterinary science. Even the latest generation of sequencing platforms can in specific conditions prove useful for diagnostic purposes for cases of novel bacterial pathogens. Thus, the need for point-of-care devices for veterinary diseases cannot be overemphasized.

Improved diagnostic tests can be applied at a number of levels. Quality assurance in the specificity of diagnosis is important for the control of the disease in the individual animal. It forms the basis for the treatment regime, and monitoring disease progression in the patient animal as well as the spread amongst other animals of the herd. Thus, early and accurate diagnosis not only ensures proper treatment of one animal, but also prevents spread to other animals and even humans.

References

Allen AL, Goupil BA and Valentine BA "A retrospective study of brain lesions in goats submitted to three veterinary diagnostic laboratories". *Journal of Veterinary Diagnostic Investigation* 25(4) (2013):482–9.

Alonzo F, III and Freitag NE "Listeria monocytogenes PrsA2is required for virulence factor secretion and bacterial viability within the host cell cytosol". *Infection and Immunity* 78 (2010):4944–57.

Alonzo F, III Port GC, Cao M and Freitag NE "The post-translocation chaperone PrsA2 contributes to multiple facets of *Listeria monocytogenes* pathogenesis". *Infection and Immunity* 77 (2009):2612–23.

Amagliani G, Giammarini C, Omiccioli E *et al.* "A combination of diagnostic tools for rapid screening of ovine listeriosis". *Research in Veterinary Science* 81 (2006):185–9.

AOAC International. *Official Methods of Analysis* (AOAC International, 16th edn, 1995).

AOAC International "Listeria species. Biochemical identification method (MICRO-ID Listeria)". In Horwitz W (ed.), *Official Methods of Analysis of AOAC International, Volume I. Agricultural Chemicals; Contaminants; Drugs* (AOAC International, 2000), 141–4.

Barbuceanu F, Diaconua C, Stamatea D *et al.* "Histopathological study of brain from cattle with nervous symptomatology". *Agriculture and Agricultural Science Procedia* 6 (2015):287–92.

Barbuddhe SB and Chakraborty T "Listeria as an enteroinvasive gastrointestinal pathogen". *Current Topics in Microbiology and Immunology* 337 (2009):173–95.

Barbuddhe SB, Malik SVS, Bhilegaonkar KN, Kumar P and Gupta LK "Isolation of *Listeria monocytogenes* and anti-listeriolysin O detection in sheep and goats". *Small Ruminant Research* 38(2) (2000):151–5.

Beauregard KE, Lee KD, Collier RJ and Swanson JA "pH dependent perforation of macrophage phagosomes by listeriolysin O from *Listeria monocytogenes*". *Journal of Experimental Medicine* 186 (1997):1159–63.

Bertsch D, Rau J, Eugster MR, Haug MC, Lawson PA *et al.* "*Listeria fleischmannii* sp. nov., isolated from cheese". *International Journal of Systemic and Evolutionary Microbiology* 63 (2013):526–32.

Bierne H, Milohanic E and Kortebi M "To be cytosolic or vacuolar: the double life of *Listeria monocytogenes*". *Frontiers in Cellular and Infection Microbiology* 8 (2018):136.

Bonazzi M, Veiga E, Pizarro-Cerda J and Cossart P "Successive post-translational modifications of E-cadherin are required for InlA-mediated internalization of *Listeria monocytogenes*". *Cellular Microbiology* 10 (2008):2208–22.

Bonnemain C, Raynaud C, Reglier-Poupet H, DubailI, Frehel C, Lety MA *et al.* "Differential roles of multiple signal peptidases in the virulence of *Listeria monocytogenes*". *Molecular Microbiology* 51 (2004):1251–66.

Borezée E, Pellegrini E, Beretti JL and Berche P "SvpA: A novel surface virulence-associated protein required for intracellular survival of *Listeria monocytogenes*". *Microbiology* 147 (2001):2913–23.

Brugere-Picoux J "Ovine listeriosis". *Small Ruminant Research* 76 (2008):12–20.

Camejo A, Carvalho AF, Reis O, Leitão E, Sousa S and Cabanes D "The arsenal of virulence factors deployed by *Listeria monocytogenes* to promote its cell infection cycle". *Virulence* 2(5) (2011): 379–94.

Campellone KG and Welch MD "A nucleator arms race: cellular control of actin assembly". *Nature Reviews Molecular Cell Biology* 11 (2010): 237–51.

Campero CM, Odeon AC, Cipolia A, Moore DP, Poso MA and Odriozola E "Demonstration of *Listeria monocytogenes* by immunochemistry in formalin-fixed brain tissues from natural cases of ovine and bovine encephalitis". *Journal of Veterinary Medicine B Infectious Diseases and Veterinary Public Health* 49 (2002): 379–83.

Chico-Calero I, Suarez M, Gonzalez-Zorn B, Scortti M, Slaghuis J, Goebel W *et al.* "Hpt, a bacterial homolog of the microsomal glucose-6-phosphate translocase, mediates rapid intracellular proliferation in Listeria". *Proceedings of the National Academy of Science* 99 (2002):431–6.

Clark, AG and McLaughlin J "Simple color tests based on an alanyl peptidase reaction which differentiate *Listeria monocytogenes* from other Listeria species". *Journal of Clinical Microbiology* 35 (1997):2155–6.

Clark, RG, Gill JM and Swanney S "*Listeria monocytogenes* gastroenteritis in sheep". *New Zealand Veterinary Journal* 52 (2004):46–7.

Cocolin L, Manzano M, Cantoni C and Comi G "A PCR-microplate capture hybridization method to detect *Listeria monocytogenes* in blood". *Molecular and Cellular Probes* 11 (1997):453–5.

Cossart P and Lebreton A "A trip in the 'New Microbiology' with the bacterial pathogen *Listeria monocytogenes*". *FEBS Letters* 588 (2014):2437–45.

Datta AR, Laksanalamai P and Solomotis M "Recent developments in molecular sub-typing of *Listeria monocytogenes*". *Food Additives and Contaminants Part A: Chemistry, Analysis, Control, Exposure and Risk Assessment* 30 (2013):1437–45.

den Bakker HC, Warchocki S, Wright EM, Allred AF, Ahlstrom C *et al.* "*Listeria floridensis* sp. nov., *Listeria aquatica* sp. nov., *Listeria cornellensis* sp. nov., *Listeria riparia sp.* nov. and *Listeria grandensis sp.* nov., from agricultural and natural environments". *International Journal of Systemic and Evolutionary Microbiology* 64 (2014):1882–9.

Dhama K, Chakraborty S, Kapoor S, Tiwari R, Kumar A, Deb R, Rajagunalan S, Singh R, Vora K and Natesan S "One world, one health veterinary perspectives". *Advances in Animal and Veterinary Sciences* 1 (2013):5–13.

Dhama K, Karthik K, Tiwari R *et al.* "Listeriosis in animals, its public health significance (food-borne zoonosis) and advances in diagnosis and control: a comprehensive review". *Veterinary Quarterly* 35–4 (2015):211–35.

Disson O, Grayo S, Huillet E *et al.* "Conjugated action of two species specific invasion proteins for fetoplacental listeriosis". *Nature* 455 (2008):1114–18.

Doijad SP, Poharkar KP, Kale SB *et al.* "*Listeria goaensis* sp. nov." *International Journal of Systemic and Evolutionary Microbiology* 68 (2018):3285–91.

Domann E, Leimeister-Wachter M, Goebel W and Chakraborty T "Molecular cloning, sequencing and identification of a metalloprotease gene from *Listeria monocytogenes* that is species specific and physically linked to the listeriolysin gene". *Infection and Immunity* 59 (1991):65–72.

Dramsi S, Biswas I, Maguin E, Braun L, Mastroeni P and Cossart P "Entry of *Listeria monocytogenes* into hepatocytes requires expression of InIB, a surface protein of the internalin multigene family". *Molecular Microbiology* 16 (1995):251–61.

Dreyer M, Aguilar-Bultet L and Rupp S "*Listeria monocytogenes* sequence type 1 is predominant in ruminant rhombencephalitis". *Nature* 6 (2016):36419.

Dussurget O, Dumas E, Archambaud C *et al.* "*Listeria monocytogenes* ferritin protects against multiple stresses and is required for virulence". *FEMS Microbiology Letters* 250 (2005):253–61.

El-Gohary AH, Mohamed AA, Ramadan HH and Abuhatab EA "Zoonotic and molecular aspects of *listeria* species isolated from some farm animals at Dakahlia province in Egypt". *Alexandria Journal of Veterinary Sciences* 58(1) (2018):208–14.

Gaillard JL, Berche P, Frehel C, Gouin E and Cossart P "Entry of *L.monocytogenes* into cells is mediated by internalin, a repeat protein reminiscent of surface antigens from Gram-positive cocci". *Cell* 65 (1991):112741.

Gasanov U, Hughes D and Hansbro PM "Methods for the isolation and identification of *Listeria* spp. and *Listeria monocytogenes*: a review". *FEMS Microbiology Reviews* 29 (2005):851–75.

Gilot P and Content J "Specific identification of Listeria welshimeri and Listeria monocytogenes by PCR assays targeting a gene encoding a fibronectin-binding protein". *Journal of Clinical Microbiology* 40 (2002):698–703.

Goldfine H and Knob C "Purification and characterization of *Listeria monocytogenes* phosphatidylinositol-specific phospholipase C". *Infection and Immunity* 60 (1992):4059–67.

Graham, TA, Golsteyn-Thomas EJ, Thomas JE and Gannon VP "Inter- and intraspecies comparison of the 16S-23S rRNA operon intergenic spacer regions of six *Listeria* spp". *International Journal of Systemic Bacteriology* 47 (1997):863–9.

Graham TA, Golsteyn-Thomas EJ, Gannon VP and Thomas JE "Genus- and species-specific detection of *Listeria monocytogenes* polymerase chain reaction assays targeting the 16S-23S intergenic spacer region of the rRNA operon". *Canadian Journal of Microbiology* 42 (1996):1155–62.

Graves LM, Helsel LO, Steigerwalt AG *et al.* "*Listeria marthii* sp. nov., isolated from the natural environment, Finger Lakes National Forest". *International Journal of Systemic and Evolutionary Microbiology* 60 (2010):1280–8.

Guillet C, Join-Lambert O, Le Monnier A *et al.* "Human listeriosis caused by *Listeria ivanovii*". *Emerging Infectious Diseases* 16(1) (2010). doi:10.3201/eid1601.091155.

Guzman CA, Rohde M, Chakraborty T *et al.* "Interaction of *Listeria monocytogenes* with mouse dendritic cells". *Infection and Immunity* 63(9) (1995):3665–73.

Halter EL, Neuhaus K and Scherer S "*Listeria weihenstephanensis sp.* nov., isolated from the water plant Lemna trisulca taken from a freshwater pond". *International Journal of Systematic and Evolutionary Microbiology* 63 (2013):641–7.

Hage E, Mpamugo O, Ohai C *et al.* "Identification of six Listeria species by real-time PCR assay". *Letters in Applied Microbiology* 58 (2014):535–40.

Henriques AR, Melo Cristino, IJ and Fraqueza MJ "Genetic characterization of *Listeria monocytogenes* isolates from industrial and retail ready-to-eat meat-based foods and their relationship with clinical strains from human listeriosis in Portugal". *Journal of Food Protection* 80(4) (2017):551–60.

Hird DW and Genigeorgis C "Listeriosis in food animals; clinical signs and livestock as a potential source of direct (non-foodborne) infection for humans". In: Miller AJ, Smith JL, Somkuti GA (eds), *Foodborne Listeriosis* (Elsevier Science Publishers B.V, 1990), 31–9.

Hitchins, AD "Chapter 10 *Listeria monocytogenes*". In US Food and Drug Administration's Bacteriological Analytical Manual (online) (2001).

Hu Q, Lyu D, Shi X *et al.* "A modified molecular beacons-based multiplex real-time PCR assay for simultaneous detection of eight foodborne pathogens in a single reaction and its application". *Foodborne Pathogens and Disease* 11 (2014):207–14.

ISO "Microbiology of food and animal feeding stuffs – Horizontal method for the detection and enumeration of Listeria monocytogenes – Part 1: Detection method. International Standard ISO 11290-1", Amendment 1, Geneva, Switzerland (2005a).

ISO "Microbiology of food and animal feeding stuffs – Horizontal method for the detection and enumeration of Listeria monocytogenes – Part 2: Enumeration method. International Standard ISO 11290-2", Amendment 1, Geneva, Switzerland (2005b).

Jaakohuhta S, Harma H, Tuomola M and Lovgren T "Sensitive Listeria spp. immunoassay based on europium (III) nanoparticulate labels using time-resolved fluorescence". *International Journal of Food Microbiology* 114 (2007):288–94.

Janakiraman V "Listeriosis in pregnancy: diagnosis, treatment, and prevention". *Reviews in Obstetrics and Gynecology* 1 (2008):179–85.

Kahn CM "Listeriosis". In Kahn CN and Line S (eds), *The Merck Veterinary Manual* (Merck and Co., 9th edn, 2005), 2240–1.

Kawasaki S, Fratamico PM, Horikoshi N *et al.* "Evaluation of a multiplex PCR system for simultaneous detection of *Salmonella* spp., *Listeria monocytogenes*, and *Escherichia coli O157:H7* in foods and in food subjected to freezing". *Foodborne Pathogens and Disease* 6 (2009):81–9.

Khan JA, Rathore RS, Khan S and Ahmad I "In vitro detection of pathogenic *Listeria monocytogenes* from food sources by conventional, molecular and cell culture method". *Brazilian Journal of Microbiology* 44(3) (2013):751–8.

Lecuit M "Human listeriosis and animal models". *Microbes and Infection* 9 (2007):1216–25.

Lee N, Kwon KY, Oh SK, Chang HJ, Chun HS and Choi SW "A multiplex PCR assay for simultaneous detection of *Escherichia coli O157:H7, Bacillus cereus, Vibrio parahaemolyticus, Salmonella spp.*, *Listeria monocytogenes*, and *Staphylococcus aureus* in Korean ready-to-eat food". *Foodborne Pathogens and Disease* 11 (2014):574–80.

Liu D, Ainsworth AJ, Austin FW and Lawrence ML "Characterization of virulent and avirulent *Listeria monocytogenes* strains by PCR amplification of putative transcriptional regulator and internalin genes". *Journal of Medical Microbiology* 52 (2003):1065–70.

Kaur S, Malik SVS, Bhilegaonkar KN, Vaidya VM and Barbuddhe SB "Use of a phospholipase-C assay, in vivo pathogenicity assays and PCR in assessing the virulence of *Listeria* spp." *Veterinary Journal* 184 (2010):366–70.

Leclercq A, Clermont D, Bizet C *et al.* "*Listeria rocourtiae sp.* nov." *International Journal of Systemic and Evolutionary Microbiology* 60 (2010):2210–14.

Mateus T, Silva J, Maia RL and Teixeira P. "Listeriosis during pregnancy: a public health concern". *ISRN Obstetrics and Gynecology* 3 (2013):851712.

McLauchlin J "Listeria and listeriosis". *Clinical Microbiology and Infection* 3(4) (1997):484–92.

Milillo SR, Stout JC, Hanning IB *et al.* "*Listeria monocytogenes* and hemolytic *Listeria innocua* in poultry". *Poultry Science* 91 (2012):2158–63.

Mraheil MA, Billion A, Mohamed W *et al.* "The intracellular sRNA transcriptome of *Listeria monocytogenes* during growth in macrophages". *Nucleic Acids Research* 39 (2011):4235–48.

Moorhead SM, Dykes GA and Cursons RT "An SNP-based PCR assay to differentiate between *Listeria monocytogenes* lineages derived from phylogenetic analysis of the *sigB* gene". *Journal of Microbiological Methods* 55 (2003):425–32.

Muñoz AI "Distribution of *Listeria monocytogenes* serotypes isolated from foods, Colombia, 2000–2009". *Biomedica* 32 (2012):408–17.

Murray EGD, Webb RA and Swann MBR "A disease of rabbits characterised by a large mononuclear leucocytosis, caused by a hitherto undescribed *bacillus* Bacterium monocytogenes (n.sp.)". *Journal of Pathology* 29 (1926):407–39.

O'Riordan M, Moors MA and Portnoy DA "Listeria intracellular growth and virulence require host-derived lipoic acid". *Science* 302 (2003):462–4.

Orsi RH, den Bakker HC and Wiedmann M "*Listeria monocytogenes* lineages: genomics, evolution, ecology, and phenotypic characteristics". *International Journal of Medical Microbiology* 301 (2011):79–96.

OIE "*Listeria monocytogenes*". Chapter 2.9.7 in *Manual of Diagnostic Tests and Vaccines for Terrestrial Animals* (2014), 1–18. Available at www.oie.int/manual-of-diagnostic-tests-and-vaccines-for-terrestrial-animals/.

Paillard, D, Dubois V, Duran R *et al.* "Rapid identification of Listeria species by using restriction fragment length polymorphism of PCR-amplified *23S rRNA* gene fragments". *Applied and Environmental Microbiology* 69 (2003):6386–6392.

Park YS, Lee SR and Kim YG "Detection of *Escherichia coli O157:H7, Salmonella spp., Staphylococcus aureus* and *Listeria monocytogenes* in kimchi by multiplex polymerase chain reaction (mPCR)". *Journal of Microbiology* 44 (2006):92–7.

Rawool DB, Malik SVS, Barbuddhe SB, Shakuntala I and Aurora R "A multiplex PCR for detection of virulence associated genes in *Listeria monocytogenes*". *Internet Journal of Food Safety* 9 (2007):56–62.

Réglier-Poupet H, Pellegrini E, Charbit A and Berche P "Identification of LpeA, a PsaA-like membrane protein that promotes cell entry by *Listeria monocytogenes*". *Infection and Immunity* 71 (2003):474–82.

Rossmanith P, Krassnig M, Wagner M and Hein I "Detection of *Listeria monocytogenes* in food using a combined enrichment/real-time PCR method targeting the *prfA* gene. *Research in Microbiology* 157 (2006):763–71.

Sabet C, Toledo-Arana A, Personnic N *et al.* "The *Listeria monocytogenes* virulence factor InlJ is specifically expressed in vivo and behaves as an adhesin". *Infection and Immunity* 76 (2008):136878.

Schär J, Stoll R, Schauer K *et al.* "Pyruvate carboxylase plays a crucial role in carbon metabolism of extra- and intracellularly replicating *Listeria monocytogenes*". *Journal of Bacteriology* 192 (2010):1774–84.

Scortti M, Monzo HJ, Lacharme-Lora L, Lewis DA and Vazquez-Boland JA "The PrfA virulence regulon". *Microbes and Infection* 9 (2007):1196–1207.

Scott PR "Clinical diagnosis of ovine listeriosis". *Small Ruminant Research* 110 (2013):138–41.

Shoukat S, Malik SVS, Rawool DW *et al.* "Comparison of indirect based ELISA by employing purified LLO and its synthetic peptides and cultural method for diagnosis of ovine listeriosis". *Small Ruminant Research* 113 (2013):301–6.

Simon MC, Gray DI and Cook N "DNA extraction and PCR methods for the detection of *Listeria monocytogenes* in cold-smoked salmon". *Applied and Environmental Microbiology* 62(3) (1996):822–4.

Stavru F, Bouillaud F, Sartori A, Ricquier D and Cossart P "*Listeria monocytogenes* transiently alters mitochondrial dynamics during infection". *Proceedings of the National Academy of Science* 108 (2011):3612–17.

Suarez M and Boland J "The bacterial actin nucleated protein ActA involved in epithelial cell invasion by Listeria monocytogenes". *Cellular Microbiology* 3 (2001):853–64.

Suo B, He Y, Paoli G, Gehring A, Tu SI and Shi X "Development of an oligonucleotide-based microarray to detect multiple foodborne pathogens". *Molecular and Cellular Probes* 24 (2010):77–86.

Swetha, C, Madhava, T, Krishnaiah, N and Kumar, V "Detection of *Listeria monocytogenes* in fish samples by PCR". *Annals of Biological Research* 3(4) (2013):1880–4.

Talon R, Lebert I, Lebert A *et al.* "Traditional dry fermented sausages produced in small-scale processing units in Mediterranean countries and Slovakia. 1: Microbial ecosystems of processing environments" *Meat Science* 77 (2007):570–9.

Tang MJ, Zhou S, Zhang XY, Pu JH, Ge QL, Tang XJ and Gao YS "Rapid and sensitive detection of Listeria monocytogenes by loop-mediated isothermal amplification". *Current Microbiology* 63 (2011):511–16.

US Department of Agriculture (USDA). *Microbiology Laboratory Guidebook*, Chapter 8.11, Revision, January (2019) (online).

US Food and Drug Administration (USFDA). *Guidance for Industry: Bioanalytical Method Validation* (US Department of Health and Human Services, 2001).

Vazquez-Boland, JA, Dominguez L, Fernandez, JF, Rodriguez-Ferri, EF, Briones, V, Blanco M and Suarez G "Revision of the validity of CAMP tests for *Listeria* identification. Proposal of an alternative method for the determination of haemolytic activity by Listeria strains". *Acta Microbiologica et Immunologica Hungarica* 37 (1990):201–6.

Vazquez-Boland JA, Kuhn M, Berche P *et al.* "Listeria pathogenesis and molecular virulence determinants". *Clinical Microbiology Reviews* 14(3) (2001):584–640.

Vera A, Gonzalez G, Domınguez M and Bello H "Main virulence factors of *Listeria monocytogenes* and its regulation". *Revista chilena de infectologia* 30 (2013):407–16.

Vines A, Reeves MW, Hunter S and Swaminathan B "Restriction fragment length polymorphism in four virulence- associated genes of *Listeria monocytogenes*". *Research in Microbiology* 143 (1992):281–94.

Walker SJ, Archer P and Banks JG "Growth of *Listeria monocytogenes* at refrigeration temperatures". *Journal of Applied Bacteriology* 68 (1990):157–62.

Walker JK, Morgan JH, McLauchlin J, Grant KA and Shallcross JA "Listeria innocua isolated from a case of ovine Meningoencephalitis". *Veterinary Microbiology* 42 (1994):245–53.

Wang RF, Cao WW and Johnson MG "16S rRNA based probes and polymerase chain reaction method to detect *Listeria monocytogenes* cells added to foods". *Applied and Environmental Microbiology* 58 (1992):2827–31.

Welch MD, Iwamatsu A and Mitchison TJ "Actin polymerization is induced by Arp2/3 protein complex at the surface of *Listeria monocytogenes*". *Nature* 85 (1997):265–9.

Weller D, Andrus A, Wiedmann M and den Bakker HC "*Listeria booriae sp.* nov. and *Listeria newyorkensis sp.* nov., from food processing environments in the USA". *International Journal of Systemic and Evolutionary Microbiology* 65 (2015):286–92.

Wernars K, Heuvelman CJ, Chakraborty T and Notermans SH "Use of the polymerase chain reaction for direct detection of *Listeria monocytogenes* in soft cheese". *Journal of Applied Bacteriology* 70 (1991):121–6.

Wesley IV. "Listeriosis in animals". In Ryser ET and Marth EH (eds), *Listeria, Listeriosis and Food Safety* (CRC Press, 3rd edn, 2007), 55–84.

Winters DK, Maloney TP and Johnson MG "Rapid detection of *Listeria monocytogenes* by a PCR assay specific for an aminopeptidase". *Molecular and Cellular Probes* 13 (1999):127–31.

Yang Y, Liu B, Dai J, Srivastava PK, Zammit DJ, Lefrançois L and Li Z "Heat shock protein gp96 is a master chaperone for toll-like receptors and is important in the innate function of macrophages". *Immunity* 26 (2007):215–26.

Zhao J, Jedlicka SS, Lannu JD, Bhunia AK and Rickus JL "Liposome-doped nanocomposites as artificial-cell-based biosensors: detection of listeriolysin O". *Biotechnology Progress* 22 (2006):32–7.

10

Pyroptosis Prevalence in Animal Diseases and Diagnosis

Praveen P. Balgir and Suman Rani
Department of Biotechnology, Punjabi University, Patiala-147002, Punjab, India
Corresponding author: Praveen P. Balgir, *balgirbt@live.com*

10.1 Introduction

Pyroptosis is classified as regulated programmed cell death that is inherently associated with inflammation. The first observation of pyroptosis was in macrophages infected by bacteria that underwent a rapid lytic cell death dependent on caspase-1 activity, described in 1992 (Fink *et al.*, 2005). The name pyroptosis was coined from *pyro* in Greek (meaning "fire" or "fever") and ptosis ("to fall"). Most recently, based on the recommendations of the Nomenclature Committee on Cell Death in 2018, pyroptosis has been defined as "a type of Regulated Cell Death (RCD) that critically depends on the formation of plasma membrane pores by members of the gasdermin protein family, often (but not always) as a consequence of inflammatory caspase activation" (Galluzzi *et al.*, 2018).

RCD occurs in response to various signals transduced into the cell, which modulate its activity accordingly. Pyroptosis is the response of the cell to number of danger signals such as invading bacteria, intracellular pathogens, toxins, oxidative stress, etc. (Figure 10.1). It has been observed that over-activation of this pathway leads to extensive cell death that may be the underlying cause of pathological conditions like tissue damage, lethal septic shock, organ failure, inflammatory bowel disease, neuronal damage, bladder muscular hyperplasia, hepatitis, auto-inflammatory diseases, brucella joint infection, acute lung injury, acute respiratory distress syndrome, inflammatory demyelination, cognitive impairment, sepsis, osteoarthritis, and many others.

10.2 Characteristic Features of Pyroptosis

Pyroptosis differs from other types of cell death such as apoptosis and necrosis morphologically and mechanistically due to the involvement of inflammatory caspases-1, -3, -4, -5, and -11 (Chen *et al.*, 2016; Wang *et al.*, 2017; Rogers *et al.*, 2017; Frank *et al.*, 2018). Instead of membrane blebbing, as in apoptosis, pyroptosis is characterized by pore formation in the plasma membrane. It includes disruption of the cell membrane and the release of its cellular content such as cytokines and chemokines to the outside. These cytokines act as activators of immune cells and are able to trigger the recruitment of inflammatory molecules from different cells. Before the discovery of gasdermin as a pore-forming protein, this mechanism was thought to be fully dependent on caspase-1 activity. This pore-forming causes alteration of ionic gradients across the membrane, which in turn causes water and ionic influx, cell swelling and rupture in that order (Bergsbaken *et al.*, 2009; Ding *et al.*, 2016). DNA cleavage is also observed in pyroptosis although the nuclei remain intact (Aglietti *et al.*, 2017).

Caspases are originally expressed as procaspases which are then activated by proteolysis, cleavage, and oligomerization into mature functional enzymes. They are the members of the cysteine-dependent protease family and cleave substrate at the C-terminal of aspartic acid with nucleophilic attack. Some of them, such as those found in humans, caspase-1, -4, -5, and -12, and in mice, caspase-1, -11, and -12 (Martinon *et al.*, 2004), are also known as inflammatory caspases as they mediate innate immunity and inflammation (Aglietti *et al.*, 2017).

The detailed molecular mechanism involving inflammasome pathways has been established with studies carried out in various animals like mice, rats, rhesus monkeys, etc., modeling for diseases like cognitive impairment, muscular hyperplasia, hepatitis, brucella infection, osteomyelitis, sepsis, and neonatal-onset multisystem inflammatory disease.

10.3 Molecular Mechanism of Pyroptosis

Pyroptosis includes two pathways: the canonical inflammasome pathway and the non-canonical inflammasome pathway. Inflammasomes are large oligomeric complexes and were first described in 2002 by Jurg Tschopp (Schroder and Tschopp, 2010) as a complex of molecules that activate caspases. Now under the term "inflammasome", a large number of types have emerged that only differ in their sensor and adaptor proteins. In most types of inflammasomes, sensor proteins are pattern recognition receptors (PRRs) that bind a specific set of pathogen-associated molecular patterns (PAMPs) ligands. Due to this specificity a number of PRRs are shown to form a distinct set of inflammasomes in response to different stimuli (Bergsbaken *et al.*, 2009). Different types of PRRs include the NLR (nod-like receptor) family, PYRIN (PYD domain)-domain-containing-1, such as nod-like receptor protein-1 (NLRP1), etc. The NLR family of proteins contains two domains, one a nucleotide-binding oligomerization domain (NOD) and the second a leucine-rich repeat (LRR)-containing protein domain. Other inflammasomes complexes include PRRs like nod-like receptor protein-3 (NLRP3), which is activated by diverse stimuli, NAIP (NLR family of apoptosis inhibitory proteins; another subset of NLR family proteins), AIM2 (absent in melanoma 2), and PYRIN. NLRP1 has been observed to be activated by *Toxoplasma gondii* and the anthrax toxin of *Bacillus anthracis*, whereas NLRP3 responds to particulate and crystalline matter like pore-forming protein toxins, various pathogens, and extracellular ATP by forming highly characterized inflammasomes (Liu *et al.*, 2010). A study by Sharif *et al.* (2019) suggests that NEK7 (mitotic ser-thr kinase) makes connections between adjacent subunits of NLRP3 with bipartite interactions to mediate the activation of the NLRP3 inflammasome. NAIP is activated by recognition of bacterium flagella. AIM2 responds to the presence of double-stranded DNA in the cytosol and gets activated. PYRIN responds to the presence of inactivated RhoA, brought about by bacterial toxin.

10.3.1 Canonical Inflammasome Pathway

After activation, PRRs oligomerize with adaptor proteins (making a bridge between PRR and pro-caspase-1) and apoptosis-associated speck-like proteins (ASCs)—containing a caspase activation and recruitment domain (CARD), which contains both a PYRIN and CARD domain, and forms an inflammasome. ASCs interact with the inflammasome sensor through PYRIN and CARD, and recruit procaspase-1 to the complex, which leads to activated caspase-1 and initiates downstream processing of proteins, which leads to the release of cytokines such as IL-1b, and pyroptosis (Aglieti *et al.*, 2017; Bergsbaken *et al.*, 2009).This pathway depends on caspase-1 activity.

Caspase-1 is expressed as a 44-kDa pro-caspase-1 consisting of a pro domain of 10-kDa CARD, a large subunit (p20) and a small subunit (p10). Within the inflammasome procaspase-1 undergoes auto-processing, releasing the CARD domain, followed by tetramerization of two small and two large subunits, which constitute the active caspase-1 enzyme. The active site of the enzyme is formed of residues from both the p10 and the p20 subunits. Within the p20 subunit is located the catalytic cysteine, Cys285, and histidine, His237, while substrate specificity is localized in the p10 residues. In accordance with the basic characteristic of caspases, caspase-1 also requires Asp in the P1 position of its substrates, immediately the N-terminal of the cleavage site. The consensus caspase-1 amino acid recognition sequence is comprised of the sequence Tyr (P4)–Val(P3)–Ala(P2)–Asp(P1). Activity of caspase-1 involves cleavage and conversion of a unique set of proteins into their biologically active and secretory forms, for example, pro-IL-1b and pro-Il-18. These activated cytokines are known to be highly inflammatory, having an important role in immune response propagation by recruiting and activating immune cells. Cytokines are known to act as intercellular messengers, communicating between various types of cells near the site of infection, tissue damage, or inflammation along with relaying the message to distal parts of the body. Thus, cytokines are able to instruct cells of the immune system as well as non-immune cells as to the nature, form, and length of innate inflammation response.

Along with cytokines, caspase-1 also takes GSDMD as a substrate and cuts it into N-terminal (GSDMD-N) and C-terminal gasdermin (GSDMD-C). This GSDMD-N terminal oligomerizes and creates pores in the plasma membrane of cells that lead to the release of inflammatory factors, cell membrane swelling, bursting, and ultimately pyroptosis (Davis *et al.*, 2019; Zhaolin *et al.*, 2019).

10.3.2 Non-canonical Inflammasome Pathway

The non-canonical pathway is a caspase-1-independent pathway, depending instead on caspase-4, -5, and -11 activity (Figure 10.1). These caspases directly recognize bacterial lipopolysaccharides (LPSs) and cleave GSDMD (Zhaolin *et al.*, 2019) into GSDMD-N and GSDMD-C, as described above in the case of caspase-1, and induce pyroptosis. As in the canonical pathway, NLRP3 inflammasome is activated in this pathway also, but maturation of IL-Iß and IL-18 occurs only by caspase-1. In the case of any pathogen attack, LPSs like ligand association recruits adapter proteins to receptors. Here, myeloid differentiation 88 (MyD88) protein acts as an adaptor and the receptors are IL-1 (IL-1R) and IL-18 (IL-18R). MyD88 is recruited to the TIR domain within the cytoplasmic region of receptors, leading to auto-phosphorylation of IRAK (IL-1R-associated kinase). This phosphorylated IRAK is now free to bind with E3 ubiquitin

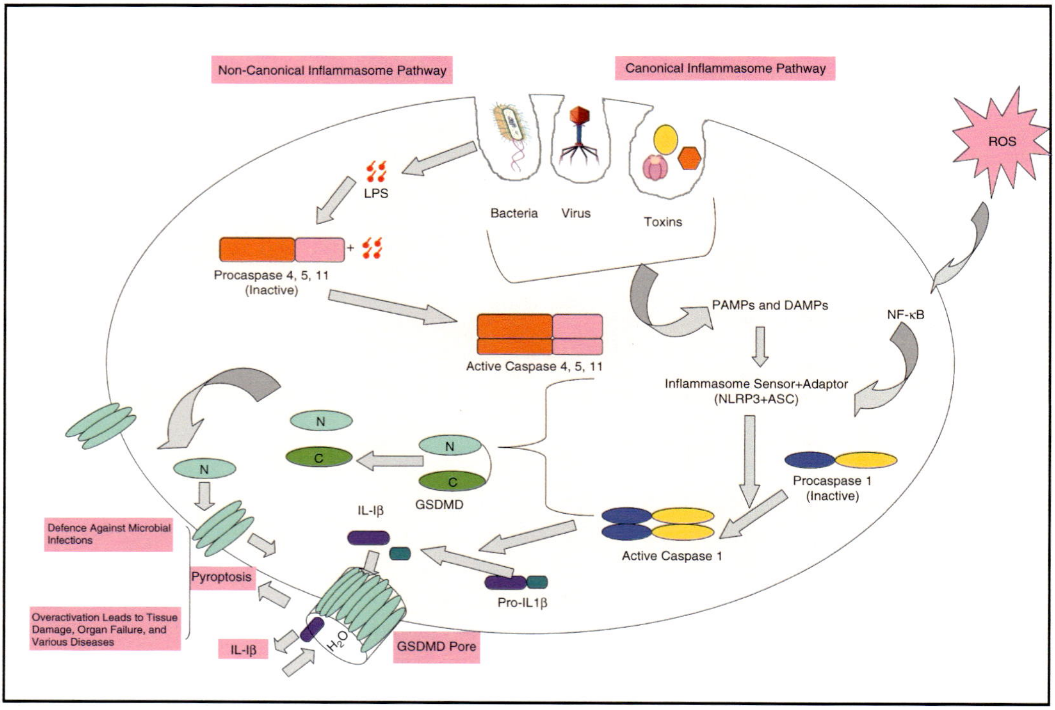

FIGURE 10.1 Canonical and non-canonical inflammasome pathways of pyroptosis. Pore-forming activity of GSDMD executes inflammatory caspase-induced pyroptosis.

ligase tumor necrosis factor (TNF) receptor-associated factor 6 (TRAF6) as it is released from the receptor-MyD88 complex. TRAF6 ubiquitinates itself and TAK1 (TGFβ-activated kinase-1), which leads to activation of IκB (inhibitor of κB) kinase complex. IκB kinase releases NF-κB from IκBα- mediated inhibition, which in turn leads to activation of NLRP3 inflammasome and ultimately pyroptosis (Zhaolin *et al.*, 2019).

Besides *GSDMD*, the gasdermin family includes five more genes in humans (and ten genes in mice): *GSDMA*, *GSDMB*, *GSDMC*, *GSDME* (*DFNA5*), and *DFNB59*. Mice lack GSDMB but have three GSDMAs, viz. GSDMA1–3, and four GSDMCs, viz. GSDMC1–4. For induction of pyroptosis, caspase-1/-4/-5/-11 carries out cleavage of its target GSDMD (Kayagaki *et al.*, 2015; Shi *et al.*, 2015), caspase -3/-6/-7 for GSDMB (Yuan *et al.*, 2018), and caspase-3 targets GSDME. Although caspases/proteases that might target GSDMA and GSDMC are unknown to date, expression of the gasdermin-N domain alone from these gasdermins can signal cell death (Frank & Vince, 2018). Dominant mutations in *GSDMA3* (Porter *et al.*, 2002; Runkel *et al.*, 2004; Saeki *et al.*, 2011; Sato *et al.*, 1998; Tanaka *et al.*, 2013) have been associated with hyperkeratosis in mice and its homologue *GSDMA* with alopecia in humans. *GSDME* mutation was implicated by Ding *et al.* (2016) in the causation of non-syndromic hearing loss in humans. It was reported in mice studies that mutations in the *GSDMA3* gene or even those within the gasdermin-N domain alone lead to activation of pyroptosis due to loss of auto-inhibition between the N- and C-domains.

Studies by Davis *et al.* (2019) revealed that during pyroptosis, major cytoskeleton constituents were cleaved and this disrupted the membrane. The process was calpain-dependent, leading to cleavage of vimentin, with degradation of intermediate filaments. Further, they reported that while smaller molecules like IL-1β, HMGB1, and lactate dehydrogenase (LDH) were released without breaching of the membrane, such breakage was needed for the release of larger inflammation stimulatory complexes like mitochondria, ASC specks, nuclei, and whole bacteria.

10.4 Pyroptosis Prevalence in Animal Diseases

In many animals cats, dogs, pigs, cattle, horses, and wild animals, a number of inflammatory, septic, and degenerative conditions, like pancreatitis, sepsis, acute kidney damage, mammary carcinoma, autoimmune disorders, complications of the reproductive system, and cardiovascular disorders, have been reported to be associated with a number of acute phase protein (APPs) biomarkers reflective of underlying inflammatory conditions.

10.4.1 Neuro-inflammation and Cognitive Impairment in Aged Rodents

Fan *et al.* (2018) showed that blocking pyroptosis can lead to the inhibition of neuro-inflammation and cognitive impairment in aged rodents. From their study they found that general anesthesia (GA) isoflurane leads to activation of Nod-like receptor protein-3 (NLRP3) inflammasome. They found that isoflurane causes overactivation of NLRP3 inflammasome, caspase-1, interleukin-1b (IL-1b), and IL-18, and ultimately excessive pyroptosis that causes damage to neurons and cognitive impairment in aging mice. Their study explored how NLRP3 inflammasome inhibitor MCC950 protected the isoflurane-exposed aging mice from cognitive impairment by inhibiting pyroptosis. They intraperitoneally injected MCC950 (10 mg/kg) into 15-month-old male C57BL/6 mice. This NLRP3 inhibitor not only provided protection to neurons by inhibiting activation of inflammasome, but also prevented pyroptosis and its consequent impairment of cognition in an aging mice model that was exposed to isoflurane. Their study pointed to the utility of NLRP3 inflammasome inhibitor MCC950 in the treatment of cognitive impairment in elderly patients under general anesthesia (Fan *et al.*, 2018).

10.4.2 Osteomyelitis

Osteomyelitis is a severe infection of bone and bone marrow that causes aberrant bone neo-formation, bone destruction, and systemic inflammatory reaction. A study from Zhu *et al.* in 2019 experimentally found the cause behind osteomyelitis to be pyroptosis. The study correlated the expression of proteins such as NLRP3 and caspase-1 with the induction of pyroptosis in osteomyelitis using inhibitors of these proteins on *S. aureus*-induced osteomyelitis both *in vitro* in bone marrow macrophages (BMMs) and *in vivo* in male C57BL/6 mice. They found that expression of these proteins associated with pyroptosis in infectious bone fragments was significantly higher than in non-affected normal bone. In a murine model they could prove that administration of NLRP3 inhibitor glyburide and caspase-1 inhibitor AC-YVAD-CMK not only effectively attenuated the bacterial infection-induced pyroptosis, but also led to repair by restoring the expression of osteogenesis markers like collagen-I and Runx2 *in vitro* and prevented the activation of osteoclast *in vitro* healing the bone injury *in vivo*. This study provided potential diagnostic biomarkers as well as treatment targets for osteomyelitis (Zhu *et al.*, 2019).

10.4.3 Neonatal-onset Multisystem Inflammatory Disease

NLRP3, also known as cryopyrin, assembles an inflammasome complex after sensing danger signals generated by foreign particles. Mutations in NLRP3 make it hyperactive, which during inflammasome formation assembled as hyperactive inflammasome and was observed to cause over-secretion of cytokines such as interleukin (IL)-1β and IL-18, leading to syndromes like neonatal-onset multisystem inflammatory disease (NOMID), Muckle-Wells syndrome (MWS), and familial cold auto-inflammatory syndrome (FCAS), of which neonatal-onset multisystem inflammatory disease (NOMID) is phenotypically the most severe. Mice with the NOMID phenotype contain many features similar to that of human diseases, as they develop severe systemic inflammation. This is due to overproduction of IL-1β and IL-18 and leads to damage to multiple organs, including the liver, spleen, skeleton, and skin. This secretion of cytokines is due to over-activation of gasdermin D. The study of Xiao *et al.* (2018) in mice showed that deletion of the GSDMD gene prevented all NOMID-associated inflammatory symptoms, thus proving the GSDMD-dependent nature of pathogenesis of NOMID and related diseases (Xiao *et al.*, 2018).

10.4.4 Sepsis

Rathkey *et al.* (2018) reported that GSDMD inhibition by necro-sulfonamide led to inhibition of pyroptosis and sepsis in murine macrophages and a mice sepsis model. Sepsis is life-threatening and severe systemic inflammatory disorder is a leading cause of cell death. Gasdermin D is a pore-forming protein of pyroptosis leading to membrane lysis and secretion of inflammatory cytokines which over-activate the innate immune system. Necro-sulfonamide directly binds with GSDMD and inhibits it and was found to ultimately inhibit pyroptosis and sepsis (Rathkey *et al.*, 2018).

Another study, by Sun *et al.* (2019), experimentally found the mechanism behind the neuroprotective effect of dexmedetomidine, an α2-adrenoceptor agonist, against various brain injuries. In their study they took *in vivo* (adult male Sprague-Dawley rats) and *in vitro* (human astrocyte 1321N1 cells) sepsis models to check the effects of dexmedetomidine on activation of inflammasome leading to glial pyroptosis and death of neurons. For *in vitro* experiments they took cultured astrocytes and induced inflammasome activation and pyroptosis by LPS exposure and checked the effect of dexmedetomidine on pyroptosis. Dexmedetomidine effectively inhibited pyroptosis in cultured astrocytes. In an *in vivo* study dexmedetomidine showed its neuroprotective function by inhibiting neuronal injury caused by LPS treatment in rats that caused increased release of pro-inflammatory cytokines IL-18 and IL-1β. Experiments confirmed that the neuroprotective effect of dexmedetomidine, an α2-adrenoceptor agonist, was inhibited by α2-adrenoceptor antagonist atipamezole. This study found that dexmedetomidine was protecting glia cells via reduction in pyroptosis, which protected neurons, which in turn preserved brain function, ultimately improving the outcome of sepsis and decreasing the mortality rate caused by LPS (Sun *et al.*, 2019).

10.4.5 Inflammatory Bowel Disease

Inflammatory bowel disease (IBD) is a most commonly observed abnormal inflammatory disease of the gastrointestinal tract caused by alteration of the intestinal microbiome, affecting the intestinal mucosal immunity. IBD may be caused in dogs due to parasitic or bacterial infection, e.g., *E. coli*, *Salmonella*, or *Giardia*, or as an allergic reaction to a specific dietary protein. Similarly, in the case of horses, common intestinal factors may be feed components, parasites, or bacterial infections. Intestinal epithelial cells (IEC) keep away intestinal flora from host cells. With the over-expression of inflammasomes in IEC, imbalance between the immune system and gut microbiota is observed and the intestinal flora affect the mucosal immunity, leading to IBD. Thus, pyroptosis was observed in IBD development suggested by a high increase of inflammatory caspases. In IBD, various studies tried to target pyroptosis signaling. Cholecalciterol cholesterol emulsion (CCE), a drug that is known to effectively inhibit colitis, also experimentally attenuated pyroptosis (Xiong *et al.*, 2016). Mesalamine and corticosteroids are also therapeutic drugs that inhibit pyroptosis in IEC (Davis *et al.*, 2017; Yuan *et al.*, 2018).

10.4.6 Brucellosis

Brucella is an intracellular bacterial pathogen causing brucellosis and in human arthritis is the most common manifestation of the disease. Here, inflammatory cell death pyroptosis acts as a preventive mechanism against pathogenesis of *Brucella*. A study by Lacey *et al.* (2018) reported the formation of inflammasomes and their proteolytic effect on pyroptotic proteins like IL-18 and interleukin-1, leading to inflammation that led to control of infection during *Brucella*-induced arthritis in C57BL/6 mice (Lacey *et al.*, 2018). The disease is widespread amongst domestic and wild animals. Literature reports are available from cattle, pigs, sheep, goats, camels, foxes, etc. (OIE, 2018). Usually, young animals and non-pregnant females are asymptomatic. As observed in the case of cattle, infection with *B. abortus or B. melitensis* in pregnant females led to placentitis, which usually resulted in abortion in late pregnancy, i.e., the fifth to ninth month. Similarly, in pigs, as in ruminants, after the initial bacteraemia, *B. suis* colonizes cells of the reproductive tract in either sexes. Later in pregnant sows brucellosis is known to lead to abortion. Another manifestation of brucellosis is in the form of arthritis in animals, which may occur in various joints, and sometimes result in spondylitis.

10.4.7 Oxidative Stress in Animals

Reactive oxygen species (ROS) are generated during the course of cellular metabolism and effectively removed by antioxidants. Imbalance in ROS homeostasis may be caused by a deficiency of anti-oxidant enzymes or in other components of anti-oxidant networks, and can lead to an increase in oxidative stress. At cellular level oxidative stress leads to toxic changes in macromolecular constituents like lipids, DNA, RNA, and proteins, thereby, increasing the rate of cell death by apoptosis, necrosis, pyroptosis, etc. (Sordillo and Aitken, 2009).

Oxidative stress has been observed in pets and companion animals when exposed to stressful social situations like transportation, mixing, and abrupt weaning of young ruminants (Gupta *et al.*, 2007; Herskin *et al.*, 2007). Several reports are available in the literature pointing to the negative effects of oxidative stress as a leading cause of different pathologies in animals. Examples of bacterial sepsis and pneumonia in pigs (Basu and Eriksson, 2001) and recurrent airway obstruction in horses have been attributed to oxidative stress (Deaton *et al.*, 2004, 2005). Further ROS flare-up was observed during stressful parturition and lactation which induced metabolic disorders in cattle (Lauritzen *et al.*, 2005; Castillo *et al.*, 2005, 2006). Biomarkers used in diagnosis of cellular oxidative stress in animals include plasma and serum levels of glutathione (GSH) (L-g-glutamyl-L-cysteinylglycine), isoprostanes, and malondialdehyde (MDA) (Marchitti *et al.*, 2008). Along with these biomarkers, ROS-reducing catalytic enzymes, such as glutathione peroxidase, catalase, superoxide dismutase, and thioredoxin reductase (Ho *et al.*, 2013; Yatoo *et al.*, 2019) are also used to diagnose the extent of oxidative stress in animals.

10.4.8 Viral Diseases in Animals

10.4.8.1 Rabies

Rabies is caused by lassiviruses which can affect all warm-blooded animals, including wild animals, which act as reservoirs of the pathogen. In mammals, due to involvement of the nervous system (NS), the disease is fatal. The rabies virus (RABV) encodes a glycoprotein that is displayed on its surface and is involved in pathogenesis, the RABV-G protein. The virus causes acute encephalomyelitis, especially observed among carnivores and bats (Rupprecht *et al.*, 2006). Rabid dog bites are the main mode of transmission to domesticated animals and humans. Singh *et al.* (2017), while reviewing rabies diagnosis and control, suggested that overexpression of the RABV-G protein activates the pyroptosis pathway. Pyroptosis, which involves the activation of caspase-1, results in cell death (Ting *et al.*, 2008). The disintegration of the cell membrane and release of cytokines results in stimulation of the innate immune response that has a protective function (Kono and Rock, 2008).

10.4.8.2 Simian Immunodeficiency Virus

A study by Lu *et al.* (2016) reported pyroptosis to be crucial in the pathogenesis of simian immunodeficiency virus (SIV). The study carried out in rhesus macaques established that SIV infection induces CD4+T cell death while amplifying the inflammatory immune response (Lu *et al.*, 2016). The study found genes of the canonical pyroptosis pathway, caspase-1, and interleukin-1 to be highly expressed as compared to controls.

10.4.8.3 Classical Swine Fever

Classified as a class-A infectious disease by the World Organization for Animal Health (OIE), classical swine fever (CSF) is caused by the CSF virus (CSFV). It results in fever, leukopenia, abortion, hemorrhage, and high mortality amongst infected animals. Pig mortality by CSF is known to cause substantial financial losses to the world pig industry. Recently, Yuan *et al.* (2018) investigated CSFV-induced pyroptosis in peripheral lymphoid organs of infected pigs. They observed formation of GSDMD-N as a result of caspase-mediated cleavage of GSDMD, driving pyroptosis. The authors reported increased damage of PBMC cell membranes in CSFV-infected cells.

Fan *et al.* (2018) observed that CSFV-infected porcine PBMCs underwent pyroptosis resulting in secretion of IL-1Beta, and an inflammatory response. Most of the infected cells were observed to die, releasing intracellular content in large quantities, causing inflammation. This process induced the death of the surrounding cells, the so-called "bystanders" effect. Thus, pyroptosis is an immune response, protecting the body against viral invasion (Ma *et al.*, 2019).

10.4.9 Bladder Muscular Hyperplasia

Bladder muscular hyperplasia is a common phenomenon in inflamed muscles and is associated with muscle expansion. The primary cause behind poor bladder function is smooth muscle inflammation-induced cell death, i.e., pyroptosis. Haldar *et al.* (2015) reported that chemotherapeutic drug cyclophosphamide metabolite acrolein caused DNA damage in mice, which activates the NLRP3 inflammasome complex, activating caspase-1 and resulting in cell death and detrusor hyperplasia. In a mouse model it was observed to lead to inflammation in cultured bladder muscle cells. Bladder muscle hyperplasia resulting from NLRP3 inflammatory pathway activation can be inhibited using inhibitor of IL-1β anakinra, a rheumatoid arthritis therapeutic drug, and IGF1 (downstream of IL-1β signaling) by IGF1-neutralizing antibody. So antagonizing these molecules can prevent muscle hyperplasia resulting from chronic inflammation (Haldar *et al.*, 2015).

10.4.10 Liver Inflammation, and Fibrosis in Mice

Liver inflammation includes steatohepatitis, steatosis, and fibrosis leading to liver cirrhosis, and ultimately leads to hepatocellular carcinoma, which is the main cause of death among all chronic liver diseases. MicroRNAs (miRNAs) are reported as the major contributors in liver diseases. One study by Heo *et al.* (2019) reported that miR-148a population decreases in alcoholic hepatitis (AH) human and model animal liver samples and in hepatocytes. FOX1 (forkhead box protein O1) protein was inhibited in alcoholic mice liver samples as FOX1 acts as transcription factor for MIR148A gene that encodes MiR-148a. MiR-148a acts as an inhibitor of TXNIP (thioredoxin-interacting protein). So in liver hepatocytes, as MiR-148a population decreases, it is unable to inhibit TXNIP, resulting in overexpression of TXNIP that activates NLRP3 inflammasome and ultimately leads to caspase-1-mediated pyroptosis.

10.4.11 Exposure to Environmental Pollution

Pollutants like polychlorinated biphenyls (PCBs) are a proven cause of immunotoxicity and neurotoxicity, with potential for carcinogenesis and reproductive dysfunction in humans; these can also result in similar pathologies in animals such as bears, in which the metabolites of PCB were reported by Liu *et al.* (2010). The mechanism was elucidated by Dong *et al.* (2019), who observed the adverse effects of PCBs in an *in vitro* HeLa cell system. They recorded that PCB29-pQ induced pyroptosis via ROS activation of NLRP3 inflammasome, which in turn activated caspase-1 to induce pyroptosis.

10.5 Pyroptosis Markers in Disease Diagnosis

Recently, Keane *et al.* (2018) assessed the utility of pyroptotic inflammasome proteins in disease diagnosis and progression in multiple sclerosis patients. As per their observation, caspase-1, interleukin (IL)-18 and apoptosis-associated speck-like proteins containing caspase recruitment domain (ASC) proteins were significantly elevated in the patient blood stream as compared to controls.

Presently, both the OIE and WHO recommend a direct immunofluorescent test (dFAT) for the diagnosis of rabies in fresh brain tissue of dogs. Otherwise, a mouse inoculation test (MIT) and virus-specific polymerase chain reaction (PCR) are better and easier to perform (Singh *et al.*, 2017) in routine diagnosis. In routine diagnosis of rabies, pyroptotic-based caspase-1, and other cytokines like IL-1β, interleukin (IL)-18, high mobility group protein B1 (HMGB1), and lactate dehydrogenase (LDH), can also be tested in rabid animals to determine the extent of disease spread within the animal.

Following pore formation in the membranes of pyroptotic cells, they display characteristic cell swelling and rupture, releasing soluble inflammatory intracellular constituents, such as ATP, IL-1β, IL-18, HMGB1, and LDH (a classic marker of cellular lysis), as well as larger inflammatory content, such as insoluble material, inflammasomes, and nuclei. These all presently constitute diagnostic markers in various inflammatory diseases in animals. Promega CytoTox 96® is an enzymatic cytotoxicity assay that measures LDH released on cytolysis of cells. It is a colorimetric assay involving conversion of a tetrazolium salt (INT) into a red formazan product, which is proportional in *in vitro* assay to the number of lysed cells, and is thus useful in assessing disease progression.

Rosenberg *et al.* (2018) reported that out of all inflammation hematological markers tested routinely, like erythrocyte sedimentation rate (ESR), lactate, fibrinogen, and plasma protein electrophoresis, only lactate values showed significant difference between diseased and control tortoises (*Gopherus polyphemus*). Serum amyloid A (SAA) in horses is the biomarker of acute phase response (APR) in the animal. It is a general systemic reaction to tissue injury (Witkowska-Piłaszewicz *et al.*, 2019). It can be assessed in the blood of the animal, as it is very low in healthy horses but increases rapidly with equine digestive, reproductive, or respiratory diseases and also following surgery. As reported in the review on SAA, it is useful in detecting some subclinical inflammatory pathologies which have the potential to disrupt training and competition in equine athletes. Kirbas *et al.* (2019) evaluated routine biochemical, hematological, and microbiological analyses along with inflammatory markers for their usefulness in neonatal calves with septicemia. Samples of 13 sick and 10 normal animals' blood were analyzed. Only three were positive for *E. coli* O157 serotype. Amongst biochemical parameters, tumor necrosis factor-alpha (TNF-α), procalcitonin (PCT), haptoglobin (Hp), interleukin-6 (IL-6) and fibrinogen (Fb) concentrations were found to be higher in neonates but returned to normal after treatment, proving their utility in assessing septicemia.

Initially, tests for IBD are carried out with fecal examinations, blood testing, and imaging of the intestines by either X-ray or ultrasound. Testing of fecal infectious agents can be used for confirmation (OIE, 2018). Also, health parameters like B12 and folate tests in blood indicate the need for supplementation of vitamins and or probiotics, respectively. Amongst large animals, histopathologic similarities exist between gastroenteritis in horses, Johne's disease in cattle, and Crohn's disease in humans. In dogs and cats, most common forms of lymphocytic-plasmacytic enteritis are followed by eosinophilic inflammation. Nucleic acid assays, PCR, real-time PCR, and their variants are the current recommendations for infectious diseases (OIE, 2018). O'Brien *et al.* (2017) have developed a caspase-1 assessment assay for cultured cells. The cells are cultured in plates where a novel substrate, Z-WEHD-aminoluciferin, is added to the cells along with thermostable luciferase enzyme with a lysis reagent. The caspase enzyme activity releases the luciferin, producing a light flash that is proportional to the quantity of active enzyme present. This test can be used for diagnosis as well as high-throughput screening for inflammasome modulators. The assay is available commercially as Caspase-Glo® 1 inflammasome assay from Promega. Other companies have also produced various colorimetric (Biovision Kit) and fluorometric (Abcam, PromoCell caspase-1 assay kits tests based on caspase cleavage sequences tagged with chromophores to produce specific reaction products. All of these assays determine active enzymes from cultured cells. ImmunoChemistry Technologie's FAM-FLICA® caspase-1 assay detects caspase-1 in living cells using an inhibitor as fluorescent probe FLICA (fluorescent labeled inhibitors of caspases) labeled with FAM dye (FAM-YVAD-FMK). The inhibitor binds the active caspase enzyme in live cells and can be detected using flow cytometry or a fluorescence plate reader.

The challenges of measuring inflammasome activation and consequently pyroptosis in disease diagnosis are manifold. Normally, ELISA or western blotting are carried out to measure inflammasome activation. Both methods have been standardized and ELISA kits and western blotting protocols for the assessment of IL-1β, IL-18, and other proteins are available commercially.

However, both methods require preprocessing of the samples by making lysates, which is taxing timewise as well as requiring sophisticated facilities. The two methods detect total caspase-1 as protein present, even if it is inactive. The other difficulty is in the form of the specificity of antibodies.

Similar difficulties are faced in assessing interleukins as inflammasome markers, as they may be included or excluded from the assay as a result of the activity of other proteases or even as a result of cross-reactivity with pro-IL-1β or pro-IL-18 that is released as a cytotoxic marker.

10.6 Conclusion and Future Prospects in Diagnosis

Pyroptosis is an RCD which is highly inflammatory and occurs during infection as a stimulant of the innate immune response of an animal's immune system. The immune system of the individual recognizes foreign danger signals and results in the release of the pro-inflammatory cytokines through the action of inflammatory caspases, which further attract other immune cells and cause inflammation to fight against infection. The removal of the intracellular replication niches and effective host's immune system promotes clearance of various infections. Over-activation of this pathway leads to extensive cell death that can cause serious health issues that have been reviewed above in various animal diseases. However, apart from ELISA as a diagnostic aid for IL-1β and IL-18 assessment, the pyroptotic assessment assays are lacking. The depth of the understanding of the molecular mechanistics of pyroptosis at present opens up a great opportunity for the development and standardization of diagnostic tests for a number of animal diseases. It can also provide for the testing of drugs for such diseases in animal models that are inhibitory to pyroptosis and thus amenable to the development of novel drug moieties for use in veterinary applications.

Acknowledgement

This work was supported by ICMR-SRF grant (File No. 45/33/2018-HUM/BMS dated 13/02/2019).

References

Aglietti RA and Dueber EC. "Recent insights into the molecular mechanisms underlying pyroptosis and gasdermin family functions." *Trends in Immunology* 38, no. 4 (2017): 261–271.

Basu S and Eriksson M. "Retinol palmitate counteracts oxidative injury during experimental septic shock." *Annals of the Academy of Medicine, Singapore* 30, no. 3 (2001): 265–269.

Bergsbaken T, Fink SL, and Cookson BT. "Pyroptosis: host cell death and inflammation." *Nature Reviews Microbiology* 7, no. 2 (2009): 99–109.

Castillo C, Hernandez J, Bravo A, *et al.* "Oxidative status during late pregnancy and early lactation in dairy cows." *The Veterinary Journal* 169, no. 2 (2005): 286–292.

Castillo C, Hernandez J, and Valverde I. "Plasma malonaldehyde (MDA) and total antioxidant status (TAS) during lactation in dairy cows." *Research in Veterinary Science* 80, no. 2 (2006): 133–139.

Chen X and He W. "Pyroptosis is driven by non-selective gasdermin-D pore and its morphology is different from MLKL channel-mediated necroptosis." *Cell Research* 26, no. 9 (2016): 1007–1020.

Davis, EM, Kaufmann Y, *et al.* "Pyroptosis of intestinal epithelial cells is crucial to the development of mucosal barrier dysfunction and intestinal inflammation." *Gastroenterology* 152, no. 5 (2017): S967.

Davis, MA, Marian R, *et al.* "Calpain drives pyroptotic vimentin cleavage, intermediate filament loss, and cell rupture that mediates immunostimulation." *Proceedings of the National Academy of Sciences* 116, no. 11 (2019): 5061–5070.

Deaton CM and Marlin DJ. "Antioxidant supplementation in horses affected by recurrent airway obstruction." *The Journal of Nutrition* 134, no. 8 (2004): 2065S–2067S.

Deaton CM, Marlin DJ, Smith NC, *et al.* "Antioxidant and inflammatory responses of healthy horses and horses affected by recurrent airway obstruction to inhaled ozone." *Equine Veterinary Journal* 37, no. 3 (2005): 243–249.

Ding J, Wang K, Liu W, *et al.* "Pore-forming activity and structural autoinhibition of the gasdermin family." *Nature* 535, no. 7610 (2016): 111–116.

Dong W, Zhu Q, Yang B, Qin Q, *et al.* "Polychlorinated biphenyl quinone induces caspase-1-mediated pyroptosis through induction of pro-inflammatory HMGB1-TLR4- NLRP3-GSDMD signal axis." *Chemical Research in Toxicology* 32 (2019): 1051–1057.

Fan Y, Du L, Fu Q, *et al.* "Inhibiting the NLRP3 inflammasome with MCC950 ameliorates isoflurane-induced pyroptosis and cognitive impairment in aged mice." *Frontiers in Cellular Neuroscience* 12 (2018): 426.

Fink SL and Cookson BT. "Apoptosis, pyroptosis, and necrosis: mechanistic description of dead and dying eukaryotic cells." *Infection and Immunity* 73, no. 4 (2005): 1907–1916.

Frank D and Vince JE. "Pyroptosis versus necroptosis: similarities, differences, and crosstalk." *Cell Death & Differentiation* 26, no. 1 (2018): 99–114.

Galluzzi L, Vitale I, Aaronson SA, *et al.* "Molecular mechanisms of cell death: recommendations of the Nomenclature Committee on Cell Death 2018." *Cell Death & Differentiation* 25, no. 3 (2018): 486–541.

Gupta S, Earley B, and Crowe MA. "Effect of 12-hour road transportation on physiological, immunological and haematological parameters in bulls housed at different space allowances." *The Veterinary Journal* 173, no. 3 (2007): 605–616.

Haldar S, Dru C, Choudhury D, *et al.* "Inflammation and pyroptosis mediate muscle expansion in an interleukin-1β (IL-1β)-dependent manner." *Journal of Biological Chemistry* 290, no. 10 (2015): 6574–6583.

Heo MJ, Kim TH, You JS, *et al.* "Alcohol dysregulates miR-148a in hepatocytes through FoxO1, facilitating pyroptosis via TXNIP overexpression." *Gut* 68, no. 4 (2019): 708–720.

Herskin MS, Munksgaard L, and Andersen JB. "Effects of social isolation and restraint on adrenocortical responses and hypoalgesia in loose-housed dairy cows." *Journal of Animal Science* 85, no. 1 (2007): 240–247.

Ho E, Galougahi KK, Liu CC, *et al.* "Biological markers of oxidative stress: applications to cardiovascular research and practice." *Redox Biology* 1, no. 1 (2013): 483–491.

Kayagaki N, Stowe IB, Lee BL, *et al.* "Caspase-11 cleaves gasdermin D for non-canonical inflammasomesignalling." *Nature* 526, no. 7575 (2015): 666–671.

Keane RW, Dietrich WD, and de Rivero Vaccari JP. "Inflammasome proteins as biomarkers of multiple sclerosis." *Frontiers in Neurology* 9 (2018): 135.

Kirbas A, Kandemir FM, Celebi D, *et al.* "The use of inflammatory markers as a diagnostic and prognostic approach in neonatal calves with septicaemia." *Acta Veterinaria Hungarica* 67, no. 3 (2019): 360–376.

Kono H and Rock KL. "How dying cells alert the immune system to danger." *Nature Reviews Immunology* 8, no. 4 (2008): 279–289.

Lacey CA, William JM, Dadelahi AS, *et al.* "Caspase-1 and caspase-11 mediate pyroptosis, inflammation, and control of Brucella joint infection." *Infection and Immunity* 86, no. 9 (2018): e00361–18.

Lauritzen B, Lykkesfeldt J, and Friis C. "Evaluation of a single dose versus a divided dose regimen of amoxycillin in treatment of Actinobacilluspleuropneumoniae infection in pigs." *Research in Veterinary Science* 79, no. 1 (2005): 61–67.

Liu S, Li S, and Du Y. "Polychlorinated biphenyls (PCBs) enhance metastatic properties of breast cancer cells by activating Rho-associated kinase (ROCK)." *PLoS One* 5, no. 6 (2010): e11272.

Liu Y, Jing YY, Zeng CY, *et al.* "Scutellarin suppresses NLRP3 inflammasome activation in macrophages and protects mice against bacterial sepsis." *Frontiers in Pharmacology* 8 (2018): 975.

Lu W, Demers AJ, Ma F, *et al.* "Next-generation mRNA sequencing reveals pyroptosis-induced CD4+ T cell death in early simian immunodeficiency virus-infected lymphoid tissues." *Journal of Virology* 90, no. 2 (2016): 1080–1087.

Ma SM, Mao Q, Yi L, *et al.* "Apoptosis, autophagy, and Pyroptosis: immune escape strategies for persistent infection and pathogenesis of classical swine fever virus." *Pathogens* 8, no. 4 (2019): 239.

Marchitti SA, Brocker C, Stagos D, *et al.* "Non-P450 aldehyde oxidizing enzymes: the aldehyde dehydrogenase superfamily." *Expert Opinion on Drug Metabolism & Toxicology* 4, no. 6 (2008): 697–720.

Martinon F and Tschopp J. "Inflammatory caspases: linking an intracellular innate immune system to autoinflammatory diseases." *Cell* 117, no. 5 (2004): 561–574.

O'Brien M, Moehring D, Muñoz-Planillo R, *et al.* "A bioluminescent caspase-1 activity assay rapidly monitors inflammasome activation in cells." *Journal of Immunological Methods* 447 (2017): 1–13.

OIE. Terrestrial Manual "Chapter 3.1.4 Brucellosis (*Brucella abortus*, *B. melitensis* and *B. suis*)," pp. 355–398 (2018). www.the-icsp.org/subcoms/Brucella.htm.

Porter RM, Lunny DP, Henderson G, *et al.* "Defolliculated (dfl): a dominant mouse mutation leading to poor sebaceous gland differentiation and total elimination of pelage follicles." *Journal of Investigative Dermatology* 119, no. 1 (2002): 32–37.

Rathkey JK, Zhao J, Liu Z, *et al.* "Chemical disruption of the pyroptotic pore-forming protein gasdermin D inhibits inflammatory cell death and sepsis." *Science Immunology* 3, no. 26 (2018): eaat2738.

Rogers C, Fernandes-Alnemri T, Mayes L, *et al.* "Cleavage of DFNA5 by caspase-3 during apoptosis mediates progression to secondary necrotic/pyroptotic cell death." *Nature Communications* 8, no. 1 (2017): 1–14.

Rosenberg JF, Wellehan JF, Jr, Crevasse SE, *et al.* "Reference intervals for erythrocyte sedimentation rate, lactate, fibrinogen, hematology, and plasma protein electrophoresis in clinically healthy captive gopher tortoises (Gopherus polyphemus)." *Journal of Zoo and Wildlife Medicine* 49, no. 3 (2018): 520–527.

Runkel F, Marquardt C, Stoeger C, *et al.* "The dominant alopecia phenotypes Bareskin, Rex-denuded, and Reduced Coat 2 are caused by mutations in gasdermin 3." *Genomics* 84, no. 5 (2004): 824–835.

Rupprecht CE, Hanlon CA, and Slate D. "Control and prevention of rabies in animals: paradigm shifts." *Developments in Biologicals* 125 (2006): 103.

Saeki N, Sasaki H, Carrasco J, *et al.* "Endothelium and epithelium: composition, functions, and pathology." In *Gasdermin Superfamily: A Novel Gene Family Functioning in Epithilial Cells*, Nova Science Publishers (eds Carrasco, J. & Matheus, M, 2011), ch. IX, 193–211.

Sato H, Koide T, Masuya H, *et al.* "A new mutation Rim3 resembling Re den is mapped close to retinoic acid receptor alpha (Rara) gene on mouse chromosome 11." *Mammalian Genome* 9, no. 1 (1998): 20–25.

Sharif H, Wang L, Wang WL, *et al.* "Structural mechanism for NEK7-licensed activation of NLRP3 inflammasome." *Nature* 570, no. 7761 (2019): 338–343.

Shi J, Zhao Y, Wang K, *et al.* "Cleavage of GSDMD by inflammatory caspases determines pyroptotic cell death." *Nature* 526, no. 7575 (2015): 660–665.

Schroder K and Tschopp J. "The inflammasomes." *Cell* 140, no. 6 (2010): 821–832.

Singh R, Singh KP, Cherian S, *et al.* "Rabies–epidemiology, pathogenesis, public health concerns and advances in diagnosis and control: a comprehensive review." *Veterinary Quarterly* 37, no. 1 (2017): 212–251.

Sordillo LM and Aitken SL. "Impact of oxidative stress on the health and immune function of dairy cattle." *Veterinary Immunology and Immunopathology* 128, no. 1–3 (2009): 104–109.

Sun YB, Zhao H, Mu DL, *et al.* "Dexmedetomidine inhibits astrocyte pyroptosis and subsequently protects the brain in in vitro and in vivo models of sepsis." *Cell Death & Disease* 10, no. 3 (2019): 1–13.

Tanaka S, Mizushina Y, Kato Y, *et al.* "Functional conservation of Gsdma cluster genes specifically duplicated in the mouse genome." *G3: Genes, Genomes, Genetics* 3, no. 10 (2013): 1843–1850.

Ting JP, Willingham SB, Bergstralh DT, *et al.* "NLRs at the intersection of cell death and immunity." *Nature Reviews Immunology* 8, no. 5 (2008): 372–379.

Wang Y, Gao W, Shi X, *et al.* "Chemotherapy drugs induce pyroptosis through caspase-3 cleavage of a gasdermin." *Nature* 547, no. 7661 (2017): 99–103.

Witkowska-Piłaszewicz OD, Żmigrodzka M, Winnicka A, *et al.* "Serum amyloid A in equine health and disease." *Equine Veterinary Journal* 51, no. 3 (2019): 293–298.

Xiao J, Wang C, Yao JC, *et al.* "Gasdermin D mediates the pathogenesis of neonatal-onset multisystem inflammatory disease in mice." *PLoS Biology* 16, no. 11 (2018): e3000047.

Xiong Y, Lou Y, Su H, *et al.* "Cholecalciterol cholesterol emulsion ameliorates experimental colitis via down-regulating the pyroptosis signaling pathway." *Experimental and Molecular Pathology* 100, no. 3 (2016): 386–392.

Yatoo MI, Parray OR, Mir M, *et al.* "Comparative evaluation of different therapeutic protocols for contagious caprine pleuropneumonia in Himalayan Pashmina goats." *Tropical Animal Health and Production* 51, no. 8 (2019): 2127–2137.

Yuan YY, Xie KX, Wang SL, *et al.* "Inflammatory caspase-related pyroptosis: mechanism, regulation and therapeutic potential for inflammatory bowel disease." *Gastroenterology Report* 6, no. 3 (2018): 167–176.

Zhaolin Z, Guohua L, Shiyuan W, *et al.* "Role of pyroptosis in cardiovascular disease." *Cell Proliferation* 52, no. 2 (2019): e12563.

Zhu X, Zhang K, Lu K, *et al.* "Inhibition of pyroptosis attenuates *Staphylococcus aureus*-induced bone injury in traumatic osteomyelitis." *Annals of Translational Medicine* 7, no. 8 (2019): 170.

11

Current Diagnostic Techniques for Influenza

Aruna Punia,[1] Pooja Choudhary,[1] Sweety Dahiya,[1] Namita Sharma,[1] Meenakshi Balhara,[1] Mehak Dangi[2] and Anil Kumar Chhillar[1]
[1] *Centre for Biotechnology, Maharshi Dayanand University, Rohtak-124001, Haryana, India*
[2] *Centre for Bioinformatics, Maharshi Dayanand University, Rohtak-124001, Haryana, India*
Corresponding author: Anil Kumar Chhillar, *anil.chhillar@gmail.com*

11.1 Introduction

The influenza virus is a zoonotic virus that generally causes acute respiratory disease and infects a large number of reptiles, birds and animals. Influenza viruses belong to the orthomyxoviridae family and can be classified into four different types: alphainfluenzavirus, also known as influenza A virus (IAV); betainfluenzavirus, also known as influenza B virus (IBV); gammainfluenzavirus, also known as influenza C virus (ICV); and deltainfluenzavirus, also known as influenza D virus (IDV) (King *et al.* 2012; Hause *et al.* 2014).

IAV has a wide host range that includes cattle, horses, poultry, humans etc. The structure of IAV consists of a negative-sense ssRNA genome which encodes 11 different proteins. IAV are divided into different subtypes based on the glycoproteins found on the surface of the virus, which are hemagglutinin (HA) and neuraminidase (NA). There are 18 HA (H1–H18) and 11 NA (N1–N11) glycoproteins that are present, which potentially form 198 different combinations (Hause *et al.* 2014; Collin *et al.* 2015; Ferguson *et al.* 2015). Aquatic birds are a natural reservoir of different IAV subtypes, mainly including geese, swans and ducks. All strains of influenza viruses cause acute respiratory illness but, of the four of them, IAV virus is the most fatal with the highest rates of morbidity. Due to its segmented genome, very high levels of genetic reassortment occur in IAV, which leads to mutation and makes treatment against influenza difficult, resulting in epidemics and pandemics. There is also a high possibility that the virus is transmitted between different species without genetic reassortment. This type of transmission is generally found in H1N1, with transmission between swine and humans, or H9N2, between poultry and humans. Most of the new influenza viruses are mutants forming from antigenic drift (Drake 1993). IBV was first identified in 1940 and has the same characteristics as IAV but with a smaller host range, infecting mostly humans and rarely other species. The antigenic drift in IBV is found to be lower than that of the A-type virus (Thompson *et al.* 2003, 2004; Francis 1940). ICV was first isolated in 1947 (Taylor 1949) and naturally infects humans (Gavin and Thomson 2004), but has also been reported in feral dogs (Ohwada *et al.* 1987), pigs (Yuanji *et al.* 1983) and dromedary camels (Elias *et al.* 2017; Bailey *et al.* 2018). ICV causes acute respiratory infection in humans and other animals but due to its low prevalence, routine virological screening is discouraged. It has a shorter genome than A and B types (one segment fewer), and its major surface glycoprotein is hemagglutinin-esterase-fusion (HEF), which functions as H and N together (Subbarao *et al.* 1998). IDV is a new member of the influenza virus category that consists of a negative-sense ssRNA with seven genomic segments that encode nine proteins. Due to its structural differences it has the ability to bind to the human tracheal epithelia, which makes it a danger to health (Song *et al.* 2016). Treatment of influenza mainly involves vaccination with inactivated influenza virus (IVV), which has been in use for over 60 years (Couch 2008). Vaccines must be updated annually due to the frequent genetic drift found in different strains of influenza (Jia *et al.* 2017). However, vaccination provides only modest protection, especially in the case of children and the elderly.

11.2 Influenza Diagnosis

Influenza is a communicable respiratory disease caused by the influenza virus; symptoms of influenza are similar to those of other respiratory diseases such as legionella, chlamydia and mycoplasma. Clinically, the features of all respiratory disease are the same, so it becomes very difficult to distinguish influenza from these pathogens (Suarez *et al.* 1998).

Large numbers of the population die (including humans, animals and birds) each year because of influenza, despite the rigorous research going on in influenza prevention. Treatment can be done with antivirals, which must be given in the first one to two days of symptom appearance, otherwise the response of the patient will be lower, especially in cases of immuno-compromised patients (Drexler *et al.* 2009). Therefore, the greatest benefits of treatment can only be attained when medicines are administered within two days of symptom appearance (Chartrand *et al.* 2012). Thus, fast and precise diagnostic methods are crucial. The various methods used to diagnose influenza are discussed below.

11.2.1 Cell Culture Approaches

11.2.1.1 Virus Culture

The virus culture method is a traditional method that was introduced in the 1940s and until now has been accredited as the gold standard for the diagnosis of influenza (Diederen *et al.* 2009). Infectious samples are inoculated in tolerant cell lines or embryonated eggs, cultured for seven to ten days and observed for cytopathic effect; further viruses are detected via diverse methods like antibody staining, erythrocytes hemadsorption or immunofluorescence microscopy (Dawson *et al.* 2007). Isolation of the influenza virus via culturing is generally performed on established cell lines, such as A549, MDCK, LLC MK2, Mv1Lu and BGMK, or primary cell lines, which may be AGMK or RhMK.

11.2.1.2 Virus Shell Culture

Another virus culture approach for virus detection is shell culture, which was introduced in the 1990s. This method entails culturing of the influenza virus in mammalian cells present in shell vials, and then staining of the virus using fluorescent monoclonal antibodies specific to influenza. This method is more efficient than the traditional virus culture method and can detect the virus within one to two days. If R-mix cells (a mixture of mink lung cells and human adenocarcinoma cells) are used in contrast to mammalian cell lines, higher sensitivity is achieved compared to the SVC (shell vial culture) approach, and this modification in method has minimized the detection time to approximately 24 to 36 hours.

11.2.2 Direct Fluorescent Antibody Test

Discovered in the 1960s, the direct fluorescent antibody test is an antigen-antibody reaction-based test generally used for the diagnosis of the influenza virus, which is also known as the immune-fluorescent antibody test. In this approach, samples (respiratory epithelial cells) are collected from nasopharyngeal swabs or nasopharyngeal aspirates and allowed to react with fluorescently tagged influenza virus-specific antibodies, whose results are inspected by fluorescent microscope (Vemula *et al.* 2016). These assays are immensely popular and widely used because of their simple procedure and quick results. Currently, the FDA has approved two DFA tests kits which are available commercially on the market: Bartels Viral Respiratory Screening and Identification (Issaquqh, USA) and D3 FastPoint L-DFA (Athens, USA).

These test kits are chiefly designed for the detection of IAV and IBV and discrimination between them, but these kits cannot subtype IAV (CDC 2019a). The sensitivity of DFA tests ranges from 60 to 80%, which is high in comparison with traditional viral isolation procedures (Leonardi *et al.* 2010). The sensitivity of these tests can be increased by using a cytospin protocol which reduces insufficient smears and improves cell morphology, thus increasing the sensitivity to 92.5% (Ginocchio *et al.* 2009). These tests are now being supplanted because of the incidence of more sensitive tests like molecular approaches (Table 11.1).

11.2.3 Serological Assays

Serological assays depend on the principle of antigen-antibody interaction for the recognition of the influenza virus. These tests are rarely suggested, since they require a subsequent serum sample; the initial sample is collected just at the commencement of illness and the subsequent one after 15–20 days of infection, as the results from a single serum sample cannot be interpreted. These assays are inexpensive and effortless, but the sensitivities are substandard (CDC 2019b). Various serological assays include hemagglutination inhibition assay (HAI), virus neutralization assay (VN), single radial hemolysis (SRH), complement fixation assay, ELISA etc.

11.2.3.1 Hemagglutination Inhibition Assay

The hemagglutination inhibition assay (HAI) determines the existence of the influenza virus by a hemagglutination-specific antibodies titer. The HIA assay principle is based on the capability of HA-specific antibodies to avert attachment of the virus to erythrocytes, which are obtained from turkey, chicken, horse, guinea pigs or humans. This test is generally operated with inactivated viruses and the results are considered positive when there is a fourfold or further increase of the specific antibody titer. The increases amid sensitive and recuperative serum samples are taken as positive readings and are calculated by hemagglutination inhibition (Li *et al.* 2017). This assay is inexpensive and effortless, but its sensitivity is incredibly low, particularly in the case of H5N1 subtypes, which limits its use for virus identification (Stephenson *et al.* 2009).

TABLE 11.1

Different diagnostic techniques and their advantages

S. No.	Diagnostic Tests	Sensitivity and Specificity	Detection Time	Other Remarks
1	Cell culture approaches Virus culture Virus shell culture	40–80%	1–7 days	Needs expertise, but cheap
2	Direct fluorescent antibody test	60–80%	Within 24 hours	Fast and easy to use; does not need any expertise
3	Serological assays Hemagglutination inhibition assay Virus neutralization assay Single radial hemolysis Complement fixation assay ELISA ENIA	Variable sensitivity of various tests ranges from 40 to 80%	5–12 hours	Very cost-effective and easy to use
4	Rapid influenza diagnostic tests BD Veritor System Sofia Influenza A+B Alere i Influenza A&B GOLD SIGN FLU Quick Navi-Flu Bioline cobas® Liat®	Nearly 100%	2–8 hours	Very cost-effective and easy to use
5	Nucleic acid-based tests Reverse transcription-polymerase chain reaction Loop-mediated isothermal amplification-based assay Simple amplification-based assay	85–100%	1–12 hours	Costly and need expertise, but due to high sensitivities these are considered to be the gold standard
6	Microarray-based approaches	90–95%	4–5 hours	Show high sensitivities but involve multiple steps which make them expensive, complex, susceptible to contamination and labor-intensive
7	Electrical-based detections	80–90%	5–30 minutes	Fast, inexpensive and easy to use

11.2.3.2 Virus Neutralization Assay

The virus neutralization assay is normally used for the identification of antibody titers of each avian and seasonal IVA strain. The VN assay measures the induction of virus-specific antibodies and the ability of these antibodies for virus neutralization, as an outcome of which viral contagion can be prohibited. Despite having more sensitivity than the HAI assay, application of the VN assay is restricted due to the need for BSL2+ and BSL3-certified laboratories (active or attenuated virus required) (Haaheim 1997).

11.2.3.3 Single Radial Hemolysis

In this technique, the antigen-antibody complex instigates complement-mediated hemolysis; it is a variant of the hemolytic test in which erythrocytes are attached to influenza virus particles coated with anti-haemagglutinin. This is a frequently used technique in the detection of usual infections and vaccinations (Storch 2003; Wang *et al.* 2017). Single radial hemolysis is more sensitive than the hemagglutination inhibition assay and does not require pre-processing of the serum to disable imprecise inhibitors.

11.2.3.4 Complement Fixation

This approach is based on immune diffusion that measures antibody retaliation against interior proteins of influenza virus NP and M (Osterhaus *et al.* 2000). Complement fixation has lower sensitivity, so it is ousted by VN, EIA and HAI assays.

11.2.3.5 Enzyme-linked Immunosorbent Assay

In the early 1990s, enzyme-linked immunosorbent assay tests (Leirs *et al.* 2016) were initially inaugurated for disease diagnosis and consistently show soaring specificity and sensitivity. These assays are offered in two types: paper strips and micro titer plates. A key shortcoming of ELISA is its inferior sensitivity in contrast to nucleic acid techniques.

Some researchers are working on this shortcoming to intensify the sensitivity of ELISA by using nanoparticles. One such attempt is the europium nanoparticle-based immunoassay (ENIA), which can detect 29 different IVA and IVB subtypes and has 16-fold elevated sensitivity over the ELISA test (Zhang *et al.* 2014).

11.2.4 Rapid Influenza Diagnostic Tests

These are antigen-based tests which rapidly identify influenza virus infections in point-of-care settings. RIDTs can identify influenza virus nucleoprotein antigens directly in respiratory samples and there is no need for the preprocessing of samples. The methodology of these tests includes the targeting of viral nucleoproteins with the help of monoclonal antibodies and the detection of results involving either enzyme immunoassays via optical signals or calorimetric assays (WHO 2010). The sensitivity of these tests is reliant on the frequency of influenza in the residents (Ran *et al.* 2015). At the time of epidemics and pandemics, predictive positives are high, thus lowering the false positives, increasing the sensitivity of these tests. Still, during low influenza occurrence, negative projecting values are lofty, which lowers the positive prophetic values. Rapid tests have confirmed high specificities (≈100%) in the diagnosis of seasonal influenza. Quite a few FDA-approved rapid test kits are commercially available, including the BD Veritor System, Sofia Influenza A+B, Alere i Influenza A&B, GOLD SIGN FLU and Quick Navi-Flu, Bioline and cobas® Liat®. There are several shortcomings of rapid test kits, including that these tests can detect either IAV or IBV but cannot discriminate between them, and that none of the rapid tests kits can differentiate between diverse strains of IAV. The main advantages of these assays are the simple handling of the tests kits, their rapid results with reasonable sensitivity (50–80%) and their soaring specificity (90%) (McMullen *et al.* 2016). Although their sensitivity is not stable, for diagnosis these tests remain the primary option in many virology laboratories due to their fast results, the ease of the assay process and their low cost.

11.2.5 Nucleic Acid-based Tests

Nucleic acid-based tests (NATs, or nucleic acid amplification tests, NAATs) are based upon the polymerase chain reaction (PCR, developed by Kary Mullis in 1983) technique and detect sequences of viral DNA/RNA. These tests are very quick, taking two to four hours, and are very sensitive, making them one of the most reliable diagnosis tools. There are varieties of NAAT tests which are being used to diagnose influenza; some of them are sequencing-based tests like ligase chain reaction, simple amplification-based assay (SAMBA), reverse transcription-PCR (RT-PCR), loop-mediated isothermal amplification-based assay (LAMP) and nucleic acid sequencing-based amplification (NASBA) (FDA 2019).

11.2.5.1 Reverse Transcription-Polymerase Chain Reaction

The reverse transcription-polymerase chain reaction (RT-PCR) assay detects RNA sequences and is considered the gold-standard assay to detect influenza. There are three essential steps involved in this assay.

(1) RNA of the virus is extracted from the clinical sample.
(2) Single-stranded cDNA is generated via reverse transcription of RNA using the reverse transcriptase enzyme.
(3) The product is amplified using PCR and labeled products are detected via fluorescence.

Results analysis of RT-PCR offers soaring specificity and sensitivity that is 105-fold higher than for ELISA and cell culture techniques. The RT-PCR technique can distinguish IAV and IBV, and is also able to differentiate among different IAV subtypes, like H1N1 or H3N2 (Lee *et al.* 2001). Moreover, the sensitivity is independent of a patient's age. A modified version of RT-PCR is "multiplex RT-PCR", in which multiple primers are used in the same reaction to detect numerous respiratory viruses simultaneously. The major shortcomings of these tests are the reaction costs (RT-PCR is one of the priciest tests) and the variable time required to complete a reaction, which can be from one to eight hours (Jia *et al.* 2017; FDA 2019).

11.2.5.2 Loop-mediated Isothermal Amplification-based Assay

The loop-mediated isothermal amplification-based assay (LAMP) is a DNA amplification assay which detects numerous viruses, including coronavirus, SARS, adenovirus, rhinovirus, monkey pox virus, Newcastle disease virus, HIV and influenza virus. Originally discovered by Notomo *et al.*, it utilizes nucleic acid with two primer sets which can recognize six different regions in the cDNA of the virus. Results can be determined either by color change in a florescent dye (SYBR green) or by photometric detection of the Mg2P2O7 byproduct which is unleashed in the solution at the end of the reaction. The sensitivity of LAMP-based approaches is found to be equivalent with RT-PCR-based assays. LAMP-based assays differentiate between avian IAV subtypes, particularly H5N1, H7N7 and H7N9, and sensitivities are found to be comparable to RT-PCR-based approaches, and are sometimes even higher (Imai *et al.* 2006, 2007; Nakauchi *et al.* 2014).

11.2.5.3 Simple Amplification-based Assay

The simple amplification-based assay (SAMBA) is a dipstick isothermal nucleic acid amplification assay, freshly discovered for the recognition of human immunodeficiency virus (HIV) and influenza.

There are three steps involved in this assay:

(1) viral RNA extraction
(2) amplification of target using isothermal DNA polymerase
(3) detection of results using dipstick-based system

SAMBA is extremely sensitive, i.e., 100% and 97.9%, for influenza A and B, and it takes one to two hours for the complete procedure (Wu *et al.* 2010, 2013).

11.2.5.4 Nucleic Acid Sequence-based Amplification

Nucleic acid sequence-based amplification (NASBA) is a sensitive technique used to detect RNA targets and amplification of DNA without any need of denaturation of DNA. NASBA includes three enzymes (RNAse H, avian myeloblastosis virus reverse transcriptase (AMV-RT), T7 RNA polymerase) and two ssDNA fragment primers. The ssDNA probes attach to amplified RNA sequences, which are then separated on a microfluidic chip.

This procedure reviewed this technique in four steps.

(1) Viral RNA is extricated from clinical samples.
(2) Primers are amplified to form RNA-DNA complex.
(3) RNAse H degrade RNA from RNA-DNA complex which results in formation of ds DNA.
(4) T7 RNA polymerase enzyme generates antisense RNA that are used for amplification of DNA (Moore *et al.* 2004).

NASBA is generally used for identifying various viruses, i.e., influenza, RSV, HIV, SARS (McMullen *et al.* 2016). The sensitivity of NASBA is found to be approximately 100% and it successfully differentiates between has H5N1 and H7N9 strains of IAV (Ge *et al.* 2010).

In 2013, Wang *et al.* made some changes in the procedure to develop a new technique known as SMART (simple method for amplifying RNA targets), to detect seasonal H1N1 and H3N2. The SMART assay verified up to 106 vRNA copies/mL with a specificity and sensitivity of 95.7% and 98.3%, respectively.

11.2.6 Microarray-based Approaches

These assays are used for the recognition and subtyping of influenza viruses. For example, the FluChip can detect and differentiate H1N1, H3N2 and H5N1 strains within four to five hours (Townsend *et al.* 2006; Dawson *et al.* 2006, 2007). Similarly, an MChip microarray has shown sensitivity and specificity of 95% and 92%, respectively, to recognize IAV. The CombiMatrix Corporation developed a microarray that can detect all known subtypes of IAV within five hours (Liu et al. 2006; Lodes *et al.* 2006).

While microarrays are small and compact tests which show high sensitivity, they involve multiple steps which make them expensive, complex, susceptible to contamination, labor-intensive and generally give false positive results due to gene mutations, RNA degradation and PCR inhibitors (Gall *et al.* 2009).

11.2.7 Electrical-based Detectors

(1) Horiguchi *et al.* (2017) proposed an Au electrode electro-chemical sensor for the detection of the influenza virus. An HA-specific receptor was immobilized on Au, which attaches to the virus each time they come into contact, and the attached virus was detected with either a quartz crystal microbalance or electrically. This technique is extremely sensitive; the quartz crystal microbalance can detect 200 μHA units within ten minutes and the electrical technique can detect 2 μHA units within 30 minutes.
(2) Nidzworski *et al.* (2017) attached a layer of 4-aminobenzoic acid and anti-M1 antibodies on boron-doped diamond (BDD) electrodes. This technique achieved an exceedingly high sensitivity of 1 fg/mL with electrochemical impedance spectroscopy within five minutes.
(3) Cheng *et al.* (2017) used an immunosensor whereby a surface acoustic wave electrode chip, which is about 50 mm in length, can detect 0.25 pg per mL of HA units within 30seconds. The sensitivity and specificity of this technique are 90% and 70%, respectively.

11.2.8 Modifications of Standard Methods

(1) In a study, Yeo *et al.* (2016) combined the rapid diagnostic assay with a smart phone and developed a rapid fluorescent diagnostic system known as SRFDS which was used as a tool in chickens for diagnosis of the H9N2 virus. Two different samples were taken and for both samples sensitivity and specificity were compared. The specificity of these assays was found to be 100%; the sensitivity of the first sample, i.e., oropharyngeal specimens, was 99.44%, and for second sample, i.e., cloacal specimens, was 95.23%, comparable to RT-PCR.
(2) Zhang *et al.* (2015) used a glucometer and designed an electrochemical test. In this test the influenza virus is exposed to glucose-containing substrate (SG1). When this SGI is utilized, glucose is released, which is detected amperometrically. This technique is amazingly fast, economical

and easy to use and offers very high specificity and sensitivity, and can detect and differentiate between 19 different strains of influenza viruses (H1N1 and H3N2) within one hour.

(3) Hmila *et al.* (2017) modified standard RT-PCR by using aptamer real-time-PCR. The aptamer was selected by systematic evolution of ligands by an exponential enrichment (SELEX) procedure which were later used as ligands in virus attachment. This assay can be directly performed on direct swabs so there is no requirement for preprocessing of samples, and it demonstrates label-free results, which make it rapid and highly sensitive.

(4) Lin *et al.* (2015) conjugated PCR with electrospray ionization-mass spectrometry for the detection of various respiratory viruses. PCR conjugated ESI-MS showed elevated sensitivities and this technique was suitable for detecting co-infections. This technique can detect different virus families, including adenoviruses, alphaviruses and coronaviruses. The major disadvantage of this assay is that it is prohibitively expensive.

(5) Eboigbodin *et al.* (2016) projected an assay by joining two different techniques that include reverse transcription in the first step followed by SIBA® (strand invasion-based amplification) in isothermal surroundings. This assay allows detection of both IAV and IBV within 15–20 minutes, where conventional RT-PCR requires 50–60 minutes. This assay also shows 100-fold greater sensitivity than RT-PCR.

(6) Sepunaru *et al.* (2016) proposed an electrochemical detection method for detection of influenza virus. In this assay, tracking of the virus is attained by means of UV-Vis spectroscopy; influenza particles can absorb AgNPs which show peak absorbance at 401 nm. Furthermore, these AgNPs-labeled viruses, when absorbed on a GC electrode, generate an electrical response. The chronoamperometric signal of AgNPs oxidation was comparative to the virus number.

11.3 Conclusion

The scope of this chapter was to compile all the currently available methods to diagnose influenza and their advantages and disadvantages. The most commonly used methods for diagnosis include the conventional, also known as gold-standard, methods of RT-PCR, culturing, ELISA etc. While these methods require extensive time in the analysis of samples, which can be from 12 to 24 hours, due to their high sensitivity and specificity they remain the most commonly used tests. As a result, there is a need for various novel methods which provide quicker but similarly sensitive and specific results as those produced by these gold-standard techniques.

RIDTs and NATs can be potent substitutes for these conventional tests. RIDTs are widely used assays during epidemics, despite their low and variable sensitivity due to the speed of their responses. On the other hand, NATs have confirmed soaring sensitivity for influenza detection, but due to their high cost and complex procedure they are not regarded as the first choice. There is a need for tools and techniques that are easy to use, handy and give fast and reliable results, without requiring technicians. This kind of procedure also demands steady modernization due to the genetic assortment of different influenza viral strains.

References

Bailey, Emily S., Jessica Y. Choi, Jane K. Fieldhouse *et al.* "The continual threat of influenza virus infections at the human–animal interface: what is new from a one health perspective?" *Evolution, Medicine, and Public Health* 1 (2018): 192–198.

CDC. "Influenza signs and symptoms and the role of laboratory diagnostics. Seasonal influenza (flu)." 2019a. Accessed on June 6, 2019. www.cdc.gov/flu/professionals/diagnosis/labrolesprocedures.htm.

CDC. "Rapid Diagnostic testing for influenza: information for clinical laboratory directors. Seasonal influenza (flu)." 2019b. Accessed on June 6, 2019. www.cdc.gov/flu/professionals/diagnosis/rapidlab.htm.

Chartrand, Caroline, Mariska M.G. Leeflang, Jessica Minion, Timothy Brewer and Madhukar Pai. "Accuracy of rapid influenza diagnostic tests: a meta-analysis." *Annals of Internal Medicine* 156(7) (2012): 500–511.

Cheng, Cheng, Haochen Cui, Jayne Wu and Shigetoshi Eda. "A PCR-free point-of-care capacitive immunoassay for influenza A virus." *Microchimica Acta* 184(6) (2017): 1649–1657.

Collin, Emily A., Zizhang Sheng, Yuekun Lang, Wenjun Ma, Ben M. Hause and Feng Li. "Cocirculation of two distinct genetic and antigenic lineages of proposed influenza D virus in cattle." *Journal of Virology* 89(2) (2015): 1036–1042.

Couch, Robert B. "Seasonal inactivated influenza virus vaccines." *Vaccine* 26(4) (2008): D5–D9.

Dawson, Erica D., Chad L. Moore, Daniela M. Dankbar *et al.* "Identification of A/H5N1 influenza viruses using a single gene diagnostic microarray." *Analytical Chemistry* 79(1) (2007): 378–384.

Dawson, Erica D., Chad L. Moore, James A. Smagala *et al.* "MChip: a tool for influenza surveillance." *Analytical Chemistry* 78(22) (2006): 7610–7615.

Diederen, Bram M.W., Dick Veenendaal, Ruud Jansen, Bjorn L. Herpers, Eric E.J. Ligtvoet and Ed P.F. Ijzerman. "Rapid antigen test for pandemic (H1N1) 2009 virus." *Emerging Infectious Diseases* 16(5) (2010): 897–898.

Drake, John W. "Rates of spontaneous mutation among RNA viruses." *Proceedings of the National Academy of Sciences* 90(9) (1993): 4171–4175.

Drexler, Jan F., Angelika Helmer, Heike Kirberg *et al.* "Poor clinical sensitivity of rapid antigen test for influenza A pandemic (H1N1) 2009 virus." *Emerging Infectious Diseases* 15(10) (2009): 1662–1664.

Eboigbodin, Kevin, Sanna Filén, Tuomas Ojalehto *et al.* "Reverse transcriptionstrand invasion based amplification (RT-SIBA): a method for rapid detection of influenza A and B." *Applied Microbiology and Biotechnology* 100(12) (2016): 5559–5567.

Ferguson, Lucas, Laura Eckard, William B. Epperson *et al.* "Influenza D virus infection in Mississippi beef cattle." *Virology* 486 (2015): 28–34.

Francis, Thomas Jr. "A new type of virus from epidemic influenza." *Science* 92(2392) (1940): 405–408.

Gall, Astrid, Bernd Hoffmann, Timm Harder, Christian Grund, Dirk Höper and Martin Beer. "Design and validation of a microarray for detection, hemagglutinin subtyping, and pathotyping of avian influenza viruses." *Journal of Clinical Microbiology* 47(2) (2009): 327–334.

FDA. "Table 1. FDA-cleared RT-PCR Assays and other molecular assays for influenza viruses." 2019. Accessed on June 4, 2019. www.cdc.gov/flu/pdf/professionals/diagnosis/table1-molecular-assays.pdf.

Gavin, Patrick J. and Richard B. Thomson, Jr. "Review of rapid diagnostic tests for influenza." *Clinical and Applied Immunology Reviews* 4(3) (2004): 151–172.

Ge, Yiyue, Lunbiao Cui, Xian Qi *et al.* "Detection of novel swine origin influenza A virus (H1N1) by real-time nucleic acid sequence-based amplification." *Journal of Virological Methods* 163(2) (2010): 495–497.

Ginocchio, Christine C., Frank Zhanga, Ryhana Manji *et al.* 2009. "Evaluation of multiple test methods for the detection of the novel 2009 influenza A (H1N1) during the New York City outbreak." *Journal of Clinical Virology* 45(3) (2009): 191–195.

Haaheim, R. "Single-radial-complement-fixation: a new immunodiffusion technique. 2. Assay of the antibody response to the internal antigens (MP and NP) of influenza A virus in human sera after vaccination and infection." *Developments in Biological Standardization* 39 (1977): 481–484.

Hause, Ben M., Emily A. Collin, Runxia Liu *et al.* "Characterization of a novel influenza virus in cattle and swine: proposal for a new genus in the Orthomyxoviridae family." *mBio* 5(2) (2014): e00031–00014.

Hmila, Issam, Manoosak Wongphatcharachai, Nacira Laamiri *et al.* "A novel method for detection of H9N2 influenza viruses by an aptamer-real time-PCR." *Journal of Virological Methods* 243 (2017): 83–91.

Horiguchi, Yukichi, Tatsuro Goda, Akira Matsumoto, Hiroaki Takeuchi, Shoji Yamaoka and Yuji Miyahara. "Direct and label-free influenza virus detection based on multisite binding to sialic acid receptors." *Biosensors Bioelectronics* 92 (2017): 234–240.

Imai, Masaki, Ai Ninomiya, Harumi Minekawa *et al.* "Development of H5-RT-LAMP (loop-mediated isothermal amplification) system for rapid diagnosis of H5 avian influenza virus infection." *Vaccine* 24(44–46) (2006): 6679–6682.

Imai, Masaki, Ai Ninomiya, Harumi Minekawa *et al.* "Rapid diagnosis of H5N1 avian influenza virus infection by newly developed influenza H5 hemagglutinin gene-specific loop-mediated isothermal amplification method." *Journal of Virological Methods* 141(2) (2007): 173–180.

Jia, Weixin, Chenfu Cao, Yanxing Lin *et al.* "Detection of a novel highly pathogenic H7 influenza virus by duplex real-time reverse transcription polymerase chain reaction." *Journal of Virological Methods* 246 (2017): 100–103.

King, Andrew M.Q., Michael J. Adams, Eric B. Carstens and Elliot J. Lefkowitz. "Family—Orthomyxoviridae." In *Virus Taxonomy*, 749–761. San Diego, CA: Elsevier, 2012.

Lee, Lee Ming-Shiuh, Poa-Chun Chang, Jui-Hung Shien, Ming-Chu Cheng and Happy K. Shieh. "Identification and subtyping of avian influenza viruses by reverse transcription-PCR." *Journal of Virological Methods* 97(1–2) (2001): 13–22.

Leirs, Karen, Phalguni T. Kumar, Deborah Decrop *et al.* "Bioassay development for ultrasensitive detection of influenza A nucleoprotein using digital ELISA." *Analytical Chemistry* 88(17) (2016): 8450–8458.

Leonardi, Gary P., Ileana Mitrache, Ana Pigal and Lester Freedman. "Public hospital-based laboratory experience during an outbreak of pandemic influenza A (H1N1) virus infections." *Journal of Clinical Microbiology* 48(4) (2010): 1189–1194.

Li, Zhu-Nan, Kimberly M. Weber, Rebecca A. Limmer *et al.* "Evaluation of multiplex assay platforms for detection of influenza hemagglutinin subtype specific antibody responses." *Journal of Virological Methods* 243 (2017): 61–67.

Lin, Yong, Yongfeng Fu, Menghua Xu *et al.* "Evaluation of a PCR/ESI-MS platform to identify respiratory viruses from nasopharyngeal aspirates." *Journal of Medical Virology* 87(11) (2015): 1867–1871.

Liu, Robin Hui, Michael J. Lodes, Tai Nguyen *et al.* "Validation of a fully integrated microfluidic array device for influenza A subtype identification and sequencing." *Analytical Chemistry* 78(12) (2006): 4184–4193.

Lodes, Michael, Dominic Suciu, Mark Elliott *et al.* "Use of semiconductor-based oligonucleotide microarrays for influenza a virus subtype identification and sequencing." *Journal of Clinical Microbiology* 44(4) (2006): 1209–1218.

McMullen, Allison R., Neil W. Anderson and Carey-Ann D. Burnham. "Pathology consultation on influenza diagnostics." *American Journal of Clinical Pathology* 145(4) (2016): 440–448.

Moore, Catherine, Sam Hibbitts, Neil Owen *et al.* "Development and evaluation of a real-time nucleic acid sequence based amplification assay for rapid detection of influenza A." *Journal of Medical Virology* 74(4) (2004): 619–628.

Nakauchi, Mina, Ikuyo Takayama, Hitoshi Takahashi, Masato Tashiro and Tsutomu Kageyama. "Development of a reverse transcription loop-mediated isothermal amplification assay for the rapid diagnosis of avian influenza A (H7N9) virus infection." *Journal of Virological Methods* 204 (2014): 101–104.

Nidzworski, Dawid, Katarzyna Siuzdak, Paweł Niedziałkowski *et al.* "A rapid-response ultrasensitive biosensor for influenza virus detection using antibody modified boron-doped diamond." *Scientific Reports* 7 (2017): 15707.

Ohwada, Kazuo, Fumio Kitame, Kanetsu Sugawara, Hidekazu Nishimura, Morio Homma and Kiyoto Nakamura. "Distribution of the antibody to influenza C virus in dogs and pigs in Yamagata Prefecture, Japan." *Microbiology and Immunology* 31(12) (1987): 1173–1180.

Osterhaus, A.D., G.F. Rimmelzwaan, B.E. Martina, T.M. Bestebroer and R.A. Fouchier. "Influenza B virus in seals." *Science* 288(5468) (2000): 1051–1053.

Ran, Zhiguang, Huigang Shen, Yuekun Lang *et al.* "Domestic pigs are susceptible to infection with influenza B viruses." *Journal of Virology* 89(9) (2015): 4818–4826.

Salem, Elias, Elizabeth A.J. Cook, Hicham Ait Lbacha *et al.* "Serologic evidence for influenza C and D virus among ruminants and camelids, Africa, 1991–2015." *Emerging Infectious Diseases* 23(9) (2017): 1556–1559.

Sepunaru, Lior, Blake J. Plowman, Stanislav V. Sokolov, Neil P. Young and Richard G. Compton. "Rapid electrochemical detection of single influenza viruses tagged with silver nanoparticles." *Chemical Science* 7(6) (2016): 3892–3899.

Song, Hao, Jianxun Qi, Zahra Khedri *et al.* "An open receptor-binding cavity of hemagglutinin-esterase-fusion glycoprotein from newly-identified influenza D virus: basis for its broad cell tropism." *PLoS Pathogens* 12(3) (2016): e1005505.

Stephenson, Iain, Alan Heath, Diane Major *et al.* "Reproducibility of serologic assays for influenza virus A (H5N1)." *Emerging Infectious Diseases* 15(8) (2009): 1252–1259.

Storch, Gregory A. "Rapid diagnostic tests for influenza." *Current Opinion in Pediatrics* 15(1) (2003): 77–84.

Suarez, David L., Michael L. Perdue, Nancy Cox *et al.* "Comparisons of highly virulent H5N1 influenza A viruses isolated from humans and chickens from Hong Kong." *Journal of Virology* 72(8) (1998): 6678–6688.

Subbarao, Kanta, Alexander Klimov, Jacqueline Katz *et al.* "Characterization of an avian influenza A (H5N1) virus isolated from a child with a fatal respiratory illness." *Science* 279(5349) (1998): 393–396.

Taylor, R.M. "Studies on survival of influenza virus between epidemics and antigenic variants of the virus." *American Journal of Public Health and the Nation's Health* 39(2) (1949): 171–178.

Thompson, William W., David K. Shay, Eric Weintraub *et al.* "Mortality associated with influenza and respiratory syncytial virus in the United States." *Journal of the American Medical Association* 289(2) (2003): 179–186.

Thompson, William W., David K. Shay, Eric Weintraub *et al.* "Influenza-associated hospitalizations in the United States." *Journal of the American Medical Association* 292(11) (2004): 1333–1340.

Townsend, Michael B., Erica D. Dawson, Martin Mehlmann *et al.* "Experimental evaluation of the FluChip diagnostic microarray for influenza virus surveillance." *Journal of Clinical Microbiology* 44(8) (2006): 2863–2871.

Vemula, Sai V., Jiangqin Zhao, Jikun Liu, Xue Wang, Santanu Biswas and Indira Hewlett. "Current Approaches for diagnosis of influenza virus infections in humans." *Viruses* 8(4) (2016): 96.

Wang, Biao, Margaret L. Russell, Angela Brewer *et al.* "Single radial haemolysis compared to haemagglutinin inhibition and microneutralization as a correlate of protection against influenza A H3N2 in children and adolescents." *Influenza and Other Respiratory Viruses* 11(3) (2017): 283–288.

Wang, Jingjing, Warren Tai, Stephanie L. Angione *et al.* "Subtyping clinical specimens of influenza A virus by use of a simple method to amplify RNA targets." *Journal of Clinical Microbiology* 51(10) (2013): 3324–3330.

WHO. Use of Influenza Rapid Diagnostic Tests. Rome: WHO, 2010.

Wu, Liang-Ta, Martin D. Curran, Joanna S. Ellis *et al.* "Nucleic acid dipstick test for molecular diagnosis of pandemic H1N1." *Journal of Clinical Microbiology* 48(10) (2010): 3608–3613.

Wu, Liang-Ta, Isabelle Thomas, Martin D. Curran *et al.* "Duplex molecular assay intended for point-of-care diagnosis of influenza A/B virus infection." *Journal of Clinical Microbiology* 51(9) (2013): 3031–3038.

Yeo, Seon-Ju, Bui Thi Cuc, Haan Woo Sung and Hyun Park. "Evaluation of a smartphone-based rapid fluorescent diagnostic system for H9N2 virus in specific-pathogen-free chickens." *Archives of Virology* 161(8) (2016): 2249–2256.

Yuanji, Guo, Jin Fengen, Wang Ping, Wang Min and Zhu Jiming. "Isolation of influenza C virus from pigs and experimental infection of pigs with influenza C virus." *The Journal of General Virology* 64(1) (1983): 177–182.

Zhang, Panhe, Sai Vikram Vemula, Jiangqin Zhao *et al.* "A highly sensitive europium nanoparticle-based immunoassay for detection of influenza A/B virus antigen in clinical specimens." *Journal of Clinical Microbiology* 52(12) (2014): 4385–4387.

Zhang, Xiaohu, Abasaheb N. Dhawane, Joyce Sweeney, Yun He, Mugdha Vasireddi and Suri S. Iyer. "Electrochemical assay to detect influenza viruses and measure drug susceptibility." *Angewandte Chemie* (International ed. in English) 54(20) (2015): 5929–5932.

12

Diagnostic Tools for the Identification of Foot-and-Mouth Disease Virus

Sweety Dahiya,[1] Aruna Punia,[1] Pooja Choudhary,[1] Namita Sharma,[1] Meenakshi Balhara,[1] Mehak Dangi[2] and Anil Kumar Chhillar[1]
[1] *Centre for Biotechnology, Maharshi Dayanand University, Rohtak-124001, Haryana, India*
[2] *Centre for Bioinformatics, Maharshi Dayanand University, Rohtak-124001, Haryana, India*
Corresponding author: Anil Kumar Chhillar, *anil.chhillar@gmail.com*

12.1 Introduction

Foot-and-mouth disease (FMD) is a well-known disorder of animals which belongs to the family *Suidae*, suborder *Ruminantia*, order *Artiodactyla* and *Camelus bactrianus* (OIE 2015), and the virus that is responsible for this disorder is named foot-and-mouth disease virus (FMDV). FMDV is classified within the *Aphthovirus* genus as a member of the *Picornaviridae* family (Bachrach 1968; Belsham 1993; Desselberger *et al.* 2002; Newman *et al.* 1973). FMD came to light in the sixteenth century and so far it remains a major concern of animal health. In 1546 AD, the Italian monk Girolamo Fracastoro made the earliest written description of FMD that occurred in cattle (Fracastoro 1546). After that, in 1897, two researchers named Friedrich Loeffler and Paul Frosch demonstrated that a filterable agent is the cause for FMD (Loeffler and Frosch 1897) and this demonstration proved to be a significant commencement in the field of virology. FMD is extremely contagious in nature and can affect both ruminants and pigs globally. FMD can be symptomatically characterized by fever, salivation, anorexia and vesicular eruptions in the mouth, on the teats and on the feet (Hirsh 2004; Quinn 2002). Its broad geographical distribution, high infectiousness and wide host range make it a dreadful viral disease of livestock (Knight-Jones and Rushton 2013). Species which are vulnerable to FMD are goats, sheep, pigs, cattle and buffaloes. Ancient-world camels exhibit resistance towards some strains of FMDV and South American camelids are moderately susceptible (OIE 2011). On the other hand, horses, cats and dogs may carry the virus on their hairs but they remain non-susceptible to FMDV. The mortality rate of FMD in young animals is high but in adult animals it is low (Mazengia 2010). FMDV has a great effect on the economy because FMD causes not only loss of production but also limits the trade of animals both locally and internationally (James and Rushton 2002). The highly vulnerable provinces for FMD are Asia, Africa and the Middle East. This disease has been completely eradicated from developed nations including Japan, Australia and New Zealand (Ding *et al.* 2011). Incursions of FMDV into FMD-free nations can result in detrimental economic losses. Hence, FMD-free nations have implemented lots of measures to retain their FMD-free status.

Preliminarily, FMD is diagnosed on the basis of clinical symptoms. But it is laborious to distinguish FMD from other vesicular infections such as swine vesicular disease (SVD), vesicular stomatitis etc. because they exhibit similar symptoms. Hence, for accurate and specific detection of FMDV, laboratory diagnosis is required (Roeder and Le Blanc Smith 1987). The functional basis of laboratory diagnosis is to demonstrate viral antigens and antibodies. Serological and nucleic acid-based assays are employed for antigens, whereas for antibodies, structural proteins (SP) or non-structural proteins (NSP) are used to differentiate infected from vaccinated animals (DIVA). FMD has been successfully controlled in various regions of the world by employing ring/regular vaccination of animals. But we cannot consider the disease-control regions to be safe because FMDV is extremely contagious in nature and disseminate rapidly (Bruner and Gillespie 1973). For the efficient management of the disease, virus outbursts should be governed carefully at an early stage, and the employed diagnostic tests should give specific, sensitive and rapid results. Persistent infection should be examined adequately so that it cannot be further transmitted. Furthermore, in endemic areas, routine vaccination of animals is highly recommended. On the other hand, the disease-free nations never vaccinated their livestock, preferring instead the restriction of animal movement as well as the slaughter of infected and suspected animals whenever the outbreaks of FMD occured (James and Rushton 2002).

12.2 Etiology

FMD virus is the only member of the genus *Aphthovirus* that was identified as a viral pathogen (Loeffler and Frosch 1897). FMD virus has seven serologically distinct serotypes, namely A, O, C, Asia-1 and SAT-1, -2 and -3. These serotypes comprise of more than 65 subtypes. FMDV serotypes A and O were named after their areas of origin: type-O for Oise (France) and type-A for Allemagne (Germany). Subsequently, serotype-C was discovered in Germany. FMDV serotype Asia-1 was initially identified in Pakistan. In 1957, during an FMDV outbreak in South Africa, three novel FMDV serotypes were identified, which were named South African Territories (SAT)-1, -2 and -3 (Bruner and Gillespie 1973; Brown 2003). The FMDV virion is of icosahedral shape with a diameter of around 30 nm. The virus contains positive-sense ssRNA encapsulated by a protein shell (Bachrach 1968). The protein shell of the virus contains 60 replicas of each structural protein, namely VP1, VP2, VP3 and VP4. VP1, VP2 and VP3 are located on the surface and form the majority of the shell structure, whereas VP4 is located inside the shell. The genome of the virus is around 8.5 kb in length and contains four significant parts (5_UTR, coding region, 3_UTR and a poly "A" tail) which play an important role in genome stability, genome replication and genome translation (Jamal and Belsham 2013).

The incubation period of FMDV may range from 2 to 14 days. When susceptible livestock come into contact with diseased animals, they may develop clinical symptoms. Severity of the symptoms relies on the age of the host, breed of the host, invulnerability of the host, virus serotype and the amount of exposure. Symptoms caused by FMDV include high temperature, excessive salivation, weight loss, anorexia, lameness and the development of vesicular lesions (Blowey and Weaver 2003; Hirsh and Zee 1999). Symptoms are generally severe in pigs, constituting severe vesicular lesions damaging the coronary band and feet. Occasionally, the lesions may also appear on the rostral and dorsal surface of the snout, knees, hocks and accessory digits (Kitching and Alexandersen 2002). Cattle symptoms include salivation and severe lesions in the mouth. However, sometimes lesions can also develop on the feet or on other parts of the body. In goats and sheep, symptoms are generally mild and are characterized as superficial lesions that cure quickly (Alexandersen and Mowat 2005). Vesicular lesions can be easily detected during the acute stage by microscopical observation (Gailiunas 1968; Yilma 1980). Alexandersen *et al.* evidenced that normal skin without any kind of histopathological changes may have significant doses of the virus (Alexandersen *et al.* 2001). FMDV can also cause miscarriage in pregnant livestock but the factors and the mechanisms that are involved in it have not been described. Infectiousness of the virus serotype may vary from species to species and sometimes within the species. For example, the "O" serotype of Taiwan (1997) developed severe vesicular lesions in pigs, whereas no such symptoms were seen in ruminants (Dunn and Donaldson 1997). This variation may be due to physiological or genetic factors. Later, Knowles *et al.* explained that changes in the 3A gene of the virus were responsible for this variation (Knowles *et al.* 2001).

FMDV can be transmitted by natural methods or by artificial methods. Natural methods comprise of direct methods and indirect methods, whereas artificial methods include direct injection of the virus strain. The most efficient and common way of FMDV transmission is either the direct method (airborne), where droplets containing the virus are deposited into the respiratory tract, or the mechanical transfer of the virus from contaminated surfaces and its subsequent entry into the skin from a cut. FMDV can be transmitted over long distances if favorable conditions are available, which include a continuous and steady wind, a stable virus concentration and cloud cover. Moreover, contact transmission can be reinforced by physical contact with contaminated secretions/excretions having a huge amount of the virus (Alexandersen and Donaldson 2002; Donaldson and Alexandersen 2002; Donaldson *et al.* 2001). For airborne transmission, the primary site of infection is generally the pharyngeal area (McVicar and Sutmoller 1976). FMDV initially replicates in the mucosal membrane of the pharynx and after that it is transmitted to the secondary sites of multiplication (feet, mouth, mammary glands) via lymphatic fluid and blood (Lefèvre *et al.* 2011). Various factors, such as temperature, pH and humidity, are the main factors determining the survival of the virus in the body of a diseased animal. FMDV can be isolated from almost all body secretions, including saliva, milk, tears, vaginal discharge, nasal discharge, feces, semen and the placenta of an aborted fetus (Hirsh 2004).

The acute stage of FMDV ends at around seven days and due to the emergence of vigorous humoral antibody response the disease symptoms gradually decline. Even after the decline of disease symptoms, a number of ruminants may convert to being FMDV carriers. An FMDV carrier is an animal which carries the infectious virus for at least one month after infection (Alexandersen and Mowat 2005; Burrows 1966; Sutmoller *et al.* 1968). The original concept of the FMDV carrier was based on field experience, but later Bekkum *et al.* in 1959 confirmed the presence of infectious FMDV in the saliva of recovered cattle. The maximum duration of the carrier state is different for different species; for African buffaloes it is 5 years; for cattle 3.5 years; for sheep 9 months; for goats 4 months (Alexandersen *et al.* 2002; Condy *et al.* 1985; Thomson *et al.* 1984; Hedger 1972). FMDV carriers can be identified by using the virus isolation method from esophageal-pharyngeal fluids and for increased sensitivity RT-PCR can be used (Murphy *et al.* 1999).

12.3 Diagnostic Techniques

Initial diagnosis of FMDV is done on the basis of host symptoms. But the symptoms caused by FMDV are found to be similar to other vesicular diseases symptoms, due to which misidentification of the disease can occur, and thus there is a need for laboratory-based diagnosis which accurately identifies FMDV (Roeder and Le Blanc Smith 1987). Nowadays, various laboratory-based techniques have been employed which accurately identify the disease (i.e., FMD) and its causative agent (i.e., FMDV). These techniques are categorized into four distinct groups, which are:

(1) virus isolation assay
(2) serological assay
    (a) complement fixation test
    (b) virus neutralization test
    (c) enzyme-linked immunosorbent assay
    (d) virus infection-associated agar gel immuno-diffusion test
(3) nucleic acid-based assay
    (a) reverse transcriptase PCR
    (b) real-time qRT-PCR
    (c) multiplex-PCR
    (d) reverse transcription loop-mediated isothermal amplification
(4) novel and high-throughput assay
    (a) microarray
    (b) pen-side assay

12.3.1 Virus Isolation Assay

A virus isolation assay is generally preferred when the amount of the virus to be tested is too low (Stear 2005). In this assay, suspensions which are sensitive to FMDV are inoculated into the tissue culture (like primary pig kidney cells) and incubated at room temperature (37°C) for 24–48 hours (Kitching and Hughes 2002) and examined for CPE (cytopathic effect) production. Primary-tissue cultures which exhibit sensitivity towards FMDV are of bovine, porcine and ovine origin. Examples of some stable cell lines which are used for virus isolation are IBRS-2, MVPK-1 clone 7, LFBK and BHK-21 (Longjam 2011). There are a few limitations of this assay: 1) the requirement of a cell culture laboratory, which is laborious and expensive; 2) the need for maintenance of cells with a regular supply, which is also laborious; 3) the requirement of four to six days to demonstrate virus presence. Sometimes, the FMDVs are unable to grow in a specific tissue culture but the absence of virus growth does not mean that the virus is not present, and thus suspected samples are subjected to further testing (Jae *et al.* 2009). All these limitations can delay the initiation of control measures.

12.3.2 Serology-based Assays

Serology-based assays were invented in the early 1930s and are taken as the gold standard if there are no biologic sample/tissue specimens available for disease identification. But there are also some disadvantages of using serology-based assays, such as the requirement of highly skilled personnel, time-frame incompatibility and labor-intensiveness. These assays can be differentiated into two categories: a) antigen detection assays and b) antibody detection assays.

12.3.2.1 Complement Fixation Test

The complement fixation test (CFT) was initially used in 1929 by Ciuca for antiserum typing and to identify FMDV of guinea pig origin (Bachrach 1968). Later, CFT successfully identified an FMDV of bovine origin by using the antiserum of guinea pigs (Traub 1983). The principle of CFT is based on Ag-Ab complexes. Red blood cells of sensitized sheep are taken as indicative agents. If Ag-Ab complexes bind with the complement (i.e., derived from a guinea pig) then no hemolysis takes place. But, if the antigen (virus) does not bind with the antibody, then the free complement causes the lysis of sheep-RBCs. Furthermore, antibodies of FMDV are serotype-specific; hence, CFT can also be used to identify different FMDV serotypes (Traub 1983). To date, CFT has been extensively used to differentiate various strains of

FMDV (Longjam *et al.* 2011; Ferris *et al.* 1984; Rweyemamu *et al.* 1978). Since its introduction, micro-CFT (a modification of CFT) has been developed, in which microtiter plates (96-well plates) are used to perform the assay instead of tubes (Darbyshire 1972).

12.3.2.2 Virus Neutralization Test

The virus neutralization test (VNT) is used to identify antibodies produced against structural proteins of FMDV and also to measure viral infectivity. This test is generally prescribed for the certification/verification of animals and their products subjected for trade (OIE 2012). In the VNT, virus and serum (in equal volumes) are first reacted with each other and then injected into a sensitive cell culture/animal host and the production of cytopathic effect (CPE) is examined. If there are antibodies then no CPE will produced. This test is more prone to variability as it greatly depends upon the cell culture; therefore, bio-containment facilities are required to perform virus neutralization testing. Currently, VNTs are performed by using microtiter systems (Kibenge 2016).

12.3.2.3 Enzyme-linked Immunosorbent Assay

The enzyme-linked immunosorbent assay (ELISA) was introduced around 1975 for the diagnosis of various infectious diseases and has since been employed as one of the best serology-based assays. ELISA is used to quantify an immobilized antigen. In this assay, a specific antibody covalently coupled with an enzyme is used. ELISA overcomes the problems of low sensitivity as well as result interpretation difficulties. Abu Elzein and Crowther were the first to report the use of indirect ELISA in screening cattle for antibody production against FMDV (Abu Elzein and Crowther 1978). Since then, indirect ELISA has successfully identified FMDV antigens from contaminated tissue-culture fluids, mice carcass and cattle tongues. This assay also identified antibodies from serum samples (Rai and Lahiri 1981). Sandwich ELISA rapidly detects viral antigens. Sandwich ELISA is performed by using serotype-specific polyclonal antibodies which are produced in guinea pigs and rabbits (Crowther and Abu Elzein 1979). This assay gives results of 100% specificity and 80% sensitivity. Liquid phase-blocking ELISA is another serology-based assay to detect FMDV antibodies in the sample. This assay can differentiate FMDV serotypes. In LP-ELISA, the primary step is to block/neutralize the antibody to FMDV by using a specific FMDV serotype. After the blocking of the antibody, the remaining FMDV is identified by using ELISA (Mc Vicar and Sutmoller 1970). Some researchers compared the results of LP-ELISA and virus neutralization tests and found that LP-ELISA results were much more reproducible than those of virus neutralization testing (Kitching *et al.* 1988; Lunt *et al.* 1994; Pattnaik *et al.* 1991). Further, the results of ELISA were also found to be far better than those of complement fixation tests because a large number of samples exhibiting negative results in CFT assays were confirmed by ELISA by their inoculation into the susceptible cultures; however, this confirmation takes four additional days (Grubman and Baxt 2004).

12.3.2.4 Virus Infection-associated Agar Gel Immuno-diffusion Test

The virus infection-associated agar gel immuno-diffusion test (VIA-AGID) is mainly used to differentiate vaccinated animals from infected animals. This assay identifies antibody against VIA antigens of infected/vaccinated animals. Animals that have been vaccinated exhibit false positive (FP) results.

12.3.3 Nucleic Acid-based Assays

Each species on the earth possesses its own unique DNA/RNA sequences which differentiate it from other species, and these unique DNA/RNA sequences have generated the idea of using nucleic acid (DNA/RNA)-based methods for the differentiation of various species. Currently, various nucleic acid-based assays are well established and are most commonly used for the diagnosis of various pathogenic species (Pantawane *et al.* 2018).

12.3.3.1 Reverse Transcriptase PCR

In reverse transcriptase PCR (RT-PCR), RNA is first transcribed into cDNA and then this cDNA is used for the amplification. To date, various RT-PCR assays have been published which have successfully identified FMDV RNA from tissue culture isolates, epithelium and other tissues (Meyer *et al.* 1991). Rodriguez *et al.* were the first to demonstrate RT-PCR for the differentiation of FMDV serotypes O, A and C (Rodriguez *et al.* 1992). For the identification of all seven FMDV serotypes (A, O, C, Asia-1, SAT-1, -2 and -3), serotype-specific primers have been designed. These serotype-specific primers focus on various regions of the virus genome involving the open reading frame (ORF), the 5′ UTR and the 3′ UTR (Callens and De Clercq 1997; Vangrysperre *et al.* 1996).

12.3.3.2 Real-time qRT-PCR

Real-time PCR (r-PCR) is a modification of the conventional PCR assay. In real-time PCR, quantitative analysis of DNA sequences is possible without the use of any post-PCR processing steps. Various fluorescent dyes, such as SYBR green, TaqMan or molecular beacon probes, are used to monitor the amplification of the target cDNA sequence directly. Nowadays, real-time reverse transcriptase PCR (rRT-PCR) assays are routinely used for the diagnosis and quantification of FMDV in developed nations. At present, two different rRT-PCR TaqMan methods are generally preferred; one method targets the internal ribosomal entry site (IRES) within the 5′ UTR region (Reid *et al.* 2002) and the other targets the RNA polymerase (3D) coding region of the genome (Callahan *et al.* 2002). Both of these assays fail to discriminate between different serotypes of FMDV; the 5′ UTR assay exhibits more sensitivity for identifying FMDV serotype-A viruses, whereas the RNA polymerase assay shows greater sensitivity for the identification of FMDV serotype-SAT viruses (King *et al.* 2006). Furthermore, both assays are unable to recognize a small number of FMDV isolates because of the presence of nucleotide mismatches within the targeted regions. Therefore, no individual assay has the capability to identify FMDV serotypes with 100% sensitivity.

12.3.3.3 Multiplex PCR

Multiplex-PCR (m-PCR) is commonly used to detect multiple serotypes in a single reaction. For multiplex-PCR, two distinct sets of primer are utilized; one targets the 1D region and the other targets the 2B region. In 2009, Tam and colleagues described fluorescence-based multiplex rRT-PCR assays for the identification of FMDV (Tam *et al.* 2009). This assay shows greater sensitivity for FMDV identification. However, some cross-reactivity between a few serotypes of FMDV was found.

12.3.3.4 Reverse Transcription Loop-mediated Isothermal Amplification

The reverse transcription loop-mediated isothermal amplification (RT-LAMP) assay does not require any thermocycler because it amplifies a specific DNA/RNA sequence at a constant temperature, hence facilitating performance of the assay in the field without the use of expensive tools. The basic principle of the RT-LAMP assay is based on an autocycling strand-displacement reaction. The process of RT-LAMP requires a DNA polymerase with significant strand-displacement activity. Additionally, it requires a set of two specially designed inner primers and outer primers (Notomi *et al.* 2000). This assay comprises of different stages. During the initial stage, these primers identify six independent sequences, whereas during the latter stages they identify four independent sequences. This assay takes less than one hour for completion and the results can be visually interpreted. For FMDV diagnosis, this assay can be employed by using high-throughput systems (Dukes *et al.* 2006).

12.3.4 Novel and High-throughput Assays

12.3.4.1 Microarray

The microarray assay is an alternative to pre-existing methods for FMDV diagnosis. This assay provides the unique capability of detecting multiple strains/pathogens by using a single DNA chip. Baxi and colleagues designed a microarray-based assay comprising of 155 oligoNtd probes which were 35–45 bp in length and serotype-specific. These probes were designed from the VP1–2A and VP3 regions of the FMDV genome. Baxi and colleagues also designed a set of two forward primers and one reverse primer for the amplification of the target sequence (approximately 1100 bp in length). The amplified target sequence was tagged by a dye named Alexa-Fluor 546 and then applied to the DNA chip of FMDV. This FMDV DNA chip can successfully identify 23 different strains of FMDV belonging to all seven serotypes (Baxi *et al.* 2005). Co-application of PCR and microarray assays can result in a powerful diagnostic assay which may possess high sensitivity as well as high-throughput capability.

12.3.4.2 Pen-side Assay

The pen-side assay is crucial to disease control strategy. This assay helps field veterinarians in their clinical diagnosis and is valuable during an outbreak because it avoids degradation of viral antigen (Ag) and delays in diagnosis. A pen-side assay for rinderpest diagnosis was designed and successfully utilized during the end of the 2001 UK FMDV outbreak (Ferris *et al.* 2001). In this assay, a monoclonal antibody (Mab) bonded with a colored latex bead was employed to identify FMDV antigens. When the Mab-bead-Ag complex migrates along a chromatographic strip, the complex is trapped within the fixed band of anti-FMDV Mab and produces an easily detectable colored line over the fixed band. Results can be read within 10 minutes. A pen-side assay for non-structural and structural proteins is also being designed by using the same principles.

12.4 Prevention and Treatment

FMD is endemic in various nations of the Middle East, Southern Asia and Africa (Jamal and Belsham 2013, 2018). As FMDV can be easily transmitted from diseased animals or contaminated surfaces to healthy animals, thorough cleaning and proper disinfection of all contaminated premises and materials (bedding, contaminated animal products, implements etc.) is required (OIE 2012). FMDV is sensitive to extreme pH and, hence, exhibits susceptibility towards various disinfecting agents including both acids and bases (carbonate, sodium hydroxide, citric acid, Virkon-S etc.) (CFSPH 2020).

At present, FMDV control and treatment has become a global socio-economic problem. Susceptible host range for FMDV is not only limited to animals, but also covers humans who consume beef of contaminated animals. To date, promising treatment for FMD is not available. Traditional methods to cure diseased animals include the usage of antimicrobials, meglumine, flunuxin, mild disinfecting agents etc. (Gakuya *et al.* 2011). Small ruminants exhibiting clinical signs of FMD can be treated by giving analgesic (like Vetalgin-Intervet) and antipyretic medication; a wide-spectrum antibiotic such as Terramycine or LA Pfizer can also be preferred. A protective dressing can also be applied at the infected part of the animal (Mohamed *et al.* 2014). A variety of solutions such as normal saline, potassium permanganate (1%), citric acid (1%) and alum (2%) are generally used to rinse the ulcerative vesicles appearing on the mouth, legs, teats and claws (El-Fatah Mahmoud 2019).

For the management of FMDV outbursts, a vaccination program is carried out to strengthen the immunity of the animals. The first vaccine against FMDV was formulated in the 1930s from live FMDV with formalin and combined with aluminum hydroxide gel. The concurrent outbreak of FMD was reduced by the use of this vaccine (Brooksby 1982). Initial treatment of FMDV control is through the vaccination of animals. However, vaccines can takes a few days to induce a response and may require a booster dose with frequent vaccination. To date, there is no vaccine which fulfills all optimal criteria such as having a wide antigenic spectrum, minimal production cost, higher efficacy and low risk of FMDV escape. Two types of vaccines are generally used: inactivated vaccines and live attenuated vaccines (Paton *et al.* 2009).

12.4.1 Attenuated Vaccines

For the formulation of live attenuated vaccines, virus strains are passed through various laboratory animals (mice, rabbits etc.) until they lose their virulence and become attenuated (Grubman and Baxt 2004).

Currently, various types of FMD attenuated vaccines are under research, including nucleic acid vaccines, synthetic peptide vaccines, viral capsids vaccines, virus-like particles vaccines (VLP) and nanoparticle vaccines. There are some disadvantages to using attenuated vaccines, including that they do not enable differentiation between diseased animals and vaccinated animals; they can develop a virus carrier stage in animals; and they can also transmit the virus to non-vaccinated animals (Jamal *et al.* 2011).

12.4.2 Inactivated Vaccines

Inactivated vaccines are formulated by amplifying FMDV in BHK-21 and then inactivating it using special chemicals such as formalin. The inactivated strain is then purified and combined with the adjuvant (Knight-Joneset *et al.* 2013). Inactivated/killed FMDV vaccines successfully reduce virus outbursts globally, providing protection against FMDV for all ruminants in around one year. But there are a number of drawbacks associated with the use of inactivated vaccines in emergency control schemes, one of which is the incomplete inactivation of the strain, which can provoke disease in animals (Guo *et al.* 2013).

References

Abu Elzein, E.M. and Crowther, John R. "Enzyme-labelled immunosorbent assay techniques in foot-and-mouth disease virus research". *Journal of Hygiene*. 80 no. 3 (1978):391–399.

Alexandersen, Soren and Donaldson, Alex I. "Further studies to quantify the dose of natural aerosols of foot-and-mouth disease virus for pigs". *Epidemiology and Infection*. 128 no. 2 (2002):313–323.

Alexandersen, Soren and Mowat, Noel. "Foot-and-mouth disease: host range and pathogenesis". *Current Topics in Microbiology and Immunology*. 288 (2005):9–42.

Alexandersen, Soren, Oleksiewicz, Martin B. and Donaldson, Alex I. "The early pathogenesis of foot-and-mouth disease in pigs infected by contact: a quantitative time course study using TaqMan RT-PCR". *Journal of General Virology*. 82 no. 4 (2001):747–755.

Alexandersen, Soren, Zhang, Zhidong and Donaldson, Alex I. "Aspects of the persistence of foot-and-mouth disease virus in animals—the carrier problem". *Microbes and Infection*. 4 no. 10 (2002):1099–1110.

Bachrach, Howard L. "Foot-and-mouth disease". *Annual Review of Microbiology*. 22 (1968):201–244.

Baxi, Mohit K., Baxi, Shailja, Clavijo, Alfonso, Burton, Kimberly M. and Deregt, Dirk. "Microarray-based detection and typing of foot-and-mouth disease virus". *Veterinary Journal*. 172 no. 3 (2005):473–481.

Belsham, Graham J. "Distinctive features of foot-and-mouth disease virus, a member of the picornavirus family; aspects of virus protein synthesis, protein processing and structure". *Progress in Biophysics and Molecular Biology*. 60 no. 3 (1993):241–260.

Blowey, Roger W. and Weaver, David A. *Color Atlas of Diseases and Disorders of Cattle* (Mosby, 2nd edn, 2003).

Brooksby, John B. "Portraits of viruses: Foot-and-mouth disease virus". *Intervirology*. 18 no. 1 (1982):1–23.

Brown, Fred. "The history of research in foot-and-mouth disease". *Virus Research*. 91 no. 1 (2003):3–7.

Bruner, Dorsey W. *Hagan's Infectious Disease of Domestic Animals* (Cornell University Press, 6th edn, 1973).

Burrows R. "Studies on the carrier state of cattle exposed to foot-and-mouth disease virus". *Journal of Hygiene*. 64 no. 1 (1966):81–90.

Callahan, Johnny D, Brown, Fred, Osorio, Fernando A., Sur, Jung H., Kramer, Ed., Long, Gary W., Lubroth, Juan, Ellis, Stefanie J., Shoulars, Katina S., Gaffney, Kristin L., Rock, Daniel L., Nelson and William M. "Use of a portable real-time reverse transcriptase-polymerase chain reaction assay for rapid detection of foot-and-mouth disease virus". *Journal of the American Veterinary Medical Association*. 220 no. 11 (2002):1636–1642.

Callens, Mia and De Clercq, Kris. "Differentiation of the seven serotypes of foot and- mouth disease virus by reverse transcriptase polymerase chain reaction". *Journal of Virological Methods*. 67 no. 1 (1997):35–44.

Center for Food Security and Public Health (CFSPH). "Foot and mouth disease: prevention and control". Iowa State University, Fiebre Aftosa (2020):1–4.

Condy, J.B., Hedger, R.S., Hamblin, Christopher. and Barnett, I.T. "The duration of the foot-and-mouth disease virus carrier state in African buffalo (i) in the individual animal and (ii) in a free-living herd". *Comparative Immunology and Microbiology of Infectious Diseases*. 8 no. 3–4 (1985):259–265.

Crowther, John R. and Abu Elzein, E.M. "Application of the enzyme linked immunosorbent assay to the detection and identification of foot-and-mouth disease viruses". *Journal of Hygiene*. 83 no. 3 (1979):513–519.
Darbyshire, J.H., Hedger, R.S. and Arrowsmith, Ann E.M. "Comparative complement-fixation studies with subtype strains of foot-and-mouth disease virus". *The Journal of Hygiene*. 70 no. 1 (1972):171–180.
Desselberger, Ulrich. "*Virus Taxonomy: Classification and Nomenclature of Viruses. Seventh Report of the International Committee on Taxonomy of Viruses*, edited by M.H.V. van Regenmortel, C.M. Fauquet, D.H.L. Bishop, E.B. Carstens, M.K. Estes, S.M. Lemon, J. Maniloff, M.A. Mayo, D.J. McGeoch, C.R. Pringle and R.B. Wickner, Virology Division, International Union of Microbiological Societies, Academic Press, San Diego, 1162 pp. ISBN: 0-12-370200-3; US$159.95". *Virus Research*. 83 no. 1–2 (2002):221–222.
Ding, Yao Z., Liu, Yong S., Zhou, Jian H., Chen, Hao-Tai, Zhang, Jie, Wei, Gang and Ma, Li-Na. "A highly sensitive detection for foot-and-mouth disease virus by gold nanopariticle improved immuno-PCR". *Virology Journal*. 8 no. 1 (2011):148.
Donaldson, Alex I. and Alexandersen, Soren. "Predicting the spread of foot and mouth disease by airborne virus". *Revue Scientifique et Technique* (Office International des Epizooties). 21 no. 3 (2002):569–575.
Donaldson Alex I., Alexandersen, Soren, Sorensen, Jens H. and Mikkelsen, Torben K. "Relative risks of the uncontrollable (airborne) spread of foot-and-mouth disease by different species" *The Veterinary Record*. 148 no. 19 (2001):602–604.
Dukes, Julit P., King, Donald P. and Alexandersen, Soren. "Novel reverses transcription loop-mediated isothermal amplification for rapid detection of foot-and mouth disease virus". *Archives of Virology*. 151 no. 6 (2006):1093–1106.
Dunn, C.S. and Donaldson, Alex I. "Natural adaption to pigs of a Taiwanese isolate of foot-and-mouth disease virus". *Veterinary Record*. 141 no. 7 (1997):174–175.
Ferris, Nigel P., Donaldson, Alex I., Barnett, I.T.R. and Osborne, R.W. "Inactivation, purification and stability of 146S antigens of foot-and-mouth disease virus for use as reagent in the complement fixation test". *Revue Scientifique et Technique* (Office International des Epizooties). 3 no. 2 (1984):339–350.
Ferris, Nigel P., Reid, Scott M., Hutchings, Geoffrey, Kitching, Paul R., Danks, Christopher, Barker, Ian and Preston, S. "Pen-side test for investigating FMD" (letter). *Veterinary Record*. 148 no. 26 (2001): 823–824.
Fracastoro, Girolamo. "De sympathia et antipathia rerum liber unus. De contagione et contagiosis morbis et eorum curatione liber III" Venice, Heirs of L. A. Junta. (1546).
Gailiunas, Peter. "Microscopic skin lesions in cattle with foot-and-mouth disease". *Archiv fiir die gesamte Virusforschung*. 25 no. 2 (1968):188–200.
Gakuya, Daniel W., Mulei, Charles M. and Wekesa, Sabenzia B. "Use of ethnoveterinary remedies in the management of foot and mouth disease lesions in a dairy herd". *African Journal of Traditional, Complementary and Alternative Medicines*. 8 no. 2 (2011):165–169.
Grubman, Marvin J. and Baxt, Barry. "Foot-and-mouth disease". *Clinical Microbiology Reviews*. 17 no. 2 (2004):465–493.
Guo, Hui Chen, Sun, Shi-Qi, Jin, Ye, Yang, Shun-Li, Wei, Yan-Quan, Sun, De-Hui, Yin, Shuang-Hui, Ma, Jun-Wu, Liu, Zai-Xin, Guo, Jian-Hong, Luo, Jian-Xun, Yin, Hong, Liu, Xiang-Tao and Liu, Ding Xiang. "Foot-and-mouth disease virus-like particles produced by a SUMO fusion protein system in Escherichia coli induce potent protective immune responses in guinea pigs, swine and cattle". *Veterinary Research*. 44 no. 1 (2013):48.
Hedger, R.S. "Foot and mouth disease and the African buffalo (*Syncerus caffer*)". *Journal of Comparative Pathology*. 82 no. 1 (1972):19–28.
Hirsh, Dwight C., MacLauchlan, James N. and Walker, Richard L. *Veterinary Microbiology* (Blackwell Science, 2nd edn, 2004).
Hirsh, Dwight C. and Zee, Yuan C. *Veterinary Microbiology and Immunology* (Blackwell Science, 2nd edn, 1999).
Jamal, Syed M. and Belsham, Graham J. "Foot and mouth disease: past, present and future". *Veterinary Research*. 44 no. 1 (2013):116.
Jamal, Syed M. and Belsham, Graham J. "Molecular epidemiology, evolution and phylogeny of foot-and-mouth disease virus". *Infection Genetics and Evolution*. 59 (2018):84–98.
Jamal, Syed M., Ferrari, Giancarlo, Ahmed, Safia, Normann, Preben and Belsham, Graham J. "Molecular characterization of serotype Asia-1 foot and mouth disease viruses in Pakistan and Afghanistan; emergence of a new genetic group and evidence for a novel recombinant virus". *Infection Genetics and Evolution*. 11 no. 8 (2011):2049–2062.

James, Andrew D. and Rushton, Jonathan. "The economics of foot & mouth disease". *Revue Scientifique et Technique* (Office International des Epizooties). 21 no. 3 (2002):637–644.

Karam, Mohamed, El-Bayoumy, M.K., Abdelrahman, K.A., Allam, Ahmad M., Farag, Tarek K., Abou-Zeina, Hala A.A. and Kutkat, Mohammad A. "Molecular characterization of foot-and-mouth disease virus collected from Al-Fayoum and Beni-Suef governorates in Egypt". *Global Veterinaria*. 13 no. 5 (2014):828–835.

Kibenge, Frederick S.B., Godoy, Marcos G. and Kibenge, Molly J.T. "Diagnosis of aquatic animal viral diseases". In Kibenge, Frederick S.B. and Godoy, Marcos G. (Eds), *Aquaculture Virology* (Academic Press, 2016):49–75.

King, Donald P., Ferris, Nigel P., Shaw, Andrew E., Reid, Scott M., Hutchings, Geoff H., Giuffre, Angelica C., Robida, John M., Callahan, Johnny D., Nelson, William M. and Beckham, Tammy R. "Detection of foot-and-mouth disease virus: comparative diagnostic sensitivity of two independent real-time reverse transcription-polymerase chain reaction assays". *Journal of Veterinary Diagnostics Investigation*. 18 no. 1 (2006):93–97.

Kitching, Richard Paul and Alexandersen, Soren. "Clinical variation in foot and mouth disease: pigs". *Revue Scientifique et Technique* (Office International des Epizooties). 21 no. 3 (2002):513–518.

Kitching, Richard Paul and Hughes, Gareth J. "Clinical variation in foot & mouth disease: sheep & goats". *Revue Scientifique et Technique* (Office International des Epizooties). 21 no. 3 (2002):505–510.

Kitching, Richard Paul, Rendle, R. and Ferris, Nigel P. "Rapid correlation between field isolates and vaccine strains of foot-and-mouth disease virus". *Vaccine*. 6 no. 5 (1988):403–408.

Knight-Jones, Theodore J.D. and Rushton, Jonathan. "The economic impacts of foot and mouth disease–What are they, how big are they and where do they occur?". *Preventive Veterinary Medicine*. 112 no 3–4 (2013):161–173.

Knowles, Nick J., Davies, Paul R., Henry, Tina, O'Donnell, Vivian, Pacheco, Juan M. and Mason, Peter W. "Emergence in Asia of foot-and-mouth disease viruses with altered host range: characterization of alterations in the 3A protein". *Journal of Virology*. 75 no. 3 (2001):1551–1556.

Lefèvre, Pierre-Charles, Blancou, Jean, Chermette, Rene and Ullenberg, Gerrit. *Infectious and Parasitic Diseases of Livestock* (CABI, 2011).

Loeffler, N. and Frosch. "Summarischer Bericht uber die Ergebnisse der Untersuchungen der Commission zur Erforschung der Maul und Klauenseuche". *Deutsche Medizinische Wochenschrift*. 23 no. 39 (1897):617.

Longjam, Neeta, Deb, Rajib, Sarmah, A.K., Tayo, Tilling, Awachat, V.B. and Saxena, V.K. "A brief review on diagnosis of foot-and-mouth disease of livestock: conventional to molecular tools". *Veterinary Medicine International*. (2011):1–17.

Lunt, Ross A., Linchongsubongkoch, Wilai and Gleeson, Laurence J. "A modified liquid phase (LP) blocking ELISA used to assess type O foot-and-mouth disease virus antigenic variation in Thailand". *Veterinary Microbiology*. 42 no. 1 (1994):79–90.

Mahmoud, Mohamed Abd El-Fatah, Ghazy, Alaa Abdelmoneam and Shaapan, Raafat Mohamed. "Diagnosis and control of foot and mouth disease (FMD) in dairy small ruminants; sheep and goats". *International Journal of Dairy Science*. 14 no. 1 (2019):45–52.

Mazengia, Hailu, Taye, Mengistie, Negussie, H., Alemu, Sefinew and Tassew, Asaminew. "Incidence of foot and mouth disease and its effect on milk yield in dairy cattle at Andassa dairy farm, Northwest Ethiopia". *Agriculture and Biology Journal of North America*. 1 no. 5 (2010):969–973.

McVicar, John W. and Sutmoller, Paul. "Foot and mouth disease: the agar gel diffusion precipitation test for antibody to virus infectious associated (VIA) antigen as a tool for epizootiological surveys". *American Journal of Epidemiology*. 92 no. 4 (1970):273–278.

McVicar, John W. and Sutmoller, Paul. "Growth of foot-and-mouth disease virus in the upper respiratory tract of non-immunized, vaccinated, and recovered cattle after intranasal inoculation". *The Journal of Hygiene*. 76 no. 3 (1976):467–481.

Meyer, Richard F., Brown, Corrie C., House, Carol, House, James A. and Molitor, Thomas W. "Rapid and sensitive detection of foot-and-mouth disease virus in tissues by enzymatic RNA amplification of the polymerase gene". *Journal of Virological Methods*. 34 no. 2 (1991):161–172.

Murphy, Mariana L. Prato, Forsyth, Morag A., Belsham, Graham J. and Salt, Jeremy S. "Localization of foot-and-mouth disease virus RNA by in situ hybridization within bovine tissues". *Virus Research*. 62 no. 1(1999):67–76.

Newman, John F., Rowlands, David J. and Brown, Fred. "A physico-chemical sub-grouping of the mammalian picornaviruses". *Journal of General Virology*. 18 no. 2 (1973):171–180.

Notomi, Tsugunori, Okayama, Hiroto, Masubuchi, Harumi, Yonekawa, Toshihiro, Watanabe, Keiko, Amino, Nobuyuki and Hase, Tetsu. "Loop-mediated isothermal amplification of DNA". *Nucleic Acids Research*. 28 no. 12 (2000):E63.

Oem, Jae Ku, Ferris, Nigel P., Lee, Kwang Nyeong, Joo, Yi-Seok, Hyun, Bang Hun and Park, Jong Hyeon. "Simple and rapid lateral-flow assay for the detection of foot-and-mouth disease virus". *Clinical and Vaccine Immunology*. 16 no. 11 (2009):1660–1664.

OIE. *Terrestrial Animal Health Code* (OIE, 20th edn, 2011), chapter 4.13, p. 165.

OIE. *Terrestrial Animal Health Code. Volume II: Recommendations Applicable to OIE Listed Disease and Other Diseases of Importance to International Trade* (OIE, 24th edn, 2015), pp. 455–477.

OIE. "Foot-and-mouth disease". In *Manual of Diagnostic Tests and Vaccines for Terrestrial Animals (Mammals, Birds and Bees)* (OIE, 7th edition, 2012), pp. 145–173.

Pantawane, Pranita B., Dhanze, Himani, Kumar, Ravi G., Grace, M.R., Dudhe, Nitin C. and Bhilegaonkar, K.N. "TaqMan real-time RT-PCR assay for detecting Japanese encephalitis virus in swine blood samples and mosquitoes". *Animal Biotechnology*. 30 no. 3 (2018):267–272.

Paton, David J., Sumption, Keith J. and Charleston, Bryan. "Options for control of foot-and mouth disease: knowledge, capability and policy". *Philosophical Transactions of the Royal Society B: Biological Sciences*. 364 no. 1530 (2009):2657–2667.

Pattnaik, B., Rai, D.V. and Venkataramanan, R. "Specificity of foot-and-mouth disease virus antigen and antibody reaction in liquid phase ELISA". *Indian Journal of Animal Sciences*. 61 no. 3 (1991):235–240.

Quinn, P.J., Markey, B.K., Carter, M.E. and Leonard, F.C. *Veterinary Microbiology and Microbial Disease* (Blackwell Science, 2002), p. 405.

Rai, Anant and Lahiri, Debomoy K. "A micro-enzyme-labelled immunosorbent assay (MICROELISA) for the detection of foot and mouth disease virus antigen and antibody". *Acta Virologica*. 25 no. 1 (1981):49–52.

Reid, Scott M., Ferris, Nigel P., Hutchings, Geoffrey H., Zhang, Zhidong, Belsham, Graham J. and Alexandersen, Soren. "Detection of all seven serotypes of foot-and-mouth disease virus by real-time, fluorogenic reverse transcription polymerase chain reaction assay". *Journal of Virological Methods*. 105 no. 1 (2002):67–80.

Rodriguez, Ana, Martínez-Salas, Encarnaacion, Dopazo, Joaquin, Dávila, Mercedes, Sáiz, Juan Carlos and Sobrino, Francisco. "Primer design for specific diagnosis by PCR of highly variable RNA viruses: typing of foot and mouth disease virus". *Virology*. 189 no. 1 (1992):363–367.

Roeder, Peter L. and Le Blanc Smith, P.M. "Detection and typing of foot and mouth disease virus by enzyme linked immunoassay: a sensitive, rapid and reliable technique for primary diagnosis". *Research in Veterinary Science*. 43 no. 2 (1987):225–232.

Rweyemamu, Mark M., Booth, James C., Head, Myles and Pay, Thomas W.F. "Microneutralization tests for serological typing and subtyping of foot-and-mouth disease virus strains". *Journal of Hygiene*. 81 no. 1 (1978):107–123.

Stear, Michael J. "*OIE Manual of Diagnostic Tests and Vaccines for Terrestrial Animals (Mammals, Birds and Bees)* 5th Edn. Volumes 1 & 2. World Organization for Animal Health 2004. ISBN 92 9044 622 6. €140". *Parasitology*. 130 no. 6 (2005):727.

Sutmoller Paul, McVicar, John W. and Cottral, George E. "The epizootiological importance of foot-and-mouth disease carriers". *Archives Gesamte Virusforschung*. 23 no. 3 (1968):227–235.

Tam, Stanley, Clavijo, Alfonso, Engelhard, Eric K. and Thurmond, Mark C. "Fluorescence-based multiplex real-time RT-PCR arrays for the detection and serotype determination of foot-and-mouth disease virus". *Journal of Virological Methods*. 161 no. 2 (2009):183–191.

Thomson, G.R., Bengis, R.G., Esterhuysen, J.J. and Pini, A. "Maintenance mechanisms for foot-and-mouth disease virus in the Kruger national park and potential avenues for its escape into domestic animal populations". *Proceedings of the 13th World Congress in Buiatrics*. 13 (1984):33–38.

Tilahun, Yilma. "Morphogenesis of vesiculation in foot-and-mouth disease". *American Journal of Veterinary Research*. 41 no. 9 (1980):1537–1542.

Traub, E. *Foot-and-Mouth Disease Typing with the Complement-fixation Test First Communication* (n.p., 1983).

Vangrysperre, W. and De Clercq, K. "Rapid and sensitive polymerase chain reaction based detection and typing of foot-and-mouth disease virus in clinical samples and cell culture isolates, combined with a simultaneous differentiation with other genomically and/or symptomatically related viruses". *Archives of Virology*. 141 no. 2 (1996):331–344.

13

Synthetic Biology-based Diagnostics for Infectious Animal Diseases

Naveen Kumar,[1] **Sandeep Bhatia**[1] **and Yashpal Singh Malik**[2,3]
[1] *Diagnostics and Vaccines Group, ICAR, National Institute of High Security Animal Diseases, Bhopal-462022, Madhya Pradesh, India*
[2] *Division of Biological Standardization, ICAR, Indian Veterinary Research Institute, Izatnagar, Bareilly-243122, Uttar Pradesh, India*
[3] *College of Animal Biotechnology, Guru Angad Dev Veterinary and Animal Science University (GADVASU), Ludhiana 141004, Punjab, India*
Corresponding author: Naveen Kumar, *navyog.yadav84@gmail.com*

13.1 Introduction

Infectious diseases, including new and exotic diseases, remain a global threat to animal and public health and contribute significantly to jeopardizing food security, the global health index, and the economies of affected countries. Livestock constitutes an important sector of the economy and contributes ≈37% of the agricultural gross domestic product worldwide (Alexandratos and Bruinsma, 2012). Infectious diseases in livestock (caused by viruses, bacteria, fungi, and parasites) are responsible for huge direct losses to this sector through increased mortality and reduced productivity, as well as indirect losses incurred due to loss of trade, cost of control, decreasing market values, and food insecurity. Therefore, improved understanding of disease surveillance, ecology, and the pathogenesis of pathogens, along with rapid and accurate diagnosis, is indispensable for improving animal infectious disease outcomes worldwide. However, accurate and early diagnosis of infectious diseases is still a major challenge before the implementation of effective preventive and control measures for infectious disease management. The ASSURED (affordable, sensitive, specific, user-friendly, rapid and robust, equipment-free, and deliverable to end-users) criteria recommended by the World Health Organization (WHO) help in the selection of an appropriate and promising diagnostic test for an infectious disease. Thus, diagnostic assays that comply with the WHO ASSURED criteria could play a pivotal role in effective infectious disease containment and management, and in reducing the associated public health risk.

A synthetic biology approach which allows the exciting and promising rational design of diagnostics may offer a rapid, accurate, and cost-effective alternative to conventional infectious disease diagnostics. Besides, synthetic biology-based diagnostics are the most suited platform especially for rapidly emerging diseases because of their shorter design-to-production cycles as compared to the commonly used nucleic acid- or antibody-based platforms (Slomovic *et al.*, 2015). Synthetic biology employs a forward-engineering approach that has been utilized by researchers to create new biological materials (Kumar *et al.*, 2016b; Liu *et al.*, 2019; Kumar *et al.*, 2020) and synthetic gene regulatory circuits (Pardee *et al.*, 2016) to translate them into user-friendly and rapid diagnostic platforms.

Here, we describe how a synthetic biology-inspired approach is being applied to meet the growing demand for novel and field-deployable diagnostic tools for livestock infectious diseases. Through examples, we describe the potentials of these synthetic biology-based diagnostics to overcome the inadequacies of presently used diagnostic approaches to livestock infectious disease detection and, consequently, contribute in transforming the future of livestock infectious disease diagnostics.

13.2 *In vitro* Diagnostics

13.2.1 Phage-based Diagnostics

The ability of phages (or bacteriophages; viruses infecting bacteria) to lyse their specific host has been used for several years as a means of exclusively classifying bacteria, and this approach is commonly known as phage typing. Phage typing is still used in many reference laboratories to detect and differentiate several strains of a particular bacterial species. However, phage typing's confinement to reference laboratories due to their maintenance of a large number of phage stocks has hampered its use in identifying bacterial pathogens in clinical settings.

Diagnostics based on engineered phages (reporter phages) are gaining importance, but at a very slow pace, in the synthetic biology space and, thus, can fill this gap towards their usage in clinical settings. The prime advantage of such diagnostics is that they are simple, rapid, and do not necessitate the usage of costly equipment. A reporter phage, engineered to carry a reporter gene in its non-essential genome, specifically infects a target bacterial species and produces a measurable signal. For example, a reporter phage carrying a firefly luciferase, upon infection, generates the luciferase enzyme, yielding light in the presence of ATP and a luciferin substrate. The emitted light can be measured with the help of a luminometer or a cost-effective box that can hold a photographic film cassette.

Different variants of reporter phages carrying either firefly luciferase (FFLux), *Vibrio harveyi* luciferase (luxAB), or *Vibrio fischeri* luciferase (luxI) have been developed for the detection of a variety of bacterial species such as *Mycobacterium tuberculosis* (Dusthackeer *et al.*, 2008), *Bacillus anthracis* (Schofield and Westwater, 2009), *Yersinia pestis* (Schofield *et al.*, 2009), *Listeria monocytogenes* (Loessner *et al.*, 1996), *Escherichia coli* 0157:H7 (Brigati *et al.*, 2007), and *Salmonella Typhimurium* (Thouand *et al.*, 2008) (Table 13.1). Besides, a reporter method that utilizes the quorum sensing system has also been developed as a diagnostic tool (Ripp *et al.*, 2008). In this tool, an *E. coli* O157:H7 phage is engineered to carry the gene encoding acyl homoserine lactone (AHL) in place of luciferase, which, upon infection, generates bioluminescence in the presence of a luxRCDABE gene cassette-carrying bioreporter, without the requirement for exogenous aldehyde substrate. Additional types of reporter outlines which utilize different fluorescent binding dyes (fluorescently labeled phages) or green fluorescent proteins (green fluorescent protein-labeled phages) have also been reported for *E. coli* O157:H7 and *Salmonella* (Goodridge *et al.*, 1999; Mosier-Boss *et al.*, 2003; Oda *et al.*, 2004). The fluorescently labeled phage, upon binding to the specific bacterial cell, can be detected with the help of fluorescence microscopy.

Despite the huge diversity, host specificity, and cost-effective production of phages, the implementation of phage-based diagnostics in clinical settings has been of limited significance until now. However, the transition from traditional phage typing to engineered phages for the detection of a wide variety of bacteria in complex sample matrices is likely to uncover the untapped potential of phage-based diagnostics in the future.

13.2.2 Synthetic Peptides-based Diagnostics

In recent years, there has been growing interest in synthetic peptides for use in diverse applications such as epitope mapping (Kumar *et al.*, 2016a), therapeutics (Isidro-Llobet *et al.*, 2019), diagnostics (Kumar *et al.*, 2016b), and vaccines (Hos *et al.*, 2018). The synthesis of a typical peptide is generally carried out by solid-phase peptide synthesis in most laboratories, which involves hazardous reagents and solvents. However, the major focus has now shifted towards green chemistry and engineering for the safe synthesis of peptides (Isidro-Llobet *et al.*, 2019). There is a huge cloud of synthetic peptides that can be discussed, but we are restricting ourselves to diagnostic applications of synthetic peptides in animal infectious diseases.

Anti-peptide antibodies, with their inbuilt high specificities and affinities, have proved to be invaluable reagents for the detection of pathogen-specific surface proteins in biological specimens. The success of this anti-peptide antibody production largely depends on several factors, including the careful designing and selection of peptides, conjugation with carrier molecules or the usage of multiple antigenic peptides, and immunization protocols (Kumar *et al.*, 2016b, 2019; Trier and Houen, 2017). The anti-peptide antibodies that typically react with one or two epitopes are parallel to monoclonal antibodies in terms of specificity and are easier and more cost-effective to produce (Dyson *et al.*, 1988; Kumar *et al.*, 2016b). Furthermore, employing multiple antigenic peptides (MAPs) is advantageous for the production of highly titered anti-peptide sera in laboratory animals because it avoids the clumpy conjugation procedure that can distort/hide the native conformation or immunodominant epitopes of the peptides (Kumar *et al.*, 2016b; Posnett *et al.*, 1988; Tam, 1988). MAPs are chemically composed of three regions, viz. an amino acid (cysteine or alanine) attached to the resin (solid support), a lysine core matrix, and an outer surface layer of four or eight peptides (of the same or different sequences) attached to the lysine core matrix. The MAP format thus increases the overall molecular weight and also matches closely the native antigenic sites on the pathogen surface-exposed proteins. Because of these novel properties, synthetic peptides have been used for the detection of antibodies against infectious bursal disease virus (Saravanan *et al.*, 2004b), infectious bronchitis virus (Jackwood and Hilt, 1995), peste des petits ruminants virus (Dechamma *et al.*, 2006), Aleutian mink disease virus (Ma *et al.*, 2016), chlamydia (Sachse *et al.*, 2018), and swine influenza virus (Du *et al.*, 2019) (Table 13.1). Anti-peptide antibodies are also used for detecting cell surface markers, such as CD20 and CD34, in a flow cytometer (Maleki *et al.*, 2013; Sepehr *et al.*, 2013).

Furthermore, these anti-peptide antibodies can also be used for the detection of viral antigens along with other supporting antibodies. The author's lab has designed, developed, and validated a novel enzyme immunoassay capable of detecting the diverse rotaviruses A (RVAs) in taxonomically divergent host species (Kumar *et al.*, 2016b). The concept of the assay is based on the detection of RVA VP6 protein in sandwich ELISA format by utilizing two antibodies, viz. capture antibodies (anti-recombinant VP6 antibodies) and detector antibodies (anti-multiple antigenic peptide antibodies). The performance characteristics of this assay were comparable to VP6 gene-based diagnostic RT-PCR as well as to commercially available ELISA kits. This assay is in routine use as a screening assay for the surveillance of RVA in different animal species at the author's lab (Kumar *et al.*, 2016b) (Table 13.1).

13.2.3 Synthetic Peptide Nucleic Acid-based Diagnostics

Peptide nucleic acids (PNAs) have been demonstrated to be excellent synthetic candidates in several biomedical applications, including in the diagnostics of infectious disease. PNAs are in fact DNA mimetics where N-(2-aminoethyl) glycine units (having neutral charge) replace the typical sugar-phosphate backbone (negatively charged), and this change has infused important features to the PNAs suited for diagnostics and therapeutics purposes, for instance, formation of stable duplex structures with the complementary RNA or DNA sequences, extreme thermal stability over a range of temperatures, high stability in acidic environments, and resistance to degradation by cellular nucleases and proteases. These unique properties

TABLE 13.1

Applications of synthetic biology-based diagnostics in various animal infectious diseases

Pathogens	Phage/Target Genes	Reporter System/ Diagnostic Assay Platform	Limit of Detection	Diagnostic Sensitivity and Specificity	References
		Phage-based diagnostics			
M. tuberculosis	phAETRC201::hsp60-FFlux (TM4ts derivative)	Reporter phage (FFlux)	8×10^1 to 1×10^5 CFU/mL	-	Dusthackeer *et al.* (2008)
B. anthracis	Wβ	Reporter phage (luxAB)	~10^5 CFU/mL	-	Schofield and Westwater (2009)
Y. pestis	ϕA1122	Reporter phage (luxAB)	~10^3 CFU/mL	-	Schofield *et al.* (2009)
L. monocytogenes	A511::luxAB	Reporter phage (luxAB)	5×10^2 to 10^3 cells/mL	-	Loessner *et al.* (1996)
E. coli 0157:H7	PPOI-luxl	Reporter phage (luxI)	10^4 CFU/mL	-	Brigati *et al.* (2007)
S. enterica	P22::luxAB	Reporter phage (luxAB)	6.5×10^3 CFU/mL	-	Thouand *et al.* (2008)
		Synthetic peptides-based diagnostics			
Detection of pathogen-specific antibodies					
Feline immunodeficiency virus	Env glycoproteins- P237	Indirect ELISA	-	-	Avrameas *et al.* (1993)
Infectious bronchitis virus	S1 glycoprotein	Indirect ELISA	-	-	Jackwood and Hilt (1995)
Peste des petits ruminants virus	N protein	Indirect ELISA	-	-	Dechamma *et al.* (2006)
Porcine reproductive and respiratory syndrome virus	N protein	Indirect ELISA	-	-	Plagemann(2006)
Foot-and-mouth disease virus	Non-structural proteins (2B, 2C, 3B1, and 3B2)	Indirect ELISA	-	98.08% and 98.88%	Yang *et al.* (2010)
Peste des petits ruminants virus	N protein	Competitive ELISA	-	96.18% and 91.29%	Zhang *et al.* (2013)
Equine arteritis virus	GP5 protein—epitope C	Indirect ELISA	-	95.65% and 80.43%	Metz *et al.* (2014)
Bovine cysticercosis (*Taenia saginata*)	Oncospheric surface protein- EP1	Indirect ELISA	-	91.6% and 90%	Guimarães-Peixoto *et al.* (2016)
Aleutian mink disease virus	VP2 protein	Indirect ELISA	-	98.0% and 97.5%,	Ma *et al.* (2016)
Chlamydia (C.) spp.	52 synthetic peptides covering B-cell epitopes	Peptide microarray coupled ELISA	-	-	Sachse *et al.* (2018)
Swine influenza virus	NP specific single-domain antibodies tagged with biotin acceptor peptide	Blocking ELISA	-	-	Du *et al.* (2019)

TABLE 13.1

Applications of synthetic biology-based diagnostics in various animal infectious diseases (Cont.)

Pathogens	Phage/Target Genes	Reporter System/ Diagnostic Assay Platform	Limit of Detection	Diagnostic Sensitivity and Specificity	References
Equine infectious anemia	Envelope protein-pgp45	Indirect ELISA	-	98.6% and 95.6%	Naves *et al.* (2019)
Detection of virus antigen					
Infectious bursal disease virus	VP3 protein	Indirect ELISA		-	Saravanan *et al.* (2004a)
Rotavirus A antigen	VP6 protein	Sandwich ELISA		74.2– 94.2% and 97.7–100% in multiple hosts	Kumar *et al.* (2016b)
		Synthetic peptide nucleic acid-based diagnostics			
Swine-origin influenza A virus (H1N1)	nonstructural protein (NS) gene	Gold-conjugated antibody-assisted PNA chromatography	1.0×10^4 – 6.0×10^4 pfu	-	Kaihatsu *et al.* (2013)
Newcastle disease virus	F gene	Unmodified AuNPs	5–10 ng viral RNA	-	Joshi *et al.* (2013)
Bovine viral diarrhea virus	5′UTR	Unmodified AuNPs	10.48 ng viral RNA	98% and 100%	Askaravi *et al.* (2017)
Enterobacteriaceae family, *E. coli*, *P. aeruginosa*, and *P. mirabilis*	16S rRNA	Double-stranded PNA probes with tethered fluorophore and quencher	-	-	Mach *et al.* (2019)
Porcine reproductive and respiratory syndrome virus	ORF6	PNA probe-mediated real-time RT-PCR	1.5×10^1 to 1.1×10^1 copies	-	Park *et al.* (2019)
Influenza A virus	Matrix gene	Unmodified AuNPs	2.3 ng viral RNA	82.41% and 96.46%	Kumar *et al.* (2020)
		Aptamers-based diagnostics			
Avian influenza (H5N1) virus	HA	Surface plasmon resonance aptasensor	0.128–12.8 HAU	-	Bai *et al.* (2012)
E. coli K88	Whole bacterium	Immuno-magnetic beads separation method	1.1×10^3 CFU/ml	-	Peng *et al.* (2014)
L. monocytogenes	Whole bacterium	Aptamer-based sandwich assay	20 CFU/mL	-	Lee *et al.* (2015)
Avian influenza (H5N1) virus	HA	Impedance aptasensor with gold nanoparticles	0.25–1.0 HAU	-	Karash *et al.* (2016)
Influenza A (H1N1) virus	HA	Sandwich aptamer assay on integrated microfluidic system	0.032 HAU	-	Tseng *et al.* (2016)

(continued)

TABLE 13.1

Applications of synthetic biology-based diagnostics in various animal infectious diseases (Cont.)

Pathogens	Phage/Target Genes	Reporter System/ Diagnostic Assay Platform	Limit of Detection	Diagnostic Sensitivity and Specificity	References
S. typhimurium	Whole bacterium	Nanogold-based colorimetric detection	100 CFU/ mL	-	Lavu *et al.* (2016)
Avian influenza (H5N2) virus	Whole virus	Sandwich-type lateral-flow strip biosensor	2.09×10^5 EID_{50}/mL to 1.2×10^6 EID_{50}/mL	-	Kim *et al.* (2019)
L. monocytogenes	Whole bacterium	Lateral-flow aptamer-based sandwich assay	53 cells/mL	-	Tasbasi *et al.* (2019)
		CRISPR/Cas-based diagnostics			
S. aureus	mecA	FISH (SYBR green I as a fluorescent probe)	10 CFU/mL	-	Guk *et al.* (2017)
Avian influenza A (H7N9)	HA	A microplate reader-based CRISPR/ Cas13a assay	1 fM	-	Liu *et al.* (2019)
SARS-CoV-2	ORF1a	CRISPR/Cas13a-LFD (lateral-flow detection)	5–10 copies/ µL	90.0% and 100.0%	Arizti-Sanz *et al.* (2020)
African swine fever virus	Major capsid protein p72 (B646L gene)	CRISPR/Cas12a-LFD (lateral-flow detection)	20 copies	-	Wang *et al.* (2020)
SARS-CoV-2	E and N genes	CRISPR/Cas12a-DETECTER-LFD (lateral-flow detection)	10 copies/ µL	95.0% and 100.0%	Broughton *et al.* (2020)

of PNAs, which provide several additional advantages over nucleic acid oligomers, make them preferred synthetic agents for diagnostic assays.

PNA applications in animal disease diagnosis are still at the infant stage and some PNA-based diagnostics utilizing PNAs as probes for real-time RT-PCR (Mach *et al.*, 2019; Park *et al.*, 2019) and specific detectors in chromatography assays (Kunihiro *et al.*, 2013) have been reported (Table 13.1). However, the use of gold nanoparticles as a reporter system offers many advantages, such as simplicity of synthesis in the laboratory, the capability to interact with several biomolecules, viz. nucleic acids, PNAs, and aptamers, and high chemical stability. Therefore, combining the PNAs with gold nanoparticles as reporters can translate the applicability of PNAs into simple, cost-effective, highly sensitive, highly specific, and visual diagnostic assays, which can serve the purpose of on-site detection of pathogens (Askaravi *et al.*, 2017; Joshi *et al.*, 2013; Kumar *et al.*, 2020) (Table 13.1). The author's lab translated PNA biosensors into a simple, visual, cost-effective, and fast diagnostic method for multiple strains of influenza A virus (Kumar *et al.*, 2020). This assay utilized a simple design principle which is based on color change on account of free PNA-induced aggregation of unmodified gold nanoparticles in the presence of non-complementary RNA sequence and *vice versa*. The visual detection assay was 2.3 ng of viral RNA and achieved a diagnostic specificity of 96.46% and sensitivity of 82.41% when RT-qPCR was used as a standard test. Furthermore, it would be an ideal strategy to include an isothermal amplification step to improve the sensitivity of this assay, and, consequently, this visual assay can be applied for the on-site diagnostics of other pathogens. Available studies provide conclusive evidence that PNAs are very efficient in hybridizing with both DNA and RNA molecules and can perform stand invasion of double-stranded genomes, thus allowing the development of extremely efficient, reproducible, and sensible diagnostics. In the future, PNAs, coupled with genome amplification methods (especially isothermal amplification methods), will allow for the development of highly sensitive portable diagnostics.

13.2.4 Aptamers-based Diagnostics

Another class of synthetic biomolecules, aptamers, are small oligonucleotides composed of either single-stranded RNA or DNA and act as oligonucleotides or affinity probes to recognize the complementary nucleic acid sequences. These aptamers can fold into three-dimensional shapes and bind non-covalently to target nucleic acid sequences. The binding affinity of aptamers to a specific target is usually improved through a process called systematic evolution of ligands by exponential enrichment (SELEX) (Stoltenburg *et al.*, 2007).

Though aptamers are equivalent to antibodies in terms of specificity and affinity, they present numerous advantages over antibodies-based diagnostics, such as their stability at room temperature, longer shelf-life, cost-effective production, and potential reuse over many cycles without losing potency, making them a safe alternative. Together, these features provide exceptional qualities to aptamers, which can be transformed for use in various diagnostic platforms. Combining aptamer sensors with surface plasmon resonance (Bai *et al.*, 2012), conjugating them with gold nanoparticles for colorimetric detection (Karash *et al.*, 2016), or using them in sandwich format to capture the antigen on a lateral-flow test (Kim *et al.*, 2019; Tasbasi *et al.*, 2019) or in an integrated microfluidic system (Tseng *et al.*, 2016) are some examples that make aptamers a promising diagnostic tool for animal infectious diseases (Table 13.1). The unique features of aptamers continue to provide researchers with opportunities to infuse them into diverse diagnostic platforms, and they hold great promise for being translated into commercial applications for the on-site detection of animal pathogens in the future.

13.2.5 CRISPR/Cas-based Biosensors

The adaptive immune system in bacteria and archaea uses RNA-guided endonucleases of various clustered regularly interspaced short palindromic repeats (CRISPR) and CRISPR-associated (CRISPR/Cas) systems to recognize and cleave foreign nucleic acid (Hille *et al.*, 2018). The CRISPR/Cas nucleases remember the previously encountered pathogens through capturing the nucleic acid sequences (spacer sequences) and use these spacer sequences to direct CRISPR/Cas proteins to kill the same pathogens during subsequent exposure. These programmable endonucleases of CRISPR/Cas systems allow the targeting of any DNA or RNA sequences (protospacer sequences, positioned adjacent to the protospacer-adjacent motif, or PAM) by using specific spacer sequences within the single guide RNA (sgRNA) (Anzalone *et al.*, 2020; Jinek *et al.*, 2012). The knowledge of programmable endonucleases to target any DNA or RNA sequence along with significant advances in the understanding of the biology and function of CRISPR/Cas have been translated into diverse clinical applications, including the development of rapid and accurate infectious disease diagnostics.

CRISPR/Cas systems have been classified into two categories, viz. class I and class II. Each of these is further classified into three different subtypes, i.e., type I, III, and IV for class I, and type II, V, and VI for class II. Class I employs multi-protein complexes to target nucleic acid for cleavage, while class II employs a single protein for target cleavage (Makarova *et al.*, 2019). Class II CRISPR/Cas systems are thus widely used due to the advantages offered by the use of a single protein. The three types of class II CRISPR/Cas systems are classified based on the use of distinct Cas proteins. Of the class II Cas proteins, type II (Cas9 protein) and type V (Cas12 protein) have RNA-guided DNA endonuclease activity, while type VI (Cas13 protein) possesses RNA targeting and cleavage activity. Since the applications of class II CRISPR/Cas systems in developing infectious disease diagnostics are emerging, the translatability of these promising systems holds potential for animal infectious disease diagnostics.

13.2.5.1 Diagnostics using CRISPR/Cas9

Guk *et al.* developed a simple, fast, sensitive, and cost-efficient method for the detection of methicillin-resistant *Staphylococcus aureus* (MRSA) (Guk *et al.*, 2017). In this method, the investigators employed CRISPR/Cas9 systems as a targeting material and SYBR green I as a fluorescent probe to detect the mecA gene of MRSA by FISH (DNA fluorescent *in situ* hybridization). When the dCas9/sgRNA complex recognizes the mecA gene, dCas9 (endonuclease dead Cas9) does not cause DNA cleavage, which can easily be detected by FISH, and the concentration of MRSA can be measured by the corresponding fluorescence intensity. This method allowed the detection of the mecA gene of MRSA in 30 minutes with a high sensitivity of detection (10 CFU/mL). Theoretically, this method can also be used for the differentiation of MRSA and methicillin-susceptible *S. aureus*.

13.2.5.2 CRISPR/Cas12- and CRISPR/Cas13-based Diagnostics

The rapid, simple, and low-cost diagnostic platforms offered by the CRISPR/Cas12/13 systems have been recently translated to on-site detection for both DNA and RNA viruses (Table 13.1). The concept of molecular detection in these diagnostics relies on the DNA endonuclease-targeted CRISPR trans reporter (DETECTR), which involves target-induced non-specific endonuclease activity of Cas12 or Cas13 after specific binding to target DNA or RNA via programmable guide RNAs, respectively. The specific detection of target DNA or RNA sequences by the programmable guide RNAs Cas12/13 can be visualized by combining a reporter molecule. For example, a CRISPR/Cas12a system with programmable guide RNAs and an ssDNA reporter (labeled with digoxin and biotin at the 5' and 3' termini, respectively) has been developed for the detection of African swine fever virus (ASFV) in the lateral-flow detection (LFD) format (Wang *et al.*, 2020). In this CRISPR/Cas12a-LFD assay, rabbit anti-mouse antibodies bind and capture the cleaved ssDNA reporter-mouse anti-digoxin-gold nanoparticles and the color change at the test line is indicative of a positive result, while on the control line, coated streptavidin can capture biotin-labeled ssDNA. The analytical sensitivity of this CRISPR/Cas12a-LFD was improved to 20 copies by combining recombinase-aided amplification. In the same way, a sensitive and portable CRISPR/Cas12-DETECTR lateral-flow assay for the detection of SARS-CoV-2 has recently been developed that combines reverse transcription and loop-mediated amplification (RT-LAMP) with the Cas12 detection of coronavirus sequences (Broughton *et al.*, 2020). The Cas12 gRNAs in this assay were programmed to target both N gene (specific for SARS-CoV-2) and E gene (to detect three SARS-like coronavirus strains: SARS-CoV-2, bat-SL-CoVZC45, and SARS-CoV). A confirmatory positive result requires detection of both N and E gene targets. The analytical sensitivity of the SARS-CoV-2-CRISPR/Cas12-DETECTR assay was 10 copies/µL, almost equal to that of CDC SARS-CoV-2 qRT-PCR (one copy/µL), and was superior in terms of speed and portability (without the requirement of any sophisticated instrumentation).

A specific high-sensitivity enzymatic reporter unlocking (SHERLOCK), which conglomerates isothermal amplification methods with Cas13a cleavage, has recently been implemented for the detection of avian influenza A H7N9 (Liu *et al.*, 2019). Using this method, which gives results in five minutes, a limit of detection of 1 nM was achieved. However, by combining reverse transcription-recombinase polymerase amplification (RT-RPA) and the T7 transcription system, the limit of detection was further improved to 1 fM, but at the cost of a slight increase in the detection time of 50 minutes. Furthermore, these assays can be combined with HUDSON (heating unextracted diagnostic samples to obliterate nucleases) to detect the pathogens directly from the biological samples without the requirement of nucleic acid extraction (Myhrvold *et al.*, 2018). Recently, by combining SHERLOCK and HUDSON, a simple, specific, and sensitive integrated diagnostic tool, SHINE (SHERLOCK and HUDSON Integration to Navigate Epidemics), has been devised for the detection of SARS-CoV-2 RNA directly from samples (without the requirement of RNA extraction). The limit of detection of this assay was 5–10 copies/µL and achieved a 90% sensitivity and 100% specificity compared to RT-qPCR (Arizti-Sanz *et al.*, 2020). The CRISPR/Cas-based diagnostic assay thus provides a promising potential for the fast, sensitive, specific, and on-site identification of pathogens, and may contribute in a significant way to the control of animal infectious diseases.

13.2.6 Synthetic RNA-based Biosensors Coupled with Synthetic Gene Networks

Synthetic gene networks are decision-based circuits that are composed of a sensor element (to sense specific nucleotide sequences) and a transducer that generates a measurable and/or colorimetric output. Initially, these synthetic gene networks were restricted to uses in reprogramming and rewiring organisms within the laboratory environment. However, with the advancements and efforts made by synthetic biologists, cell-free systems are now available commercially. In simple terms, cell-free systems represent the essential transcription and translation machinery of a cell but they are sterile and abiotic. The properties of these cell-free systems that make them easily deployable in clinics and in resource-limited settings are: (i) stability at room temperature (in the freeze-dried form); (ii) ease of storage, transportation, and activation by simply adding water; and (iii) cost-effectiveness. However, converging the two synthetic biology technologies (cell-free extracts and RNA-based molecular sensors) can significantly promote portable and low-cost diagnostic platform development. In this case, an RNA toehold switch (a molecular sensor) can be designed that can bind and detect any target RNA sequence, while a cell-free transcription-translation system (freeze-dried on a paper disk) allows the detection of colorimetric output, which can be visualized with the naked eye.

RNA toehold switches are synthetic RNA mimetics having a recognition sequence (toehold) complementary to the desired target RNA sequences, followed by a hairpin loop and a ribosome binding site (RBS). Upon specific binding of the toehold sensor to a complementary RNA sequence, the hairpin loop unfolds, thereby exposing the RBS and allowing the translation of the reporter gene in the presence of the cell-free extracts. In the absence of a complementary RNA sequence, the stable hairpin loop does not open up and the reporter gene remains suppressed (switch-off mode). The designing of toehold switches requires the consideration of a series of factors: (a) a toehold switch should have exclusive sequence complementarity to the desired RNA sequence to avoid off-target detection; (b) a stable hairpin loop structure is a must to avoid translation of a reporter gene in the absence of complementary RNA sequence; (c) it should be free from stop codons; and (d) the toehold switch-pathogen RNA sequence duplex should have more favorable energy, to ensure unfolding of the hairpin loop. An online web tool for the design of toehold switches can be assessed at https://yiplab.cse.cuhk.edu.hk/toehold/ (To *et al.*, 2018).

By utilizing the potential of these two synthetic biology technologies, a portable biosensor carrying toehold switches was developed for the detection of Ebola virus RNA by assimilating a cell-free transcription-translation system on paper (Pardee *et al.*, 2014). These Ebola virus-specific toehold switches were also able to differentiate the Zaire and Sudan strains, both of which carried only a three-nucleotide difference. However, the toehold switches-based sensor showed analytical sensitivity down to 30 nM and, therefore, further improvements in the limit of detection are desirable for the deployment of this biosensor at the field level (Table 13.2). On similar grounds, the sensitivity of toehold switch-based

TABLE 13.2

Promising paper-based synthetic RNA-based biosensors

S. No.	Pathogens	Virus Enrichment	Sensor	Reporter System	Detection Limit	References
1.	Ebola virus	-	Toehold switches	Cell-free transcription-translation systems (lacZ)	30 nM	Pardee *et al.* (2014)
2.	Zika virus	Viral RNA amplification by isothermal amplification	Toehold switches	Cell-free transcription-translation systems (lacZ)	3 fM	Pardee *et al.* (2016)
3.	Norovirus	Virus enrichment by synbodies followed by viral RNA amplification by isothermal amplification	Toehold switches	Cell-free transcription-translation systems (lacZα peptide-lacZw)	270 zM	Ma *et al.* (2018)

sensors was improved by combining an isothermal amplification method, nucleic acid sequence-based amplification (NASBA), with existing synthetic biology methodologies (similar to those used for Ebola virus detection) for the detection of Zika virus (Pardee *et al.*, 2016). This improved the sensitivity of the portable biosensor to 2.8 fM. Furthermore, combining NASBA with the CRISPR/Cas9 system allowed for differentiation between the American and African Zika virus strains (Pardee *et al.*, 2016). Recently, to further improve sensitivity, norovirus GII.4 Sydney was first enriched by synbodies followed by viral RNA amplification via isothermal amplification methods (NASBA or reverse transcriptase recombinase polymerase amplification (RT-RPA)) (Ma *et al.*, 2018). This allowed a detection limit down to 270 zM, and NASBA provided an improved limit of detection as compared to RT-RPA (Table 13.2). Though these results have been demonstrated in a lab environment, the commercial scalability for direct field applications requires thorough investigation of portable biosensor efficiency and stability. Overall, these synthetic biology approaches hold promise in the future for fast, simple, accurate, and portable animal infectious disease molecular diagnostics.

13.3 *In vivo* Diagnostics

With the advancement and implementation of synthetic gene circuits and modeling, it is now possible to engineer cells (both bacterial and mammalian cells) to sense the surrounding environment. Using these engineered cells (or *in vivo* biosensors) to sense diseased conditions as well as host response in real-time holds promise for *in vivo* diagnostics in the future. However, biosafety concerns related to the use of these engineered cells or sensors in the environment need to be carefully examined before translating them into real-time *in vivo* diagnostics.

The classical example of usage of such *in vivo* diagnostics includes engineered probiotic bacteria that have recently been used to diagnose liver metastasis through detection signals in urine (non-invasive method) (Danino *et al.*, 2015). The bacteria were engineered to express the lacZ and the luxCDABE operon, where lacZ reporters produce a small molecule on cleaving the substrate which can easily be detected in urine. The stability of synthetic circuits (one challenge while designing engineered bacteria) was maintained by the expression of the *Bacillus subtilis* alp7 gene (to ensure equal plasmid segregation upon cell division) and a toxin-antitoxin system (to ensure the maintenance of plasmid). Rational engineering of bacteria can thus monitor and record health status and can warn of any changes in the environment linked to different disease status. Combining engineered bacterial strains for multiple sensing would be a more promising approach towards real-time monitoring of disease/pathogen status.

13.4 Conclusions and Future Perspectives

The advancement and implementation of synthetic biology in recent years joins the modern system of diagnostics in tackling the challenges (such as the requirement of cost-effective, simple, fast, and portable diagnostics) posed by animal infectious diseases. The diverse aforementioned synthetic biology approaches have provided convincing evidence for the translation of promising technologies into cost-effective and portable diagnostics suitable for the on-site detection of pathogens. Synthetic gene circuits coupled with RNA sensors appear to be particularly promising as a portable diagnostic platform required for animal infectious disease detection. *In vivo* diagnostics are still in their nascent stage; however, once established, they could progress towards real-time surveillance of multiple pathogens in precision medicine. The authors believe that synthetic biology-based novel diagnostics will contribute in a significant way towards efforts to control animal infectious diseases in the future.

Acknowledgments

The authors acknowledge and thank their respective institutes. Yashpal Singh Malik acknowledges the Education Division, ICAR, Ministry of Agriculture and Farmers Welfare, Government of India, for the National Fellowship.

References

Alexandratos, Nikos and Jelle Bruinsma. *World Agriculture Towards 2030/2050: The 2012 Revision*. ESA Working Paper No. 12-03. Food and Agriculture Organization of the United Nations. 2012.

Anzalone, Andrew V., Luke W. Koblan, and David R. Liu. "Genome editing with CRISPR–Cas nucleases, base editors, transposases and prime editors." *Nature Biotechnology* 38, no. 7 (2020), 824–844.

Arizti-Sanz, Jon, Catherine A. Freije, Alexandra C. Stanton, Chloe K. Boehm, Brittany A. Petros, Sameed Siddiqui, Bennett M. Shaw, *et al.* "Integrated sample inactivation, amplification, and Cas13-based detection of SARS-CoV-2." *bioRxiv* (2020). doi:10.1101/2020.05.28.119131.

Askaravi, Maryam, Seyedeh E. Rezatofighi, Saadat Rastegarzadeh, and Masoud R. Seifi Abad Shapouri. "Development of a new method based on unmodified gold nanoparticles and peptide nucleic acids for detecting bovine viral diarrhea virus-RNA." *AMB Express* 7, no. 1 (2017), 137.

Avrameas, Alexandre, Arthur Donny Strosberg, Anne Moraillon, Pierre Sonigo, and Gianfranco Pancino. "Serological diagnosis of feline immunodeficiency virus infection based on synthetic peptides from Env glycoproteins." *Research in Virology* 144 (1993), 209–218.

Bai, Hua, Ronghui Wang, Billy Hargis, Huaguang Lu, and Yanbin Li. "A SPR aptasensor for detection of avian influenza virus H5N1." *Sensors* 12, no. 9 (2012), 12506–12518.

Brigati, Jennifer R., Steven A. Ripp, Courtney M. Johnson, Polina A. Iakova, Patricia Jegier, and Gary S. Sayler. "Bacteriophage-based bioluminescent bioreporter for the detection of *Escherichia coli* O157:H7." *Journal of Food Protection* 70, no. 6 (2007), 1386–1392.

Broughton, James P., Xianding Deng, Guixia Yu, Clare L. Fasching, Venice Servellita, Jasmeet Singh, Xin Miao, *et al.* "CRISPR–Cas12-based detection of SARS-CoV-2." *Nature Biotechnology* 38, no. 7 (2020), 870–874.

Danino, Tal, Arthur Prindle, Gabriel A. Kwong, Matthew Skalak, Howard Li, Kaitlin Allen, Jeff Hasty, and Sangeeta N. Bhatia. "Programmable probiotics for detection of cancer in urine." *Science Translational Medicine* 7, no. 289 (2015), 289ra84.

Dechamma, Hosur Joyappa, Vikas Dighe, Chokkalingam Ashok Kumar, Rabindra Prasad Singh, Muddappa Jagadish, and Satish Kumar. "Identification of T-helper and linear B epitope in the hypervariable region of nucleocapsid protein of PPRV and its use in the development of specific antibodies to detect viral antigen." *Veterinary Microbiology* 118, no. 3–4 (2006), 201–211.

Du, Taofeng, Guang Zhu, Xiaoping Wu, Junyang Fang, and En-Min Zhou. "Biotinylated single-domain antibody-based blocking ELISA for detection of antibodies against swine influenza virus." *International Journal of Nanomedicine* 14 (2019), 9337–9349.

Dusthackeer, Azger, Vanaja Kumar, Selvakumar Subbian, Gomathi Sivaramakrishnan, Guofang Zhu, Balaji Subramanyam, Sameer Hassan, Selvakumar Nagamaiah, John Chan, and Narayanan Paranji Rama. "Construction and evaluation of luciferase reporter phages for the detection of active and non-replicating tubercle bacilli." *Journal of Microbiological Methods* 73, no. 1 (2008), 18–25.

Dyson, Helen Jayne, Richard A. Lerner, and Peter E. Wright. "The physical basis for induction of protein-reactive antipeptide antibodies." *Annual Review of Biophysics and Biophysical Chemistry* 17, no. 1 (1988), 305–324.

Goodridge, Lawrence, Jinru Chen, and Mansel Griffiths. "Development and characterization of a fluorescent-bacteriophage assay for detection of *Escherichia coli* O157:H7." *Applied and Environmental Microbiology* 65, no. 4 (1999), 1397–1404.

Guimarães-Peixoto, Rafaella P., Paulo S. Pinto, Marcus R. Santos, Marcelo D. Polêto, Letícia F. Silva, and Abelardo Silva-Júnior. "Evaluation of a synthetic peptide from the Taenia saginata 18 kDa surface/secreted oncospheral adhesion protein for serological diagnosis of bovine cysticercosis." *Acta Tropica* 164 (2016), 463–468.

Guk, Kyeonghye, Joo O. Keem, Seul G. Hwang, Hyeran Kim, Taejoon Kang, Eun-Kyung Lim, and Juyeon Jung. "A facile, rapid and sensitive detection of MRSA using a CRISPR-mediated DNA FISH method, antibody-like dCas9/sgRNA complex." *Biosensors and Bioelectronics* 95 (2017), 67–71.

Hille, Frank, Hagen Richter, Shi P. Wong, Majda Bratovič, Sarah Ressel, and Emmanuelle Charpentier. "The biology of CRISPR-Cas: backward and forward." *Cell* 172, no. 6 (2018), 1239–1259.

Hos, Brett J., Elena Tondini, Sander I. Van Kasteren, and Ferry Ossendorp. "Approaches to improve chemically defined synthetic peptide vaccines." *Frontiers in Immunology* 9 (2018), 884.

Isidro-Llobet, Albert, Martin N. Kenworthy, Subha Mukherjee, Michael E. Kopach, Katarzyna Wegner, Fabrice Gallou, Austin G. Smith, and Frank Roschangar. "Sustainability challenges in peptide synthesis and purification: from R&D to Production." *The Journal of Organic Chemistry* 84, no. 8 (2019), 4615–4628.

Jackwood, Mark W. and Deborah A. Hilt. "Production and immunogenicity of multiple antigenic peptide (MAP) constructs derived from the S1 glycoprotein of infectious bronchitis virus (IBV)." *Advances in Experimental Medicine and Biology* (1995), 213–219.

Jinek, Martin, Krzysztof Chylinski, Ines Fonfara, Michael Hauer, Jennifer A. Doudna, and Emmanuelle Charpentier. "A programmable dual-RNA-guided DNA endonuclease in adaptive bacterial immunity." *Science* 337, no. 6096 (2012), 816–821.

Joshi, Vinay G., Kantaraja Chindera, Arvind K. Singh, Aditya P. Sahoo, Vikas D. Dighe, Dimpal Thakuria, Ashok K. Tiwari, and Satish Kumar. "Rapid label-free visual assay for the detection and quantification of viral RNA using peptide nucleic acid (PNA) and gold nanoparticles (AuNPs)." *Analytica Chimica Acta* 795 (2013), 1–7.

Kaihatsu, Kunihiro, Shinjiro Sawada, and Nobuo Kato. "Rapid identification of swine-origin influenza A virus by peptide nucleic acid chromatography." *Journal of Antivirals & Antiretrovirals* 5, no. 4 (2013), 80–84.

Karash, Sardar, Ronghui Wang, Lisa Kelso, Huaguang Lu, Tony J. Huang, and Yanbin Li. "Rapid detection of avian influenza virus H5N1 in chicken tracheal samples using an impedance aptasensor with gold nanoparticles for signal amplification." *Journal of Virological Methods* 236 (2016), 147–156.

Kim, Sang H., Junho Lee, Bang H. Lee, Chang-Seon Song, and Man B. Gu. "Specific detection of avian influenza H5N2 whole virus particles on lateral flow strips using a pair of sandwich-type aptamers." *Biosensors and Bioelectronics* 134 (2019), 123–129.

Kumar, Naveen, Sandeep Bhatia, Richa Sood, Atul K. Pateriya, and Yashpal S. Malik. "Immunoinformatics: where immunology meets bioinformatics." *Journal of Immunology and Immunopathology* 21, no. 2 (2019), 55.

Kumar, Naveen, Sandeep Bhatia, Atul K. Pateriya, Richa Sood, S. Nagarajan, Harshad V. Murugkar, Satish Kumar, Praveen Singh, and Vijendra P. Singh. "Label-free peptide nucleic acid biosensor for visual detection of multiple strains of influenza A virus suitable for field applications." *Analytica Chimica Acta* 1093 (2020), 123–130.

Kumar, Naveen, Yashpal S. Malik, Satish Kumar, Kuldeep Sharma, Subhankar Sircar, Sharad Saurabh, Baldev R. Gulati, *et al.* "Peptide-recombinant VP6 protein based enzyme immunoassay for the detection of group A rotaviruses in multiple host species." *PLoS One* 11, no. 7 (2016b), e0159027.

Kumar, Naveen, Yashpal S. Malik, Satish Kumar, Arvind Kumar, Kuldeep Sharma, Subhankar Sircar, and Kuldeep Dhama. "Identification of immune-dominant epitopes within bovine rotavirus VP6 protein by synthetic peptide approach." *Journal of Pure and Applied Microbiology* 10 (2016a), 447–450.

Lavu, Padma S., Bhairab Mondal, Shylaja Ramlal, Harishchandra S. Murali, and Harsh V. Batra. "Selection and characterization of aptamers using a modified whole cell bacterium SELEX for the detection of *Salmonella enterica serovar typhimurium*." *ACS Combinatorial Science* 18, no. 6 (2016), 292–301.

Lee, Sang-Hee, Ji-Young Ahn, Kyeong-Ah Lee, Hyun-Ju Um, Simranjeet S. Sekhon, Tae Sun Park, Jiho Min, and Yang-Hoon Kim. "Analytical bioconjugates, aptamers, enable specific quantitative detection of Listeria monocytogenes." *Biosensors and Bioelectronics* 68 (2015), 272–280.

Liu, Yufeng, Hongpan Xu, Chang Liu, Lijun Peng, Haroon Khan, Lunbiao Cui, Rui Huang, *et al.* "CRISPR-Cas13a nanomachine based simple technology for avian influenza A (H7N9) virus on-site detection." *Journal of Biomedical Nanotechnology* 15, no. 4 (2019), 790–798.

Loessner, Martin J., Catherine E.D. Rees, Gordon S.A.B. Stewart, and Siegfried Scherer. "Construction of luciferase reporter bacteriophage A511::luxAB for rapid and sensitive detection of viable *Listeria* cells." *Applied and Environmental Microbiology* 62, no. 4 (1996), 1133–1140.

Ma, Duo, Luhui Shen, Kaiyue Wu, Chris W. Diehnelt, and Alexander A. Green. "Low-cost detection of norovirus using paper-based cell-free systems and synbody-based viral enrichment." *Synthetic Biology* 3, no. 1 (2018), ysy018.

Ma, Fanshu, Lei Zhang, Yang Wang, Rongguang Lu, Bo Hu, Shuang Lv, Xianghong Xue, *et al.* "Development of a Peptide ELISA for the Diagnosis of Aleutian Mink Disease." *PLoS One* 11, no. 11 (2016), e0165793.

Mach, Kathleen E., Aniruddha M. Kaushik, Kuangwen Hsieh, Pak K. Wong, Tza-Huei Wang, and Joseph C. Liao. "Optimizing peptide nucleic acid probes for hybridization-based detection and identification of bacterial pathogens." *The Analyst* 144, no. 5 (2019), 1565–1574.

Makarova, Kira S., Yuri I. Wolf, Jaime Iranzo, Sergey A. Shmakov, Omer S. Alkhnbashi, Stan J. Brouns, Emmanuelle Charpentier, *et al.* "Evolutionary classification of CRISPR–Cas systems: a burst of class 2 and derived variants." *Nature Reviews Microbiology* 18, no. 2 (2019), 67–83.

Maleki, Leili A., Jafar Majidi, Behzad Baradaran, Jalal Abdolalizadeh, and Aliakbar M. Akbari. "Production and characterization of murine monoclonal antibody against synthetic peptide of CD34." *Human Antibodies* 22, no. 1–2 (2013), 1–8.

Metz, Germán E., Esteban N. Lorenzón, María S. Serena, Santiago G. Corva, Carlos J. Panei, Silvina Díaz, Eduardo M. Cilli, and María G. Echeverría. "Development of a peptide ELISA for the diagnosis of Equine arteritis virus." *Journal of Virological Methods* 205 (2014), 3–6.

Mosier-Boss, Pamela A., Stephe H. Lieberman, John M. Andrews, Forest L. Rohwer, Linda E. Wegley, and Mya Breitbart. "Use of fluorescently labeled phage in the detection and identification of bacterial species." *Applied Spectroscopy* 57, no. 9 (2003), 1138–1144.

Myhrvold, Cameron, Catherine A. Freije, Jonathan S. Gootenberg, Omar O. Abudayyeh, Hayden C. Metsky, Ann F. Durbin, Max J. Kellner, *et al.* "Field-deployable viral diagnostics using CRISPR-Cas13." *Science* 360, no. 6387 (2018), 444–448.

Naves, João H., Fernanda G. Oliveira, Juliana M. Bicalho, Paula S. Santos, Ricardo A. Machado-de-Ávila, Carlos Chavez-Olortegui, Rômulo C. Leite, and Jenner K. Reis. "Serological diagnosis of equine infectious anemia in horses, donkeys and mules using an ELISA with a gp45 synthetic peptide as antigen." *Journal of Virological Methods* 266 (2019), 49–57.

Oda, Masahito, Masatomo Morita, Hajime Unno, and Yasunori Tanji. "Rapid detection of *Escherichia coli* O157:H7 by using green fluorescent protein-labeled PP01 bacteriophage." *Applied and Environmental Microbiology* 70, no. 1 (2004), 527–534.

Pardee, Keith, Alexander A. Green, Tom Ferrante, D. Ewen Cameron, Ajay DaleyKeyser, Peng Yin, and James J. Collins. "Paper-based synthetic gene networks." *Cell* 159, no. 4 (2014), 940–954.

Pardee, Keith, Alexander A. Green, Melissa K. Takahashi, Dana Braff, Guillaume Lambert, Jeong W. Lee, Tom Ferrante, *et al.* "Rapid, low-cost detection of Zika virus using programmable biomolecular components." *Cell* 165, no. 5 (2016), 1255–1266.

Park, Ji-Young, Seong-Hee Kim, Kyoung-Ki Lee, Yeon-Hee Kim, Bo-Yeon Moon, ByungJae So, and Choi-Kyu Park. "Differential detection of porcine reproductive and respiratory syndrome virus genotypes by a fluorescence melting curve analysis using peptide nucleic acid probe-mediated one-step real-time RT-PCR." *Journal of Virological Methods* 267 (2019), 29–34.

Peng, Zhihui, Min Ling, Yi Ning, and Le Deng. "Rapid fluorescent detection of *Escherichia coli* K88 based on DNA aptamer library as direct and specific reporter combined with immuno-magnetic separation." *Journal of Fluorescence* 24, no. 4 (2014), 1159–1168.

Plagemann, Peter G. "Peptide ELISA for measuring antibodies to N-protein of porcine reproductive and respiratory syndrome virus." *Journal of Virological Methods* 134, no. 1–2 (2006), 99–118.

Posnett David N., Helen McGrath, and James P. Tam. "A novel method for producing anti-peptide antibodies. Production of site-specific antibodies to the T cell antigen receptor beta-chain." *Journal of Biological Chemistry* 263 (1988), 1719–1725.

Ripp, Steven, Patricia Jegier, Courtney M. Johnson, Jennifer R. Brigati, and Gary S. Sayler. "Bacteriophage-amplified bioluminescent sensing of Escherichia coli O157:H7." *Analytical and Bioanalytical Chemistry* 391, no. 2 (2008), 507–514.

Sachse, Konrad, Kh. S. Rahman, Christiane Schnee, Elke Müller, Madlen Peisker, Thomas Schumacher, Evelyn Schubert, Anke Ruettger, Bernhard Kaltenboeck, and Ralf Ehricht. "A novel synthetic peptide microarray assay detects Chlamydia species-specific antibodies in animal and human sera." *Scientific Reports* 8, no. 1 (2018), 4701.

Saravanan, Ponnusamy, Satish Kumar, and J.M. Kataria. "Use of multiple antigenic peptides related to antigenic determinants of infectious bursal disease virus (IBDV) for detection of anti-IBDV-specific antibody in ELISA—quantitative comparison with native antigen for their use in serodiagnosis." *Journal of Immunological Methods* 293, no. 1–2 (2004b), 61–70.

Saravanan, Ponnusamy, Satish Kumar, J.M. Kataria, and Thaha Jamal Rasool. "Detection of Infectious bursal disease virus by ELISA using an antipeptide antibody raised against VP3 region." *Acta Virologica* 48, no. 1 (2004a), 39–45.

Schofield, David A., Ian J. Molineux, and Caroline Westwater. "Diagnostic bioluminescent phage for detection of *Yersinia pestis*." *Journal of Clinical Microbiology* 47, no. 12 (2009), 3887–3894.

Schofield, David A. and Caroline Westwater. "Phage-mediated bioluminescent detection of Bacillus anthracis." *Journal of Applied Microbiology* 107, no. 5 (2009), 1468–1478.

Sepehr, Koushan S., Behzad Baradaran, Jafar Majidi, Jalal Abdolalizadeh, Leili Aghebati, and Fatemeh Z. Shahneh. "Development and characterization of monoclonal antibodies against human CD20 in Balb/c mice." *Human Antibodies* 21, no. 3–4 (2013), 57–64.

Slomovic, Shimyn, Keith Pardee, and James J. Collins. "Synthetic biology devices for in vitro and in vivo diagnostics." *Proceedings of the National Academy of Sciences* 112, no. 47 (2015), 14429–14435.

Stoltenburg, Regina, Christine Reinemann, and Beate Strehlitz. "SELEX—A (r)evolutionary method to generate high-affinity nucleic acid ligands." *Biomolecular Engineering* 24, no. 4 (2007), 381–403.

Tam, James P. "Synthetic peptide vaccine design: synthesis and properties of a high-density multiple antigenic peptide system." *Proceedings of the National Academy of Sciences* 85, no. 15 (1988), 5409–5413.

Tasbasi, B. B., Buket C. Guner, Mert Sudagidan, Samet Ucak, Murat Kavruk, and Veli C. Ozalp. "Label-free lateral flow assay for *Listeria monocytogenes* by aptamer-gated release of signal molecules." *Analytical Biochemistry* 587 (2019), 113449.

Thouand, Gerald, Patricia Vachon, Shiliang Liu, Marcelle Dayre, and Mansel William Griffiths. "Optimization and validation of a simple method using P22::luxAB bacteriophage for rapid detection of *Salmonella enterica* serotypes A, B, and D in poultry samples." *Journal of Food Protection* 71, no. 2 (2008), 380–385.

To, Andrew C., David H. Chu, Angela R. Wang, Frances C. Li, Alan W. Chiu, Daisy Y. Gao, Chung H. Choi, *et al.* "A comprehensive web tool for toehold switch design." *Bioinformatics* 34, no. 16 (2018), 2862–2864.

Trier, Nicole H. and Gunnar Houen. "Peptide antibodies in clinical laboratory diagnostics." *Advances in Clinical Chemistry* (2017), 43–96.

Tseng, Yi-Ting, Chih-Hung Wang, Chih-Peng Chang, and Gwo-Bin Lee. "Integrated microfluidic system for rapid detection of influenza H1N1 virus using a sandwich-based aptamer assay." *Biosensors and Bioelectronics* 82 (2016), 105–111.

Wang, Xinjie, Pinpin Ji, Huiying Fan, Lu Dang, Wenwei Wan, Siyuan Liu, Yanhua Li, *et al.* "CRISPR/Cas12a technology combined with immunochromatographic strips for portable detection of African swine fever virus." *Communications Biology* 3, no. 1 (2020), 62.

Yang, Ji-fei, Su-zhen Yang, Yan-yan Yang, Ai-min Zhi, Dong Zhao, Yu-bao Zhi, Guang-xu Xing, Rui-guang Deng, Shu-jun Chai, and Gai-ping Zhang. "Development of a synthetic peptide ELISA assay for the detection of foot-and-mouth disease virus nonstructural protein antibodies." *Agricultural Sciences in China* 9, no. 11 (2010), 1677–1683.

Zhang, Guo-Rui, Rui-Song Yu, Jiang-Yong Zeng, Yu-Min Zhu, Shi-Juan Dong, Luobu Dunzhu, Se Zhu, Ciren Duoji, Zhi-Hai Lei, and Zhen Li. "Development of an epitope-based competitive ELISA for the detection of antibodies against Tibetan peste des petits ruminants virus." *Intervirology* 56, no. 1 (2013), 55–59.

14

Recent Trends in Diagnosis of Campylobacter *Infection*

Pooja Choudhary,[1] Aruna Punia,[1] Sweety Dahiya,[1] Namita Sharma,[1] Meenakshi Balhara,[1] Mehak Dangi[2] and Anil Kumar Chhillar[1]
[1] *Centre for Biotechnology, Maharshi Dayanand University, Rohtak-124001, Haryana, India*
[2] *Centre for Bioinformatics, Maharshi Dayanand University, Rohtak-124001, Haryana, India*
Corresponding author: Anil Kumar Chhillar, *anil.chhillar@gmail.com*

14.1 Introduction

Zoonotic diseases are a classification of infectious disease that spreads from animals to humans by various pathogens such as viruses, bacteria and fungus. The majority of animals associated with these diseases are vertebrates. Zoonotic diseases are estimated as a significant human health concern globally, as more than 60% of human pathogens have zoonotic pedigree (WHO, 2011). Viruses and bacteria are more prominent zoonotic functionaries as compared to other microbes as they are readily transmitted from the day-to-day, routine interactions of humans and animals.

Campylobacteriosis is a zoonotic disease for which *Campylobacter* bacteria is responsible. These bacteria are extensively present in nature with a global existence and are capable of colonizing at mucosal surfaces, so the intestines of avian and mammalian species are the most common site of occurrence. In recent years, these microorganisms have caught more and more attention from researchers as a causative agent of anything from gastroenteritis to Guillain-Barre syndrome (Levin, 2007; Lindmark *et al.*, 2009; WHO, 2011; Kirkpatrick and Tribble, 2011). Lately, the relevance of *Campylobacter* as a diarrhoeagenic agent in human beings has attained more consideration. Thermophilic *Campylobacter* species are known to cause foodborne infections and *Campylobacter jejuni* has been the most regularly reported (80–90%) causative agent (Food Net, 2012). Surveys conducted in various regions of the globe have suggested that the incidence rate is about 70% in sheep, cattle and pigs, whereas it is 100% in chickens (Food Net, 2012). Poultry are the largest carriers of *Campylobacter* bacteria, especially *Campylobacter jejuni*, while pigs are the most remarkable source of *Campylobacter coli*.

14.2 Morphological Characteristics of *Campylobacter*

Members of the *Campylobacter* genus are non-spore-forming, gram-negative and shaped as a spirally curved rod of small size, ranging from 0.5 to 5 µm in length and 0.2 to 0.9 µm in width (Silva *et al.*, 2011), but *Campylobacter gracilis* and *Campylobacter hominis* are straight rods. Most of them are motile via a polar unsheathed flagellum attached at one or both the ends of the bacteria. The exceptions to this phenomenon are *Campylobacter showae*, with its five unipolar flagella, and *Campylobacter gracilis*, without a single flagellum, due to which it is non-motile (Debruyne *et al.*, 2008). Their motion is darting and rapid, such that *Campylobacter* spin about their long axis in a corkscrew-like manner. Due to their minute structure and great motility, *Campylobacter* species are easily capable of passing through membrane filters ranging from 0.45 to 0.65 µm. This property is utilized for the isolation of *Campylobacter* species from experimental trials (Steele and McDermott, 1984; Bolton *et al.*, 1988).

14.3 Pathogenesis of *Campylobacter*

Out of 34 species and 14 subspecies of *Campylobacter*, four species have the most zoonotic significance (*Campylobacter jejuni*, *Campylobacter coli*, *Campylobacter upsaliensis* and *Campylobacter fetus*). Contaminated environment, food, semen, water and pieces of equipment are key sources of its transmission. Widespread isolation reports are available from sheep, cattle, swine and dogs (Kumar *et al.*, 2012a, 2012b), horses, mice, cats and from avian species (quails, turkeys, psittacines, passerines, pigeons, waterfowl etc.) (Jay-Russell *et al.*, 2012). Isolation reports from wild animals (Cape hyrax, llama, chimpanzee, orangutan, Japanese macaque, African elephant and gorilla) are also available. In poultry, the isolation rate is observed to be as high as 90–100% but, on average, it is estimated that around the world 50% of poultry meat is contaminated with *Campylobacter*.

At present, *Campylobacter* is acknowledged as one of the most prevalent causes of illness associated with bacteria, responsible for various diseases, such as early embryonic mortality, abortion, diarrhoea and infertility (Doyle and Erickson, 2006). *Campylobacter* is a key factor of gastroenteritis all over the world; the Netherlands reports around 59,000 cases annually (Kemmeren *et al.*, 2006) and more than 50,000 cases of *Campylobacter* were detected in Wales and England in 1997 (CDSC, 1998). In the United States, the *Campylobacter* species affects 1.5 million people each year (CDC, 2019a). In a recent outbreak in Spain, multidrug-resistant *Campylobacter jejuni* caused diarrhoea in 30 people, with the source of the infection attributed to dogs (CDC, 2019b). Human beings suffering from campylobacteriosis exhibit symptoms such as abdominal cramps, watery or bloody diarrhoea and nausea (Blaser and Engberg, 2008), and in some cases it results in potentially life-threatening complications like arthritis, Guillain-Barre syndrome, abortion, meningitis, haemolytic uremic syndrome etc. In developing countries, there is the chance that many cases may not be detected and, accordingly, it has now become a great concern of food safety agencies that *Campylobacter* should be controlled in the food chain.

14.4 Diagnosis of *Campylobacter* Infection (Campylobacteriosis)

As an essential part of any disease prevention and control strategy, quick and confirmatory diagnosis of the initial clinical infection is required. For *Campylobacter*, diagnosis is of particular importance, since its symptoms match with two other important foodborne pathogens, viz. *Salmonella* and pathogenic *Escherichia*. Diagnosis of *Campylobacter* is generally based on cultural isolation/identification of the causative agent, biochemical characterization and the employment of recent molecular tools and techniques (Sails *et al.*, 2003a; Persson and Olsen 2005; Al-Amri *et al.*, 2007; Lindmark *et al.*, 2009; Wassenaar *et al.*, 2009; Ahmed *et al.*, 2012; Eberle and Kiess, 2012). Preliminary identification is carried out by microscopic examination of stained smears for characteristic morphology and observing typical motility patterns using phase-contrast microscopy, or using a hanging drop method to keenly observe curved or spiral-shaped slender rods exhibiting corkscrew-like motility. This primary testing is followed by biochemical testing that confirms the genus and species of isolates. Molecular techniques of PCR, RFLP, RAPD, multiplex PCR, real-time PCR, PFGE, ALFP, MLST and others are being utilized for diagnostic and typing purposes.

14.4.1 Conventional Methods for Detection of the Pathogen

14.4.1.1 Direct Demonstration of the Pathogen

The organism can be identified by its characteristic morphology and motility pattern in fresh semen/vaginal/mucal/faecal/stool samples using phase-contrast/dark-field microscopy (with phase-contrast microscopy usually being preferred). Microscopical examination is done by mixing a small amount of sample material with saline; the prepared smear is stained with 1% carbol-fuchsin, which leads to the observation of all the different shapes of cells (comma-shaped, gull-wing-shaped, curved, C-shaped and long spiral).

14.4.1.2 Culture and Identification

Campylobacter species are sensitive to oxidizing radicals and oxygen, making it important to develop a selective media that comprises of one or more oxygen scavengers, like pyruvate, ferrous, iron, blood and selective agents such as antibiotics in particular. *Campylobacter* requires a microaerophilic atmosphere that contains 3–5% oxygen, 85% nitrogen and 10% carbon dioxide for optimal growth and some species require hydrogen. Before plating on agar, most procedures incorporate some sort of pre-enrichment in a liquid medium. Corry *et al.* (1995) have given a detailed account of the advancements of procedures for *Campylobacter*. *Campylobacter* can be isolated from faecal samples via plating on selective media or purification techniques using non-selective agar. Also, augmentation may be incorporated for increasing the culture sensitivity of naturally stained bacteria, or if the concentration of bacteria is low in the faeces/semen of domestic and pet animals.

14.4.1.3 Selective Media for Campylobacter *Isolation*

The recovery of *Campylobacter* species can be carried out using a variety of media and the selective media for *Campylobacter* may be bifurcated into two groups: charcoal-based media and blood-based media. Both charcoal and blood constituents are useful in removing oxygen derivatives. Antibiotics used in selective media determine the selectivity of the media. Some of the antibiotics used include cephalosporins (cefoperazone), trimethoprim, vancomycin, cycloheximide (actidione) and amphotericin B. A notable characteristic of all available selective agents is that they allow growth of both *Campylobacter*

TABLE 14.1

Selective media for Campylobacter cultivation

Sr. No.	Blood-Containing-Media	Charcoal-Containing-Media
1	Preston-Agar	mCCDA (modified-charcoal-cefoperazone-deoxycholate-agar) a little improved variety of original CCDA
2	Skirrow-Agar	Karmali-Agar or CSM (charcoal-selective-medium)
3	Butzler-Agar	CAT-Agar (cefoperazone-amphotericin-teicoplanin) for the growth of Campylobacter upsaliensis
4	Campy-Cefex	

jejuni and *Campylobacter coli* and none of the existing media can distinguish between these two species. The use of two or more media has been suggested to increase the chances of *Campylobacter* detection from samples compared to the use of a single medium and a few additional supplements (Oyarzabal *et al.*, 2005). Also, it should be noted that other *Campylobacter* species (e.g., *Campylobacter hyointestinalis*, *Campylobacter helveticus*, *Campylobacter lari*, *Campylobacter fetus* and *Campylobacter upsaliensis*) can be grown on the medium for more to less extent, and growth is more probable on a less-selective temperature range of 37°C.

A few examples of selective blood-containing media and charcoal-containing media for the culturing of *Campylobacter* are listed in Table 14.1.

14.4.2 Confirmation of *Campylobacter*

Generally, any bacteria are confirmed after isolating them in pure culture, but preliminary confirmation of *Campylobacter* is done by microscopic examination of a suspected colony sample. *Campylobacter* is a gram-negative, non-spore-forming, thermophilic, microaerobic spiral- or S-shaped bacterium. These organisms are oxidase-/catalase-positive and do not ferment carbohydrates, grow optimally at a pH between 6.5 and 7.5 and are more sensitive to hostile conditions than *Salmonella* and *Escherichia coli*.

14.4.2.1 Colony Characteristics

Colonies typically appear after two to four days and are smoothly circular (usually of 1 mm diameter), slightly raised, grey-coloured and glistening. If *Campylobacter* is grown on Skirrow agar or other supplementary blood-containing agars, then its colonies appear slightly pink, circular, convex, smooth and shiny, while on charcoal-based media like mCCDA, the colonies are greyish, even, moistened, with or without a metallic lustre and have a tendency to spread across the plate.

14.4.2.2 Enzyme Immune Assays

Enzyme immune assays (EIA) such as Premier CAMPY assay (Meridian) and ProsSpecT *Campylobacter* Microplate (Remel) are available that take about 2.5 hours to perform but are accessible only for the recognition of *Campylobacter* in human stool samples. Similarly, lateral-flow assays like Immunocard STAT! CAMPY (Meridian) and the Xpect *Campylobacter* assay (Remel) are also available that take about 20 minutes to perform, but with the same limitation. The immune-based methodology for the identification of foodborne pathogens is well-known and comprises of enzyme-linked immunosorbent assays (ELISA), flow cytometry and quantitative immunofluorescence (Yolken, 1982; Maciorowski *et al.*, 2006; Baker *et al.*, 2016; Alahi and Mukhopadhyay, 2017). To increase specificity and sensitivity of these immune-based assays, monoclonal and polyclonal antibodies are used (Yolken, 1982; Preiner *et al.*, 2014; Alahi and Mukhopadhyay, 2017); these generally targeted epitopes include lipopolysaccharides, flagellin and many more protein antigens (Nachamkin and Hart, 1986; Lamoureux *et al.*, 1997). A well-known example is demonstrated by Nachamkin and Hart (1986); in their work they concluded the production of murine monoclonal antibodies for one of two different *Campylobacter* flagellin epitopes, which then became able to detect *Campylobacter* species and also distinguish *Campylobacter jejuni* or *Campylobacter coli*.

14.4.3 Molecular Tools and Techniques for *Campylobacter* Diagnosis

Molecular approaches for the identification and detection of foodborne pathogens are highly specific and sensitive. These techniques exploit genetic-level information which is continuously increasing day by day (Gharst *et al.*, 2013; Park *et al.*, 2014; Baker *et al.*, 2016). These diagnostic techniques are the most advanced, cost-efficient and time-efficient, for example, mPCR, RT-PCR etc.

Molecular tools include phenotypic methods (which exploit the metabolites which are expressed via bacteria) and genotypic methods (which use tools like PCR and electrophoresis and detect specific genes found in particular bacteria).

14.4.3.1 Phenotypic Methods

The phenotypic methods used in the discrimination of *Campylobacter* species comprise mainly of bio-typing and phage-typing. Even though they have a low power of discrimination, they are still in use and are moderately competent for the characterization of foodborne bacterial pathogens (Wiedmann, 2002).

14.4.3.1.1 Bio-typing

Campylobacter jejuni and *Campylobacter coli* can be grouped into extensive groups via bio-typing. This scheme is constructed on the idea of the detection of bacteria via their expression of metabolic activities, the morphological characteristics of the colony, environmental tolerances or bio-chemical reactions (Vandenberg *et al.*, 2006; Eberle and Kiess, 2012). This technique includes methods like hippurate hydrolysis tests and indoxyl acetate hydrolysis tests.

Hippurate hydrolysis test. *Campylobacter jejuni* can be differentiated from other *Campylobacter* species by a hippurate hydrolysis test because only *Campylobacter jejuni* is hippurate-positive among all *Campylobacter* species. Nowadays, commercia hippurate hydrolysis test disks are available from various manufacturers. However, the distinction of *Campylobacter jejuni* and *Campylobacter coli* by hippurate hydrolysis testing (Barrett *et al.*, 1988) is not always accurate (Nicholson and Patton, 1993); Steinhauserová *et al.* in 2001 also reported the incidence of hippurate-negative *Campylobacter jejuni*, which poses a difficulty in differentiation with this test.

Indoxyl acetate hydrolysis test. This test is based on the principle of the release of the indoxyl group of indoxyl acetate after its reaction with bacterial esterase. This method is used for the detection of *Campylobacter* and its related genera (Mills and Gherna, 1987). The bacteria hydrolyze the indoxyl acetate within five to ten minutes and it is indicated by the appearance of a dark-blue colour.

14.4.3.1.2 Phage-typing

Phage-typing is a method in which bacteriophages are used to detect a specific strain of bacteria in a single species. It depends on the principle that one type of bacteriophage infects one type of bacterium and consumes it. It is generally used in addition with serotyping for the characterization of *Campylobacter jejuni* (Grajewski *et al.*, 1985). This method uses a virulent phage on a bacterial host regardless of any kind of receptor for adhesion. When the phage is able to attach to the cell to cause infection in the bacteria, the phage disrupts the bacterial cell by following a characteristic pattern of lysis in the culture, a condition referred to as 'plaque' formation (Grajewski *et al.*, 1985). Similar to with serotyping, due to the presence of cross-reactivity the use of phage-typing is also restricted (Sails *et al.*, 2003b).

14.4.3.2 Genotyping Methods

Genotyping methods are mainly differentiated into two main groups: macro-restriction-mediated analyses and PCR methods.

14.4.3.2.1 Macro-restriction-mediated Analyses

Multilocus enzyme electrophoresis (MLEE). In this technique, a bacterial isolate is differentiated based on variations found among the electrophoretic mobility in different constitutive enzymes under non-denaturing environments (Wiedmann, 2002). The mobilities of enzymes are directly related to the mutations (Aeschbacher and Piffaretti, 1989). Using these benefits of MLEE, it can be used for epidemiological studies of *Campylobacter* outbreaks.

Multilocus sequence typing (MLST). MLST is frequently used in studies of population biology, epidemiological investigations and the pathogenic evolution of bacteria (Noormohamed and Fakhr, 2014). In this technique, first cDNA is amplified and then these amplified sequences are compared. Sequences that are found to be exactly the same are assigned the same allele number and vice versa (Maiden *et al.*, 1998). MLST has often been used to characterize *Campylobacter* species in milk, pork, duck, chicken and beef.

14.4.3.2.2 Polymerase Chain Reaction (PCR)-based Assays

Most genotypic techniques are based on polymerase chain reaction (PCR) since it is specific, quick and cost-effective (Asakura *et al.*, 2017). PCR transforms epidemiological studies at the molecular level; it is versatile and can detect the occurrence and non-occurrence of an organism in any kind of sample via recognizing a gene which is exclusive and specific for the pathogen of interest (Mohan, 2011). Several variations of the PCR technique have been developed and are in use for the detection of *Campylobacter* species, including RT-PCR, multiplex-PCR and QRT-PCR. To increase the specificity of PCR, it can also be combined with enzyme immunoassay (EIA) (Eberle and Kiess, 2012; Park *et al.*, 2014). Basically, monoplex-PCR, which was used in the past for the detection and distinction of *Campylobacter* species, has now been substituted by multiplex-PCR for a synchronized distinction of *Campylobacter* species (Asakura *et al.*, 2017).

Amplified length polymorphism (AFLP) and random amplified polymorphic DNA analysis (RAPD) are other two PCR-based techniques which are used for *Campylobacter* genotyping that provide a moral discriminatory power. However, due to some limitations, these techniques cannot be used successfully in routine genotyping (Mohan, 2011). On *et al.* (2013) highlighted that it is indeed necessary to revalidate the already-present PCR methods for *Campylobacter jejuni* and *Campylobacter coli* for the confirmation of strain specificity, and to avoid incorrect detection when a new species of *Campylobacter* is detected.

Multiplex PCR. This is a rapid and trustworthy process for the determination of the occurrence and non-occurrence of multiple gene targets in a sample that discriminates at both species and subspecies level. Zhao *et al.* (2001) screened various *Campylobacter* isolates extracted from chicken, turkey, pork and beef by using mPCR and efficiently discriminated *Campylobacter jejuni* and *Campylobacter coli*; but a residual *Campylobacter* species isn't confirmed by multiplex-PCR. Like immune-based techniques, it does not have any complications in the determination of cognate strains.

Real-time quantitative PCR (qPCR). This was developed for the mutual determination of *Campylobacter* between various samples. Park *et al.* (2011) analyzed numerous water samples by utilizing multiple melting temperatures for the quantification of *Campylobacter jejuni* (80.1°C), *Escherichia coli* (83.3°C) and *Salmonella* (85.9°C) in one reaction. qPCR and culturing techniques show a visible drop in the living cell count in a spiked watershed sample after cold treatment at 4°C for seven days. This method avoids the duplicity of results and 100%-positive results were detected.

Digital PCR (dPCR). Baker (2012) described that dPCR uses a segment of negative replicates to find a complete sequence of gene targets which is calculated using the Poisson statistical algorithm. This can be done by separation of the sample into small fragments. The result of positive versus negative reactions tells the accurate copy number for a special gene in one sample, whereas qPCR tracks fluorescence during the process; consequently, dPCR is expressively particular and more specific than qPCR.

14.4.3.2.3 Ribotyping

There are multiple copies of rRNA gene loci (5S, 16S and 23S rRNA) that are found at several positions in different bacteria; these regions are highly conserved sequences and have highly variable flanking non-coding sequences which are used for the subtyping of various bacteria as well as *Campylobacter*. This technique is used for genotyping as well as identifying the evolutionary relationship between bacterial isolates, by using agarose gel electrophoresis and southern blot hybridization. However, there is a drawback of ribotyping in *Campylobacter* species, which is that it contains only three copies of rRNA gene, so it is not able to differentiate between several other *Campylobacter* species such as *Campylobacter fetus* subspecies *fetus* and *Campylobacter fetus* subspecies *venerealis* (Denes *et al.* 1997). The relatively low discriminatory power of ribotyping and the elaborative nature of the technique make it a relatively unsuitable method for routine genotyping.

14.4.3.2.4 Fla-typing

Fla-typing is a simple and cost-effective technique of *Campylobacter* identification which can distinguish many strains of *Campylobacter* species, including *Campylobacter lari* strains, *Campylobacter coli* strains, *Campylobacter helveticus*, and *Campylobacter jejuni* subspecies *doylei*. Fla-typing is a reliable and relatively simple diagnostic technique but there are drawbacks, like the various protocols for different strains, and this makes it less user-friendly for certain laboratories.

14.4.4 Metagenomics as a Diagnostic Tool

Metagenomics is a commanding, significant and valuable tool for decrepitation of the diversity and dynamic of microbes such as bacteria, viruses and fungus in tissues and samples from different animals/humans. This approach is used as a substitute for the sequencing of the genomes of different microbiota. Nowadays, metagenomics approaches are gaining importance in clinical studies with diagnostic purposes. Metagenomics and highly sensitive sequencing methodology allow an increase in studies related to zoonotic diseases like *Campylobacter* and other microbes in animals/humans. Conventional diagnostics of *Campylobacter* recognizes species, strains and serotypes of curiosity in independent colonies through the isolation of *Campylobacter*. These methodologies can produce millions of small sequences (150 bp) and enable their scrutiny because they are culture-independent so no cloning procedure is required. The two main and important ranges in metagenomics are structural and functional metagenomics.

14.4.4.1 Structural Metagenomics

Structural metagenomics includes the study of the conformation of microbiomes and groups which describes the classes and types of implementation in tissues of organisms. It also offers applicable shreds of evidence about the ecological niches of microorganisms and hypothesizes about relations among pathogens, hosts and native microbiomes.

14.4.4.2 Functional Metagenomics

Functional metagenomics is an attractive approach in diagnosis; as a result, some proteins can be perceived and identified in definite circumstances in precise tissues. The first step in metagenomics analysis is the extraction of high-quality DNA. A large quantity of bacterial DNA from human tissue or animal tissue is isolated and then microbiomes of *Campylobacter* are studied. Other studies of microbiomes such as metatranscriptomics, metaproteomics and lipidomics also have importance. High-throughput sequencing methods allow the attainment of a large sequencing database which includes genes, transcripts and proteins and allows the establishment of metabolic networks for the identification and understanding of host-pathogen relations. The techniques used in the detection of foodborne pathogens are fast, species-specific, accurate and efficient.

14.5 Conclusion and Future Perspectives

Campylobacteriosis has become the leading foodborne disease worldwide and is a major cause of disease in animals and birds. Cattle, pigs, dogs, cats, sheep, poultry and poultry products are the main source of infection to human beings, especially of *Campylobacter coli*, *Campylobacter jejuni* and *Campylobacter fetus*. Controlling campylobacteriosis in the food chain should be the primary objective for reducing human health hazards, which requires the development of innovative and sequential intervention strategies. Early and timely diagnosis of infection, along with effective biosecurity measures, proper hygiene and sanitation and suitable treatment, are important for the prevention and control of *Campylobacter*, and therefore a lot of effort is being put into achieving early diagnosis of human cases using a wide variety of direct and indirect detection methods along with specific identification tests. Epidemiological studies, particularly in outburst researches, are profited by developments in rapid diagnostics and molecular-level typing methods. Epidemiological investigations of campylobacteriosis outbreaks are increasingly being conducted using the innovative and constantly developing typing and subtyping systems available, providing evidence for the recognition of outbreaks of the disease and improving attempts to relate them with vectors for disease outbreaks. Safe food/water supply and the adaptation of good kitchen hygiene and proper cooking practices are helpful in reducing foodborne illness. Currently, there are no effective commercial vaccines available to control *Campylobacter* infection. No sole technique is perfect, and thus the development of a novel typing method that combines efficiency with efficacy, while overcoming the shortcomings of currently used methods, is considered crucial. Strengthening of the diagnostic facilities globally for this important pathogen is suggested, along with necessary R&D measures for the prevention and control of *Campylobacter* and their emerging zoonoses.

References

Aeschbacher, Martin and Jean-Claude Piffaretti. "Population genetics of human and animal enteric *Campylobacter* strains." *Infection and Immunity* 57 no.5 (1989): 1432–37.

Ahmed, Monir U., Louise Dunn and Elena P. Ivanova. "Evaluation of current molecular approaches for genotyping of *Campylobacter jejuni* strains." *Foodborne Pathogens and Disease* 9 no.5 (2012): 375–85.

Alahi, Md Eshrat E. and Subhas C. Mukhopadhyay. "Detection methodologies for pathogen and toxins: a review." *Sensors* 17 no.8 (2017): 1–20.

Al-Amri, Aisha, Abiola C. Senok, Abdulrahman Y. Ismaeel, Ali E. Al-Mahmeed and Giuseppe A. Botta. "Multiplex PCR for direct identification of *Campylobacter spp.* in human and chicken stools." *Journal of Medical Microbiology* 56 no.10 (2007): 1350–55.

Asakura, Hiroshi, Naoto Takahashi, Shiori Yamamoto and Hiroyuki Maruyama. "Draft genome sequence of *Campylobacter jejuni* CAM970 and *C. coli* CAM962, associated with a large outbreak of foodborne illness in Fukuoka, Japan, in 2016." *Genome Announcements* 5 no.24 (2017): e00508–17.

Baker, Christopher A., Peter M. Rubinelli, Si H. Park and Steven C. Ricke. "Immuno-based detection of shiga toxin-producing pathogenic *Escherichia coli*: a review on current approaches and potential strategies for optimization." *Journal Critical Reviews in Microbiology* 42 no.4 (2016): 656–75.

Baker, Monya. "Digital PCR hits its stride." *Nature Methods* 9 (2012): 541–4.

Barrett, Timothy J., Charlotte M. Patton and George K. Morris. "Differentiation of *Campylobacter* species using phenotypic characterization." *Lab Medicine* 19 no.2 (1988): 96–102.

Blaser, Martin J. and Jørgen Engberg. "Clinical aspects of *Campylobacter jejuni* and *Campylobacter coli* infections." In Nachamkin, Irvin, Christine M. Szymanski and Martin J. Blaser (eds), *Campylobacter* (Washington, DC: American Society for Microbiology Press, 3rd edn, 2008), 99–121.

Bolton, Frederick J., D.N. Hutchinson and G. Parker. "Reassessment of selective agars and filtration techniques for isolation of *Campylobacter* species from faeces." *European Journal of Clinical Microbiology & Infectious Diseases* 7 no.2 (1988): 155–60.

CDC. National Center for Emerging and Zoonotic Infectious Diseases (NCEZID), Division of Foodborne, Waterborne, and Environmental Diseases (DFWED). December 23, 2019a. www.cdc.gov/campylobacter/outbreaks/puppies-12-19/index.html.

CDC. "Outbreak of multidrug-resistant campylobacter infections linked to contact with pet store puppies." CDC, December 17, 2019b. www.cdc.gov/campylobacter/outbreaks/puppies-12-19/index.html.

CDSC. "Common gastrointestinal infections, England and Wales." *Communicable Disease Report* 8 (1998): 14.

Corry, Janet E.L., David E. Post, Pierre Colin and Marie J. Laisney. "Culture media for the isolation of campylobacters." *International Journal of Food Microbiology* 26 no.1 (1995): 43–76.

Debruyne, Lies, Dirk Gevers and Peter Vandamme. "Taxonomy of the family Campylobacteraceae." In Nachamkin, Irvin, Christine M. Szymanski and Martin J. Blaser (eds), *Campylobacter* (Washington, DC: American Society for Microbiology Press, 3rd edn, 2008), 3–25.

Denes, A.S., Cheryl L. Lutze-Wallace, Marianne L. Cormier and Manuel M. Garcia. "DNA fingerprinting of *Campylobacter fetus* using cloned constructs of ribosomal RNA and surface array protein genes." *Veterinary Microbiology* 54 no.2 (1997): 185–93.

Doyle, Michael P. and Marilyn C. Erickson. "Reducing the carriage of foodborne pathogens in livestock and poultry." *Poultry Science* 85 no.6 (2006): 960–73.

Eberle, Krista N. and Aaron S. Kiess. "Phenotypic and genotypic methods for typing *Campylobacter jejuni* and *Campylobacter coli* in poultry." *Poultry Science* 91 no.1 (2012): 255–64.

Gharst, Gregory, Omar A. Oyarzabal and Syeda K. Hussain. "Review of current methodologies to isolate and identify *Campylobacter* spp. from foods." *Journal of Microbiological Methods* 95 no.1 (2013): 84–92.

Grajewski, Barbara A., John W. Kusek and Henry M. Gelfand. "Development of a bacteriophage typing system for *Campylobacter jejuni* and *Campylobacter coli*." *Journal of Clinical Microbiology* 22 no.1 (1985): 13–18.

Jay-Russell, Michele T., Anna H. Bates, Leslie A. Harden, William G. Miller and Robert E. Mandrell. "Isolation of *Campylobacter* from feral swine (*Sus scrofa*) on the ranch associated with the 2006 *Escherichia coli* O157:H7 spinach outbreak investigation in California." *Zoonoses Public Health* 59 no.5 (2012): 314–19.

Kemmeren, Jeanet M., Marie-Josée J. Mangen, Yvonne T.H.P. van Duynhoven and Arie H. Havelaar. "Priority setting of foodborne pathogens." *Rijksinstituut voor Volksgezondheid en Milieu (RIVM)*. Report (2006).

Kirkpatrick, Beth and David Tribble. "Update on human *Campylobacter jejuni* infections." *Current Opinion Gastroenterology* 27 no.1 (2011): 1–7.

Kumar, Rajesh, Amit K. Verma, Amit Kumar, Mukesh Srivastava and H.P. Lal. "Prevalence of *Campylobacter sp.* in dogs attending veterinary practices at Mathura, India and risk indicators associated with shedding." *Asian Journal of Animal and Veterinary Advances* 7 no.8 (2012a): 754–60.

Kumar, Rajesh, Amit K. Verma, Amit Kumar, Mukesh Srivastava and H.P. Lal. "Prevalence and antibiogram of *Campylobacter* infections in dogs of Mathura, India." *Asian Journal of Animal and Veterinary Advances* 7 no.5 (2012b): 434–40.

Lamoureux, Maryse, Anna Mackay, Serge Messier *et al.* "Detection of *Campylobacter jejuni* in food and poultry viscera using immunomagnetic separation and microtitre hybridization." *Journal of Applied Microbiology* 83 no.5 (1997): 641–51.

Levin, Robert E. "*Campylobacter jejuni:* a review of its characteristics, pathogenicity, ecology, distribution, subspecies characterization and molecular methods of detection. *Food Biotechnology* 21 no.4 (2007): 271–347.

Lindmark, Barbro, Pramod K. Rompikuntal, Karolis Vaitkevicius *et al.* "Outer membrane vesicle-mediated release of cytolethal distending toxin (CDT) from *Campylobacter jejuni*." *BMC Microbiology* 9 (2009): 220.

Maciorowski, Kenneth G., Paul Herrera, Frank T. Jones, Suresh D. Pillai and Steve C. Ricke. "Cultural and immunological detection methods for detection of *Salmonella* spp. in animal feeds: a review." *Veterinary Research Communications* 30 no.2 (2006): 127–37.

Maiden, Martin C. J., Jane A. Bygraves, Edward Feil *et al.* "Multilocus sequence typing: a portable approach to the identification of clones within populations of pathogenic microorganisms." *Proceedings of the National Academy of Sciences of the United States of America* 95 no.6 (1998): 3140–5.

Mills, Charles K. and Robert L. Gherna. "Hydrolysis of indoxyl acetate by *Campylobacter* species." *Journal of Clinical Microbiology* 25 no.8 (1987): 1560–1.

Mohan, Vathsala. "Molecular epidemiology of campylobacteriosis and evolution of *Campylobacter jejuni* ST-474 in New Zealand: a thesis presented in partial fullfilment [sic] of the requirements for the degree of Doctor of Philosophy at Massey University, Institute of Veterinary, Animal and Biomedical Sciences, Massey University, Palmerston North, New Zealand." 2011.

Nachamkin, Irving and Andrea M. Hart. "Common and specific epitopes of *Campylobacter* flagellin recognized by monoclonal antibodies." *Infection and Immunity* 53 no.2 (1986): 438–40.

Nicholson, Mabel A. and Charlotte M. Patton. "Application of Lior biotyping by use of genetically identified *Campylobacter* strains." *Journal of Clinical Microbiology* 31 no.12 (1993): 3348–50.

Noormohamed, Aneesa and Mohamed K. Fakhr. "Molecular typing of *Campylobacter jejuni* and *Campylobacter coli* isolated from various retail meats by MLST and PFGE." *Foods* 3 no.1 (2014): 82–93.

On, Stephen L.W., Jørgen Brandt, Angela Cornelius *et al.* "PCR revisited: a case for revalidation of PCR assays for microorganisms using identification of *Campylobacter* species as an exemplar." *Quality Assurance Safety Crops Foods* 5 no.1 (2013): 49–62.

Oyarzabal, Omar, Ken Macklin, James M. Barbaree and Robert S. Miller. "Evaluation of agar plates for direct enumeration of *Campylobacter* spp. from poultry carcass rinses." *Applied and Environmental Microbiology* 71 no.6 (2005): 3351–4.

Park, Si H., Irene Hanning, Robin Jarquin *et al.* "Multiplex PCR assay for the detection and quantification of *Campylobacter* spp., *Escherichia coli* O157:H7, and *Salmonella* serotypes in water samples." *FEMS Microbiology Letters* 316 no.1 (2011): 7–15.

Park, Si H., Muhsin Aydin, Anita Khatiwara *et al.* "Current and emerging technologies for rapid detection and characterization of *Salmonella* in poultry and poultry products." *Food Microbiology* 38 (2014): 250–62.

Persson, Søren and Katharina E. P. Olsen. "Multiplex PCR for identification of *Campylobacter coli* and *Campylobacter jejuni* from pure cultures and directly on stool samples." *Journal of Medical Microbiology* 54 no.11 (2005): 1043–7.

Preiner, Johannes, Noriyuki Kodera, Jilin Tang *et al.* "IgGs are made for walking on bacterial and viral surfaces." *Nature Communications* 5 no.4394 (2014): 1–8.

Sails, Andrew D., Andrew J. Fox, Frederick J. Bolton, David R. A. Wareing and David L.A. Greenway. "A real-time PCR assay for the detection of *Campylobacter jejuni* in foods after enrichment culture." *Applied and Environmental Microbiology* 69 no.3 (2003a): 1383–90.

Sails, Andrew D., Bala Swaminathan and Patricia I. Fields. "Utility of multilocus sequence typing as an epidemiological tool for investigation of outbreaks of gastroenteritis caused by *Campylobacter jejuni*." *Journal of Clinical Microbiology* 41 no.10 (2003b): 4733–39.

Silva, Joana, Daniela Leite, Mariana Fernandes, Cristina Mena, Paul A. Gibbs and Paula Teixeira. "*Campylobacter* spp. as a foodborne pathogen: a review." *Frontiers in Microbiology* 2 (2011): 200.

Steele, Trevor W. and Sean N. McDermott. "The use of membrane filters applied directly to the surface of agar plates for the isolation of *Campylobacter jejuni* from feces." *Pathology* 16 no.3 (1984): 263–5.

Steinhauserová, Iva, J. Ceskova, Klára Fojtíková and Iveta Obrovská. "Identification of thermophilic *Campylobacter* spp. by phenotypic and molecular methods." *Journal of Applied Microbiology* 90 no.3 (2001): 470–5.

Vandenberg, Olivier, Kurt Houf, Nicole Douat *et al.* "Antimicrobial susceptibility of clinical isolates of non-*jejuni/coli* campylobacters and arcobacters from Belgium." *The Journal of Antimicrobial Chemotherapy* 57 no.5 (2006): 908–13.

Wassenaar, Trudy M., Aurora Fernández-Astorga, Rodrigo Alonso *et al.* "Comparison of *Campylobacter fla*-SVR genotypes isolated from humans and poultry in three European regions." *Letters in Applied Microbiology* 49 no.3 (2009): 388–95.

WHO. "Campylobacter Factsheet". World Health Organization, 2011. www.who.int/mediacentre/factsheets/fs255/en/index.html.

Wiedmann, Martin. "Subtyping of bacterial foodborne pathogens." *Nutrition Reviews* 60 no.7 Pt.1 (2002): 201–8.

Yolken, Robert H. "Enzyme immunoassays for the detection of infectious antigens in body fluids: current limitations and future prospects." *Reviews of Infectious Diseases* 4 no.1 (1982): 35–68.

Zhao, Cuiwei, Beilei Ge, Juan F. de Villena *et al.* "Prevalence of *Campylobacter* spp., *Escherichia coli*, and *Salmonella* serovars in retail chicken, turkey, pork, and beef from the greater Washington, D.C., area." *Applied and Environmental Microbiology* 67 no.12 (2001): 5431–6.

15

Recent Trends in Bovine Tuberculosis Detection and Control Methods

Monika
Department of Zoology, Government College Bahadurgarh, Jhajjar, Haryana
Corresponding author: Monika, joonmonika@gmail.com

15.1 Introduction

The World Organization for Animal Health (OIE) is an intergovernmental organization that is recognized by the World Trade Organization (WTO). It is responsible for the worldwide improvement of animal health and describes bTB as a chronic bacterial disease of animals with the etiological agents being members of the *Mycobacterium tuberculosis* complex, primarily *M. bovis*. bTB can practically affect many species of mammals by causing a general state of illness, coughing, and eventually death. Bovine TB is a contagious zoonotic disease that might potentially spread from infected animals to other animals and humans. bTB is not only a major infectious disease among cattle, but is also reported in many other domesticated, non-domesticated, and various wildlife species, including African buffaloes, bison, equines, badgers, raccoons, sheep, goats, camels, pigs, wild boars, possums, deer, rhinoceroses, antelopes, minks, dogs, squirrels, cats, foxes, ferrets, rats, primates, llamas, tapirs, elks, elephants, otters, seals, moles, coyotes, lions, leopards, and tigers. Today, bTB is listed in the OIE Terrestrial Animal Health Code, and must be reported to the OIE as per protocol (OIE, 2009).There is no denying the fact that bTB not only threatens human livelihoods by posing a risk to food safety and human health, but it potentially may impact economic and trade relations amongst countries. According to the WHO Global Tuberculosis Report of 2019, an estimated 143,000 recent cases of zoonotic TB (caused by *M. bovis*) were reported in the year 2018. The report also emphasizes the need for better detection strategies for zoonotic TB that require enhanced awareness and expertise among health care providers, improved laboratory research capacity, and effective access to accurate as well as rapid diagnostic tools.

This chapter aims at describing newer technological advances in the prevailing diagnostic approaches and detection methods for *M. bovis* infection in animals, especially in cattle, and to discuss major surveillance programs.

15.1.1 Bovine TB: The Causative Organism and the Disease

TB in cattle has been reported worldwide, except in Antarctica. The analysis of *M. bovis* phylogeography indicates that a considerable extent of the worldwide distribution of the bovine pathogen has resulted from anthropogenic factors like the cattle trade within the last 200 years (Smith, 2012). *M. bovis* is a member species of the *M. tuberculosis* complex (MTBC) and is an acid-fast, non-motile, aerobic, rod-shaped, slow-growing intracellular bacterial pathogen. It is the principal etiological agent of bovine TB, although in several cases other species, such as *M. caprae* or *M. tuberculosis*, have been reported to infect cattle (Rodriguez *et al.*, 2011). bTB is a chronic, debilitating disease that may frequently be asymptomatic in the early stages. As the disease progresses, progressive weight loss, fluctuating fever, weakness, loss of appetite, prominent lymph nodes, anorexia, and an intermittent cough are observed (Kumar *et al.*, 2014). Anatomically, the disease causes a chronic granulomatous, caseous necrosis in the lungs and the associated lymph nodes. There are various routes to infection, such as the aerogenous route (via inhalation), enterogenous route, or the alimentary route via ingestion (raw milk ingestion by suckling calves), congenital route (less common), genital route (during artificial insemination or copulation in the case of vaginitis in females or orchitis in males), and infection through the skin (wounds) or teat canal (not common). Of these, the most common mode is found to be through inhalation; hence, cattle density in dairy farms is a determining factor in controlling transmission (Cousins, 2001).

Following infection, the host mounts an immune response which is characterized by the predominance of the cell-mediated immunity (CMI) component. As the disease progresses over time, the humoral response amplifies and the CMI drops (Kumar *et al.*, 2014; Ratledge and Dale, 2009). The knowledge of host immune response components is an important aspect used in bovine TB diagnostic methods, as we shall see below.

15.1.2 Host Genetics

*M. bovis*is a complex pathogen that not only infects multiple species but also varies in its pathogenic potential in different host species. Some studies have reported considerable differences in susceptibility to *M. bovis* infection between different species and even cattle subspecies, for example, increased disease severity and higher prevalence of bTB in the Holstein breed as compared to the Zebu breeds in Central Ethiopia (Ameni *et al.*, 2007). It has also been reported that *M. bovis* with different genotypes and from different hosts showed variable virulence in a mouse model of tuberculosis, and naturally occurring *M. bovis* cases across Northern Ireland over nine years have reported that the various genotypes differed in their virulence (Aguilar *et al.*, 2009; Wright *et al.*, 2013).

15.1.3 Surveillance Strategies, Prevention, and Control Methods

Bovine TB is also a major human health concern, particularly in developing countries and rural areas due to the high risk of transmission to farm workers (dairy and agricultural) and also because of the consumption of unpasteurized milk in many countries. Since *M. bovis* is a zoonotic disease that has a huge host repertoire, its control becomes a more serious issue. bTB control is a multi-factorial problem that requires significant specialist input across various disciplines. Ideally, to move from control to eradication it also requires the inclusive efforts of public bodies with all stakeholders in society (Byrne *et al.*, 2019).

> Surveillance is the group of activities which provide early warning of animal health and welfare problems, allowing tracking and analysis of the way diseases spread.
>
> (Animal & Plant Health Agency (APHA), GOV.UK website)

Surveillance is a main component of a disease's prevention and control, with some common objectives that include case-finding, i.e., detection of bovine tuberculosis in a program species animal, estimation of prevalence and incidence, providing data to help in estimating the compliance with program standards, and giving stakeholders and decision-makers relevant actionable information. Surveillance usually mainly comprises of two approaches, classed as "active" or "passive". Active surveillance is achieved by conducting a targeted routine testing program of clinically normal animals using OIE-approved testing methods like TST and INF-gamma assays. However, the testing programs may be different for different countries. Passive surveillance is the examination of suspected infection in an animal with *M. bovis*, either clinically or *postmortem*. It involves the continuous monitoring of the populations surveyed for existing disease status (APHA).

Different countries follow different strategies according to their local socio-economic parameters. For example, in low-prevalence regions or countries, targeted risk-based surveillance may prove to be a better management strategy in terms of cost-effectiveness as compared to the conventional surveillance strategies in use. In risk-based surveillance, as the name suggests, the focus is on the subset of the animal population with higher risk of infection. This approach improves sensitivity of the surveillance system and minimizes economic and labor investments (VanderWaal *et al.*, 2017). Bovine TB is successfully controlled in most of the developed world (including the UK, the USA, and much of Europe), owing to serious implementation of national bovine TB control programs, through spill-over from wildlife reservoir hosts is a challenge in maintaining their TB-free status. This success is partially due to the adoption of the "test and cull" strategy. Contrastingly, bovine TB remains a serious problem in developing countries like India due to lack of a strict disease control program, lack of its sincere implementation, economic costs, and social barriers against "test and cull" strategies (Srinivasan *et al.*, 2018). Therefore, different countries use different approaches, such as "test and segregation" strategies in the early stages, and "test-and-slaughter" methods in the later stages of control and eradication programs. This minimizes the problems associated with human resources, financial limitations, and socio-cultural hindrances. Several disease eradication programs in various countries have been successful in reducing or eliminating the disease in cattle by following a multi-faceted approach. Some important aspects of the prevention and control of the disease are:

- a regular sanitation and disinfection drive to prevent spread within the herd
- the pasteurization of milk
- detailed *postmortem* meat inspection of diverse tissues like lungs, lymph nodes, liver, spleen, intestines, pleura, and peritoneum

- an intensive surveillance approach (including on-farm visits)
- the systematic testing of each individual suspected animal
- the adoption of "test and slaughter" or "test and segregate" policies
- a quarantine program for infected herds
- DNA fingerprinting on pathogen isolates
- vaccination
- adequate local legislation
- regular monitoring of the prevention and control program

It is a well-accepted fact that an efficient surveillance system critically depends on detection and diagnostic tests that are rapid, sensitive, specific, and reliable (Mishra *et al.*, 2005).

15.2 Some Basics of Performance Characteristics of Diagnostic Tests

A diagnostic test is any approach used to gather clinical information to make a clinical decision (i.e., diagnosis). For any diagnostic test to be adopted, it must be evaluated for at least the following four attributes.

Sensitivity. This is defined as the proportion of diseased animals that are correctly identified by the test.
Specificity. This means the proportion of healthy animals that are correctly identified amongst the tested animals.
Accuracy. This is the ability of a test to give a true measurement of the analyte (the substance being measured).
Precision. This is the ability of a test to give consistent results on the same sample.

It should be noted that a lack of sensitivity may lead to false-negative outcomes/results and a lack of specificity may lead to false-positive readings/results. Both sensitivity and specificity together determine the apparent prevalence of the disease and the proportion of test-positive animals that are diseased. For establishing the sensitivity and specificity of a particular test, the results of one test are compared to those of another test, called the *standard test*. Hence, this does not establish sensitivity or specificity, but only *relative sensitivity* and *relative specificity*. Therefore, much caution must be taken while choosing the standard test in such comparisons. Ideally, the sensitivity and specificity of the standard test are known and approach 100%.

Accuracy and precision are the measures of quality control. Also, both influence the above two factors, i.e., sensitivity and specificity of a test. Importantly, errors, inaccuracies, and inconsistencies during testing may arise due to several factors such as the test itself, the technician (sample handlers), and the nature of the analyte or sample. Therefore, it is important to ensure that any inaccuracies or inconsistencies in results do not exceed "acceptable limits", which are determined by careful application of suitable statistical tests (Martin, 1977). Hence, for different samples and situations, different tests may be employed to achieve efficient testing parameters.

15.2.1 Purpose of Diagnostic Tests

Before we delve into the details of diagnostic methods, let us contemplate the actual purpose(s) of diagnosis. The classical literature on the subject suggests three main purposes of diagnostic tests, namely:

- discovery of the infection (by screening test, generally used on apparently healthy livestock populations to detect infected animals. It is desirable to choose a test with high sensitivity. This needs to be followed by a confirmatory test)
- confirmation (by confirmatory tests conducted on animals strongly suspected to be infected. This must exhibit a specificity approaching 100%; however, lower sensitivity is acceptable)

- exclusion (these tests rule out the presence of *M. bovis* infection in the suspects. Thus, these tests must have a sensitivity approaching 100%) (Adams, 2001)

Hence, since the discovery of infection is conventionally the first step, an ideal screening test is desired to be so sensitive that it identifies all the diseased animals tested, and necessarily avoids identifying non-diseased animals as diseased, i.e., no false-positives (National Research Council, 1994). However, a single test may cater to more than one of these purposes. Also, all these three objectives are usually achieved in a population by a combination of various *in vivo* and *in vitro* tests that fulfil the abovementioned purposes.

15.2.2 Attributes of an Ideal Diagnostic Test

The WHO in its Bulletin has published a guide to aid the selection of diagnostic tests, wherein criteria termed "ASSURED (affordable, sensitive, specific, user-friendly, rapid and robust, equipment-free, and deliverable to end-users)" are suggested to be used as a benchmark for identifying the diagnostic test that is most appropriate in a given setting (WHO, 2017). The Bulletin further describes steps before one should adopt a particular diagnostic test, such as:

- defining the test's purpose
- reviewing the market for the availability of the product, additional equipment, and maintenance thereof
- reviewing the regulatory approval by international and national bodies
- analyzing sufficient authentic literature to determine the test's optimal diagnostic accuracy
- determining the test's diagnostic accuracy in practice under real-life conditions
- monitoring the test in routine use for quality control

Hence, in the light of these guidelines, it is imperative in our present context to also discuss the typical characteristics that an ideal diagnostic test for *M. bovis* should have. According to the existing literature and the National Research Council (1994), the result of the ideal diagnostic test should have the following attributes.

- It should be able to be detected throughout the course of infection (irrespective of early or late stages).
- It should have sufficient intensity that can be consistently detected or amplified to detectable levels without distorting the signal/noise ratio.
- It should be reproducible across diverse populations, genotypes, and varied samples.
- It should have the highest levels of specificity, and hence able to be uniquely and specifically associated with *M. bovis* infection.

It is on these lines that the conventional tests as well as the newer innovative approaches have been developed, tested, and adopted worldwide for the detection of bTB. Often, it is found that a single test may not suffice for all the above-mentioned requirements. Hence, a combinatorial approach is followed wherein the conventional gold-standard tests are supplemented with the rapid and more accurate innovative tests. We shall see many such instances in the following sections.

15.3 Detection Methods and Strategies

To make a diagnosis, certain methods may be used (generally in combination) such as health history, physical examination, and tests like blood tests, imaging tests, and biopsies. Some of these methods result in findings that are distinctive or characteristic of a particular disease or condition and are hence called *pathognomonic* tests. Other tests may indirectly indicate the etiological agent or the disease and are hence

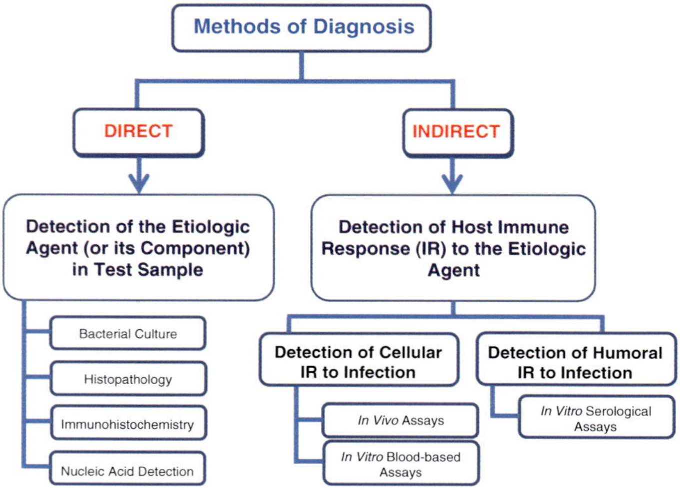

FIGURE 15.1 Approaches for bTB diagnosis based on different methodologies.

also called *surrogate* tests (Adams, 2001). For decades, many methods have been used to diagnose bovine TB as effectively as possible.

Based on their methodologies, these methods have been classified into two broad categories, which further branch into diverse groups, as shown in Figure 15.1. The two categories are as follows.

- *Direct detection methods*. These lead to detection of the causative agent (via acid-fast staining of the pathogen or nucleic acid detection-based assays) in the biological sample sourced from the diseased animal.
- *Indirect detection methods*. In these methods, detection is based on the identification of a host immune response (via measuring the cell-mediated or humoral responses) to the etiologic agent.

Both approaches have their advantages and disadvantages. Over the decades, detection methodologies have evolved progressively with improved testing technologies and rapid industrial advances. Many newer improvements have arisen, catering to both direct and indirect detection methods, especially in culture-based assays, PCR, RFLP, spoligotyping, ELISA, interferon-gamma, and molecular assays. Some major conventional diagnostic tests and newer advancements therein are described in the following sections.

15.3.1 Direct Detection of the Pathogen

15.3.1.1 Postmortem Examination

Postmortem diagnosis involves a thorough systematic necropsy examination of the suspected or diseased animal carcass. It is a tentative diagnostic method based on the detection and recognition of typical lesions caused by mycobacterial infection. If the histopathological analysis of the lungs, associated lymph nodes, and the mesenteric lymph nodes shows characteristic lesions (i.e., caseous necrosis, epithelioid cells, mineralization, multinucleated giant cells, and macrophages), it can be treated as a presumptive diagnosis of mycobacteriosis. A thorough and careful necropsy examination can identify more than 90% of cases with macroscopic lesions. However, bovine tuberculosis is a chronic disease that requires a variable period of a few weeks to years following exposure to *M. bovis* for the development of lesions to an extent that they can be recognized by *postmortem* examination. Moreover, there could be non-visible lesions (NVLs) because of the early infection stage. Therefore, a more definitive diagnosis requires the *postmortem* examination to be supplemented with bacterial isolation and culture-based detection methods. In such cases, it has been reported that immunohistological examination is quite sensitive as compared to the traditional Ziehl-Neelsen (ZN) technique and can be a good supplementary diagnostic tool (Medeiros *et al.*, 2010). With the discovery of newer specific antigenic determinants and proteins, techniques based on immunohistochemistry may provide for improved diagnosis. Purohit *et al.* (2007) showed that anti-MTP-64, which is a specific antigen for *M. tuberculosis* complex, may serve as a promising detection marker. Newer confirmatory direct detection methods based on immunohistochemical methods, immunoassays, nucleic detection-based methods, and chemical analysis of specific metabolic by-products of *M. bovis* play a significant role in bTB diagnosis that may or may not have been predicted by *postmortem* examination (Corner, 1994).

15.3.1.2 Direct Microscopic Detection

Staining the smears or prepared tissue material obtained during *postmortem* or *antemortem* clinical examination of the suspected animal with acid-fast dye and then visualizing *Mycobacteria* under a compound microscope has long been a popular and reliable method. This is a cost-effective method especially in developing countries. The staining is typically done with a Ziehl-Neelsen (ZN) stain which reveals the pink-stained typical rod-shaped bacilli. Alternatively, fluorescent stains such as auramine- rhodamine have also been used for better visualization (Willey *et al.*, 2008). The acid-fast bacilli need to be further confirmed specifically to identify *M. bovis* by immunohistochemical staining with specific antibodies and/or nucleotide amplification of *M. bovis*-specific genomic regions by polymerase chain reaction (PCR) (Adams, 2001).

15.3.1.3 Bacteriological Culture

According to the OIE, the laboratory bacteriological culture of *M. bovis* bacilli isolated from clinical samples is still recognized as the gold-standard test for diagnosis of infection. Typically, microorganisms have specific growth patterns and biochemical properties which are popularly exploited for their identification. Generally, bacterial growth can be observed on solid or liquid media as the development of colonies or turbidity, respectively. The period required by the inoculated culture to manifest visible growth for detection is an important variable. For example, *Mycobacteria* are slow-growing organisms that may take a few weeks to develop visible colonies on solid media or detectable turbidity in liquid media. In the case of *Mycobacteria*, an agar-based medium (Middlebrook 7H11) or egg-based medium (Stonebrink or Löwenstein-Jensen with pyruvate) are suitable for the primary isolation of pure culture from clinical samples. Usually, by using these suitable media, the growth of *M. bovis* occurs within three to six weeks of incubation (OIE, 2009). The pure cultures thus obtained are used for microscopic and growth characteristic analysis. Once a culture is obtained, it can be used for further confirmatory tests based on morphology, biochemical tests, or molecular biology identification techniques. These conventional culture-based techniques are laborious, time-consuming, and require extensive biosafety laboratory culture facilities. However, innovations have led to the development of radiometric methods like the BACTEC system, which is capable of detecting the early growth of *Mycobacteria* in culture (Middlebrook *et al.*, 1977). The BACTEC 460 TB system (Becton Dickinson, Sparks, MD, USA) is a detection system for the growth of *Mycobacteria* and is carried out by the quantitative measurement of $^{14}CO_2$ liberated by the metabolism of ^{14}C-labeled substrate in the culture medium. This is a comparatively rapid test that gives results within 10–14 days. There have been tremendous innovations in automatable radiometric detection for monitoring the mycobacterial species in terms of their growth, detection, and susceptibility testing (Rodrigues *et al.*, 2007). More recently, a non-radiometric technology, the BD BACTEC™ MGIT™ automated mycobacterial detection system, has been devised that uses fluorometric technology for considerably accurate detection of O_2 consumption and is useful for liquid culture and susceptibility testing studies. It is a popular method because of its high levels of sensitivity and accuracy.

15.3.1.4 Nucleic Acid Detection-based Molecular Assays

Nucleic acid-based detection tests are robust methods of diagnosis that are generally used as confirmatory tests for *M. bovis*. In these tests, there are two broad principles, namely, *amplification-based* tests and *hybridization-based* tests. In these tests, the basic strategy is to exploit the specific unique features of the *M. bovis* genome that are capable of differentiating it from the genomes of *Mycobacterium tuberculosis* complex (MTC) organisms which show a high degree of homology with its genome. A significant achievement in the form of elucidation of the *M. tuberculosis* genome sequence by Cole *et al.* (1998) allowed researchers to perform comparative analyses that provided significant insights into the *M. bovis* genome. Subsequently, apath-breaking advance in our knowledge of *M. bovis* has been brought about by the elucidation of its whole genome sequence by Garnier *et al.* in 2003 (Ramos *et al.*, 2015). Later on, whole-genome sequencings and high-throughput analysis of more and more mycobacterial genomes have given impetus to efforts towards the discovery of newer unique *M. bovis* genomic regions which can be used to detect the organism unambiguously. Since then, several genomic regions of *M. bovis* have been developed as targets for its detection and typing, with the list of potential targets being enriched every few years. There are certain *M. bovis* genomic regions which are conventionally used as diagnostic targets (Shah and Rauf, 2001; Kwaghe *et al.*, 2011; Ramos *et al.*, 2015). Let us discuss a few of these major targets.

- *Insertion sequences (ISs).* These are mobile genetic elements known to occur in many bacteria, in variable copy numbers in the genome, and are used as common markers for epidemiological studies. Commonly used IS elements for typing *M. bovis* are IS6110 (single copy number in *M. bovis* genome) and IS1081.
- *Direct-repeat regions (DRs).* These are interspersed regions occurring between non-repetitive sequences called spacers. These are also used for typing different bacterial strains.
- *Polymorphic GC-repeat sequences (PGRSs).* PGRSs are many tandem repeats of a 96-bp GC-rich consensus sequence and are used as targets for typing. These are quite abundant amongst the repetitive sequences like IS or DR genetic elements.
- *Variable number of tandem repeats (VNTRs).* These are repetitive elements occurring in tandem in the genome with highly variable copy numbers. Typing these is also known as "DNA fingerprinting" of the genomes.
- *Ribosomal RNA (rRNA) genes.* These are highly conserved regions in genomes. Amplification and analysis of the spacer region between the genes coding for 16S and 23S rRNA is achieved by using primers against conserved regions. These variable spacer sequences are specific for different species of *Mycobacteria* and are hence used as markers.
- *Protein-encoding genes.* Some protein-encoding genes (such as 65-kDa) and secreted proteins (such as Ag85, MPB70) are conserved in *Mycobacteria* and also bear certain unique regions which are utilized as a marker for detection.

Two types of nucleic acid detection assays are used for the analysis of the genomic targets (as discussed above). A brief account of each of these is provided below.

Polymerase chain reaction (PCR) and its modifications. Since its discovery by K.B. Mullis in 1987, PCR has emerged as a standard genotyping and epidemiological detection tool. The basic principle in PCR is the polymerase-catalyzed *in vitro* amplification of target DNA fragments using specific primers. The repetitive cycles of temperature-based steps of denaturation, annealing, and extension weave thousands of copies of the target DNA that, on purification, can be used for several molecular biology techniques (Mullis and Falsona, 1987). Polymerase chain reaction-based tests are a convenient and popular choice due to their successful application on formalin-fixed paraffin-embedded tuberculous lesions sections, and fresh tissue, blood, and milk samples (Miller *et al.*, 1997; Wards *et al.*, 1995; Mishra *et al.*, 2005). In recent times, there have been tremendous advances in PCR technology in terms of methodology and the resultant signals. Table 15.1 depicts some important applications of PCR and its modifications. It shows how technological innovations have shaped the current status of molecular diagnosis in *M. bovis*.

Due to the versatility of PCR methodology, the OIE recommends its use for the diagnosis of tuberculosis in animals as an auxiliary method.

Hybridization-based methods. Nucleic acid hybridization is also used as a conventional gold-standard assay and is a robust, rapid, accurate, and widely used technique. It is based on the principle of binding

TABLE 15.1

PCR and its advanced modifications that are used for bTB diagnostics

PCR or its Modification	Result/Finding	Reference
PCR	A method for rapid identification of *Mycobacteria* to species level by using PCR of the gene encoding for the 65-kDa heat shock protein	Telenti *et al.* (1993)
RAPD-PCR	Identification of the use of the random amplified polymorphic DNA (RAPD) technique for a species-specific *M. bovis* genomic fragment and species-specific identification of *M. bovis* by single-step PCR assay which can be used in epidemiological studies	Rodriguez *et al.* (1995)
Fluorescence resonance energy transfer PCR(FRET-PCR)	The first report of the detection of *M. bovis* in clinical tissues using real-time fluorescence technology involving the use of an *M. tuberculosis* complex-specific FRET in combination with rapid-cycle PCR. It opens avenues for the development of a high-throughput molecular diagnostic test for bovine tuberculosis	Taylor *et al.* (2001)
Nested-PCR	*hupB* encoding gene(the histone-like protein annotated as *Mb3010c* in *M. bovis*)-based nested PCR assay (N-PCR) for the direct detection of *M. bovis* in bovine samples is a reliable test	Mishra *et al.* (2005)
Real-time PCR	Development of multiplex real-time PCR assay for the rapid detection of *Mycobacterium bovis* DNA in cattle lymph nodes	Koh *et al.* (2011)
Nested-PCR	Development of nested-PCR (targeting IS6110) assay that was found to be more rapid than the mycobacterial culture method and is unhindered by any contaminating organisms in the bacterial culture	Adams *et al.* (2013)
Multiplex-PCR	Development of multiplex-PCR assays that can detect *M. bovis* DNA directly in tissue samples has the potential to be a valid additional tool for *postmortem* diagnosis of bovine TB	Carvalho *et al.* (2015)
PCR and ELISA	Use of multiple diagnostic tests, i.e., PCR and ELISA, to detect late-stage disease which fails to be detected by TST	Prakash *et al.* (2015)
One-tube multiplex PCR	Development of one-tube multiplex-PCR for targeting 16S rRNA, Rv3873, and a 12.7-kb fragment in the genomes of an MTC organism. Found to be a useful tool to differentiate *M. bovis* from other members of MTC.	Quanz *et al.* (2016)
Real-time PCR	The study shows promising results based on real-time PCR assay for *mpb70*. The authors propose that it has great potential as a detection tool for MTBC in animal tissues and is comparable to the efficacy of the culture method	Lorente-Leal *et al.* (2019)

of complementary nucleotide sequences to form heteroduplexes or homoduplexes. The probe is generally a suitably labeled complementary sequence that binds to an immobilized single-stranded target nucleotide sequence and reveals its presence by producing a signal on binding (Kwaghe *et al.*, 2011). Restriction fragment length polymorphism (RFLP) is a gold-standard molecular technique with high discriminative power and reproducibility which is also used for molecular typing of mycobacterial species. Various studies show that nucleic acid probe-based assays comprise a useful adjunct to culture-based confirmation assays in bovine TB diagnosis. Fluorescent probes and *in situ* hybridization assays may be employed to decrease the time consumed and for ease of handling as compared to radioactively labeled probes (Shah and Rauf, 2001).

As technological innovation has progressed, both amplification-based and hybridization-based techniques are coupled to achieve a rapid, convenient, "in-house", and high-sensitivity assay such as the widely used spoligotyping technique. By this approach, researchers have been able to amalgamate the advantages of the two methods for achieving a technique having better potential than both the original methods. The probe is generated or labeled by the PCR steps and then hybridized to the sample nucleic acid. Kamerbeek *et al.* in 1997 developed a simple method for the detecting and typing (simultaneously) of *M. tuberculosis* in clinical specimens. It depends on the polymorphism of the chromosomal DR locus. The DR locus is a region in the genome containing a variable number of short direct repeats interspersed with non-repetitive spacers. Hence, it was named "spacer oligo typing", or "spoligotyping", based on the hybridization patterns (strain-dependent) of *in vitro*-amplified DNA with multiple spacer oligonucleotides. It was found that spoligotyping could differentiate *M. bovis* from *M. tuberculosis*, which had hitherto been a difficult task in which even the traditional methods failed. Hence, it has proven to be a convenient and important method in standard detection and typing protocols across the globe (Medeiros *et al.*, 2010).

Despite their obvious advantages of being rapid, versatile, and economically suitable, nucleotide-based assays have their limitations due to their varying specificity and sensitivity depending on factors like the target under study, the quality and quality of genomic DNA extracted from a clinical sample, contamination of cross-reacting nucleotides introduced during genomic DNA extraction, and their requirement of standardization for each probe/primer. Also, nucleotide-based assays may not indicate the presence of a live viable pathogen, as they are based on DNA, which is quite a stable molecule. Therefore, the OIE recommends that laboratory culture is used in parallel withnucleotide-based assays to confirm viable *M. bovis*.

15.3.2 Detection of Cell-mediated Immunity in Host

This is an indirect method of detection which can reveal infection by *M. bovis*. It has been well documented that in tuberculosis, cell-mediated immunity (CMI) plays a significant role as a predominant factor in controlling the disease (Medeiros *et al.*, 2010; Pollock and Neill, 2002). CMI is a complex set of mechanisms that result from complex interactions between antigen-presenting cells and T lymphocytes. The recognition of the pathogen is followed by the initiation of cell activation, secretion of soluble mediators, cell proliferation, and cytotoxic activity to combat the infection.

Assessment of the various components of the CMI pathway is exploited for indirect detection methods such as *in vivo* assays like tuberculin DTH skin testing or *in vitro* blood-based assays. Figure 15.2 shows the cell-mediated response pathway steps that are useful in bTB diagnosis in cattle. The blood assays monitor host-produced inflammatory markers (e.g., cytokines) that can be easily detected and quantified.

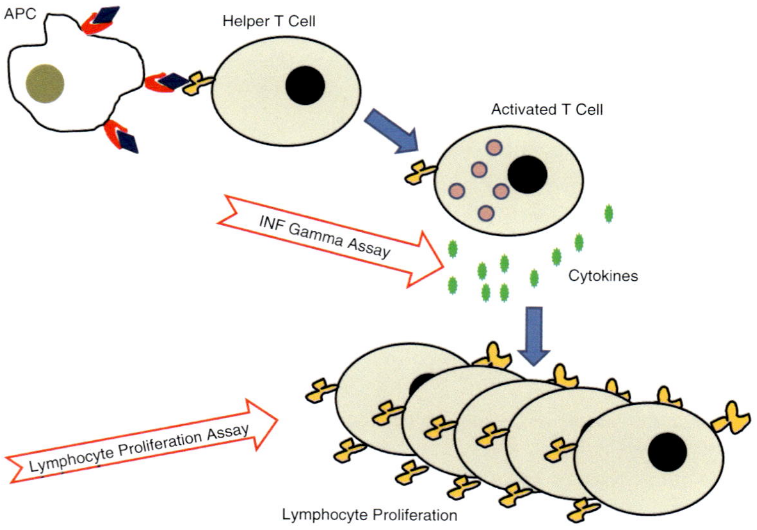

FIGURE 15.2 A small part of cell-mediated immune response is represented that is usually exploited for bTB diagnosis via interferon-gamma assay and lymphocyte proliferation assay (LPA); APC-antigen-presenting cell.

15.3.2.1 Tuberculin DTH Skin Test

The tuberculin DTH skin test is a convenient and cost-effective *in vivo* test which has been conventionally used as a gold standard for diagnostic testing and screening purposes, especially in new and asymptomatic MTC infections. Ever since it was recommended by Robert Koch in 1890, it has been extensively used for diagnosis. The test is based on the measurement of cell-mediated immunity by the detection of a delayed-type hypersensitivity (DTH) response to the components of *Mycobacteria* (tuberculin) injected intradermally in the suspected animal. Cell-mediated hypersensitivity is a function of specifically sensitized T lymphocytes that activate macrophages to cause an inflammatory response. The response is delayed (and hence its naming as a delayed-type test), usually starting two or three days after contact with the antigen, and often lasts for several days or weeks. A positive skin test shows that the animal has been infected with the agent but may not imply the presence of current disease (Brooks *et al.*, 2010). Using PPD (purified protein derivative of tuberculin) products are recommended over heat-concentrated synthetic medium tuberculins due to their higher specificity and easier standardization (OIE, 2009). In DTH skin testing, a specified amount of tuberculin is administered by intradermal inoculation into the skin of the mid-neck or in the caudal fold of the tail by a trained health care worker. Since the skin of the neck is more sensitive than the caudal fold, a higher dose may be used in the latter for compensation. After the injection, an infected animal generally shows reaction, i.e., redness, a raised and hardened area (induration) around the injection site. Test result interpretation is based on the size of the reaction site and certain characteristics of the tested individual like body temperature. As per OIE guidelines, skin thickness is measured with the help of calipers before and after inoculation (72 hours). The presence of DTH is indicated by an increase in skin thickness, which is interpreted using the "CDC Recommendations for Interpreting Reactions to the Tuberculin Skin Test" (www.nap.edu/catalog/10045.html).

Some major limitations of detection of DTH response by various methods (Table 15.2) include difficulties in administration and interpretation of results, cross- reactivity, the need for multiple visits, low degree of standardization, risk of anaphylaxis, and sensitization of the animal by environmental

TABLE 15.2

Modifications of the tuberculin skin test (Mishra *et al.*, 2005; Birhanu *et al.*, 2015)

TST Modification	Methodology and Reactivity Testing	Limitations
Single intradermal test (SID)	Intradermal injection of bovine tuberculin PPD into the caudal fold or the cervical fold is administered. Skin thickness is measured before inoculation and 48–72 hours post-inoculation	Prone to false-positives; poor sensitivity
Comparative intradermal test (CID)	PPDs from *M. avium* (PPD-A) and *M. bovis* (PPD-B) are injected intradermally in the side of the neck into separate clipped sites approximately 10–12 cm apart. Skin thickness is measured between the two injection sites before injection and 72 hours after injection. The results are used to differentiate between *M. bovis*-infected animals and others that those responding to PPD-B due to exposure to other *Mycobacteria*	More complex process and result interpretation than SID
Short thermal test	Tuberculin is injected intradermally into the neck of cattle that have a rectal temperature of not more than 39°C (or 102°F) at the time of injection and for two hours after. The animal gives a positive result if the body temperature at four, six and eight hours rises above 40°C	Risk of anaphylaxis and death of the animal being tested
Stormont test	The test is performed on the same lines as the SID test with a second injection at the same site seven days later. Skin thickness is measured before inoculation and 24 hours after the second injection	Multiple visits required; more than one inoculation at the same site required

Mycobacteria and variations due to the genetic background of the animal (Ramos *et al.*, 2015; Field, 2001). There is also a problem of occurrence of false-negatives due to variable factors like animals being at an advanced stage of the disease, or at an early stage of infection (i.e., six weeks); cows having recently delivered; the old age of cattle; and the purity, potency, and dosage of the tuberculin preparation used for testing (Mishra *et al.*, 2005). Therefore, there is an urgent need for the development of more robust assays to decrease the rates of false-negatives and false-positives. The *in vitro* blood-based assays are a step forward in this direction.

15.3.2.2 Gamma-interferon Assay

This *in vitro* assay is based on measuring the release of IFNγ (an immunological hormone or messenger protein) after stimulation of sensitized lymphocytes during the 16–24-hour incubation period with avian and bovine PPD in a whole-blood culture system. Since this assay requires viable white blood cells, blood samples are recommended to be transported to the laboratory as soon as is practical under proper storage conditions, to be tested within a day of blood sample collection (Shah and Rauf, 2001; Kwaghe *et al.*, 2011). It has been found that the choice of defined mycobacterium antigens (e.g., ESAT-6 and CFP-10) influences the specificity and efficacy of this test. The result of the test is obtained by conducting a sandwich ELISA in which two separate monoclonal antibodies are used against bovine gamma-interferon. Figure 15.3 represents a schematic diagram of different types of ELISA.

IFN-gamma ELISA has been found to be quite useful as a complement to skin testing. The major advantages of this test are its capability to detect early infections, hence allowing for the detection of many infected animals before they can be a potential source of infection for other animals or contamination of the environment; the possibility of rapid repeat testing; and the need for only a one-time visit to a farm or animal to collect the sample. However, it has certain limitations, such as high logistic demands in terms of laboratory resources, instrumentation, sample collection and transport, possible non-specific response in young animals, high cost, and low specificity.

The major advancement in the accurate and highly sensitive detection of gamma-interferon is the development of kit-based assays, i.e., the BOVIGAM assay (Vordermeier *et al.*, 2001), which is now an OIE-registered diagnostic kit for bTB in cattle, sheep, goats, and buffaloes.

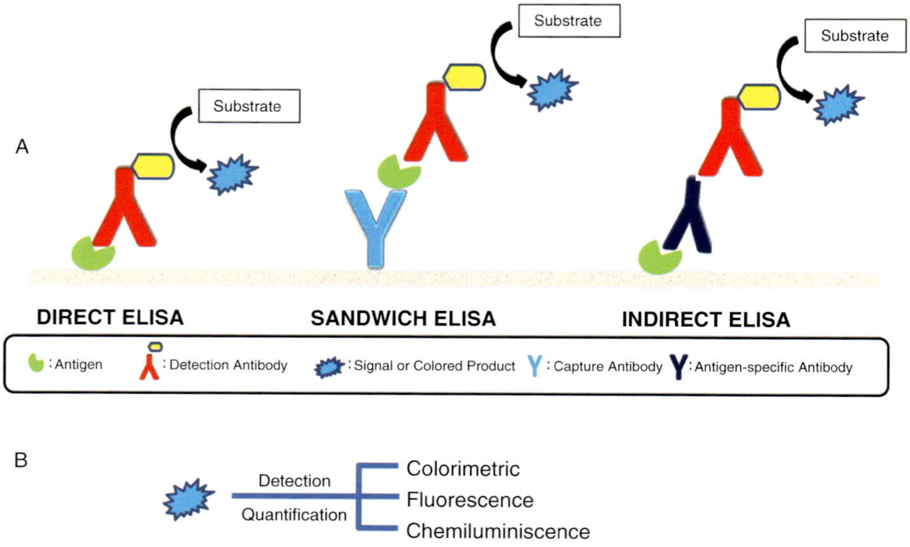

FIGURE 15.3 (A) The various modifications of the ELISA technique for detection and quantification of the antigen (direct and sandwich ELISA) or for antigen-specific antibody (indirect ELISA); (B) the detection and quantification of the signal may be carried out by colorimetric-, fluorescence-, or chemiluminescence-based methods.

15.3.2.3 Lymphocyte Proliferation Assay

The lymphocyte proliferation assay (LPA) is an *in vitro* assay that compares the reactivity of peripheral blood lymphocytes to a tuberculin PPD from *M. bovis* (PPD-B) and a PPD from *M. avium* (PPD-A). The assay can be performed on whole blood or purified lymphocytes from peripheral blood samples. The blood lymphocytes are grown in a standard mammalian cell culture set up and stimulated with specific antigens (i.e., PPD-A and PPD-B) separately. After a few days of incubation, cells are harvested and analyzed for proliferated lymphocytes. The results are generally analyzed as the response to PPD-B minus the response to PPD-A (Kwaghe *et al.*, 2011). This technique is advantageous as it has greater specificity by removing the response to cross-reactive antigens of other *Mycobacteria* to which the animal may have been exposed. However, it has its limitations, which are common to gamma-interferon assays, in terms of logistics, sample handling, the requirement of laboratory facilities, long incubation period, and the potential requirement of radioactive nucleotides or their expensive alternatives.

15.3.2.4 Enzyme-linked Immunosorbent Spot (ELISPOT) Assay

Czerkinsky *et al.* described a solid-phase enzyme-linked immunosorbent spot (ELISPOT) assay for the enumeration of B cells secreting a specific antibody and T cells secreting cytokinesin response to antigen activation (Czerkinsky *et al.*, 1983, 1988). Since then, ELISPOT has been extensively used as a robust, simple, and effective detection and enumeration tool for analyzing antigen-specific B cells and subsets of T cells. In this assay, the culture plate floor is coated with a specific capture antibody. The procedure is simple and requires basic laboratory facilities. Immune cells are cultured on this antibody-coated surface in the presence or absence of stimuli. The molecules secreted by the cultured cells (antibodies in the case of B cells and cytokines from T cells) are captured by the specific antibodies. After optimum incubation, cells and culture media are removed through a washing step and the specific antibody-bound molecules are detected using a detection procedure similar to that used in a typical ELISA. Detection is carried out by using a reaction based on a precipitating product so that the result is a visible spot on the surface of the plate, and each spot corresponds to an individual B cell or T cell. The spots are counted manually or using an automated reader. An ELISPOT assay specific for bovine interferon-gamma (BoIFN-γ) has been developed and subsequently applied for the diagnosis of bovine tuberculosis. Monoclonal antibodies against native BoIFN-γ are used as capture antibodies, as well as detecting antibodies (Xu *et al.*, 2015). There have been significant modifications and innovations to the ELISPOT technology to further fine-tune and enhance its specificity as well as sensitivity. Innovation in the detection steps has resulted in the FluoroSpot assay, which is essentially a variant of ELISPOT technology that uses fluorescence-based detection entities (Gazagne *et al.*, 2003). The detection is based on the principle that a fluorophore emits light at a specific wavelength on excitation by a light source. Each fluorophore is analyzed in an automated reader which is equipped with filters for different wavelengths and a separate image is captured for each fluorophore in case more than one fluorophore is used. Subsequently, the images are combined digitally to enable multiplex analysis. Efforts by Gazagne *et al.* gave rise to a FluoroSpot assay for the detection of single T lymphocytes simultaneously secreting several cytokines. The advantage of simultaneous detection of several cytokines lies in enhanced qualitative analysis of functionally distinct T cell subpopulations. More recently, multilevel analysis in FluoroSpot assays has been developed which enables not only multiple analysis but also detection of co-positioned spots, allowing for the detection of secretion patterns of two or more different samples in a single well (Janetzki *et al.*, 2014). Most recently, a FluoroSpot assay has been developed by Steinbach *et al.* (2019) which enumerates individual antigen-specific IFN-γ+ and IL-2+ T cell subsets. The assay suggests that greater levels of IL-2-secreting T cells could act as biomarkers for active TB in cattle.

15.3.3 Detection of the Host Antibody Response to Infection

It has been found that in tuberculosis, antibody-mediated defense mechanisms such as complement fixation and antibody-dependent cytotoxicity play a relatively minor role, whereas cell-mediated immunity (CMI) is of much greater importance. Moreover, looking at the temporal profile of the host immune

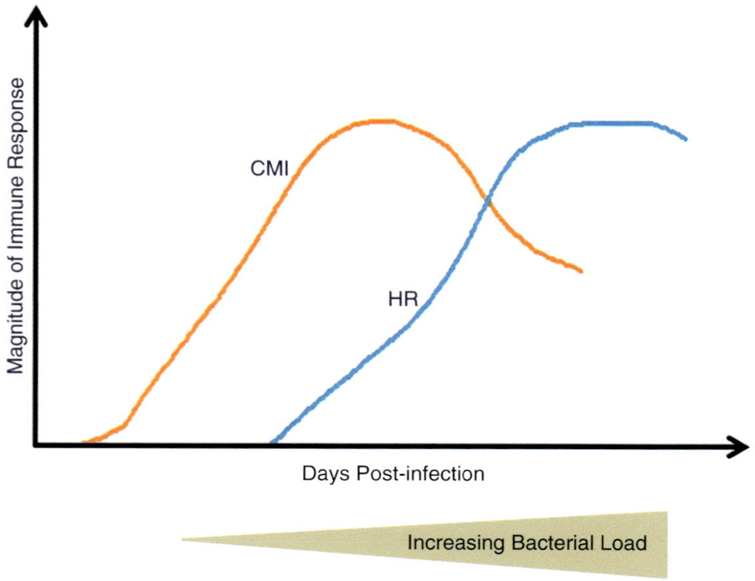

FIGURE 15.4 During the progression of the disease (bTB), after infection, indicators of cell-mediated immune (CMI) response are detected much earlier as compared to humoral response (HR). The bacterial load increases with the progression of time after infection.

This figure is for representation only, and is not to scale.

response to *M. bovis* during the disease, itis developed later and in rather a more irregular manner as compared to CMI (Figure 15.4).

In fact, it has been reported that an inverse relationship between cellular and humoral immune responses to *M. bovis* was found in cattle with natural infection (Ritacco *et al.*, 1991). Diagnosis based on humoral responses to *M. bovis* infection is often fraught with challenges since immunological responses are dependent on antigen presentation and the subsequent lymphocyte differentiation. There is often a variable time period following infection by *M. bovis* during which the humoral response of the host cannot be detected. Also, the first antibody response signal detection is weak. With the increasing growth of *M. bovis* in the host over time, the antigenic stimulation increases, and hence the intensity of the response signal generally increases during the later period of infection. There are also other reasons for failure to detect humoral responses, such as differential biological and genetic variability. Due to the above-mentioned issues, serological tests should not be used as substitute or alternative diagnostic tests for the detection of bovine tuberculosis but rather as complementary tests for detecting the more advanced stages of infection. Nonetheless, there have been immense technological advancements in serological diagnostics of bovine tuberculosis. Various humoral diagnostic tests are described below.

15.3.3.1 Enzyme Immunoassay or Enzyme-linked Immunosorbent Assay

As the name suggests, the technique of enzyme immunoassay (EIA) or enzyme-linked immunosorbent assay (ELISA) requires an antibody conjugated with an enzyme (called a *detection antibody*) that catalyzes a reaction in which the substrate is usually colorless and the generated product is a colored entity. Such a substrate giving rise to a colored product is called a *chromogenic substrate*. Several enzymes have been utilized for ELISA, such as alkaline phosphatase (AP), horseradish peroxidase (HRP), and β-galactosidase. The working principle of ELISA is based on detecting a target molecule using highly specific antibody-antigen interactions. For detection, the target molecule must be immobilized on a surface either directly or by using an already surface-immobilized *capture antibody*. The target molecule is then allowed to bind with a *detection antibody* which is conjugated with an enzyme. Typically, ELISA is performed in a multi-well plate. Several modifications of ELISA have been developed for qualitative or quantitative measurement of the target antigen (via direct ELISA or sandwich ELISA) as well as for the antibody against the target antigen (via indirect ELISA), which may be an antigen or antibody, as shown in Figure 15.3. Indirect ELISA is used for serological detection of antibodies raised in host serum against the pathogen (Owen *et al.*, 2013). ELISA has been one of the most promising and rapidly evolving technologies for the detection of *M. bovis* because of its obvious advantages. It can be packaged in economically suitable and standardized ready-to-use kits with stable reagents, e.g., Bio-X Diagnostics. The detection method is flexible as it can be carried out by using colorimetric-, fluorescence-, or chemiluminescence-based methods.

15.3.3.2 Multi-antigen Print Immunoassay

Lyashchenko *et al.* (2000) developed a new method called multi-antigen print immunoassay (MAPIA) for serological diagnosis of infectious diseases such as tuberculosis, which generates a heterogeneous antibody repertoire in the host. The test is based on a cocktail of protein antigens specific to the pathogen. Briefly, the assay involves the impregnation of nitrocellulose membranes with antigens by micro-aerosolization (this step is also called printing), followed by incubation along with test serum samples, and finally signal detection is done as in any standard immunological procedure using a conjugated secondary antibody. This technique is found to have greater diagnostic sensitivity when compared to enzyme-linked immunosorbent assay (ELISA) for a cocktail of protein antigens of *M. tuberculosis*. Hence, MAPIA is considered a better choice compared to conventional ELISA for the serological diagnosis of diseases that involve a heterogeneous antibody immune response. Waters *et al.* (2017) have demonstrated a MAPIA-based method that could identify many TST non-reactive bovine tuberculosis-affected cattle. The use of their method could be employed for efficient bTB surveillance and control methods.

15.3.3.3 Dual-path Platform Assay

A novel chromatographic immunoassay called the dual-path platform (DPP) assay has been developed by Chembio Diagnostic Systems, Medford, New York, USA. It utilizes a modification of the lateral-flow technology and has been recently used for serological analysis for *M. bovis* infections. Briefly, in this assay, the test sample and the conjugate (or the colorimetric marker) are delivered separately and independently to each other on perpendicular nitrocellulose membranes. It is this design that increases the sensitivity of the assay by reducing non-specific interaction between the conjugate and immunoglobulin in the test sample. Studies have shown promising results with a high diagnostic accuracy of the DPP test (Lyashchenko *et al.*, 2013).

15.3.3.4 Fluorescent Polarization Assay

The fluorescent polarization assay (FPA) is a highly versatile and advanced technology which was first described by Perrin in 1926. The principle behind FPA is that on being excited by polarized light, fluorescent molecules will emit polarized light. The basic method is that a fluorophore is excited by linearly polarized light followed by the measurement of the emitted fluorescence (of the fluorophore) by two polarizing filters, of which one is oriented parallel to and the other is oriented perpendicular to the plane of the polarized light excitation source. Now, the polarization values for any fluorophore molecule or complex are inversely related to its speed of molecular rotation. Since the speed of rotation is also inversely related to the size of the molecule, it implies that the polarization values are proportional to the molecular size of the fluorophore. For its application as a diagnostic test for *M. bovis*, FPA may be used to detect specific antigen-antibody complexes. One such assay was described for the detection of antibodies to *M. bovis* MPB70 protein in bovine sera by Jolley *et al.* (2007). This technology has also been used in a diagnostic kit by the Diachemix Corporation in which a fluorescein-labeled peptide conjugate corresponding to a small polypeptide (epitope) derived from *M. bovis*-specific MPB70 protein is used. On binding of the epitope-specific antibodies (from the serum of an infected animal) to the fluorescein-peptide conjugate, the polarization increases as compared to the values obtained by fluorescein-labeled peptide conjugate measured alone. The fluorescence is detected by an automated micro-plate reader capable of multi-mode fluorescence polarization measurements. The major advantage of this technology is that the procedure does not require any washing steps and hence is fast and convenient with comparable sensitivity and specificity to existing methods.

15.3.3.4 The SeraLyte-Mbv (PriTest Inc) Assay

This is a highly sensitive chemiluminescence-based assay for detection of the immune responses to a single *M. bovis* antigen, MPB83, a protein that is one of the most consistently recognized antigens in *M. bovis*-infected animals. The major advantage of using a single-antigen-based assay is that screening multiple antigens not only increases the cost of an assay but also the risk of cross-reactivity (Green *et al.*, 2009). The method requires the use of magnetic iron beads covalently attached to the MPB83 antigen which on incubation with the test serum bind to a specific antibody in infected animals. The ferrite conjugates are first collected at a magnetic port and processed with anti-bovine primary antibody, a biotinylated secondary antibody, and further processed for chemiluminescent reagent, and the signal is detected by an automated machine. The intensity of the emitted signal corresponds to the concentration of MPB83-specific serum antibody bound to the ferrite conjugate. This technique has shown a high degree of specificity, as is desired of a single-antigen test.

15.4 Futuristic Approaches

15.4.1 Detection of the Host Enzyme Adenosine Deaminase

Adenosine deaminase (ADA) is an essential enzyme that catalyzes the deamination reaction of adenosine to inosine in the purine catabolic pathway. ADA has a role in the proliferation and differentiation of T lymphocytes, in the maturation of monocytes into macrophages. Hence, ADA is considered to be a significant indicator of active cellular immunity. The assays based on the determination of serum ADA levels have been widely used for the diagnosis of human TB (Barua and Hossain, 2014; Shah and Rauf, 2001). The study by Barua and Hossain (2014) aimed to evaluate the role of ADA enzyme activity in the diagnosis of bTB. A recent study by Dhaliwal *et al.* (2020) has reported that serum ADA activity was significantly higher in bTB-infected cattle. This study opens up a newer avenue for host enzymatic factor determination as a diagnostic test.

15.4.2 Detection of Humoral Response Based on IgA (With or Without IgG)

Using serological assays as detection tools is attractive to researchers and clinicians owing to their simplicity, versatility, and economic benefits. Despite limitations to the method, the detection of humoral response is an important indicator in the diagnosis of mycobacterial diseases. Most serodiagnostic studies on cattle have majorly focused on the assessment of the immunoglobulin G (IgG) antibody. However, certain studies on active human TB have revealed immunoglobulin A (IgA) antibody to have a promising diagnostic role (Conde *et al.*, 2004). Further, Jeon *et al.* (2015) investigated the usefulness of IgA antibodies in bovine TB diagnosis. Their results show the suitability of using IgA antibodies against MPB70 and MPB83 to detect bovine TB. This study also suggests ways to improve the sensitivity and specificity of detection systems by using more than one type of immunoglobulin.

15.4.3 Use of Recombinant Molecules as Markers

Rapid advances in molecular biology have provided an immense boost to the emerging technologies for disease detection, diagnosis, surveillance, and control methods. One such remarkable improvement has been the ability to create fusion proteins (or bio molecules).

Studies have shown ELISA with the ESAT-6/MPB70/MPB83 chimera to be useful for the discrimination of BTB-positive and -negative cattle in herds before a tuberculin skin test (Souza *et al.*, 2012). In yet another recent study by Parthasarathy *et al.* (2012), the use of a recombinant ESAT-6-CFP-10 fusion protein as compared to ESAT-6, CFP-10, or a combination of both proteins in an IFN-gamma ELISPOT assay has shown higher specificity and sensitivity for detecting bTB.

15.4.4 High-throughput Technological Advances for Detection of Conventional Targets

Studies have shown that HPLC analysis of the mycolic acid esters can be used for the separation of BCG from *M. tuberculosis* and *M. bovis* in mycobacterial reference laboratory (Floyd *et al.*, 1992). In another study, Butler *et al.* (1991) reported the effective use of high-performance liquid chromatography (HPLC) analysis of the mycolic acids for the rapid identification of *Mycobacterium* species. The advantage of this technology is that it is rapid, reproducible, and enables species to be identified within 2 to 18 hours. However, the major disadvantage is the need for expensive equipment, software, and skilled technical support.

In yet another approach reported by Stewart *et al.* (2013) and known as immunomagnetic separation (IMS) technology, magnetic bead-based separation is used to selectively isolate and concentrate *M. bovis* cells from lymph node tissue samples for subsequent detection by PCR (IMS-PCR) or culture (IMS-MGIT).

Also, Hadi *et al.* (2018) have reported high-resolution multidimensional mass spectrometry analysis of DPP-captured immune complexes in cattle. By adopting this approach, the authors have tried to identify the captured *M. bovis*-specific peptides, which may further aid in the development of more accurate tuberculosis diagnostics for animals and humans (Bryne *et al.*, 2019).

15.4.5 Combinatorial Approaches

For effective bovine TB management, the development of accurate diagnostic tests that apply to a wide spectrum of susceptible hosts is desirable. Despite all the developments, it is difficult to archive 100% efficacy in the specificity, sensitivity, and accuracy of the diverse methods of detection. Each method has its limitations and cannot be used in isolation as a confirmatory test and called an "ideal diagnostic test". Hence, there is consensus that a combinatorial approach is the best one, in which more than one diagnostic test is used for the detection of *M. bovis*. Various studies have given different combinations, preserving the gold-standard methods (culture and DTH) as a component. Prakash *et al.* (2015) reported that ELISA and PCR could detect infection at the advanced stage that fails detection by tuberculin skin testing.

15.5 Conclusion

Encouraging advancements have been made in the diagnostic methods and detection tools (as shown in Table 15.3) that can potentially bring about more effective disease prevention and control programs. The immense development of molecular techniques due to technological advances has broadened the horizons for newer diagnostic methods for bovine tuberculosis. Although to date the gold-standard test of TST holds its prominence, there have been additions to the repertoire of auxiliary tests, such as IFN-gamma and PCR-based approaches as surrogate methods. Still, the race to develop less expensive, highly specific, versatile, and significantly reliable tests that can easily be adopted in less-developed countries continues.

TABLE 15.3

Summary of some significant advances in bTB diagnostics

S. No.	Detection Technique	References	Title of Research Paper	Remarks
1.	IFN-gamma detection-based assay (BOVIGAM)	Vordermeier, *et al.* (2001)	Use of synthetic peptides derived from the antigens ESAT-6 and CFP-10 for differential diagnosis of bovine tuberculosis in cattle	The study reports the reactivity of five peptides of CFP-10 and ESAT-6, each as a peptide cocktail for T cell assays and whole-blood gamma interferon assays. It further shows that the peptide cocktail can discriminate between *M. bovis* infection and BCG vaccination with considerable sensitivity and specificity
2.	Lymphocyte proliferation assay (LPA)	Spohr *et al.* (2015)	A new lymphocyte proliferation assay for potency determination of bovine tuberculin PPDs	The study presents an alternative *in vitro* method that reliably quantifies tuberculin PPD potency using flow cytometry-based LPA. Individual PPD preparations were assayed for potency estimates with reference to an international standard. The results revealed that this *in vitro* LPA method may replace the current guinea pig skin testing in the future and hence reduce animal suffering without compromising on the efficacy of the disease detection system
3.	FluoroSpot assay	Steinbach *et al.* (2019)	Potential of the dual IFN-γ/IL-2 fluorescence-immunospot assay to distinguish different stages in bovine tuberculosis	The study presents a FluoroSpot method to enumerate individual antigen-specific (IFN-γ/IL-2) T cell subsets *ex vivo*. The active TB cases in cattle can be identified by considering T cells producing IL-2 in greater amounts as a potential biomarker
4.	Serological assays: multi-antigen print immunoassay (MAPIA) and dual-path platform (DPP) assay	Waters *et al.* (2017)	Potential for rapid antibody detection to identify tuberculous cattle with nonreactive tuberculin skin test results	Using serologic assays in series with TST can identify a significant number of TST non-reactive tuberculous cattle for more efficient removal from TB-affected herds
5.	Fluorescent polarization assay (FPA)	Jolley *et al.* (2007)	Fluorescence polarization assay for the detection of antibodies to *Mycobacterium bovis* in bovine sera	The study reports the use of FPA for detection of antibodies against a small polypeptide derived from the *M. bovis* MPB70 protein. The study shows encouraging results that can be potentially applied for surveillance programs
6.	Combinatorial approach	Hadi *et al.* (2018)	Development of a multidimensional proteomic approach to detect circulating immune complexes in cattle experimentally infected with *Mycobacterium bovis*	This study describes the development of an assay wherein a dual-path platform (DPP) assay and LC-MS/MS are used in combination to discover *M. bovis*-specific peptides in serum samples from calves

References

Adams, A.P., Bolin, S.R., Fine, A.E., Bolin, C.A., and Kaneene, J.B. 2013. Comparison of PCR versus culture for detection of *Mycobacterium bovis* after experimental inoculation of various matrices held under environmental conditions for extended periods. *Appl. Environ. Microbiol.* 79(20):6501–6.

Adams, L.G. 2001. In vivo and in vitro diagnosis of *Mycobacterium bovis* infection. *Rev. Sci. Tech. Off. Int. Epiz.* 20(1):304–24.

Aguilar, L.D., Zumárraga, M.J., Jiménez, O.R., *et al.* 2009. *Mycobacterium bovis* with different genotypes and from different hosts induce dissimilar immunopathological lesions in a mouse model of tuberculosis. *Clin. Exp. Immunol.* 157:139–147.

Ameni, G., Aseffa, A., Engers, H., *et al.* 2007. High prevalence and increased severity of pathology of bovine tuberculosis in Holsteins compared to zebu breeds under field cattle husbandry in central Ethiopia. *Clin. Vaccine Immunol.* 14:1356–61.

APHA. The Animal and Plant Health Agency Vet Gateway. http://apha.defra.gov.uk/External_OV_Instructions/TB_Instructions/Passive_Surveillance/index.htm (accessed on March 12, 2020).

Barua, R. and Hossain, M.A. 2014. Adenosine deaminase in diagnosis of tuberculosis: a review. *Anwer Khan Mod. Med. Coll. J.* 5(2):43–8.

Birhanu, T., Mezgebu, E., Eyasu Ejeta, E., and Gizachew, A. 2015. Review on diagnostic techniques of bovine tuberculosis in Ethiopia. *Rep Opinion.* 7(1):7–14.

Brooks, G.F., Jawetz, E., Melnick, J.L., and Adelberg, E.A. 2010. *Jawetz, Melnick, & Adelberg's Medical Microbiology*. New York: McGraw Hill Medical.

Butler, W.R., Jost, K.C., and Kilburn, J.O. 1991. Identification of mycobacteria by high performance liquid chromatography. *J. Clin. Microbiol.* 29:2468–72.

Byrne, A.W., Allen, A.R., O'Brien, D.J., and Miller, M.A. 2019. Editorial: bovine tuberculosis—international perspectives on epidemiology and management. *Front. Vet. Sci.* 6:202.

Carvalho, R.C.T., Castro, V.S., Silva, F.G.S., *et al.* 2015. Detection of *Mycobacterium bovis* in bovine carcasses by multiplex-PCR. *Afr. J. Microbiol. Res.* 9(35):1978–83.

Cole, S.T., Brosch, R., Parkhill, J., *et al.* 1998. Deciphering the biology of *Mycobacterium tuberculosis* from the complete genome sequence. *Nature.* 393(6685):537–44.

Conde, M.B., Suffys, P., Silva, J.R.L.E., Kritski, A.L., and Dorman, S.E. 2004. Immunoglobulin A (IgA) and IgG immune responses against P-90 antigen for diagnosis of pulmonary tuberculosis and screening for *Mycobacterium tuberculosis* infection. *Clin. Diagn. Lab. Immunol.* 11:94–7.

Corner, L.A. 1994. Post mortem diagnosis of *Mycobacterium bovis* infection in cattle. *Vet. Microbiol.* 40(1–2):53–63.

Cousins, D.V. 2001. *Mycobacterium bovis* infection and control in domestic livestock. *Rev. Sci. Tech. Off. Int. Epiz.* 20(1):71–85.

Czerkinsky, C.C., Nilsson, L.A., Nygren, H., Ouchterlony, O., and Tarkowski, A. 1983. A solidphase enzyme-linked immunospot (ELISPOT) assay for enumeration of specific antibody-secreting cells. *J. Immunol. Methods.* 65:109–21.

Czerkinsky, C., Andersson, G., Ekre, H.-P., Nilsson, L.-Å., Klareskog, L., and Ouchterlony, Ö. 1988. Reverse ELISPOT assay for clonal analysis of cytokine production. I. Enumeration of gamma-interferon-secreting cells. *J. Immunol. Methods.* 110:29–36.

Dhaliwal, N.K., Narang, D., Chandra, M., Filia, G., and Tejinder, S. 2020. Evaluation of adenosine deaminase activity in serum of cattle and buffaloes in the diagnosis of bovine tuberculosis. *Vet. World.* 13(1):110–13.

Field, M.J. 2001. *Tuberculosis in the Workplace*. Washington, DC: The National Academies Press.

Floyd, M.M., Silcox, V.A., Jones, W.D. Jr., Butler, W.R., and Kilburn, J.O. 1992. Separation of *Mycobacterium bovis* BCG from *Mycobacterium tuberculosis* and *Mycobacterium bovis* by using high-performance liquid chromatography of mycolic acids. *J. Clin. Microbiol.* 30(5):1327–30.

Garnier, T., Eiglmeier, K., Camus, J.C., *et al.* 2003. The complete genome sequence of*Mycobacterium bovis*. *Proc. Natl. Acad. Sci. USA.* 100(13):7877–82.

Gazagne, A., Claret, E., and Wijdenes, J. 2003. A fluorospot assay to detect single T lymphocytes simultaneously producing multiple cytokines. *J. Immunol. Methods*. 283:91–8.

Green, L.R., Jones, C.C., and Sherwood, A.L. 2009. Single-antigen serological testing for bovine tuberculosis. *Clin. Vaccine Immunol.* 16(9):1309–13.

Hadi, S.A., Waters, W.R., Palmer, M., Lyashchenko, K.P., and Sreevatsan, S. 2018. Development of a multidimensional proteomic approach to detect circulating immune complexes in cattle experimentally infected with *Mycobacterium bovis*. *Front. Vet. Sci.* 5:141.

Janetzki, S., Rueger, M., and Dillenbeck, T. 2014. Stepping up ELISpot: multi-level analysis in FluoroSpot assays. *Cells*. 3:1102–15.

Jeon, H.S., Shin, A-R., and Son, Y-J. 2015. An evaluation of the use of immunoglobulin A antibody response against mycobacterial antigens for the diagnosis of *Mycobacterium bovis* infection in cattle. *J. Vet. Diagn. Invest*. 27(3):344–51.

Jolley, M.E., Nasir, M.S., and Suruballi, O.P. 2007. Fluorescence polarization assay for the detection of antibodies to *Mycobacterium bovis* in bovine sera. *Vet. Microbiol.* 120:113–21.

Kamerbeek, J., Schouls, L., Kolk, A., *et al.* 1997. Simultaneous detection and differentiation of *Mycobacterium tuberculosis* for diagnosis and epidemiology. *J. Clin. Microbiol.* 35(4):907–14.

Koh, B.-R.-D., Jang, Y.-B., Ku, B.-K., Cho, H.-S., *et al.* 2011. Development of real-time PCR for rapid detection of *Mycobacterium bovis* DNA in cattle lymph nodes and differentiation of *M. bovis* and *M. tuberculosis*. *Korean J. Vet. Serv*. 34(4):321–31.

Kumar, A., Tiwari, R., Chakraborty, S., *et al.* 2014. Insights into bovine tuberculosis (bTB), various approaches for its diagnosis, control and its public health concerns: an update. *Asian J. Anim. Vet. Adv.* 9(6):323–44.

Kwaghe, A.V., Geidam, Y.A., and Egwu, G.O. 2011. Diagnostic techniques for bovine tuberculosis: an update. *Am. J. Sci.* 7(11):204–15.

Lorente-Leal, V., Liandris, E., Castellanos, E., *et al.* 2019. Validation of a real-time PCR for the detection of *Mycobacterium tuberculosis*complex members in bovine tissue samples. *Front. Vet. Sci.* 6:61.

Lyashchenko, K.P., Greenwald, R., Esfandiari, J., *et al.* 2013. Rapid detection of serum antibody by dual-path platform VetTB assay in white-tailed deer infected with *Mycobacterium bovis*. *Clin. Vaccine Immunol.* 20(6):907–11.

Lyashchenko, K.P., Singh, M., Colangeli, R., and Gennaro, M.L. 2000. A multi-antigen print immunoassay for the development of serological diagnosis of infectious diseases. *J. Immunol. Method.* 242:91–100.

Martin, S.W. 1977. The evaluation of tests. *Can. J. Comp. Med.* 41(1):19–25.

Medeiros, L.S., Marassi, C.D., Figueiredo, E.E.S., and Lilenbaum, W. 2010. Potential application of new diagnostic methods for controlling bovine tuberculosis in Brazil. *Brazilian J. Microbiol.* 41(3):531–41.

Middlebrook, C., Reggiardo, Z., and Tigert, W.D. 1977. Automatable radiometeric detection of growth of mycobacterium tuberculosis in selective media. *Amer. Rev. Resp. Dis.* 115:1066–9.

Miller, J., Jenny, A., Rhyan, J., Saari, D., and Suarez, D. 1997. Detection of *Mycobacterium bovis* in formalin-fixed, paraffin-embedded tissues of cattle and elk by PCR amplification of an IS6110 sequence specific for *Mycobacterium tuberculosis* complex organisms. *J. Vet. Diagn. Invest.* 9(3):244–9.

Mishra, A., Singhal, A., Chauhan, D.S., *et al.* 2005. Direct detection and identification of *Mycobacterium tuberculosis* and *Mycobacterium bovis* in bovine samples by a novel nested PCR assay: correlation with conventional techniques. *J. Clin. Microbiol.* 43:5670–8.

Mullis, K.B. and Falsona, F.A. 1987. Specific syntheses of DNA in vitro via a polymerase catalysed chain reaction. *Methods Enzymol.* 155:350–5.

National Research Council. 1994. *Livestock Disease Eradication: Evaluation of the Cooperative State-Federal Bovine Tuberculosis Eradication Program.* Washington, DC: The National Academies Press.

OIE. 2009. *Manual of Diagnostic Tests and Vaccines for Terrestrial Animals*. www.oie.int (accessed March 12, 2020).

Owen, J.A., Punt, J., Stranford, S.A., Jones, P.P., and Kuby, J. 2013. *Kuby Immunology*. New York: W.H. Freeman.

Parthasarathy, S., Veerasami, M., Appana, G., *et al.* 2012. Use of ESAT-6-CFP-10 fusion protein in the bovine interferon gamma ELISPOT assay for diagnosis of *Mycobacterium bovis* infection in cattle. *J. Microbiol. Methods*. 90(3):298–304.

Perrin, F. 1926. Polarization de la Lumiere de Fluorescence. Vie Moyenne de Molecules dans L'etat Excite. *J. Phys. Radium*. 7:390.

Prakash, C., Kumar, P., Joseph, B., *et al.* 2015. Evaluation of different diagnostics tests for detection of tuberculosis in cattle Indian. *J. Vet. Pathol.* 39(1):1–4.

Pollock, J.M. and Neill, S.D. 2002. *Mycobacterium bovis* infection and tuberculosis in cattle. *Vet. J.* 163(2):115–27.

Purohit, M.R., Mustafa, T.T., Wiker, H.G., Mørkve, H.G.O., and Sviland, L. 2007. Immunohistochemical diagnosis of abdominal and lymph node tuberculosis by detecting *Mycobacterium tuberculosis* complex specific antigen MPT64. *Diag. Pathol.* 2(1):36.

Quan, Z., Haiming, T., Xiaoyao, C., Weifeng, Y., Hong, J., and Hongfei, Z. 2016. Development of one-tube multiplex polymerase chain reaction (PCR) for detecting *Mycobacterium bovis*. *J. Vet. Med. Sci.* 78(12):1873–6.

Ramos, D.F., Silva, P.E.A., and Dellagostin, O.A. 2015. Diagnosis of bovine tuberculosis: review of main techniques. *Braz. J. Biol.* 75:830–7.

Ratledge, C. and Dale, J.W. 2009. *Mycobacteria Molecular Biology and Virulence*. New York: John Wiley & Sons.

Ritacco, V., Lopez, B., De Kantor, I.N., Barrera, L., Errico, F., and Nader, A. 1991. Reciprocal cellular and humoral immune responses in bovine tuberculosis. *Res. Vet. Sci.* 50(3):365–7.

Rodriguez, J.G., Mejia, G.A., Portillo, P.D., Patarroyo, M.E., and Murillo, L.A. 1995. Species-specific identification of *Mycobacterium bovis* by PCR. *Microbiol.* 141:2131–8.

Rodriguez, S., Bezos, J., Romero, B., *et al.* 2011. *Mycobacterium caprae* infection in livestock and wildlife, Spain. *Emerg. Infect. Dis.* 17:532–5.

Rodrigues, C.S., Shenai, S.V., Almeida, D., *et al.* 2007. Use of bactec 460 TB system in the diagnosis of tuberculosis. *Indian J. Med. Microbiol.* 25:32–6.

Shah, A. and Rauf, Y. 2001. Newer methods for the laboratory diagnosis of tuberculosis. *JK-Practioner.* 8(4):266–9.

Smith, N.H. 2012. The global distribution and phylogeography of *Mycobacterium bovis* clonal complexes. *Infect. Genet. Evol.* 12:857–65.

Srinivasan, S., Easterling, L., and Bipin, R., *et al.* 2018. Prevalence of bovine tuberculosis in India: A systematic review and meta-analysis. *Transbound Emerg. Dis.* 65:1627–1640.

Steinbach, S.H., Vordermeier, M., and Jones, G.J. 2019. Potential of the dual IFN-γ/IL-2 fluorescence-immunospot assay to distinguish different stages in bovine tuberculosis. *Vet. Immunol. Immunopathol.* 217:109930.

Stewart, L.D., McNair, J., McCallan, L., Gordon, A., and Grant, I.R. 2013. Improved Detection of *Mycobacterium bovis* infection in bovine lymph node tissue using immunomagnetic separation (IMS)-based methods. *PLoS One* 8(3):e58374.

Spohr, C., Kaufmann, E., Battenfeld, S., *et al.* 2015. A new lymphocyte proliferation assay for potency determination of bovine tuberculin PPDs. *Altex.* 32(3).

Souza, I.I.F., Melo, E.S.P., Ramos, C.A.N., *et al.* 2012. Screening of recombinant proteins as antigens in indirect ELISA for diagnosis of bovine tuberculosis. *SpringerPlus.* 1:77.

Taylor, M.J., Hughes, M.S., Skuce, R.A., and Neill, S.D. 2001. Detection of *Mycobacterium bovis* in bovine clinical specimens using real-time fluorescence and fluorescence resonance energy transfer probe rapid-cycle PCR. *J. Clin. Microbiol.* 39(4):1272–8.

Telenti, A., Marchesi, F., Balz, M., Bally, F., Bottger, E.C., and Bodmer, T. 1993. Rapid identification of mycobacteria to the species level by polymerase chain reaction and restriction enzyme analysis. *J. Clin. Microbiol.* 31(2):175–8.

VanderWaal, K., Enns, E.A., Picasso, C., *et al.* 2017.Optimal surveillance strategies for bovine tuberculosis in a low prevalence country. *Sci. Rep.* 7:4140.

Vordermeier, H.M., Whelan, A., Cockle, P.J., Farrant, L., Palmer, N., and Hewinson, R.G. 2001. Use of synthetic peptides derived from the antigens ESAT-6 and CFP-10 for differential diagnosis of bovine tuberculosis in cattle. *Clin. Diagn. Lab. Immunol.* 8(3):571–8.

Wards, B.J., Collins, D.M., and de Lisle, G.W. 1995. Detection of *Mycobacterium bovis* in tissues by polymerase chain reaction. *Vet. Microbiol.* 43(2–3):227–40.

Waters, W.R., Vordermeier, H.M., and Rhodes, S. 2017. Potential for rapid antibody detection to identify tuberculous cattle with nonreactive tuberculin skin test results. *BMC Veterinary Research.* 13:164.

WHO. 2017. *Bulletin of the World Health Organization.* 95: 639–645.

WHO. 2019. *WHO Global Tuberculosis Report*. www.who.int/tb/publications/global_report/en/ (accessed March 12, 2020).

Willey, J.M., Sherwood, L., Woolverton, C.L., and Prescott, L.M. 2008. *Prescott, Harley, and Klein's Microbiology*. New York: McGraw-Hill Higher Education.

Wright, D.M., Allen, A.R., Mallon, T.R., *et al.* 2013. Field-isolated genotypes of *Mycobacterium bovis* vary in virulence and influence case pathology but do not affect outbreak size. *PloS One* 8(9):e74503.

Xu, Z., Shan, F., Shan, F., *et al.* 2015. Development of an interferon-gamma ELISPOT for bovine tuberculosis. *Sheng Wu Gong Cheng Xue Bao*. 31(2):183–94.

16

Livestock Enteric Viruses: Latest Diagnostic Techniques for their Easy and Rapid Identification

Sushila Maan,[1] Renu Singh,[1] Monika Punia[2] and Kanisht Batra[1]
[1] *College of Veterinary Sciences, Lala Lajpat Rai University of Veterinary and Animal Sciences, Hisar-125004, Haryana, India*
[2] *Department of Biotechnology, Chaudhary Devi Lal University, Sirsa-125055, Haryana, India*
Corresponding author: Sushila Maan, ***sushilamaan105@gmail.com; sushilamaan105@luvas.edu.in***

16.1 Introduction

Viral gastroenteritis has been recognized as an important condition of animals and is considered to be one of the biggest threats to the health of animals throughout the world, especially in emergent nations including India. Severe diarrhoea, vomition and pyrexia indicate for the clinical illness associated with enteric infections. Frequent infection outbreaks because of enteric viruses are responsible for the affecting the overall health and wellbeing of humans and animals, which in turn causes huge financial loses (Wu *et al.*, 2016). These financial losses are mainly because of increased morbidity, mortality and cost involving labour and medication. Several intestinal pathogens including bacteria, viruses and protozoa are responsible for this disease development. The most important infectious agents responsible for causing neonatal calf diarrhoea are rotavirus, coronavirus, enteropathogenic *E. coli*, *Salmonella* and *Cryptosporidium* species. Those viruses which induce gastrointestinal diseases are named enteric viruses (Figure 16.1). Among enteric pathogens, viruses constitute the major threat as there is a lack of proper therapeutic interventions. These enteric viruses enter the body through the faecal-oral route and can infect even in very low concentrations. They multiply and reproduce inside the gastro-intestinal tract of the

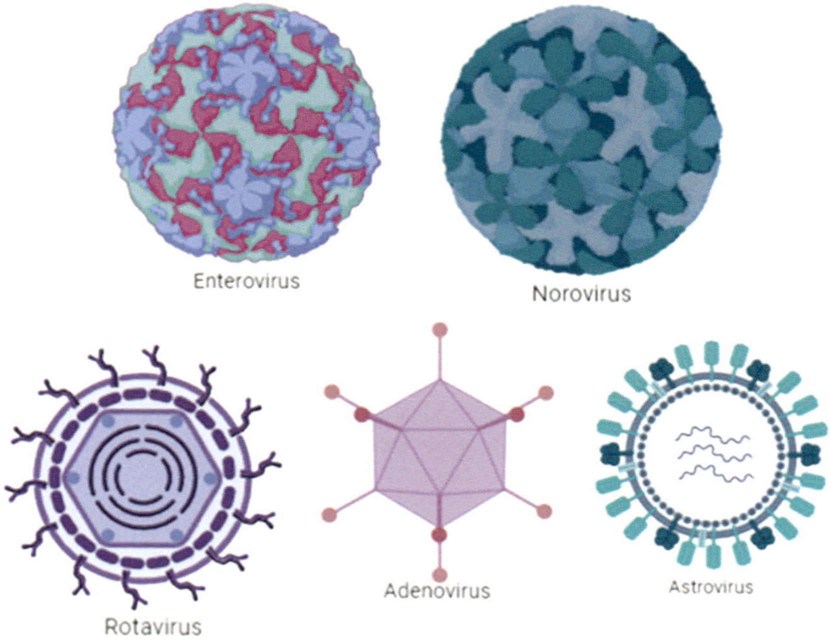

FIGURE 16.1 Major enteric viruses of livestock.

patient. Studies by Mullis *et al.* (2012) and Lekshmi *et al.* (2018) showed the presence of a high number of virus particles (10^5–10^{11} virus particles per gram) in stools of patients suffering from enteric virus infection. Spread of these viruses is even possible via food, water, fomites and human contact. They even can spread long distances underwater and through estuarine water, rivers, seawater, aerosols emitted from sewage treatment plants, insufficiently treated water, drinking water and private wells that receive treated or untreated wastewater either directly or indirectly.

Enteric viruses have been recognized since 1970, including viruses mainly belonging to the four families, i.e., *Reoviridae* (rotaviruses), *Caliciviridae* (calciviruses), *Astroviridae* (astroviruses) and *Adenoviridae* (adenoviruses), and are known to cause millions of cases of enteric viral infection each year (Table 16.1). Other common viral agents responsible for causing enteric infections are picobirnavirus, norovirus, sapovirus, hepatitis E virus, kobuvirus, parechovirus etc. (Dhama *et al.*, 2009; Malik *et al.*, 2014a; Sircar *et al.*, 2016).

Before the onset of advanced molecular techniques, the cell culture system was the preferred practice for the identification of enteric virus infections. In the present scientific era, a broad range of commercial products have been generated and several of these are available as handy and user-friendly kits that can be supplied at the point of care. These tests are simple to perform and can be conducted outside of the test centre to provide fast disease testing. The only drawback is that they cannot distinguish infective viruses unlike cell culture-based assays. In the last few years, development of the various molecular techniques has greatly improved the limit of detection of enteroviruses compared to that of the cell culture system. Except for adenoviruses and parvoviruses, the majority of enteric viruses are RNA viruses, and most molecular techniques therefore rely on detecting specific viral RNA sequences. Detailed studies of the viral genome and advances in molecular tools/techniques can improve selectivity and reactivity remarkably.

These molecular diagnostic techniques are setting a new path from which the scientific community can explore and gather more information regarding these life-threatening enteric viruses. Therefore, the major aim of this chapter is to focus on the latest developments made in the molecular diagnostic techniques for the easy and fast detection of major enteric viruses.

TABLE 16.1

Major effects of enteric viruses on livestock species

Virus Family	Species	Genus	Host Species	Disease/Symptoms	References
Picornaviridae	Bovine enterovirus	*Enterovirus*	*Bos taurus* (cattle)	Diarrhea, abortion	Fong and Lipp (2005)
	Porcine enterovirus/ teschovirus		*Sus scrofadomesticus* (pig)	Teschen-Talfan disease, pneumonia, polioencephalomyelitis, vesicular diseases, myocarditis, diarrhoea, fertility disorders and skin abrasion	Fong and Lipp (2005)
	Swine vesicular disease virus		*Sus scrofadomesticus* (pig)	Highly contagious lesions identical to those caused by FMD (foot-and-mouth disease) virus	Fong and Lipp (2005)
Reoviridae	Rotavirus	*Rotavirus*	Virtually all livestock species, lambs, goat, camelids etc.	Acute diarrhoea	Papp H *et al.* (2014)
Caliciviridae	Bovine noroviruses	*Norovirus*	*Bos Taurus* (cattle)	Anorexia, diarrhoea, lethargy, loss of appetite, ataxia, decreased milk production, fever and lesions in intestine	CDC (2016); Vildevall (2011)
	Porcine noroviruses		Pigs	Mostly diarrhoea, lesions in small intestine (little is known about sub-clinical and persistent infections)	Bank-Wolf *et al.* (2010)
	Avian nephritis virus	*Astrovirus*	Poultry, especially *Gallus domesticus* (chicken)	Chicken diarrhoea, duck hepatitis, turkey enteritis and avian nephritis	Perot *et al.* (2017)
	Porcine sapoviruses	*Sapovirus*	*Sus scrofadomesticus* (pig)	Vomiting and diarrhoea in young pigs	Proietto *et al.* (2016)
Adenoviridae	Bovine adenovirus	*Adenovirus*	*Bos taurus* (cattle)	Diarrhoea with mucus, melena or haemoatochezia, anorexia, possible dysphagia, pyrexia, dyspnoea and tachypnoea	Smyth *et al.* (1996); CABI (2019)
	Porcine adenovirus		*Sus scrofadomesticus* (pigs)	Watery diarrhoea, occasionally accompanied by vomiting, emaciation and severe dehydration	Honark and Larson (2016)

16.2 Latest Diagnostic Techniques for Identification of Major Enteric Viruses Affecting Livestock

As stated above, enteric diseases cause major health problems, with the most common symptoms being diarrhoea, dehydration and weight loss. The gravity of these symptoms largely depends on the etiology, which includes a number of enteropathogens. Enteric virus infection is responsible for many diseases of livestock and ever since the emergence of these viruses, continuous efforts have been made to diagnose and treat them. Since then, many diagnostic techniques have been developed, including cell culture assays, immunological detection protocols and advanced molecular assays (Table 16.2). The following section of this chapter is focused on discussing the important enteric viruses of livestock species and the latest diagnostic developments made towards the accurate and rapid detection of enteric viruses.

16.2.1 Bovine Coronaviruses

Bovine coronaviruses (BCoVs) are enveloped viruses with a (positive, single-stranded) RNA genome (27~32 kb). They belong to the genus *Betacoronavirus*, previously classified as group 2a coronaviruses (Cho and Yoon, 2014). Three different formats of the infection can be seen in bovines: a) calf diarrhoea (enteritis) in newborn calves in the first two weeks of age; b) winter dysentery with haemorrhagic diarrhoea in adult animals; and c) bovine respiratory disease complex (BRDC) in cattle of all age groups. These viruses replicate in gut epithelial cells, causing severe bloody diarrhoea, loss of electrolytes and malnutrition. Decaro *et al.* (2008) also reported that these viruses can affect lungs together with intestines in bovines BCoVs can also jump the species boundary, giving rise to bovine-like CoVs infecting various mammals. BCoVs are rarely isolated using cell culture methods but in a study by Hansa *et al.* (2013), BCoVs were successfully cultured in Vero cell lines that were confirmed using fluorescence antibody testing (FAT) and RT-PCR studies.

Weather conditions also put serious impact on the spread of infections caused by BCoVs. The increased receptor-destroying enzyme (RDE) activity against mouse erythrocytes in strains of virus isolated in winter helps in the elution of mature virions from the surfaces of infected cells and is thus responsible for enhancing the virulence of BCoV (Park *et al.*, 2006).

One improved technique used in animal diagnostic laboratories is multiplex RT-PCR. Multiplexing of an RT-PCR panel can simultaneously detect multiple infection-causing agents directly from stool samples and is faster and more responsive in comparison to the conventional diagnostic tests (Cho *et al.*, 2012). The PCR results are in accordance with those of traditional diagnostic tests (~97%) and exhibit testing sensitivity on a par with and even finer than that of established tests. Cho *et al.* (2012) concluded that the multiplexing of a PCR panel can be a tool for a prompt and valid diagnosis of calf diarrhoea associated with BCoVs, group A BRV, *E. coli* K99+, *Salmonella* and/or *Cryptosporidium*. Continuous efforts are being made to develop more robust and high-throughput-performing assays, e.g., the groundbreaking two-step, SYBR Green I-based real-time RT-PCR assay. This technology uses two sets of primers targeting the highly conserved sequences of the nucleocapsid (N) gene of BCoV. It was observed that the assay is highly specific in distinguishing between positive and negative samples (Amer and Almajhdi, 2011). Technically, the SYBR Green RT-PCR used the binding of the fluorescent dye to dsDNA. This dye emits a considerable amount of fluorescence. The amount of dsDNA is in direct proportion to the emitted fluorescence. Thus, the ease of usage and the cost-effectiveness of this technology make it quite noted among the scientific community.

16.2.2 Bovine Enteroviruses

Bovine enteroviruses (BEVs) have a 7.5-kb, positive-sense (+) ssRNA genome which belongs to the family *Picornaviridae*, genus *Enterovirus*, species *Enterovirus E*. The virus is non-enveloped with icosahedral symmetry. The viral genome has a single open reading frame (ORF) flanked by 5' and 3' untranslated regions (UTRs). The single ORF encodes a single long polyprotein having four structural proteins (VP1, VP2, VP3 and VP4 encoded in P1) and seven non-structural proteins (2A, 2B and 2C encoded in

TABLE 16.2

Different techniques used for detection and identification of livestock enteric viruses

	Method	Advantage	Disadvantage	Reference
Cell culture assays	Plaque assay	Unambiguous method for the direct quantification of infectious virons	Ameliorated and graded plaque assay protocol not available for every condition	Baer and Kehn-Hall (2014)
	Tissue culture infective dose	More amenable to standardization, fewer crucial steps that may impact the results	More qualitative than quantitative	Smitther *et al.* (2013)
	Immunofluorescence and flow cytometry	Highly reproducible, moderately time-consuming	Expensive technique, technically demanding	Kumar (2013)
	ELISA	Reproducibility of results, inexpensive	Technically demanding, can read only one analyte at a time	Kumar (2013)
Molecular assays	Conventional PCR	Responsive, quick and easy to perform	Can access all nucleic acids present in a sample, including extra genomes	Smither *et al.* (2013); Richards (1999)
	RT-PCR	Specific primers for specific virus, increased specificity, frozen samples can be used in RT-PCR	RT-PCR inhibitors can hamper the reaction (false negative), decreased sensitivity when low level of virus in samples	Rose *et al.* (1997)
	Multiplex PCR	Reduction in cost of testing due to simultaneous detection of many pathogens	Limited number of detector channels, sensitivity may differ with change in a primer-probe set lot, preferential amplification of the stronger target	Hajia (2017)
	Integrated cell culture PCR	Excludes inactivated virus amplification, higher level of sensitivity and specificity	Technically demanding, time-consuming	Lee and Jeong (2004)
	Real-time PCR	Simple set-up with increased confidence in results	Requires expertise in interpretation of results and occasionally can't distinguish between infectious and non-infectious particles	Chigor and Okoh (2012)
	Luminex-based assay	Can quantify multiple samples at a time, i.e., multiplexing and customizable	Occasional uncertainty of results due to use of multiple ligands, requirement of specialized equipment	Elshal and McCoy (2006)
Next-generation sequencing	Next-generation sequencing	Enormously high-throughput, ultra-deep sequencing	Expensive technique, technically demanding	Hert *et al.* (2008)

P2 as well as 3A, 3B, 3C and 3D encoded in P3). The genus *Enterovirus* (EV) has 12 species defined as *Enterovirus A–H* and *J* (EV-A, -B, -C, -D, -E, -F, -G, -H and -J) while *Rhinovirus* has three species, *A–C* (RV-A, -B and -C). BEVs belonging to EV-E and EV-F and can be differentiated from other EVs by the unique secondary structure of their RNA genome. The structure of BCoV RNA is a 5′ cloverleaf and the internal ribosome entry site (IRES) is linked by additional nucleotide sequences at the 5′ UTR. Though BEVs were isolated from cattle in the late 1950s, studies have detected BEVs in other animal species like possums, bottlenose dolphins, camels and alpacas, along with cattle (Tsuchiaka *et al.*, 2017).

BEV RNA has been utilized in tracking environmental pollution with animal origin. Highly sensitive real-time PCR has been developed which can detect BEV RNA adjacent to cattle herds acting as an environmental contaminant (Jiménez-Clavero *et al.*, 2005). This optimized qPCR can detect as low as 12 copies of RNA per 4.6×10^3 to 4.6×10^4 $TCID_{50}$. Moreover, a highly conserved 3D gene-based SYBR Green-based real-time PCR assay has been used for speedy and effectual diagnosis of viral RNA (Zhu *et al.*, 2015). It can detect enteroviruses with a sensitivity of 7.13×10^1 plasmid copies/μL with 100% specificity.

In order to study the whole genome of BEV, other cutting-edge technologies have been used. These include shotgun metagenomics by MinION sequencing and NextSeq500 (Illumina). MinION is a compact and portable device. Even though MinION technology is still at the evolving stage, its portability and compactness make it an extremely acceptable method. MinION is a true long-read sequence technology which is based on estimating the variation in ionic current. When the single-stranded nucleic acid passes through the biological nanopores, it disrupts the flow of ionic current, which in turn is measured by MinION. Thus, the difference in current pattern will prove helpful in knowing the whole genome sequence of the desired samples. Beato *et al.* (2018) identified and characterized a BEV strain extracted from a calf diarrhoea sample using both the sequencing platforms. Portable MinION sequence technology, which is fast, reliable and user-friendly, can be used successfully in veterinary diagnostic laboratories.

16.2.3 Rotaviruses

Among all enteric viral infections, rotaviruses (RV) are the leading cause of mortality and loss. They were first identified in 1969 and 1973 in faecal samples of diarrheic cattle and stool extracts of diarrheic children, respectively (Bishop *et al.*, 1973). The genus *Rotavirus* falls in the *Reoviridae* family, comprising of eight groups (RVA, RVB to RVH) and two tentative groups, I (RVI) and J (RVJ). Group-A rotaviruses are further divided into 50P or 35G types depending upon variation in their VP4 (a protease-sensitive protein) and VP7 (glycoprotein) outer capsid proteins of the virion, which are responsible for inducing neutralizing antibodies (Rojas *et al.*, 2017). Genotypes G6, G8 or G10, in combination with either P [1], P [5] and/or P [11] and genotypes G6 P [5], G6 P [1] and G10 P [11] are among the most frequent in BoRV-A (Ramos Caruzo *et al.*, 2010). The G6 and G10 types are widespread in cattle and other domestic animals, warranting crucial and timely control measures to reduce disease affliction.

Towards the finding of novel viral strains of rotaviruses, samples from horses, canines, chiropterans, bovines, birds, felines, pigs and small rodents were tested by RT-PCR with specially designed consensus primers N-VP4F1/N-VP4R1. In RT-PCR the cDNA copies of RNA were made using a reverse-transcriptase enzyme. As this PCR is converting unstable RNA to more stable and robust cDNA, thus with this PCR technology *in vitro* expression studies are attainable. After amplification of the consensus sequence a nested PCR was performed using another set of primers, i.e., N-VP4F2 and N-VP4R2 specific for VP4 gene.

Additionally, conventional sequencing can also be used. The sequence fragments generated from the DNA sequencer can be assembled and edited using bioinformatics software. Further sequence comparison and studies revealed that there is frequent transmission of these viruses among various species ("jump"), as well as the presence of genome segment rearrangements in rotaviruses (reassortment) (De Barros *et al.*, 2018).

Similarly, in India many diversified strains of rotavirus are prevalent and their epidemiology has been widely studied, presenting them as the most prevailing cause of gastroenteritis among various host species (Basera *et al.*, 2010; Kattoor *et al.*, 2013; Malik *et al.*, 2014b). Bovine, porcine and equine rotavirus strains have exhibited antigenic similarities to human strains, observed using RNA–RNA hybridization assays (Van Der Heide *et al.*, 2005). Phylogenetic analysis of human and animal rotavirus genetic make-up shows frequent intersections among the strains' evolution, which is probably a consequence of multiple gene re-assortments. The inter-species spread and ensuing re-assortments are among the major processes resulting in enhanced diversity within the rotaviruses, and are thus responsible for the origination of new pathogenic strains with altered virulence. Ongoing efforts in the field of cell culture assays are helping in the development of well-grounded and efficient cell culture-based identification methods. Lee *et al.* (2013) ameliorated an assay for effective and rapid detection of samples taken from the environment for the presence of viable enteric viruses. They studied six enteric viruses, i.e., rotavirus G1, poliovirus, coxsackie virus A9, coxsackie virus B5, hepatitis A virus and adenovirus type 41. The MA104 cell line was found to be the most suitable for the identification of disease-causing enteric viruses. Gautam *et al.* (2016) showed that the single-step multiplex qRT-PCR assay allows fast and reliable rotavirus genotype identification for monitoring prevalent rotavirus wild-type strains.

RT-qPCR has become a benchmark technology in pathogen detection, genetic testing, disease research, microarray validation, RNAi validation and gene expression technology. Real-time PCR has an edge over other PCRs as it keeps an eye on the progress of the PCR reaction as it occurs in real time, precisely assessing the amount of amplicon at each cycle, which in turn allows highly accurate estimation of the amount of a virus in a sample. Another advantage is that the two reactions, i.e., amplification and identification, both occur in one tube, thus there is no need for post-PCR testing. In RT-qPCR, after every cycle of PCR the amount of DNA is quantified with the amount of florescent produced. The fluoroprobe attached to the added probe produces fluorescence, which in turn is directly proportional to the amplicon generated. Information gathered from the growing phase of the multiplying cycle gives insight into the number of targeted sites present in the tested sample. The dsDNA-binding fluorophores, or light-emitting molecules attached to PCR primers or small nucleotide molecules that hybridize with PCR products during amplification, are among the different fluorescent reporters which are successfully used in RT-PCR. By plotting fluorescence against cycle number, the q-PCR machine produces an amplification curve that shows the cumulation of by-product over the course of the whole PCR reaction. More advanced technologies were used for the identification of rotavirus from clinical samples. The next-generation sequencing (NGS) technology used by Anis *et al.* (2018) showed that often a mixed infection was present, thus making it difficult to identify the disease-causing agent. Thus, NGS is among the most fitting ways to check such samples, saving the time required for testing samples for different viruses. Through building a library focusing on pathogen genomic regions of interest, thus the selective enrichment and sequencing of clinical samples will result in amplification of the targeted region. NGS technology has the potential to perform millions of sequencing reactions at once, referred to as massively parallel sequencing. Initially, NGS technology requires DNA fragmentation, its ligation with distinctly designed adapters, followed by its denaturation. Following the denaturation step, the denatured fragments are allowed to bind to complementary adapters which are in turn bound to the flow cell. Subsequently, the amplification step is carried out. By tracking the addition of the complementary labelled nucleotides one can find the base. After the incorporation of the single fluorescent dye-labelled dNTP, the dye is enzymatically cleaved. At the end of the reactions all the data is gathered from every cycle involving the three following steps, namely enzyme-based addition, imaging and cleavage. All gathered data, i.e., reads, are aligned using available bioinformatic software to get a contiguous DNA sequence (Maan *et al.*, 2018). The researcher found this futuristic technology to be very reliable, flexible, fast and efficient, able to solve problems which require in-depth information beyond the reach of conventional DNA techniques.

16.2.4 Astroviruses

Like rotaviruses, belonging to the family *Astroviridae*, astroviruses are also equally important. Madeley and Cosgrove were the first to use the term astrovirus, in 1975. They used electron microscopy and reported astroviruses as tiny, round viruses (approximately 28 nm diameter) with a star-like appearance (Kurtz and Lee, 1987). Astroviruses have an uncapped, single-stranded (ss), positive-sense (+) RNA genome of 6.8 to 7.9 kb long and a poly-A tail at the 3' end. The family *Astroviridae* comprises of two genera, *Avastrovirus* and *Mamastrovirus*, detected in avians and mammals, respectively. They have shown high genetic diversity along with affecting a broad host range including humans, bovines, swines, ovines, minks, dogs, cats, mice, chickens and turkeys (De Benedictis *et al.*, 2011).

Astroviruses are mainly transmitted via contaminated food and water and the major symptoms of such infection in animals include diarrhoea, scours, haemorrhagic hepatitis, gastroenteritis etc. In the 1970s the first description of astrovirus was made from clinical samples of children; it was subsequently reported in cattle, pigs, sheep, minks, dogs, cats, mice, sea lions, whales, chickens and turkeys (Li *et al.*, 2013). Li *et al.* carried out metagenomics studies on cattle brain tissue samples and their NGS studies revealed that bovine astrovirus (BoAstV-NeuroS1) is genetically closer to an ovine astrovirus, supposing it to be associated with neurologic disease, emphasized through real-time testing and genomic analysis of bovine faecal isolates.

In a study on turkeys, efforts were made for concurrent identification of turkey astrovirus-2 (TAstV-2), avian rotavirus and avian reovirus. In order to identify these viruses, specially designed primers were used. These primers were designed to focus on the conserved sequences of the NSP4 gene of avian rotavirus, the polymerase gene of TAstV-2 and the S4 gene of avian reovirus. Using these primer pairs, multiplexed RT-PCR was performed and it was concluded that this method is quite efficient in the simultaneous detection of these enteroviruses (Jindal *et al.*, 2012). In another study on rabbits, with the assistance of an advanced molecular technique, i.e., qRT-PCR, a novel astrovirus was identified. Samples were taken from rabbits with enterocolitis. For analysis of the rabbit enterovirus, specific and targeted primer-probes were used. They interpreted that astroviruses show frequent appearance in the intestinal contents of both ill rabbits and even in those rabbits that are symptomless (Martella V. *et al.*, 2011).

16.2.5 Caliciviruses

During the last two decades, members of the family *Caliciviridae*, including the genera *Vesivirus*, *Lagovirus*, *Norovirus* (NoV) and *Sapovirus* (SaV), have appeared as a cause of widespread gastroenteritis and food-borne illness. Caliciviruses get their name from the cup-shaped depressions present on the outer surface of the virons. These viruses first received attention during the 1940s in the US, and in the year 2002 delineation and isolation of a "vesicular exanthema of swine-like calicivirus" from an aborted bovine foetus magnified the concern of the scientific community about the role of calciviruses in the development of animal diseases.

The *Norovirus* genome is about 7.5 kbp in size and comprises of linear, non-segmented positive-sense (+) RNA. The virus replicates in the small intestine and causes gastroenteritis, whose major symptoms include diarrhoea leading to dehydration, vomiting and stomach pain. The *Norovirus* genus comprises of viruses that can cause infection in a large range of hosts including humans, pigs, cattle and mice of all ages, and in closed surroundings can lead to huge outbreaks. This wide range of hosts increases the possibility of the spread of viral infections from animals to humans, i.e., zoonotic transmission (Johnson *et al.*, 2015). Infection can be transmitted either indirectly or directly, through the food chain or via animal contact, and cross-species transfer of animal viruses to humans is possible. In a report by the CDC (2017), *Norovirus* was found to affect impoverished populations of the world, responsible for an average of 200,000 deaths globally in a year. In a detailed study by Villabruna *et al.* (2019) on animal noroviruses, it was revealed that interspecies transmission is present and this situation is responsible for causing infectious diseases in humans. The major animal hosts are bats, rodents, birds and other wildlife. Prior to genome sequencing of *Norovirus*, electron microscopy was the exclusive technique available for its detection. Later on, more cost-effective and practical methods came into existence, i.e., conventional and reverse-transcriptase PCR. The assays were targeted at the conserved area in ORF1 (region A) of the POL gene. Other PCR-dependent operating procedures that have been used for the sensing of noroviruses include digital PCR (dPCR) (Haramoto *et al.*, 2018). For differentiating pathogenic viruses from non-pathogenic viruses, the most suitable process is to combine a cell culture method with a molecular method. Molecular methods alone are, however, considered less efficient in differentiating infective from non-infective viruses as both types of virus have the same structural protein but differ in virulence. Hence, integrated cell culture-polymerase chain reaction (ICC-PCR) combines the best of both methods to overcome the shortfalls of each.

One of the most responsive and suitable methods of target DNA amplification is isothermal amplification, such as NASBA (nucleic acid sequence-based amplification) and LAMP (loop-mediated isothermal amplification). With the integration of a reverse-transcription (RT) step, isothermal amplification can be used for the detection of viruses like noroviruses. These reliable methods were used by Chen and Hu (2016) for the identification of noroviruses. However, RT-qPCR aiming at the ORF1-ORF2 junction region is found to be the fastest and most reliable, specific and sensitive technique for the detection of noroviruses (Vinjé, 2015).

In a single reaction, multiplex molecular diagnostic technologies (MMDTs) can concurrently identify all the genetic material present in the sample, thus markedly reducing time, labour and cost. A multiplex involving a single-tube real-time reaction has been developed for the detection of different genogroups of *Norovirus* (Hoehne and Schreier, 2006). Real-time multiplex technology can even detect noroviruses from other enteric viruses associated with gastroenteritis, like sapoviruses, adenoviruses and rotaviruses (Jiang *et al.*, 2014). Recently, several MMDTs such as BioFireFilm Array Gastrointestinal (GI) Panel (Salt Lake City, UT, USA), Luminex xTAG Gastrointestinal Pathogen Panel (GPP) (Toronto, Canada) and the Nanosphere Verigene Enteric Pathogens (EP) Test (Northbsrook, IL, USA) have obtained permission from the United States Food and Drug Administration (USFDA) (Chen and Hu, 2016). These diagnostic kits are being used for the fast and reliable testing and identification of disease-causing enteric viruses such as noroviruses.

DNA microarray is a reliable technique which can concurrently identify and sequence major enteric viruses including noroviruses. For identification and sequencing, specially designed targeted primers are used, but because of the limited amount of genetic diversity in the viruses this technique is still not widely used. Using next-generation sequencing approaches, many diverse sequences were identified among the ORF2 region of the *Norovirus* genome. In order to obtain precise virus genotyping, one method is to have sequencing of the major capsid region. Another method includes complete or partial sequencing of the ORF1 and ORF2 regions. These methods of viral genotyping were proposed by Kroneman *et al.* (2013).

The *Caliciviridae* family has another genus, named *Sapovirus* (SaV), which contains a single species (also named *Sapovirus*). The *Sapovirus* genome size is equivalent to that of *Norovirus*, i.e., 7.7 kb. The virus is without an envelope, having a positive-sense (+) ssRNA with a 3'-end poly (A) tail but not a 5' cap. It has the capability of infecting both humans and animals. The major symptoms include vomition, diarrhoea, chills, nausea, headache, abdominal cramps and muscle pain (myalgia). Using electron microscopy, it was first identified in 1980 in the USA (Saif *et al.*, 1980) and later, based on its polymerase (RdRp) and viral protein 1 (VP1), was divided into seven genogroups, namely I to VII, where groups I, II, IV and V infect humans and groups III, VI and VII infects pigs, cows and mink (Jun *et al.*, 2016). In one study, *Sapovirus* was identified from faecal samples of cats and dogs (Soma *et. al.*, 2015).

SYBR Green-based qRT-PCR was successfully developed by Mauroy *et al.* (2012) using a p289-p290 primer pair (p290: GATTACTCCAAGTGGGACTCCAC; p289: TGACAATGTAATCATCACCATA), which allows for easy, fast and reliable detection of SaV from pig stool samples. One of the most reliable and responsive techniques for gene expression analysis is q-PCR. This technique is broadly used for pathogen identification and quantification along with determination of transgenic copy numbers. From this experiment it was deduced that qRT-PCR is equally sensitive to but more specific than conventional PCR. Metagenomic study has also been used for the identification of novel groups of canine SaV in the genus *Sapovirus* (Li *et al.*, 2011).

16.2.6 Picobirnaviruses

Picobirnaviruses (PBVs) are group of viruses which fall under the newly classified family *Picobirnaviridae*. PBVs are one of the major causes of many enteric viral diseases in animals and humans. The *Picobirnavirus* name was derived from two Latin words, i.e., *pico*, meaning "small", and *bi*, meaning "two". The "rna" stands for the nature of genetic material (RNA). These are tiny, unenveloped viruses with bi-segmented dsRNA with genome size ranging from 2.4 to 2.6 kbp (slow-migrating segments) and 1.5 to 1.8 kbp (fast-migrating segments) (Malik *et al.*, 2014a). Pereira *et al.* (1988) were the first to report PBVs, from faecal samples of children, and later the virus was retrieved from the faeces of various mammals including rats, rabbits, cattle and giant anteaters (Woo *et al.*, 2016). The virus is often observed as a co-infection along with other diarrhoeal agents like rotaviruses, caliciviruses and astroviruses (Ganesh *et al.*, 2012). In porcine and other animal hosts, matching patterns of PBV infection have also been detected (Geng *et al.*, 2011). RT-PCR based on its replication gene (RNA-dependent RNA polymerase) has been utilized for detection of this virus from diarrheic piglets (Carruyo *et al.* ,2008; Wilburn *et al.*, 2017). Available evidence shows high sequence similarity between porcine and human PBVs, equine and human PBVs, and rodent and human PBVs. These similarities show that new viruses are evolving because of surviving crossing points in the ecology and evolution of heterologous PBV strains (Malik *et al.*, 2014b; Kattoor *et al.*, 2016).

Very recently, based on complete genome sequence 2, *Picobirnavirus* has also been detected in bats, dogs, vervet monkeys and wolves (Conceicao-Neto *et al.*, 2016). One of the latest techniques is metagenomics study. Under this approach, direct environmental samples such as factory streams, faecal samples etc. are studied to measure diversity and genetic relatedness. Thus, genetically divergent and novel viruses have been identified, including picobirnaviruses. Picornaviruses have been isolated from faecal samples of many animals, like roe deer, weaned female foals, bovines, cattle, horses, pigs and rhesus macaques (Malik *et al.*, 2018), demonstrating their wide host range and diversity. Further, in order to explore their diversity, traditional DNA sequencing technologies (sanger sequencing, shotgun sequencing etc.) are insufficient. To obtain more in-depth information and for better understanding of complex genomic research, the next-generation system (NGS) system is being used. High-throughput and massively parallel 454 pyrosequencing have been used initially to carry out metagenomics studies of this virus.

Thus, NGS has tremendous potential and can assists in fulfilling the research gap, and is thus becoming an everyday research tool in veterinary diagnostic laboratories.

16.3 Conclusion

These latest molecular diagnostic techniques, which are more precise, sensitive and reliable, help in faster, easier and accurate diagnosis of enteric viruses of veterinary importance. These techniques have given new insights into the viral etiologies of acute gastroenteritis; however, the rapid revolution and emergence of novel strains of these viruses present constant challenges in their detection. The latest studies carried out in the advanced molecular field suggest that NGS can be used as a one of the most versatile diagnostic tools without putting much monetary pressure on veterinary diagnostic laboratories. As we know that most enteric viruses are responsible for causing serious food-borne and waterborne diseases in both humans and livestock, there is an urgent need to direct future research perspectives to focus on the adoption of these new methods in a portable format to ensure their wide use in clinical settings as well as in the food industry and under different environmental conditions.

References

Amer, H.M. & Almajhdi F.N. (2011). Development of a SYBR Green I based real-time RT-PCR assay for detection and quantification of bovine coronavirus. *Molecular and Cellular Probes*, 25, 101–107.

Anis, E., Hawkins, I.K., Ilha, M., Woldemeskel, M.W., Saliki, J.T. & Wilkes, R.P. (2018). Evaluation of Targeted next-generation sequencing for detection of bovine pathogens in clinical samples. *Journal of Clinical Microbiology*, 56(7), e00399-18.

Baer, A. & Kehn-Hall, K. (2014). Viral concentration determination through plaque assays: using traditional and novel overlay systems. *Journal of Visualized Experiments*, 93, e52065.

Bank-Wolf, B.R., Konig, M. & Thiel, H.J. (2010). Zoonotic aspects of infections with norovirus and sapoviruses. *Veterinary Microbiology*, 140(3–4), 204–212.

Basera, S.S., Singh, R., Vaid, N., Sharma, K., Chakravarti, S. & Malik, Y.P.S. (2010). Detection of rotavirus infection in bovine calves by RNA-PAGE and RT-PCR. *Indian Journal of Virology*, 21(2), 144–147.

Beato, M.S., Marcacci, M., Schiavon, E., Bertocchi, L., Di Domenico, M., Peserico, A., Mion, M., Zaccaria, G., Cavicchio, L., Mangone, I., Soranzo, E., Patavino, C., Cammà, C. & Lorusso, A. (2018). Identification and genetic characterization of bovine enterovirus by combination of two next generation sequencing platforms. *Journal of Virological Methods*, 260, 21–25.

Bishop, R.F., Davidson, G.P., Holmes, I.K., Ruck, B.J. (1973). Virus particles in epithelial cells of duodenal mucosa from children with acute nonbacterial gastroenteritis. *The Lancet*, 2, 1281–1283.

CABI (2019). Bovine adenoviruses infections. CABI Datasheet. www.cabi.org/isc/datasheet/91695.

Carruyo, G.M., Mateu, G., Martínez, L.C., Pujol, F.H., Nates, S.V., Liprandi, F. & Ludert, J.E. (2008). Molecular characterization of porcine picobirnaviruses and development of a specific reverse transcription-PCR assay. *Journal of Clinical Microbiology*, 46(7), 2402–2405.

CDC. (2016). Norovirus symptoms. Archived from the original on 6 December 2018.

CDC. (2017). Norovirus worldwide. 15 December 2017. www.cdc.gov/norovirus/downloads/global-burden-report.pdf

Chen, H. & Hu, Y. (2016). Molecular diagnostic methods for detection and characterization of human noroviruses. *Open Microbiology* Journal, 10, 78–89.

Chigor, V.N. & Okoh, A.I. (2012). Quantitative RT-PCR detection of hepatitis A virus, rotaviruses and enteroviruses in the Buffalo River and source water dams in the Eastern Cape Province of South Africa. *International Journal of Environmental Research and Public Health*, 9(11), 4017–4032.

Cho, Y.I. & Yoon, K.J. (2014). An overview of calf diarrhea – infectious etiology, diagnosis, and intervention. *Journal of Veterinary Science*, 15(1), 1–17.

Cho, Y.I., Kim, W.I., Liu, S., Kinyon, J.M. & Yoon, K.J. (2012). Ecology of calf diarrhea in cow-calf operations. *Journal of Veterinary Diagnostic Investigation*, 22, 509–517.

Conceicao-Neto, N., Mesquita, J.R., Zeller, M., Yinda, C.K., Álvares, F., Roque, S., Petrucci-Fonseca, F., Godinho, R., Heylen, E., Van Ranst, M. & Matthijnssens, J. (2016). Reassortment among picobirnavi-ruses found in wolves. *Archives of Virology*, 161(10): 2859–2862.

De Barros, B.d.C.V., Chagas, E.N., Bezerra, L.W., Ribeiro, L.G., Duarte Júnior, J.W.B., Pereira, D. *et al.* (2018) Rotavirus A in wild and domestic animals from areas with environmental degradation in the Brazilian Amazon. *PLoS ONE*, 13(12): e0209005.

De Benedictis, P., Schultz-Cherry, S., Burnham, A. & Cattoli, G. (2011). Astrovirus infections in humans and animals: molecular biology, genetic diversity, and interspecies transmissions. *Infection, Genetics and Evolution*, 11, 1529–1544.

Decaro, N., Campolo, M., Desario, C., Cirone, F., D'abramo, M., Lorusso, E., Greco, G., Mari, V., Colaianni, M.L., Elia, G., Martella, V. & Buonavoglia, C. (2008). Respiratory disease associated with bovine coronavirus infection in cattle herds in Southern Italy. *Journal of Veterinary Diagnostic Investigation*, 20, 28–32.

Dhama, K., Chauhan, R.S., Mahendran, M. & Malik, S.V.S. (2009). Rotavirus diarrhea in bovines and other domestic animals. *Veterinary Research Communications*, 33, 1–23.

Elshal, M.F. & McCoy, J.P. (2006). Multiplex bead array assays: performance evaluation and comparison of sensitivity to ELISA. *Methods*, 38(4), 317–323.

Fong, T.T. & Lipp, E.K. (2005). Enteric viruses of humans and animals in aquatic environments: health risks, detection, and potential water quality assessment tools. *Microbiology and Molecular Biology Reviews*, 69(2), 357–371.

Ganesh, B., Bányai, K., Martella, V., Jakab, F., Masachessi, G. & Kobayashi, N. (2012). Picobirnavirus infections: viral persistence and zoonotic potential. *Reviews in Medical Virology*, 22: 245–256.

Gautam, R., Mijatovic-Rustempasic, S., Esona, M.D., Tam, K.I., Quaye, O. & Bowen, M.D. (2016). One-step multiplex real-time RT-PCR assay for detecting and genotyping wild-type group A rotavirus strains and vaccine strains (Rotarix® and RotaTeq®) in stool samples. *PeerJ*, 4, e1560.

Geng, J., Wang, L., Wang, X., Fu, H., Bu, Q., Liu, P., Zhu, Y., Wang, M., Sui, Y. & Zhuang, H. (2011). Potential risk of zoonotic transmission from young swine to human: seroepidemiological and genetic characterization of hepatitis E virus in human and various animals in Beijing, China. *Journal of Viral Hepatitis*, 18: e583–590.

Hajia, M. (2017). Limitations of different PCR protocols used in diagnostic laboratories: a short review. *Modern Medical Laboratory Journal*, 1(1), 1–6.

Hansa, A., Rai, R.B., Dhama, K., Wani, M.Y., Saminathan, M. & Ranganath, G.J. (2013). Isolation of bovine coronavirus (BCoV) in vero cell line and its confirmation by direct FAT and RT-PCR. *Pakistan Journal of Biological Sciences*, 16, 1342–1347.

Haramoto, E., Kitajima, M., Hata, A., Torrey, J.R., Masago, Y., Sano, D. & Katayama, H. (2018). A review on recent progress in the detection methods and prevalence of human enteric viruses in water. *Water Research*, 135: 168–186.

Hert, D., Fredlake, C. & Barron, A. (2008). Advantages and limitations of next-generation sequencing technologies: A comparison of electrophoresis and non-electrophoresis methods. *Electrophoresis*, 29, 4618–4626.

Hoehne, M. and Schreier, E. (2006). Detection of *Norovirus* genogroup I and II by multiplex real-time RT- PCR using a 3'-minor groove binder-DNA probe. *BMC Infectious Diseases*, 6, 69.

Honark, S. & Leedom Larson, K.R. (2016). Porcine adenovirus. Swine Health Information Center and Center for Food Security and Public Health, Iowa State University.

Jiang, Y., Fang, L., Shi, X., Zhang, H., Li, Y., Lin, Y. Qiu, Y., Chen, Q., Li, H., Zhou, L. & Hu, Q. (2014). Simultaneous detection of five enteric viruses associated with gastroenteritis by use of a PCR assay: a single real-time multiplex reaction and its clinical application. *Journal of Clinical Microbiology*, 52(4), 1266–1268.

Jiménez-Clavero, M.A., Escribano-Romero, E., Mansilla, C., Gómez, N., Córdoba, L., Roblas, N., Ponz, F., Ley, V. & Sáiz, J.C. (2005). Survey of bovine enterovirus in biological and environmental samples by a highly sensitive real-time reverse transcription-PCR. *Applied and Environmental Microbiology*, 71(7): 3536–3543.

Jindal, N., Chander, Y., Pathnayak, D.P., Mor, S.K., Ziegler, A.F. & Goyal, S.M. (2012). A multiplex RT-PCR for the detection of astrovirus, rotavirus, and reovirus in turkeys. *Avian Diseases*, 56, 592–596.

Johnson, C., Hitchens, P.L., Smiley Evans, T., Goldstein, T., Thomas, K., Clements, A., Joly, D.O., Wolfe, N.D., Daszak, P., Karesh, W.B. & Mazet, J.K. (2015). Spillover and pandemic properties of zoonotic viruses with high host plasticity. *Scientific Reports*, 5, 14830.

Jun, Q., Lulu, T., Qingling, M., Xingxing, Z., Haiting, L., Shasha, G., Zibing, C., Xuepeng, C., Jinsheng, Z., Zaichao, Z., Kuojun, C. & Chuangfu, C. (2016). Serological and molecular investigation of porcine sapovirus infection in piglets in Xinjiang, China. *Tropical Animal Health and Production*, 48. 10.1007/s11250-016-1023-8.

Kattoor, J.J., Malik, Y.S., Sharma, K., Kumar, N., Batra, M., Jindal, N. & Yadav, A.S. (2013). Molecular evidence of group D rotavirus in commercial broiler chicks in India. *Avian Biology Research*, 6, 313–316.

Kattoor, J.J., Sircar, S., Saurab, S., Subramaniyan, S., Dhama, K. & Malik, Y.S. (2016). Picobirnavirus: A putative emerging threat to human and animals. *Advances in Animal and Veterinary Sciences*, 4: 327–331.

Kroneman, A., Vega, E., Vennema, H., Vinjé, J., White, P.A., Hansman, G., Green, K., Martella, V., Katayama, K. & Koopmans, M. (2013). Proposal for a unified norovirus nomenclature and genotyping. *Archives of Virology*, 158(10), 2059–2068.

Kumar, P. (2013). Methods for rapid virus identification and quantification. *Materials and Methods*, 3, 10.13070/mm.en.3.207.

Kurtz, J.B. & Lee, T.W. (1987). Astroviruses: human and animal. In Bock, G. & Whelan, J. (eds), *Ciba Foundation Symposium 128. Novel Diarrhoea Viruses*. John Wiley & Sons.

Lee, H.K. & Jeong, Y.S. (2004). Comparison of total culturable virus assay and multiplex integrated cell culture-PCR for reliability of waterborne virus detection. *Applied and Environmental Microbiology*, 70(6), 3632–3636.

Lee, J.H., Lee, G.C., Kim, J.I., Yi, H.A. & Lee, C.H. (2013). Development of a new cell culture-based method and optimized protocol for the detection of enteric viruses. *Journal of Virological Methods*, 191(1), 16–23.

Lekshmi, M., Oishi Das, S.K. & Nayak, B.B. (2018). Occurrence of human enterovirus in tropical fish and shellfish and their relationship with fecal indicator bacteria. *Veterinary World*, 11(9), 1285.

Li, L., Diab, S., McGraw, S., Barr, B., Traslavina, R., Higgins, R., Talbot, T., Blanchard, P., Rimoldi, G., Fahsbender, E., Page, B., Phan, T.G., Wang, C., Deng, X., Pesavento, P. & Delwart, E. (2013). Divergent astrovirus associated with neurologic disease in cattle. *Emerging Infectious Diseases*, 19(9), 1385–1392.

Li, L., Pesavento, P.A., Shan, T., Leutenegger, C.M., Wang, C. & Delwart, E. (2011). Viruses in diarrhoeic dogs include novel kobuviruses and sapoviruses. *The Journal of General Virology*, 92(Pt 11), 2534–2541.Maan, S., Dalal, S., Kumar, A., Dalal, A., Bansal, N., Chaudhary, D., Gupta, A. & Maan, N.S. (2018). Novel molecular diagnostics and therapeutic tools for livestock diseases. In Gahlawat, S., Duhan, J., Salar, R., Siwach, P., Kumar, S. & Kaur, P. (eds), *Advances in Animal Biotechnology and its Applications*. Springer.

Malik, Y.S., Kumar, N., Sharma, K., Dhama, K., Shabbir, M.Z., Ganesh, B., Kobayashi, N. & Banyai, K. (2014a). Epidemiology, phylogeny, and evolution of emerging enteric Picobirnaviruses of animal origin and their relationship to human strains. *Biomed Research International*, 780752.

Malik, Y.S., Kumar, N., Sharma, K., Sircar, S., Dhama, K., Bora, D.P., Dutta, T.K., Prasad, M. & Tiwari, A.K. (2014b). Rotavirus diarrhea in piglets: A review on epidemiology, genetic diversity and zoonotic risks. *Indian Journal of Animal Sciences*, 84, 1035–1042.

Malik, Y.S., Sircar, S., Saurabh, S., Kattoor, J.J., Singh, R., Ganesh, B., Ghosh, S., Dhama, K. & Singh, R.K. (2018). Epidemiologic status of picobirnavirus in India, a less explored viral disease. *Open Virology Journal*, 12, 99–109.

Martella, V., Moschidou, P., Pinto, P., Catella, C., Desario, C., Larocca, V., Circella, E., Bànyai, K., Lavazza, A., Magistrali, C., Decaro, N. & Buonavoglia, C. (2011). Astroviruses in rabbits. *Emerging Infectious Diseases*, 17(12), 2287–2293.

Mauroy, A., Van der Poel, W.H.M., Hakze-Van der Honing, R., Thys, C. & Thiry, E. (2012). Development and application of a SYBR Green RT-PCR for first line screening and quantification of porcine sapovirus infection. *BMC Veterinary Res*earch, 8, 193.

Mullis, L., Saif, L.J., Zhang, Y., Zhang, X. & Azevedo, M.S.P. 2012. Stability of bovine coronavirus on lettuce surfaces under household refrigeration conditions. *Food Microbiol*ogy, 30(1), 180–186.

Papp, H., Malik, Y.S., Farkas, S.L., Jakab, F., Martella, V. & Banyai, K. (2014). Rotavirus strains in neglected animal species including lambs, goats and camelids. *Virus Diseases*, 25(2), 215–222.

Park S.J., Jeong C, Yoon S.S., Choy H.E., Saif L.J., Park S.H., Kim Y.J., Jeong J.H., Park S.I., Kim H.H., Lee B.J., Cho H.S., Kim S.K., Kang M.I. and Cho K.O. (2006). Detection and characterization of bovine coronaviruses in fecal specimens of adult cattle with diarrhea during the warmer seasons, *Journal of Clinical Microbiology*, 44(9), 3178–3188.

Pereira, H.G., Fialho, A.M., Flewett, T.H., Teixeira, J.M. & Andrade Z.P. (1988). Novel viruses in human faeces. *The Lancet*, 2, 103–104.

Perot, P., Lecuit, M. & Eloit, M. (2017). Astrovirus diagnostics. *Viruses*, 9(1): 10.

Proietto, S., Killoran, K. & Leedom Larson, K.R. 2016. Porcine sapovirus. Swine Health Information Center and Center for Food Security and Public Health, Iowa University.

Ramos Caruzo, T.A., Diederichsen de Brito, W., Elsner, M., Munford, V. & Rácz, M.L. (2010). Molecular characterization of G and P-types bovine rotavirus strains from Goiás, Brazil: high frequency of mixed P-type infections. *Memórias do Instituto Oswaldo Cruz, Rio de Janeiro*, 105, 1040–1043.

Richards, G.P. (1999) Limitations of molecular biological techniques for assessing the virological safety of foods. *Journal of Food Protection*, 62, 691–697.

Rojas, M.A., Gonçalves, J.L.S., Dias, H.G., Manchego, A. & Santos, N. (2017). Identification of two novel Rotavirus A genotypes, G35 and P [50], from Peruvian alpaca faeces. *Infection, Genetics and Evolution*, 55, 71–74.

Rose, J.B., Zhou, X., Griffin, D.W. & Paul J.H. (1997). Comparison of PCR and plaque assay for detection and enumeration of coliphage in polluted marine waters. *Applied and Environmental Microbiology*, 63, 4564– 4566.

Saif, L.J., Bohl, E.H., Theil, K.W., Cross, R.F. & House, J.A. (1980). Rotavirus-like, calicivirus-like, and 23-nm virus-like particles associated with diarrhea in young pigs. *Journal of Clinical Microbiology*, 12, 105–111.

Sircar, S., Saurabh, S., Kattoor, J.J., Deol, P., Dhama, K., Khurana, S.K. & Malik, Y.S. (2016). Evolving views on enteric viral infections of equines: An appraisal of key pathogens. *Journal of Experimental Biology and Agriculture Science*, 4(Spl-4-EHIDZ): S182–195.

Smither, S.J., Lear-Rooney, C., Biggins, J., Pettitt, J., Lever, M.S. & Olinger, G.G., Jr. (2013). Comparison of the plaque assay and 50% tissue culture infectious dose assay as methods for measuring filovirus infectivity. *Journal of Virological Methods*, 193(2), 565–571.

Smyth, J.A., Benko, M., Moffett, D.A. & Harrach, B. (1996). Bovine adenovirus type 10 identified in fatal cases of adenovirus-associated enteric disease in cattle by in situ hybridization. *Journal of Clinical Microbiology*, 34(5), 1270–1274.

Soma, T., Nakagomi, O., Nakagomi, T. & Mochizuki, M. (2015). Detection of *Norovirus* and *Sapovirus* from diarrheic dogs and cats in Japan. *Microbiology and Immunology*, 59(3), 123–128.

Tsuchiaka, S., Rahpaya, SS., Otomaru, K. *et al.* (2017). Identification of a novel bovine enterovirus possessing highly divergent amino acid sequences in capsid protein. *BMC Microbiology*, 17, 18.

Van der Heide, R., Koopmans, M.P.G., Shekary, N., Houwers, D.J., Van Duynhoven, Y.T.H.P. & Van der Poel, W.H.M. (2005). Molecular characterizations of human and animal group a rotavirus in the Netherlands. *Journal of Clinical Microbiology*, 43(2), 669–675.

Vildevall, M. (2011). The *Norovirus* puzzle: characterization of human and bovine norovirus susceptibility patterns (thesis). Linkoping University Medical Dissertations No. 1244, Sweden.

Villabruna, N., Koopmans, M.P.G. & de Graaf, M. (2019). Animals as reservoir for human *Norovirus*. *Viruses*, 11(5), 478.

Vinjé, J. (2015). Advances in laboratory methods for detection and typing of *Norovirus*. *Journal of Clinical Microbiology*, 53(2), 373–381.

Wilburn, L., Yodmeeklin, A., Kochjan, P., Saikruang, W., Kumthip, K., Khamrin, P. & Maneekarn, N. (2017). Molecular detection and characterization of picobirnaviruses in piglets with diarrhea in Thailand. *Archives Virology*, 162(4), 1061–1066.

Woo, P.C., Teng, J.L., Bai, R., Wong, A.Y., Martelli, P., Hui, S.W., Tsang, A.K., Lau, C.C., Ahmed, S.S., Yip, C.C., Choi, G.K., Li, K.S., Lam, C.S., Lau, S.K. & Yuen, K.Y. (2016). High diversity of Genogroup I Picobirnaviruses in mammals. *Frontiers in Microbiology*, 7, 1886.

Wu, J., Cao, Y., Young, B., Yuen, Y., Jiang, S., Melendez, D., Stewart, J.R. *et al.* (2016). Decay of coliphages in sewage-contaminated freshwater: uncertainty and seasonal effects. *Environmental Science and Technology*, 50(21), 11593–11601.

Zhu, T., Zhao, G., Shen, F., Hou Peili, Wang, H., Li, J. & He, H. (2015). Establishment and preliminary application of the SYBR Green I real-time PCR assay for detection of the bovine enterovirus. *Bing Du Xue Bao*, 31(5), 488–493.

17

Coronaviruses: Recent Trends and Approaches in Diagnosis and Management

Samander Kaushik,[1] **Yashika Sharma,**[1] **Sulochana Kaushik,**[2] **Jaya Parkash Yadav**[2] **and Minakshi Prasad**[3]

[1] *Centre for Biotechnology, Maharshi Dayanand University, Rohtak-124001, Haryana, India*

[2] *Department of Genetics, Maharshi Dayanand University, Rohtak-124001, Haryana, India*

[3] *Department of Animal Biotechnology, Lala Lajpat Rai University of Veterinary and Animal Sciences, Hisar-125004, Haryana, India*

Corresponding author: Samander Kaushik, *samanderkaushik@gmail.com*

17.1 Introduction

Human health and wealth are highly influenced by a number of dangerous emerging viruses, of which the severe acute respiratory syndrome coronavirus (SARS-CoV), Middle East respiratory syndrome coronavirus (MERS-CoV), and coronavirus infectious disease-19 (COVID-19) viral outbreaks are recent examples. SARS-CoV, MERS-CoV, and COVID-19 belong to the family *Coronaviridae*. SARS-CoV emerged in China in 2003; MERS-CoV emerged in 2012 in Jordan; COVID-19 is a newly emerging coronavirus initiating in Wuhan, China, which has spread throughout the world. SARS-CoV and MERS-CoV were limited to a few places only, while COVID-19 has infected a large part of the human population throughout the globe (Lu, H., 2013). COVID-19 has become adaptive to human infection with the potential for easy transmission between persons or communities, due to the absence of immunity against it. Therefore, COVID-19 has become highly contagious in nature. The modern human life-style of fast travel and trade systems has been a great helper for the quick spreading of COVID-19, which became a pandemic very soon after its emergence. In a few months, COVID-19 had successfully spread to more than 215 countries and was responsible for more than 10 million laboratory-confirmed cases, with 0.5 million deaths up to 26 June 2020. Although COVID-19 has high spreading or infection power, its mortality rate (death rate) is 4.80%, which is lower than for other dangerous coronaviruses like SARS-CoV (10%) and MERS-CoV (37.1%) (www.worldometers.info/coronavirus, accessed on 30 June 2020). To stop the further expansion of it or to gain effective control over COVID-19 infection, scientists, the health fraternity, employees, and other persons related to health and management should co-operate at national as well as international level, exchanging information and strategies, developing various management protocols, and sharing their experiences (Yoo, 2019).

17.2 Virus, Virology, and Pathogenesis

The family *Coronaviridae* is one of the biggest virus families, containing many viruses responsible for respiratory and enteric tract diseases in various animals. Some coronaviruses have evolved themselves for human infection. Coronaviruses are comparatively large viruses, with a size range of 100–160 nm. All coronaviruses are spherical in shape, surrounded by a lipoprotein envelope. The genome of coronaviruses is single-stranded RNA in the range of 27–32 kb, which is positive-sense in nature, assembled on a proteinous capsid and protected by a lipoprotein envelope (Lai, 1997). The spikes are the important out-growth portion of coronaviruses; during electron microscopy, their specific spike patterns are very helpful for the identification of coronaviruses up to some level. There are different types of spikes: a) long (20 nm) glycoprotein S-spikes present in every coronavirus in large numbers; b) small hemagglutinin-esterase (HE) spikes, found only in a few coronaviruses; c) trans-membrane glycoproteins and envelope protein spikes found in small numbers in many coronaviruses (Escors *et al.*, 2001; Locker *et al.*, 1992). The viruses belonging to the *Coronaviridae* family can be broadly divided into three serogroups according to their genome structure. The members of the serogroups 1 and 2 are able to infect various mammalian species. 229E-CoV, NL63-CoV, OC43-CoV, HKU1-CoV, SARS-CoV, MERS-CoV, and COVID-19 belong to serogroups 1 and 2, with a capacity for human infection. Those viruses belonging to serogroup 3 can infect birds only.

229E-CoV, NL63-CoV, OC43-CoV, and HKU1-CoV are self-limit coronaviruses that can cause 30% or more upper-respiratory-tracheal viral diseases in humans, but they are responsible for only mild infections, and therefore they have little medical significance. SARS-CoV, MERS-CoV, and COVID-19 are well known for their dangerous human infection. Recently, these three coronaviruses have adapted from animals and have become responsible for mild to fatal diseases in humans (Snijder *et al.*, 2003; Su *et al.*, 2016). Generally, coronaviruses are species-specific, but sometimes a particular virus can break the species barrier, via expanding its genetic variability through mutation or recombination in its genome while replicating in the host during animal infection. Accidently, a mutant coronavirus may be originated, which can jump the species barrier and start an infection in humans directly or through another intermediate animal (Paules *et al.*, 2020). The recent outbreak of the novel coronavirus (COVID-19) could have been adapted from an animal because the majority of initial human cases were noted in a group associated with the live animal market of Wuhan, China. After some time, the virus may have acquired the capacity of human infection, spreading via person to person through droplets or direct contact as well as nosocomial infection (Li *et al.*, 2020; Wang *et al.*, 2020; Chang *et al.*, 2020; Carlos *et al.*, 2020). Transmission from asymptomatic carriers or COVID-19 patients, over a longer period, provides the chance of rapid expansion of the virus among the public. Good stability, an easy spreading route (the respiratory system), a high infection rate, the absence of immunity in the public, a fast travel system, and the inter-connected nature of the world are responsible factors for the high potential of COVID-19 infection. Due to these high potential factors, COVID-19 has become pandemic agent with high morbidity and considerable mortality (Zhao *et al.*, 2020; Biscayart *et al.*, 2020; Munster *et al.*, 2020).

Viruses are species-specific; like other viruses, coronaviruses can be infectious to a particular host. The first step of viral infection is entry into the specific host or, more precisely, into a particular cell or tissue system. Viruses will interact with their specific receptor on the basis of the complementary nature of the viral spike and cellular receptors. Large numbers of particular types of receptors are present on the specific cells of their host. COVID-19 and other coronaviruses interact with specific receptors present on their target cells in the respiratory tracts of humans. Bioinformatics analysis of COVID-19 spike and cellular receptors indicates that COVID-19 and SARS-CoV utilize the same receptors in humans (Lu, R. *et al.*, 2020). The spikes of SARS-CoV and COVID-19 interact with the angiotensin-converting enzyme-2 (ACE-2) cellular receptor and enter the cells. The ACE-2 receptors are present in a variety of cells belonging to the lungs, heart, kidney, various parts of the small intestine, and other important tissues of the body. MERS-CoV enters into human cells through dipeptidyl peptidase-4 (DPP4), a transmembrane glycoprotein, in place of ACE-2 receptors (Li *et al.*, 2003; Qian *et al.*, 2013; Lu, G. *et al.*, 2013; Raj *et al.*, 2013). Like other viruses, after binding with their specific host receptors, human coronaviruses also enter into the cells of an infected person through the fusion of the coronavirus envelope along with the host cell plasma membrane, or via endosomal membranes. After entry into the host cytoplasm, the components of the virus are enabled and hijack cellular machinery for their own purpose. Coronaviruses contain positive-sense RNA which, after releasing into the host cytoplasm, translates into pp1a and pp1ab poly-proteins (De Wilde *et al.*, 2017). The translations produce structural and non-structural proteins and form the replication-transcription complex (RTC) in double-membrane vesicles (Sawicki *et al.*, 2005). The RTC of the virus replicates continuously to synthesize a nested set of sub-genomic RNAs. These RNAs are translated into the accessory and structural proteins of the viruses (Hussain *et al.*, 2005; Perrier *et al.*, 2019). The newly synthesized viral genomic RNA, capsid proteins, envelope glycol-proteins, and other compulsory viral components are assembled in sequence and in a specific manner to form a complete virus.

After complete assembly of the coronavirus, the virion-containing vesicles fuse with the plasma membrane of the host cell, from where the virus buds out from the host cell. When coronavirus was inoculated in an animal cell culture for virus isolation, it produced a variety of cytopathic effects (CPEs). The pattern and extent of CPEs are dependent upon the coronaviral strain as well as the host cell. Various factors are responsible for the pattern and extent of CPEs. They interfere with cellular internal signal pathways, cause the derangement of various cytoplasmic functions, stimulate production of cytokines/chemokines, and affect the transcription rate and translation of various important cellular proteins or factors. Many coronaviruses are responsible for host cell fusion, while some are responsible for apoptosis.

17.3 Global Epidemiology

Easy and quick modes of transmission, viral nature, high population densities, and suitable environmental conditions are major factors contributing to the rapid spreading of SARS-CoV, MERS-CoV, and COVID-19. The majority of respiratory viruses produce similar clinical symptoms; therefore, they should be accurately diagnosed by standardized laboratory-based assays, not merely on the basis of their clinical symptoms. Unfortunately, only a few developed countries have the proper viral diagnostic capacity through laboratory-based methods. Without specific laboratory-confirmed data or a reliable surveillance system, authenticity and accuracy of estimates over their prevalence is doubtful. The viral reproductive number (R0) can be used for calculation of the average number of viral infections induced by infected persons to other susceptible persons in their vicinity. The R0 of SARS-CoV is 1.4–5.5, for MERS-CoV is < 1, while for newly emerging COVID-19 it is 2.2–2.6; for influenza viruses, it is higher (5–25). Therefore, the R0 suggests that SARS-CoV, MERS-CoV, and COVID-19 are less infectious than influenza viruses (Prompetchara *et al.*, 2020; Riley *et al.*, 2003).

17.4 Virus Diagnosis

The effective management of any viral outbreak requires the use of rapid, highly sensitive, agent-specific, and economical diagnosis assays. There is no routine specific surveillance or continuous diagnosis system for coronaviruses in the majority of the world, especially in developing parts. The diagnosis of coronaviruses is somehow difficult, as many of them cannot be cultured in *in vitro* conditions or identified by well-standardized immunological reagents, and their genomic sequences are not available. Human coronaviruses 229E, NL63, OC43, and HKU1 cause only self-limited mild infections. There is no need for a diagnosis of 229E, NL63, OC43, or HKU1. On the other hand, life-threatening SARS-CoV, MERS-CoV, and COVID-19 should be accurately diagnosed for effective management and prevention of further spreading. Keen interest in the diagnosis of SARS-CoV, MERS-CoV, and COVID-19 has also led to the discovery of other previously unrecognized human and animal coronaviruses. The identification of these life-threatening coronaviruses has stimulated virologists for the detailed study of their origin, evolution, pathogenesis, and virology. For their accurate diagnosis, virologists have developed fast, highly sensitive, agent-specific, and cost-effective diagnostic assays. The clinical symptoms of coronaviruses and other respiratory viral infections are very similar to each other. Therefore, the accurate diagnosis of coronaviruses is possible only through reliable virology laboratory-based assays. In the initial, emerging phase of a coronavirus or any other virus outbreak, genomic sequences are unavailable for molecular diagnosis. The diagnosis of the majority of emerging viruses is initiated via virus isolation in cell-line/animal models or sometimes via electron microscopy/immune electron microscopy. As soon as a serum or specific antibodies are available, serological diagnosis is also possible. Once genomic sequence data of emerging viruses are available, then molecular assays like conventional PCR, RT-PCR, and real-time RT-PCR become the best methods for diagnosis.

Coronaviruses are typical viruses causing respiratory and gastro-intestinal infection in both animals and humans. According to the nature of coronaviruses, respiratory secretion and fecal samples can be collected for diagnostic purposes. The appropriate samples should be collected during a particular stage of infection, in sterile conditions, following the WHO bio-safety guidelines for that particular coronavirus. Nasopharyngeal aspirates, nasopharyngeal swabs, throat and nose swabs, or broncho-alveolar lavages should be collected for coronavirus isolation and antigen detection via molecular assays. An appropriate amount of fecal specimen should be collected for gastro-dominant coronaviruses. A pair of blood samples from different phases of the disease should be collected for the serological diagnosis or sero-surveillance of coronaviruses. The collected samples should be transported immediately to a virology laboratory in specified and sterile conditions. The collected sample material should be processed immediately at a specified condition at a designated bio-safety level. Appropriate and standardized diagnostic assays should be applied to clinical samples or their components for the accurate diagnosis of coronaviruses. SARS-CoV, MERS-CoV, and COVID-19 detection or diagnosis was initiated with virus isolation and electron microscopy, both classical virological techniques, due to the non-availability of their genome sequences. With time, various reagents for the molecular and serological diagnosis of coronaviruses were developed, accelerating their detection. Molecular diagnosis assays are more useful in every respect; therefore, trends shift from classic to molecular diagnosis after the availability of reagents and genomic sequences of emerging or novel coronaviruses (Drosten *et al.*, 2003; Ksiazek *et al.*, 2003; Peiris *et al.*, 2003). Historically, SARS-CoV was isolated in an animal cell culture, and then identified with the help of microarrays (Wang *et al.*, 2003). The partial sequence information of a novel virus can be obtained with the help of conventional RT-PCR via random primers and consensus primers (Drosten *et al.*, 2003; Ksiazek *et al.*, 2003; Peiris *et al.*, 2003). A novel human coronavirus (NL63) could be identified during animal cell culture isolation via virus discovery based on the cDNA-AFLP (VIDISCA) approach with the help of deriving the genetic sequence of its fragments (Van der Hoek *et al.*, 2007). In another outbreak, HKU1 and novel bat coronaviruses were identified by RT-PCR with the help of consensus primer methods (Poon *et al.*, 2005; Woo *et al.*, 2005). Microarrays may be a very useful technique in the future for identification and diagnosis (Kistler *et al.*, 2007). Coronaviruses can be detected or diagnosed through virus isolation (cell-line, embryonated egg, and animal models), electron microscopy/immune electron microscopy, various serological techniques, and modern molecular assays.

17.4.1 Virus Isolation

Among various methods of virus isolation, like animal cell culture, embryonated egg, and animal models, virus isolation is considered to be the gold standard. Virus isolation is a time-consuming procedure and higher containment facilities are required for it. Due to the time-consuming, virus isolation cannot consider as the best method for viral diagnostic purposes but produced plenty of viruses in the end. These amounts of viruses can be utilized for antigenic and molecular characterizations of emerging or any further mutant viruses. HCoV-OC43 and its related strains of coronaviruses are very difficult to cultivate in the cell culture system. HCoV-OC43 cannot be cultured in a continuous cell-line but instead requires organ cultures, hence the "OC" in HCoV-OC43, which stands for "organ culture". In contrast, HCoV-229E and its related strains can be cultivated to some extent. Recently, few strain-specific cell-lines have become available for the cultivation of both (HCoV-OC43 and HCoV-229E) laboratory-adapted human coronaviruses strains, but isolation from clinical samples still remains a challenging task. HCoV-229E and its related strains of coronaviruses can be isolated with the help of the roller culture monolayers technique by using human embryonic lung fibroblasts (W-138 and MRC-5 cells) and human embryonic intestinal fibroblast cells (MA-177). During the course of virus isolation in their recommended cell-line, viruses are absorbed from the inoculums to the cell-line through their specific receptors during incubation periods. After viral entry, the virus is replicated in the host cells. In response to viral replication, cells become small, granular, and round in appearance, known as cytopathic effects (CPEs). CPEs can be seen in the whole monolayer or the peripheral region. The extent of CPEs depends upon the severity of viruses; a complete monolayer of cells can be destroyed rarely in the initial isolation phase but after repeated inoculation extent of CPEs increase (Myint, 1995). Vero E6 cells or fetal rhesus kidney cells have been used for the isolation of SARS-CoV (Drosten *et al.*, 2003; Ksiazek *et al.*, 2003; Peiris *et al.*, 2003b). The several passages of SARS-CoV in the cell-line cause mutations in the genome. The substitutions of amino acids in the spike and M genes may be responsible for the adaptation of the virus (Poon *et al.*, 2005). HCoV-NL63 can be cultured in tertiary monkey kidney cells and in LLC-MK2 cells. HCoV-HKU1 is difficult to grow but has been isolated in HuH7 cells (Vabret *et al.*, 2006).

17.4.1.1 Advantages of Virus Isolation

- Virus isolation helps in the initial diagnosis of a novel virus.
- It is a gold-standard test and can be used to compare the sensitivity and specificity of other diagnostic methods.
- It eventually produces a good amount of viruses, which can be utilized for further antigenic and molecular characterizations.
- It is helpful for vaccine development.

17.4.1.2 Disadvantages of Virus Isolation

- Virus isolation is time-consuming.
- It is very prone to contamination.
- It cannot cultivate many viruses.
- A high-containment-level facility is required for virus isolation.
- It is not a good method of diagnosis.

17.4.2 Electron Microscopy

Electron microscopy cannot be considered a good diagnosis technique, as the majority of viruses have a similar appearance. Cellular debris along with other unwanted materials also hampers viral identification in the sample via an electron microscope. Coronaviruses have a specific crown-like appearance; therefore, microscopy can provide some clue for the initial identification of coronaviruses at the emerging stage. Due to their specific appearance, coronaviruses can be identified in clinical samples containing epithelial cells from the nasopharynx, cell culture isolates (229E, SARS-CoV), and organ culture (OC43). All coronaviruses have a similar appearance to one another and to some other viruses, but a specific antibody combines with a specific virus; therefore, immune electron microscopy can be utilized for diagnosis by using a convalescent serum or virus-specific monoclonal antibody. Some strains of coronaviruses causing enteric infection discharge in stool samples can be diagnosed with the help of immune electron microscopy (Duckmanton *et al.*, 1997). If two viruses have the same size and shape, they can be confused during electron microscopy, and therefore immune electron microscopy should be combined with other techniques (Cornelissen *et al.*, 1997).

17.4.2.1 Advantages of Electron Microscopy

- Electron microscopy is very helpful in initial diagnosis during viral emerging.
- The shape and size of viruses can be calculated with the help of electron microscopy.
- It gives information on the number and shape of viral spikes.
- Viral pleomorphic nature can be studied by electron microscopy.

17.4.2.2 Disadvantages of Electron Microscopy

- The cost and maintenance of the electron microscope is very high.
- Electron microscopy cannot differentiate between two viruses with the same size and similar shape.
- It cannot diagnose pleomorphic viruses on the basis of their appearance.
- The spikes present on coronaviruses are not always clearly visible through negative staining.

17.4.3 Serology

Serology is one of the most common diagnostic methods used for various viral groups. The various immunological assays (CFT, ELISA, RIA, IFA, or neutralization) are based upon the basic principle that "a specific antigen can combine with a specific antibody". These methods have been utilized for sero-diagnosis or seroprevalence of coronaviruses (Myint, 1995). Sero-epidemiological studies of SARS-CoV are done on ice-cold acetone-fixed virus-infected cells of patients, with the help of immunofluorescence or virus neutralization assays. In a serological study, neutralizing antibodies against SARS-CoV attained peak titer at about four months after infection; gradually, titer decreased, and about 16% of survivors do not have detectable levels of neutralizing antibody after three years (Cao *et al.*, 2007). Like for flavivirus, coronavirus-specific antibodies can also show cross-reactivity. For example, a SARS-CoV-specific antibody is cross-reactive with other human coronaviruses (OC43, 229E) during the immune-fluorescent assay, while the reverse is not true (Chan *et al.*, 2005). The sensitivity and specificity of ELISA are also poor; therefore, positive results must be confirmed by other assays like immunofluorescence or micro-neutralization tests (Woo *et al.*, 2004).

17.4.3.1 Advantages of Serology

- Serological assays are rapid, sensitive, and specific.
- They are cost-effective.
- They can be performed even on the bad-side without laboratory.
- They are very useful in studying the efficacy of a vaccine.
- A low bio-containment level is required for serological assays.
- They are useful for the diagnosis of infections of viruses that cannot be cultivated.

17.4.3.2 Disadvantages of Serology

- Serological assays are less sensitive and specific than molecular assays.
- They can be applied to blood samples only.
- A specific pairing of antigen and antibody is required.

- Diagnosis in the acute phase via serology is very limited.
- A lag-phage is required in antibody development.

17.4.4 Molecular Diagnosis

The accurate diagnosis of coronaviruses is possible with reliable laboratory diagnosis assays. Initially, coronaviruses can be diagnosed in culture by electron microscopy or immune electron microscopy through their shape, size, and morphology. Sometimes serological methods may be helpful for diagnosis at the initial stage of the viral outbreak. In later stages, as genomic sequences of emerging viruses become available and primers and probes are designed, molecular assays become the prime method of diagnosis. In the modern era, virology is developing in every respect and molecular diagnosis assays have become the priority because they are rapid, highly sensitive, antigen-specific, and economical for viral diagnosis.

Conventional PCR is a very famous molecular diagnostic technique, which produces millions of copies of amplicons with the help of target-specific primers and other reagents, like dNTPs and thermo-stable Taq DNA polymerase. Taq DNA polymerase is a heat-stable enzyme able to exponentially amplify the target DNA in co-operation with a thermo-cycler. The process involves three steps: denaturation of target DNA; annealing temperature for combining the primers at their specific sites; extension temperature for synthesizing the complementary DNA. These steps should be repeated 40–45 times to get a sufficient amount of DNA amplicon. Conventional PCR/RT-PCR is extensively utilized for the amplification of small quantities of extracted target DNA into the desired amount. Which can be further utilized for laboratory diagnosis, analysis, or other purposes? PCR can amplify only DNA molecules, and therefore in the case of RNA viruses, their RNA should be converted into DNA before PCR with the help of a reverse-transcriptase enzyme. Conventional PCR is very simple, with good sensitivity and sequence specificity, and has highly influenced modern diagnostic procedures. Convectional PCR/RT-PCR-based assays can be routinely and reliably utilized for the diagnosis of various types of coronavirus infection in patients (Shen *et al.*, 2020; Balboni *et al.*, 2012; Uhlenhaut *et al.*, 2012). In all the three above-mentioned assays, coronavirus-excreted RNA is converted into complementary DNA with the help of reverse-transcription enzymes, random hexamer, dNTPs, and buffer compounds. The complementary cDNA is amplified with the help of a PCR thermo-cycler and further detected or analyzed with the help of electrophoresis or sequencing (Shen *et al.*, 2020; Adachi *et al.*, 2004; Setianingsih *et al.*, 2019). As compared to other diagnostic techniques, RT-PCR is significantly more sensitive than conventional methods (Wan *et al.*, 2016; Noh *et al.*, 2017), and is the predominantly used diagnostic method for various coronaviruses, including newly emerging COVID-19 (Corman *et al.*, 2012; Lu X *et al.*, 2014; Corman et al., 2020).

Conventional RT-PCR gives only the positive and negative status of the patient, without quantitative information. Real-time RT-PCR is an advanced version of conventional PCR, which can be considered as a gold-standard molecular technique to detect COVID-19 and other coronaviruses. Real-time RT-PCR is a well-established technique, needing only a specific primer-probe, with the rest of the components of the reaction remaining the same as or similar to those used for other viruses. There are two types of real-time RT-PCR: fluorescence dye-based or Taqman probe-based assays. Taqman probe-based real-time RT-PCR is more sensitive, specific, and less time-consuming than conventional RT-PCR. The reagents for a real-time RT-PCR assay are costly and high-cost equipment is also required.

Loop-mediated isothermal amplification (LAMP) is another molecular DNA/RNA amplification technique with high specificity, efficiency, and rapidity under isothermal conditions. LAMP uses a set of four specially designed primers along with a DNA polymerase enzyme, which has strand displacement activity to synthesize target DNA. LAMP is specific, highly sensitive, very simple, and requires no special instrumentation. LAMP has become a very famous isothermal amplification diagnosis assay in molecular biology since its initial development. LAMP uses strand-displacement polymerases instead of heat denaturation to generate a single-stranded template; hence, it has the advantage of running at a constant temperature, simultaneously reducing the cumbersomeness of a thermo-cycler as well as the energy required. LAMP technology is proven to be more stable and more sensitive than rapid commercial kits, virus isolation and other molecular detection assays. A disadvantage of LAMP is its tendency to sometimes produce false-positive results.

17.5 Management of Coronaviruses

A viral infection can be easily prevented through an effective vaccine or specific antiviral therapy. When there is no vaccine or antiviral, then prevention and symptomatic therapy are somewhat helpful. Of the several coronaviruses, only seven (229E, NL63, OC43, HKU1, SARS-CoV, MERS-CoV, and COVID-19) are responsible for natural infections in human beings. 229E-CoV, NL63-CoV, OC43-CoV, and HKU1-CoV cause self-limited mild infections in the upper respiratory region, without requiring any specific treatment. SARS-CoV, MERS-CoV, and COVID-19 infections range from asymptomatic to life-threatening, and they have a considerably high death rate. Due to high morbidity and mortality, SARS-CoV, MERS-CoV, and COVID-19 need clinical management, which depends upon the clinical symptoms and severity of these diseases. A number of therapeutic agents have been identified due to several outbreaks of dangerous coronaviruses. The more specific, sensitive and economical drug comes after the understanding of molecular virology of these viruses in the available of cell culture or animal model system (Holmes, 2003). As these are emerging viruses, there is no specific vaccine or effective antiviral available to treat them. Supportive and symptomatic care is the only treatment strategy for these dangerous coronaviruses. Their management depends upon clinical symptoms and the severity of infection, and is sometimes carried out with the help of a combination of several broad-spectrum antibiotics, antivirals, and corticosteroids. Convalescent plasma therapy along with management therapy has also been tried in various parts of the world (Jin *et al.*, 2020).

17.5.1 Ribavirin

Ribavirin is one of the purine nucleoside analog types of antiviral, and is responsible for interference with the RNA polymerases of viruses, reducing polymerase activity (Parker, 2005). Ribavirin is already used in the therapy of respiratory syncytial virus (RSV) and hepatitis C virus (HCV), reducing viral RNA synthesis and helping in viral clearance (Jordan *et al.*, 2018; Thomas *et al.*, 1999). Although it has long been in continuous use, it has some side effects, such as hemolytic anemia (Knowles *et al.*, 2003). During a control experimental study, results were not satisfactory; therefore, it was not recommendable for the treatment of SARS-CoV (Knowles *et al.*, 2003; van Vonderen *et al.*, 2003). However, ribavirin was used extensively during the SARS-CoV and MERS-CoV outbreaks in the absence of any alternative (Zumla *et al.*, 2016). Whether ribavirin can be an effective antiviral against COVID-19 must be studied in a controlled clinical trial.

17.5.2 Other Antiviral Drugs

Glycyrrhizin and its derivatives can be utilized as an antiviral for the treatment of SARS-CoV and other coronaviruses (Cinatl *et al.*, 2003; Wu *et al.*, 2004; Hoever *et al.*, 2005). The mechanism of glycyrrhizin and its derivatives is to interact with cellular signaling pathways, transcription factors, and up-regulation to induce nitrous oxide syntheses (Cinatl *et al.*, 2003). Glycyrrhizin and its derivatives can reduce plasma membrane fluidity, delaying viral entry into the cell (Harada, 2005). A well-known anti-malarial drug, chloroquine, was shown to have anti-SARS-CoV activity when an *in vitro* study was done on a Vero E6 cell-line (Savarino *et al.*, 2003; Keyaerts *et al.*, 2004; Vincent *et al.*, 2005). Chloroquine increases the pH of the endosomal of virus that can interfere with the terminal glycosylation on the ACE2 receptor (Vincent *et al.*, 2005), which may be responsible for its antiviral activities against all related viruses that enter through the ACE2 receptor, such as SARS-CoV, MARS-CoV, and COVID-19. The protease inhibitor 3CLpro has the capacity to prevent the formation of the functional replication complex, which may inhibit the replication of SARS-CoV, MARS-CoV, and COVID-19 (Bacha *et al.*, 2004; Lee *et al.*, 2005; Martina *et al.*, 2005; Renu *et al.*, 2020). 3CLpro has some conserve region found in genome of various coronaviruses, can be commonly used as an antiviral against the protease of all these viruses (Yang *et al.*, 2005; Lau *et al.*, 2005). During bioinformatics studies, homology modeling has suggested that there are enough similarity in the substrate-binding conservation regions present in the genomes of SARS-CoV, HCoV-229E, and PEDV (Anand *et al.*, 2003). Lopinavir was a widely used antiviral in the treatment of MERS-CoV at the initial stage, in the absence of a vaccine. Combined therapy of ribavirin and interferon shows more useful results in comparison to individual therapy (Al-Tawfiq *et al.*, 2014). A combination of cyclosporin A (CsA), cycloheximide, mycophenolate, IFN-b, omacetaxinemepe succinate, anisomycin, and emetine dihydrochloride hydrate is best in comparison to other individual or combined anti-viral therapies in the treatment of MERS-CoV (Al-Hazmi *et al.*, 2016).

17.5.3 Monoclonal Antibody Therapy

In the absence of a vaccine and a specific antiviral, a monoclonal antibody can be an alternative to treat an emerging infection. Pure viruses are the primary requirement, as monoclonal antibodies cannot be produced without the availability of viruses in their pure form. Production and purification of monoclonal antibodies requires significant time. Monoclonal antibodies should be produced against some surface parts or components of the pathogen or virus. 229E-CoV, NL63-CoV, OC43-CoV, and HKU1-CoV cause self-limited mild infections, without requiring any specific monoclonal therapy. SARS-CoV, MERS-CoV, and COVID-19 have emerged as high-potential viruses requiring immediate attention. In order to effectively control a particular viral infection, as monoclonal antibodies are strain-specific, therefore, virus specific monoclonal antibodies can be useful for therapeutic purposes. SARS and other virus-specific monoclonal antibodies are available; these are helpful for patient recovery (Zhang *et al.*, 2005). In animal experimentation, monoclonal antibodies produced in response to SARS-CoV were able to protect ferrets from infection (ter Meulen *et al.*, 2004). Respiratory syncytial virus (RSV) is a well-known virus that causes childhood pneumonia. There is no vaccine or specific antiviral against RSV, but a monoclonal antibody can be utilized for therapeutic purposes to control neonatal pneumonia caused by RSV (Johnson *et al.*, 1997). Plasma or convalescent serum therapy has also been tried in some parts of the world to treat SARS-CoV patients, but these are unplanned emergency treatments to save lives whose efficacy is unknown. When plasma or convalescent serum therapy was studied on a mice model, the therapy helped to ease their recovery, which may have been due to the interference of antibodies in plasma or convalescent serum with SARS-CoV (Wong *et al.*, 2004b; Traggiai *et al.*, 2004; Yeh *et al.*, 2005).

In another therapeutic effort, a B-cell immortalization procedure was applied using CpG oligonucleotide (CpG, 2006) as the polyclonal B-cell activator, along with Epstein-Barr virus. The B-cell immortalization effect was studied in irradiated allogeneic mononuclear cells to study their memory in convalescent SARS-CoV patients. Neutralizing monoclonal antibodies were produced in response to the stable B-cell clone (S3.1). These monoclonal antibodies were able to prevent SARS-CoV infection in the lungs of mice during an animal experimental study (Traggiai *et al.*, 2004). Monoclonal antibodies are new therapeutic agents, and more than 35 different types of monoclonal antibodies that can neutralize SARS-CoV have been isolated through studies. For neutralizing the receptor-binding region of the S protein of SARS-CoV, several recombinant human single-chain variable region fragments (scFvs) have been identified (Sui *et al.*, 2004, 2005). *In vitro* and animal experimentation models with genetically engineered monoclonal antibodies showed some promising neutralization behavior against SARS-CoV.

17.5.4 Interferon

SARS-CoV affects the interferon signaling pathway (Cheung *et al.*, 2005; Law *et al.*, 2005; Spiegel *et al.*, 2005). Interferon one of the important host factors, which are very helpful in the protection of host cells from the coronaviruses as well as other viral infections. In the case of SARS-CoV, interferon types IFN-a and IFN-b (but not interferon type Ig) are found to be effective. Interferon types IFN-a and IFN-b have shown potent inhibition against the infection and replication of SARS-CoV (Zheng *et al.*, 2004). In an *in vitro* study conducted by a Swedish scientist, IFN-a and IFN-b produced via a natural procedure were more useful and effective against SARS-CoV than IFN-b produced through recombinant technology (Chen *et al.*, 2004). In another study, CpG oligodeoxynucleotide (BW001) activated the dendritic and other peripheral blood mononuclear cells for the production of IFN (A type interferon). When a Vero cell-line was treated by supernatant fluid or interferon was produced by stimulated dendritic cells and mononuclear cells, these cells showed more protection from SARS-CoV infection (Bao *et al.*, 2006). Animal experimental studies have revealed that macaques were protected from pneumocytes due to SARS-CoV infection when pre-treated with paginated IFN-a (Haagmans *et al.*, 2004), while post-exposure treatment with IFN-a has shown only intermediate protection from SARS-CoV infection. However, a randomized double-blind controlled trial study for the uses of interferon in SARS-CoV infection is yet to be conducted. A few clinical trials from various regions of the world have reported on the treatment of SARS-CoV with interferon, but the majorities of these were conducted in uncontrolled studies and were only used in emergencies to save lives.

In conclusion, recent emerging viruses like Dengue, Chikungunya, Nipah, Zika, and COVID-19 have raised a very serious health concern (Bos *et al.*, 2018; Russo *et al.*, 2020; Sharma *et al.*, 2019a; Sharma *et al.*, 2020; Kaushik *et al.*, 2020a). For these emerging viral agents, there should be effective and reliable diagnostic methods. Presently, viral can be diagnoses through electron microscopy, virus isolations, serological methods, and molecular diagnosis. Virus isolation is the gold standard but has many problems. Molecular diagnostic assays are comparatives better than other diagnostic methods for viral agents (Broor *et al.*, 2009; Bhararj *et al.*, 2009; Broor *et al.*, 2011; Sharma *et al.*, 2018; Divya *et al.*, 2019) and their effective management; vaccines or antiviral treatment are essential. In the absence of vaccines or antiviral, ethnomedicine is gaining interest because of its safety and broad-spectrum activity over synthetic drugs. Medicinal plants play a significant role in controlling various viral infections of herpes simplex viruses, Chikungunya, and Dengue (Vachirayonstien *et al.*, 2010; Kaushik *et al.*, 2018; Sharma *et al.*, 2019b; Kaushik *et al.*, 2020b; Kaushik *et al.*, 2020c; Kaushik *et al.*, 2021). *In silico*-based screening approaches provided more rational metabolites with high and specific potential and reduced futile exercises as compared to conventional *in vitro* methods (Ammendolia *et al.*, 2012; Mo and Li., 2015; Jakhar *et al.*, 2020).

References

Adachi, D., Johnson, G., Draker, R., Ayers, M., Mazzulli, T., Talbot, P. J. and Tellier, R. "Comprehensive detection and identification of human coronaviruses, including the SARS-associated coronavirus, with a single RT-PCR assay." *Journal of Virological Methods* 122, no. 1 (2004): 29–36.

Al-Hazmi, Ali. "Challenges presented by MERS corona virus, and SARS corona virus to global health." *Saudi Journal of Biological Sciences* 23, no. 4 (2016): 507–511.

Al-Tawfiq, Jaffar A., Hisham Momattin, Jean Dib, and Ziad A. Memish. "Ribavirin and interferon therapy in patients infected with the Middle East respiratory syndrome coronavirus: an observational study." *International Journal of Infectious Diseases* 20 (2014): 42–46.

Ammendolia, Maria Grazia, Mariangela Agamennone, Agostina Pietrantoni, Fabio Lannutti, Rosa Anna Siciliano, Beatrice De Giulio, Carla Amici, and Fabiana Superti. "Bovine lactoferrin-derived peptides as novel broad-spectrum inhibitors of influenza virus." *Pathogens and Global Health* 106, no. 1 (2012): 12–19.

Anand, Kanchan, John Ziebuhr, Parvesh Wadhwani, Jeroen R. Mesters, and Rolf Hilgenfeld. "Coronavirus main proteinase (3CLpro) structure: basis for design of anti-SARS drugs." *Science* 300, no. 5626 (2003): 1763–1767.

Bacha, Usman, Jennifer Barrila, Adrian Velazquez-Campoy, Stephanie A. Leavitt, and Ernesto Freire. "Identification of novel inhibitors of the SARS coronavirus main protease 3CLpro." *Biochemistry* 43, no. 17 (2004): 4906–4912.

Balboni, Andrea, Laura Gallina, Alessandra Palladini, Santino Prosperi, and Mara Battilani. "A real-time PCR assay for bat SARS-like coronavirus detection and its application to Italian greater horseshoe bat faecal sample surveys." *The Scientific World Journal* (2012). doi:10.1100/2012/989514

Bao, Musheng, Yi Zhang, Min Wan, Li Dai, Xiaoping Hu, Xiuli Wu, Li Wang *et al.* "Anti-SARS-CoV immunity induced by a novel CpG oligodeoxynucleotide." *Clinical Immunology* 118, no. 2–3 (2006): 180–187.

Bharaj, Preeti, Wayne M. Sullender, Sushil K. Kabra, Kalaivani Mani, John Cherian, Vikas Tyagi, Harendra S. Chahar, Samander Kaushik, Lalit Dar, and Shobha Broor. "Respiratory viral infections detected by multiplex PCR among pediatric patients with lower respiratory tract infections seen at an urban hospital in Delhi from 2005 to 2007." *Virology Journal* 6, no. 1 (2009): 1–11.

Biscayart, Cristian, Patricia Angeleri, Susana Lloveras, Tânia do Socorro Souza Chaves, Patricia Schlagenhauf, and Alfonso J. Rodríguez-Morales. "The next big threat to global health? 2019 novel coronavirus

(2019-nCoV): what advice can we give to travellers? Interim recommendations January 2020, from the Latin-American Society for Travel Medicine (SLAMVI)." *Travel Medicine and Infectious Disease* 33 (2020): 101567.

Bos, Sandra, Gilles Gadea, and Philippe Despres. "Dengue: a growing threat requiring vaccine development for disease prevention." *Pathogens and Global Health* 112, no. 6 (2018): 294–305.

Broor, Shobha, Harendra Singh Chahar, and Samander Kaushik. "Diagnosis of influenza viruses with special reference to novel H1N1 2009 influenza virus." *Indian Journal of Microbiology* 49, no. 4 (2009): 301–307.

Broor, Shobha, Swati Gupta, Sarita Mohapatra, Samander Kaushik, Muneer A. Mir, Priti Jain, Lalit Dar, and Renu B. Lal. "Emergence of 2009A/H1N1 cases in a tertiary care hospital in New Delhi, India." *Influenza and Other Respiratory Viruses* 5, no. 6 (2011): e552–e557.

Cao, Wu-Chun, Wei Liu, Pan-He Zhang, Fang Zhang, and Jan H. Richardus. "Disappearance of antibodies to SARS-associated coronavirus after recovery." *New England Journal of Medicine* 357, no. 11 (2007): 1162–1163.

Carlos, W. Graham, Charles S. Dela Cruz, Bin Cao, Susan Pasnick, and Shazia Jamil. "COVID-19 disease due to SARS-CoV-2 (novel coronavirus)." *American Journal of Respiratory and Critical Care Medicine* 201, no. 4 (2020): 7–8.

Chan, Wai S., Wu, Chun, Chow, Sammy C., Cheung, T., To, Ka-Fai, Leung, Wai-Keung, Chan, Paul. K., Lee, Kam-Cheong, Ng, Ho-Keung, Au, Deborah M. and Lo, Anthony W. "Coronaviral hypothetical and structural proteins were found in the intestinal surface enterocytes and pneumocytes of severe acute respiratory syndrome (SARS)." *Modern Pathology* 18, no. 11 (2005): 1432–1439.

Chang, De, Minggui Lin, Lai Wei, Lixin Xie, Guangfa Zhu, Charles S. Dela Cruz, and Lokesh Sharma. "Epidemiologic and clinical characteristics of novel coronavirus infections involving 13 patients outside Wuhan, China." *Journal of the American Medical Association* 323, no. 11 (2020): 1092–1093.

Chen, Luni, Peng Liu, He Gao, Bing Sun, Desheng Chao, Fei Wang, Yuanjue Zhu, Göran Hedenstierna, and Chen G. Wang. "Inhalation of nitric oxide in the treatment of severe acute respiratory syndrome: a rescue trial in Beijing." *Clinical Infectious Diseases* 39, no. 10 (2004): 1531–1535.

Chung, Grace T. Y., Rossa W. K. Chiu, Jo L. K. Cheung, Yongjie Jin, Stephen S. C. Chim, Paul K. S. Chan, and Y. M. Dennis Lo. "A simple and rapid approach for screening of SARS-coronavirus genotypes: an evaluation study." *BMC Infectious Diseases* 5, no. 1 (2005): 87.

Cinatl, J., Morgenstern, B., Bauer, G., Chandra, P., Rabenau, H., and Doerr, H. W. "Glycyrrhizin, an active component of liquorice roots, and replication of SARS-associated coronavirus." *The Lancet* 361, no. 9374 (2003): 2045–2046.

Corman, V. M., Müller, M. A., Costabel, U., Timm, J., Binger, T., Meyer, B., Kreher P., Lattwein, E., Eschbach-Bludau, M., Nitsche, A., Bleicker, T., Landt, O., Schweiger, B., Drexler, J. F., Osterhaus, A.D., Haagmans, B. L., Dittmer, U., Bonin, F., Wolff, T., Drosten, C. "Assays for laboratory confirmation of novel human coronavirus (hCoV-EMC) infections." *Eurosurveillance* 17, no. 49 (2012): 20334.

Corman, Victor M., Olfert Landt, Marco Kaiser, Richard Molenkamp, Adam Meijer, Daniel KW Chu, Tobias Bleicker *et al.* "Detection of 2019 novel coronavirus (2019-nCoV) by real-time RT-PCR." *Eurosurveillance* 25, no. 3 (2020): 2000045.

Cornelissen, L. A., Wierda, C. M., Van Der Meer, F. J., Herrewegh, A. A., Horzinek, M. C., Egberink, H. F. and De Groot, R. J. "Hemagglutinin-esterase, a novel structural protein of torovirus." *Journal of Virology* 71, no. 7 (1997): 5277–5286.

de Wilde, Adriaan H., Eric J. Snijder, Marjolein Kikkert, and Martijn J. van Hemert. "Host factors in coronavirus replication." In *Roles of Host Gene and Non-coding RNA Expression in Virus Infection, Ralph A. Tripp S. Mark Tompkins Editors* pp. 1–42. Springer, Cham, 2017.

Dhull, Divya, Vikrant Sharma, Yashika Sharma, and Samander Kaushik. "Applicability of molecular assays for detection and typing of herpes simplex viruses in encephalitis cases." *Virusdisease* 30, no. 4 (2019): 504–510.

Drosten, Christian, Stephan Günther, Wolfgang Preiser, Sylvie Van Der Werf, Hans-Reinhard Brodt, Stephan Becker, Holger Rabenau *et al.* "Identification of a novel coronavirus in patients with severe acute respiratory syndrome." *New England Journal of Medicine* 348, no. 20 (2003): 1967–1976.

Duckmanton, Lynn, Bo Luan, John Devenish, Raymond Tellier, and Martin Petric. "Characterization of torovirus from human fecal specimens." *Virology* 239, no. 1 (1997): 158–168.

Escors, David, Javier Ortego, Hubert Laude, and Luis Enjuanes. "The membrane M protein carboxy-terminus binds to transmissible gastroenteritis coronavirus core and contributes to core stability." *Journal of Virology* 75, no. 3 (2001): 1312–1324.

Haagmans, Bart L., Thijs Kuiken, Byron E. Martina, Ron A. M. Fouchier, Guus F. Rimmelzwaan, Geert Van Amerongen, Debby Van Riel *et al.* "Pegylated interferon-α protects type 1 pneumocytes against SARS coronavirus infection in macaques." *Nature Medicine* 10, no. 3 (2004): 290–293.

Harada, Shinji. "The broad anti-viral agent glycyrrhizin directly modulates the fluidity of plasma membrane and HIV-1 envelope." *Biochemical Journal* 392, no. 1 (2005): 191–199.

Hoever, Gerold, Lidia Baltina, Martin Michaelis, Rimma Kondratenko, Lia Baltina, Genrich A. Tolstikov, Hans W. Doerr, and Jindrich Cinatl. "Antiviral activity of glycyrrhizic acid derivatives against SARS–coronavirus." *Journal of Medicinal Chemistry* 48, no. 4 (2005): 1256–1259.

Holmes, Kathryn V. "SARS coronavirus: a new challenge for prevention and therapy." *The Journal of Clinical Investigation* 111, no. 11 (2003): 1605–1609.

Hussain, Snawar, Yu Chen, Yalin Yang, Jing Xu, Yu Peng, Ying Wu, Zhaoyang Li, Ying Zhu, Po Tien, and Deyin Guo. "Identification of novel subgenomic RNAs and noncanonical transcription initiation signals of severe acute respiratory syndrome coronavirus." *Journal of Virology* 79, no. 9 (2005): 5288–5295.

Jakhar, Renu, Samander Kaushik, and Surendra K. Gakhar. "3CL hydrolase-based multiepitope peptide vaccine against SARS-CoV-2 using immunoinformatics." *Journal of Medical Virology* 92, no. 10 (2020): 2114–2123.

Jin, Ying-Hui, Lin Cai, Zhen-Shun Cheng, Hong Cheng, Tong Deng, Yi-Pin Fan, Cheng Fang *et al.* "A rapid advice guideline for the diagnosis and treatment of 2019 novel coronavirus (2019-nCoV) infected pneumonia (standard version)." *Military Medical Research* 7, no. 1 (2020): 4.

Johnson, Syd, Cynthia Oliver, Gregory A. Prince, Val G. Hemming, David S. Pfarr, Sheau-Chiann Wang, Melissa Dormitzer *et al.* "Development of a humanized monoclonal antibody (MEDI-493) with potent in vitro and in vivo activity against respiratory syncytial virus." *Journal of Infectious Diseases* 176, no. 5 (1997): 1215–1224.

Jordan, Paul C., Sarah K. Stevens, and Jerome Deval. "Nucleosides for the treatment of respiratory RNA virus infections." *Antiviral Chemistry and Chemotherapy* 26 (2018): 2040206618764483.

Kaushik, Samander, Sulochana Kaushik, Yashika Sharma, Ramesh Kumar, and Jaya Parkash Yadav. "The Indian perspective of COVID-19 outbreak." *Virusdisease* 31, no. 2 (2020a): 146–153.

Kaushik, Sulochana, Ginni Jangra, Vaibhav Kundu, Jaya Parkash Yadav, and Samander Kaushik. "Anti-viral activity of Zingiber officinale (Ginger) ingredients against the Chikungunya virus." *Virusdisease* 31, no. 3 (2020b): 270–276.

Kaushik, Sulochana, Lalit Dar, Samander Kaushik, and Jaya Parkash Yadav. "Identification and characterization of new potent inhibitors of Dengue virus NS5 proteinase from *Andrographis paniculata* supercritical extracts on in animal cell culture and in silico approaches." *Journal of Ethnopharmacology* 267 (2021): 113541.

Kaushik, Sulochana, Samander Kaushik, Ramesh Kumar, Lalit Dar, and Jaya Parkash Yadav. "In-vitro and in silico activity of Cyamopsis tetragonoloba (Gaur) L. supercritical extract against the dengue-2 virus." *Virusdisease* 31, no. 4 (2020c): 470–478.

Kaushik, Sulochana, Samander Kaushik, Vikrant Sharma, and Jaya Yadav. "Antiviral and therapeutic uses of medicinal plants and their derivatives against dengue viruses." *Pharmacognosy Reviews* 12, no. 24 (2018): 177–185.

Keyaerts, Els, Leen Vijgen, Piet Maes, Johan Neyts, and Marc Van Ranst. "In vitro inhibition of severe acute respiratory syndrome coronavirus by chloroquine." *Biochemical and Biophysical Research Communications* 323, no. 1 (2004): 264–268.

Kistler, Amy, Pedro C. Avila, Silvi Rouskin, David Wang, Theresa Ward, Shigeo Yagi, David Schnurr, Don Ganem, Joseph L. DeRisi, and Homer A. Boushey. "Pan-viral screening of respiratory tract infections in adults with and without asthma reveals unexpected human coronavirus and human rhinovirus diversity." *Journal of Infectious Diseases* 196, no. 6 (2007): 817–825.

Knowles, Sandra R., Elizabeth J. Phillips, Linda Dresser, and Larissa Matukas. "Common adverse events associated with the use of ribavirin for severe acute respiratory syndrome in Canada." *Clinical Infectious Diseases* 37, no. 8 (2003): 1139–1142.

Ksiazek, Thomas G., Dean Erdman, Cynthia S. Goldsmith, Sherif R. Zaki, Teresa Peret, Shannon Emery, Suxiang Tong *et al.* "A novel coronavirus associated with severe acute respiratory syndrome." *New England Journal of Medicine* 348, no. 20 (2003): 1953–1966.

Lai, Michael M. C. and David Cavanagh. "The molecular biology of coronaviruses." *Advances in Virus Research*, vol. 48, (1997): 1–100.

Lau, Susanna K. P., Patrick C. Y. Woo, Kenneth S. M. Li, Yi Huang, Hoi-Wah Tsoi, Beatrice H. L. Wong, Samson S. Y. Wong, Suet-Yi Leung, Kwok-Hung Chan, and Kwok-Yung Yuen. "Severe acute respiratory syndrome coronavirus-like virus in Chinese horseshoe bats." *Proceedings of the National Academy of Sciences* 102, no. 39 (2005): 14040–14045.

Law, Helen K. W., Chung Yan Cheung, Hoi Yee Ng, Sin Fun Sia, Yuk On Chan, Winsie Luk, John M. Nicholls, J. S. Peiris, and Yu Lung Lau. "Chemokine up-regulation in SARS-coronavirus-infected, monocyte-derived human dendritic cells." *Blood* 106, no. 7 (2005): 2366–2374.

Lee, Ting-Wai, Maia M. Cherney, Carly Huitema, Jie Liu, Karen Ellis James, James C. Powers, Lindsay D. Eltis, and Michael N. G. James. "Crystal structures of the main peptidase from the SARS coronavirus inhibited by a substrate-like aza-peptide epoxide." *Journal of Molecular Biology* 353, no. 5 (2005): 1137–1151.

Li, Qun, Xuhua Guan, Peng Wu, Xiaoye Wang, Lei Zhou, Yeqing Tong, Ruiqi Ren *et al.* "Early transmission dynamics in Wuhan, China, of novel coronavirus-infected pneumonia." *New England Journal of Medicine*, 382 (2020): 1199–1287.

Li, Wenhui, Michael J. Moore, Natalya Vasilieva, Jianhua Sui, Swee Kee Wong, Michael A. Berne, Mohan Somasundaran *et al.* "Angiotensin-converting enzyme 2 is a functional receptor for the SARS coronavirus." *Nature* 426, no. 6965 (2003): 450–454.

Locker, J. Krijnse, John K. Rose, Marian C. Horzinek, and P. J. Rottier. "Membrane assembly of the triple-spanning coronavirus M protein. Individual transmembrane domains show preferred orientation." *Journal of Biological Chemistry* 267, no. 30 (1992): 21911–21918.

Lu, Guangwen, Yawei Hu, Qihui Wang, Jianxun Qi, Feng Gao, Yan Li, Yanfang Zhang *et al.* "Molecular basis of binding between novel human coronavirus MERS-CoV and its receptor CD26." *Nature* 500, no. 7461 (2013): 227–231.

Lu, Roujian, Xiang Zhao, Juan Li, Peihua Niu, Bo Yang, Honglong Wu, Wenling Wang *et al.* "Genomic characterisation and epidemiology of 2019 novel coronavirus: implications for virus origins and receptor binding." *The Lancet* 395, no. 10224 (2020): 565–574.

Lu, Xiaoyan, Brett Whitaker, Senthil Kumar K. Sakthivel, Shifaq Kamili, Laura E. Rose, Luis Lowe, Emad Mohareb *et al.* "Real-time reverse transcription-PCR assay panel for Middle East respiratory syndrome coronavirus." *Journal of Clinical Microbiology* 52, no. 1 (2014): 67–75.

Martina, Erika, Nikolaus Stiefl, Björn Degel, Franziska Schulz, Alexander Breuning, Markus Schiller, Radim Vicik, Knut Baumann, John Ziebuhr, and Tanja Schirmeister. "Screening of electrophilic compounds yields an aziridinyl peptide as new active-site directed SARS-CoV main protease inhibitor." *Bioorganic & Medicinal Chemistry Letters* 15, no. 24 (2005): 5365–5369.

Mo, Jinyu and Jian Li. "In silico analysis for structure, function and T-cell epitopes of a hypothetical conserved (HP-C) protein coded by PVX_092425 in Plasmodium vivax." *Pathogens and Global Health* 109, no. 2 (2015): 61–67.

Munster, Vincent J., Marion Koopmans, Neeltje van Doremalen, Debby van Riel, and Emmie de Wit. "A novel coronavirus emerging in China: key questions for impact assessment." *New England Journal of Medicine* 382, no. 8 (2020): 692–694.

Myint, Steven H. "Human coronavirus infections." In *The Coronaviridae*, pp. 389–401. Springer, Boston, MA, 1995.

Noh, Ji Yeong, Sun-Woo Yoon, Doo-Jin Kim, Moo-Seung Lee, Ji-Hyung Kim, Woonsung Na, Daesub Song, Dae Gwin Jeong, and Hye Kwon Kim. "Simultaneous detection of severe acute respiratory syndrome, Middle East respiratory syndrome, and related bat coronaviruses by real-time reverse transcription PCR." *Archives of Virology* 162, no. 6 (2017): 1617–1623.

Parker, William B. "Metabolism and antiviral activity of ribavirin." *Virus Research* 107, no. 2 (2005): 165–171.

Paules, Catharine I., Hilary D. Marston, and Anthony S. Fauci. "Coronavirus infections: more than just the common cold." *Journal of the American Medical Association* 323, no. 8 (2020): 707–708.

Peiris, J. S. M., Lai, S. T., Poon, L. L. M., Guan, Y., Yam, L. Y. C., Lim, W., Nicholls, J., Yee, W. K. S., Yan, W. W., Cheung, M. T. and Cheng, V. C. C., "Coronavirus as a possible cause of severe acute respiratory syndrome." *The Lancet* 361, no. 9366 (2003): 1319–1325.

Perrier, Anabelle, Ariane Bonnin, Lowiese Desmarets, Adeline Danneels, Anne Goffard, Yves Rouillé, Jean Dubuisson, and Sandrine Belouzard. "The C-terminal domain of the MERS coronavirus M protein contains a trans-Golgi network localization signal." *Journal of Biological Chemistry* 294, no. 39 (2019): 14406–14421.

Poon, Leo L. M., Daniel K. W. Chu, Kwok-Hung Chan, On Kei Wong, Trevor M. Ellis, Y. H. C. Leung, Susanna K. P. Lau *et al.* "Identification of a novel coronavirus in bats." *Journal of Virology* 79, no. 4 (2005): 2001–2009.

Prompetchara, Eakachai, Chutitorn Ketloy, and Tanapat Palaga. "Immune responses in COVID-19 and potential vaccines: lessons learned from SARS and MERS epidemic." *Asian Pacific Journal of Allergy and Immunology* 38, no. 1 (2020): 1–9.

Qian, Zhaohui, Emily A. Travanty, Lauren Oko, Karen Edeen, Andrew Berglund, Jieru Wang, Yoko Ito, Kathryn V. Holmes, and Robert J. Mason. "Innate immune response of human alveolar type ii cells infected with severe acute respiratory syndrome–coronavirus." *American Journal of Respiratory Cell and Molecular Biology* 48, no. 6 (2013): 742–748.

Raj, V. Stalin, Huihui Mou, Saskia L. Smits, Dick H. W. Dekkers, Marcel A. Müller, Ronald Dijkman, Doreen Muth *et al.* "Dipeptidyl peptidase 4 is a functional receptor for the emerging human coronavirus-EMC." *Nature* 495, no. 7440 (2013): 251–254.

Riley, Steven, Christophe Fraser, Christl A. Donnelly, Azra C. Ghani, Laith J. Abu-Raddad, Anthony J. Hedley, Gabriel M. Leung *et al.* "Transmission dynamics of the etiological agent of SARS in Hong Kong: impact of public health interventions." *Science* 300, no. 5627 (2003): 1961–1966.

Russo, Gianluca, Lorenzo Subissi, and Giovanni Rezza. "Chikungunya fever in Africa: a systematic review." *Pathogens and Global Health* 114, no. 3 (2020): 111–119.

Savarino, Adrea, John R. Boelaert, Antonio Cassone, Giancario Majori, and Roberto Cauda. "Effects of chloroquine on viral infections: an old drug against today's diseases." *The Lancet Infectious Diseases* 3, no. 11 (2003): 722–727.

Sawicki, S. G. and D. L. Sawicki. "Coronavirus transcription: a perspective." In *Coronavirus Replication and Reverse Genetics*. Enjuanes L. (Ed.), pp. 31–55. Springer, 2005.

Setianingsih, Tri Yuli, Ageng Wiyatno, Teguh Sarry Hartono, Evi Hindawati, Aghnianditya Kresno Dewantari, Khin Saw Myint, Vivi Lisdawati, and Dodi Safari. "Detection of multiple viral sequences in the respiratory tract samples of suspected Middle East respiratory syndrome coronavirus patients in Jakarta, Indonesia 2015–2016." *International Journal of Infectious Diseases* 86 (2019): 102–107.

Sharma, Vikrant, Dhruva Chaudhry, and Samander Kaushik. "Evaluation of clinical applicability of reverse transcription-loop-mediated isothermal amplification assay for detection and subtyping of Influenza A viruses." *Journal of Virological Methods* 253 (2018): 18–25.

Sharma, Vikrant, Manisha Sharma, Divya Dhull, Yashika Sharma, Sulochana Kaushik, and Samander Kaushik. "Zika virus: an emerging challenge to public health worldwide." *Canadian Journal of Microbiology* 66, no. 2 (2020): 87–98.

Sharma, Vikrant, Sulochana Kaushik, Ramesh Kumar, Jaya Parkash Yadav, and Samander Kaushik. "Emerging trends of Nipah virus: A review." *Reviews in Medical Virology* 29, no. 1 (2019a): e2010.

Sharma, Vikrant, Sulochana Kaushik, Pooja Pandit, Divya Dhull, Jaya Parkash Yadav, and Samander Kaushik. "Green synthesis of silver nanoparticles from medicinal plants and evaluation of their antiviral potential against chikungunya virus." *Applied Microbiology and Biotechnology* 103, no. 2 (2019b): 881–891.

Shen, Minzhe, Yin Zhou, Jiawei Ye, Abdu Ahmed Abdullah Al-Maskri, Yu Kang, Su Zeng, and Sheng Cai. "Recent advances and perspectives of nucleic acid detection for coronavirus." *Journal of Pharmaceutical Analysis* (2020). https://doi.org/10.1016/j.jpha.2020.02.010.

Snijder, Eric J., Peter J. Bredenbeek, Jessika C. Dobbe, Volker Thiel, John Ziebuhr, Leo L. M. Poon, Yi Guan, Mikhail Rozanov, Willy J. M. Spaan, and Alexander E. Gorbalenya. "Unique and conserved features of genome and proteome of SARS-coronavirus, an early split-off from the coronavirus group 2 lineage." *Journal of Molecular Biology* 331, no. 5 (2003): 991–1004.

Spiegel, Martin, Andreas Pichlmair, Luis Martínez-Sobrido, Jerome Cros, Adolfo García-Sastre, Otto Haller, and Friedemann Weber. "Inhibition of beta interferon induction by severe acute respiratory syndrome coronavirus suggests a two-step model for activation of interferon regulatory factor 3." *Journal of Virology* 79, no. 4 (2005): 2079–2086.

Su, Shuo, Gary Wong, Weifeng Shi, Jun Liu, Alexander C. K. Lai, Jiyong Zhou, Wenjun Liu, Yuhai Bi, and George F. Gao. "Epidemiology, genetic recombination, and pathogenesis of coronaviruses." *Trends in Microbiology* 24, no. 6 (2016): 490–502.

Sui, Jianhua, Wenhui Li, Akikazu Murakami, Azaibi Tamin, Leslie J. Matthews, Swee Kee Wong, Michael J. Moore *et al.* "Potent neutralization of severe acute respiratory syndrome (SARS) coronavirus by a human mAb to S1 protein that blocks receptor association." *Proceedings of the National Academy of Sciences* 101, no. 8 (2004): 2536–2541.

Sui, Jianhua, Wenhui Li, Anjeanette Roberts, Leslie J. Matthews, Akikazu Murakami, Leatrice Vogel, Swee Kee Wong, Kanta Subbarao, Michael Farzan, and Wayne A. Marasco. "Evaluation of human monoclonal antibody 80R for immunoprophylaxis of severe acute respiratory syndrome by an animal study, epitope mapping, and analysis of spike variants." *Journal of Virology* 79, no. 10 (2005): 5900–5906.

Ter Meulen, Jan, Alexander BH Bakker, Edward N. Van Den Brink, Gerrit J. Weverling, Byron EE Martina, Bart L. Haagmans, Thijs Kuiken, *et al.* "Human monoclonal antibody as prophylaxis for SARS coronavirus infection in ferrets." *The Lancet* 363, no. 9427 (2004): 2139–2141.

Thomas, H. C., Török, M. E., Forton, D. M. and Taylor-Robinson, S. D., "Possible mechanisms of action and reasons for failure of antiviral therapy in chronic hepatitis C." *Journal of Hepatology* 31 (1999): 152–159.

Traggiai, Elisabetta, Stephan Becker, Kanta Subbarao, Larissa Kolesnikova, Yasushi Uematsu, Maria Rita Gismondo, Brian R. Murphy, Rino Rappuoli, and Antonio Lanzavecchia. "An efficient method to make human monoclonal antibodies from memory B cells: potent neutralization of SARS coronavirus." *Nature Medicine* 10, no. 8 (2004): 871–875.

Uhlenhaut, Christine, Jeffrey I. Cohen, Steven Pavletic, Gabor Illei, Juan Carlos Gea-Banacloche, Mones Abu-Asab, Tammy Krogmann, Larisa Gubareva, Shasta McClenahan, and Philip R. Krause. "Use of a novel virus detection assay to identify coronavirus HKU1 in the lungs of a hematopoietic stem cell transplant recipient with fatal pneumonia." *Transplant Infectious Disease* 14, no. 1 (2012): 79–85.

Vabret, Astrid, Julia Dina, Stéphanie Gouarin, Joëlle Petitjean, Sandrine Corbet, and François Freymuth. "Detection of the new human coronavirus HKU1: a report of 6 cases." *Clinical Infectious Diseases* 42, no. 5 (2006): 634–639.

Vachirayonstien, Thaveechai, Duanthanorm Promkhatkaew, Malee Bunjob, Asawachai Chueyprom, Pranee Chavalittumrong, and Pathom Sawanpanyalert. "Molecular evaluation of extracellular activity of medicinal herb Clinacanthus nutans against herpes simplex virus type-2." *Natural Product Research* 24, no. 3 (2010): 236–245.

Van der Hoek, Lia. "Human coronaviruses: what do they cause?" *Antiviral Therapy* 12, no. 4 B (2007): 651–658.

Van Vonderen, M. G., Bos, J. C., Prins, J. M., Wertheim-van Dillen, P. and Speelman. "Ribavirin in the treatment of severe acute respiratory syndrome (SARS)." *Netherlands Journal of Medicine* 61, no. 238 (2003): 42.

Vincent, Martin J., Eric Bergeron, Suzanne Benjannet, Bobbie R. Erickson, Pierre E. Rollin, Thomas G. Ksiazek, Nabil G. Seidah, and Stuart T. Nichol. "Chloroquine is a potent inhibitor of SARS coronavirus infection and spread." *Virology Journal* 2, no. 1 (2005): 1–10.

Wan, Zhenzhou, Ya'nan Zhang, Zhixiang He, Jia Liu, Ke Lan, Yihong Hu, and Chiyu Zhang. "A melting curve-based multiplex RT-qPCR assay for simultaneous detection of four human coronaviruses." *International Journal of Molecular Sciences* 17, no. 11 (2016): 1880.

Wang, David, Anatoly Urisman, Yu-Tsueng Liu, Michael Springer, Thomas G. Ksiazek, Dean D. Erdman, Elaine R. Mardis, *et al.* "Viral discovery and sequence recovery using DNA microarrays." *PLoS Biology* 1, no. 2 (2003): e2.

Wang, Wenling, Yanli Xu, Ruqin Gao, Roujian Lu, Kai Han, Guizhen Wu, and Wenjie Tan. "Detection of SARS-CoV-2 in different types of clinical specimens." *Journal of the American Medical Association* 323, no. 18 (2020): 1843–1844.

Woo, Patrick C. Y., Susanna K. P. Lau, Chung-ming Chu, Kwok-hung Chan, Hoi-wah Tsoi, Yi Huang, Beatrice H. L. Wong *et al.* "Characterization and complete genome sequence of a novel coronavirus, coronavirus HKU1, from patients with pneumonia." *Journal of Virology* 79, no. 2 (2005): 884–895.

Woo, Patrick C. Y., Susanna K. P. Lau, Beatrice H. L Wong, Kwok-Hung Chan, Wai-Ting Hui, Grace S. W. Kwan, J. S. Malik Peiris, Robert B. Couch, and Kwok-Yung Yuen. "False-positive results in a recombinant severe acute respiratory syndrome-associated coronavirus (SARS-CoV) nucleocapsid enzyme-linked immunosorbent assay due to HCoV-OC43 and HCoV-229E rectified by Western blotting with recombinant SARS-CoV spike polypeptide." *Journal of Clinical Microbiology* 42, no. 12 (2004): 5885–5888.

Wu, Chung-Yi, Jia-Tsrong Jan, Shiou-Hwa Ma, Chih-Jung Kuo, Hsueh-Fen Juan, Yih-Shyun E. Cheng, Hsien-Hua Hsu *et al.* "Small molecules targeting severe acute respiratory syndrome human coronavirus." *Proceedings of the National Academy of Sciences* 101, no. 27 (2004): 10012–10017.

Yang, Haitao, Weiqing Xie, Xiaoyu Xue, Kailin Yang, Jing Ma, Wenxue Liang, Qi Zhao *et al.* "Design of wide-spectrum inhibitors targeting coronavirus main proteases." *PLoS Biology* 3, no. 10 (2005): e324.

Yeh, Kuo-Ming, Tzong-Shi Chiueh, L. K. Siu, Jung-Chung Lin, Paul KS Chan, Ming-Yieh Peng, Hsiang-Lin Wan *et al.* "Experience of using convalescent plasma for severe acute respiratory syndrome among healthcare workers in a Taiwan hospital." *Journal of Antimicrobial Chemotherapy* 56, no. 5 (2005): 919–922.

Yoo, Jin-Hong. "The fight against the 2019-nCoV outbreak: an arduous march has just begun." *Journal of Korean Medical Science* 35, no. 4 (2019): e56.

Zhang, Mei-Yun, Vidita Choudhry, Xiaodong Xiao, and Dimiter S. Dimitrov. "Human monoclonal antibodies to the S glycoprotein and related proteins as potential therapeutics for SARS." *Current Opinion in Molecular Therapeutics* 7, no. 2 (2005): 151–156.

Zhao, Shi, Qianyin Lin, Jinjun Ran, Salihu S. Musa, Guangpu Yang, Weiming Wang, Yijun Lou *et al.* "Preliminary estimation of the basic reproduction number of novel coronavirus (2019-nCoV) in China, from 2019 to 2020: a data-driven analysis in the early phase of the outbreak." *International Journal of Infectious Diseases* 92 (2020): 214–217.

Zheng, B., He, M. L., Wong, K. L., Lum, C. T., Poon, L. L., Peng, Y., Guan, Y., Lin, M. C. and Kung, H. F. Potent inhibition of SARS-associated coronavirus (SCOV) infection and replication by type I interferons (IFN-alpha/beta) but not by type II interferon (IFN-gamma). *Journal of Interferon and Cytokine Research* 24 (2004): 388–390.

Zumla, Alimuddin, Jasper F. W. Chan, Esam I. Azhar, David S. C. Hui, and Kwok-Yung Yuen. "Coronaviruses: drug discovery and therapeutic options." *Nature Reviews Drug Discovery* 15, no. 5 (2016): 327–347.

18

Recombinase Polymerase Amplification: A New Approach for Disease Diagnosis

Monika Punia,[1] Nidhi Saini,[1] Suresh Kumar Gahlawat[1] and Sushila Maan[2]
[1] *Department of Biotechnology, Chaudhary Devi Lal University, Sirsa-125055, Haryana, India*
[2] *Department of Animal Biotechnology, Lala Lajpat Rai University of Veterinary and Animal Sciences, Hisar-125004, Haryana, India*

18.1 Introduction

Recombinase polymerase amplification (RPA) is a single-channel (tube) method of DNA detection by isothermal amplification. For RPA, only the addition of a reverse transcriptase enzyme is required to detect RNA. cDNA generation is not required as a separate step. Also, RPA only needs a thermal cycler, water bath or heat batch in order to maintain a constant temperature. RPA reactions can be conducted rapidly simply by holding the tube, as they work best from room temperature (20–25°C) to 42°C. These properties make it an excellent candidate for low-cost and fast molecular tests for the detection of infectious agents.

TwistDx Ltd., situated in Cambridge, UK, launched and developed this technique. Niall Armes from ASM Scientific Ltd. introduced RPA in 2006, which was used to detect a wide range of targets including bacteria, parasites and fungi, genetic alterations in cancer cells, viruses and GMOs (Daher *et al.*, 2016). This technique amplifies both DNA as well as RNA strands and is therefore applied to various fields like food safety, medicine, animal sciences, agriculture etc. (Zheng *et al.*, 2015). Detection time and amplification vary according to the target sequences, primers, amplicon size and sample type used. Over the past decade, the development and adaptation of new and existing isothermal amplification technologies for molecular diagnostics has expanded greatly.

RPA assays have the following important parameters.

RPA primer size. This should be between 30 and 35 bases long for optimum efficiency. Longer primers (> 45 bases) have a high likelihood of the formation of primer dimers and hence are not recommended. The best RPA results can be achieved by using long sequences with short amplicons of size 100–200 bp. Also, less than 30% or greater than 70% GC content should be avoided (Lobato & Sullivan, 2018) (www.twistdx.co.uk).

Time and temperature. Various strategies are used to maintain temperatures such as the use of incubators, heaters and even body heat. Most RPA procedures operate between 37 and 41°C with no need for tight temperature control (Lobato & Sullivan, 2018) (www.twistdx.co.uk).

18.2 Methodology and Different Parameters Controlling RPA

The recombinase enzyme and oligonucleotide primer bind together to make a complex. These primers then bind to their homologous sequences present in the DNA duplex. After this, a single-stranded DNA binding (SSB) protein binds to the displaced DNA strand to form a stabilized D-loop. DNA amplification is initiated by enzyme polymerase if only the target sequence exists. Amplification then progresses and, being extremely precise, can be identified within minutes, beginning with a small number of target copies of DNA. RPA uses two primers and one optional probe with easy design demands. Recombinase enzyme along with accessory proteins are used in RPA to unwind the DNA. RPA has high efficiency and specificity (10^{-4} fold amplification in ten minutes) and does not require an additional temperature step for DNA denaturation (www.twistdx.co.uk). There are various factors involved in RPA which are elaborated below.

18.2.1 Primer and Probe Design

18.2.1.1 Primer Design

Initial studies suggested that RPA requires specifically designed primers with a length of 30–35 bases, whereas later studies suggested that normal PCR primers can be used, and efficient amplification can be achieved (Mayboroda *et al.*, 2015). Longer primers may be used for up to 45 nucleotides, but longer primers lead to the formation of secondary structures. Therefore, it is also recommended that long traces of guanines at 5' ends should be avoided, while cytidines may be beneficial, with guanines and cytidines at 3' appearing to boost efficiency. It is not recommended to use GC content below 30% or above 70% as with PCR primers because sequences that facilitate primers, secondary structures or hairpins should not be used. RPA performs best with amplicons between 100 and 200 bp and can amplify targets up to 1–5 kb (Sharma *et al.*, 2014).

The process for primer selection involves four steps:

a) target area selection
b) design of primer
c) screening of experiments
d) screening of secondary and tertiary applicants

Software for the design of RPA primers like with LAMP and PCR is not available (Sharma *et al.*, 2014).

18.2.1.2 Probe Design

Typically, three types of probes are provided to support the various kits. The TwistAmp™ exo probe (typically between 46 and 52 nucleotides) and the TwistAmp® fpg probe (typically between 32 and 35 nucleotides) are used for fluorogenic real-time detection. These probes are usually labelled with a fluorophore, a quencher (e.g., a region quencher) that is in close proximity to the fluorophore to temporarily inhibit the fluorescent signal, and a blocker (e.g., C3-spacer, a phosphate, a biotin-TEG or an amine) at the 3'-end serving to stop polymerase extension from there. The real-time detection is predicated on the cleavage of fluorogenic probes at an abasic site between the fluorophore and the quencher. The abasic site can either be tetrahydrofuran (THF), a dSpacer (a derivative of the THF) or a dR group (the deoxyribose of the abasic site via a C-O-C linker). The TwistAmp™ exo probe cleaves by the *E. coli* exonuclease III at a THF or a dSpacer site, while the TwistAmp™ fpg probe cleaves by the glycosylase/lyase *E. coli* fpg at the dR position. After the enzymatic cleavage, the TwistAmp® exo probe can function a forward primer. However, the TwistAmp™ fpg probe cannot function a primer because of different catalytic mode (beta-elimination) of the glycosylase/lyase *E. coli* fpg protein, which does not generate an extendable 3'-OH group but a 3'-phosphate group.

A third probe, TwistAmp™ LF (typically between 46 and 52 nucleotides), is employed for lateral-flow strip detection. This probe is labelled at the 5'-end (e.g., with fluorescein) and features a blocker at the 3'-end, and an inside abasic site (THF or dSpacer). The Nfo endonuclease IV cleaves at this a basic site of the TwistAmp™ LF probe, and generates an extendable 3'-OH group for polymerization. However, unlike the *E. coli* exonuclease III, which degrades most of the amplicons during RPA reaction, the Nfo endonuclease IV generates a slower signal and incomplete cleavage to avoid amplicon degradation. Therefore, the TwistAmp™ LF probe can also be used for cases when gel electrophoresis (GE) is chosen as a detection method (Piepenburg *et al.*, 2011; Li *et al.*, 2018).

18.2.2 Temperature

Various studies have showed that RPA works at ambient temperatures in warm areas, e.g., 30°C, and various apparatus are employed to control reaction temperatures, which range from 22 to 45°C and do not require narrow control. Most published studies are optimized for temperatures between 37 and 42°C (Kersting *et al.*, 2014; Lillis *et al.*, 2014).

18.2.3 Effect of Crowding Agent and Mixing

The crowding agent plays an important role in the main RPA biochemical process by preventing the spontaneous breakdown of the recombinase enzyme in the presence of SSB proteins needing amplification. Viscosity has a negative effect on RPA which hampers the diffusion of reagents through the reaction mixture, which can be reduced by including a mixing step of five minutes after the initiation of RPA. The mixing cycle can be prevented by reducing the total reaction volume to 5 ml (Lillis *et al.*, 2016). The mixing time reduces from hours to one minute by the use of a phase-guided passive batch microfluid chamber actuated by a syringe (Hakenberg *et al.*, 2012).

18.2.4 Incubation Time

The time required to amplify the template to detectable levels is called the incubation time, which depends on the number of starting DNA copies; 20 minutes are sufficient for amplification but the lowest amplification time was observed to be 3–4 minutes. In most applications, a long incubation period is not beneficial because at the solution phase of RPA the recombinase consumes all available ATP within 25 minutes (Xia *et al.*, 2014).

18.2.5 Types of Samples

The types of samples used in amplification are dsDNA, methylated DNA, ssDNA, DNA produced through reverse transcription of DNA or miRNA (Wee & Trau, 2016). Some reverse transcriptase enzymes used with RPA are SensiscriptR (Qiagen), TranscriptorR (Roche) and MuLVR (Applied Biosystems). Initial studies showed TranscriptorR performs best and cDNA can be produced before RPA or in the same reaction; RT-Freeze is also available from TwistD (Wahed *et al.*, 2013).

Different types of kits are available for better RPA reactions, provided by the manufacturer according to the type of research method (as shown in Table 18.1). In general, the manufacturer provides two types of kit: freeze-dried, suitable for the field and at the point of attention; and other sets with a minimum of lyophilized reactions. The kits contain all of the reagents needed to increase nucleic acids by the use of different end-user primers. Another liquid form is given in bulk by all available reagents so that users can combine them to create master mixes for their own applications in different scales. Users can use the reagents in the same way as the pre-made PCR master mixes found in every molecular biology laboratory freezer. Various types of RPA kits are available on the market, each with specific characteristics. Some are discussed in Table 18.1.

Based on the use of kits, RPA reactions adopt various detection systems; for instance, a few kits need a simple downstream agarose gel detection system. Efficient time detection kits use two samples of RPA-exo or fpg (probe). The use of RPA is incompatible with standard samples like TaqMan and PCR Taq polymerases. In certain RPA kits, lateral-flow detection (LF) is required. A THF residue of E and 5"- fluorophore (e.g., FAM) are required for the design of the LF sample. Recognizing and slicing *E. coli* endonuclease IV (Nfo), primers are identical for kits based on Nfo to exo samples. Exonuclease III can then be replaced by the Nfo endonuclease as the same substrate is used. All kits developed for RPA use lateral-flow experiments, biotin-labelled reverse primers, and bind a double-labelled amplicon with the Nfo probe, which is then collected in golden nanoparticles by the species-specific anti-FAM antibody. Biotin is detected by another immobilized analyte, forming a detection line on MGHD 1 (TwistDx). The lateral-flow cycle is tracked via a control line with immobilized anti-species antibodies (Daher *et al.*, 2016).

18.3 RPA Reaction Conditions

The TwistAmp™ Basic Kit (TwistDx) is used to perform the RPA. All instructions are given by the manufacturing company. Single-plex requires preparation of the reaction mix in a 1.5-ml tube. Add primer A and primer B (10 μM) 2.4 μl, then add free rehydration buffer 29.5 μl, template and water (13.2 μl) to make a total volume of 47.5 μl. Vortex and spin briefly. Then mix properly by pipette and add 2.5 μl of 280-mM magnesium acetate (MgOAc) (supplied) and mix well to start reaction. Incubate at 39°C for 20 minutes. For a low template copy number, remove the strip after four minutes, vortex and spin briefly and replace in the heating device. After 20 minutes, clean amplicons before running on agarose gels (www.twistdx.com.uk).

Templates with a dried enzyme pellet bind to the RPA strips and fluorescence measurements are performed at 470 nm detectable at 520 nm in the FAM channel. This was done in the ESE Quant tube scanner (Qiagen) at 42°C for 20 minutes (Euler *et al.*, 2012). Signal slope and the combined threshold analysis are done using tube scanner software for signal interpretation.

18.3.1 Multiplexing in RPA

Multiplexing with RPA majorly depends on target sequence, amplicon size and primer design. Therefore, for every multiplexing assay, careful optimization of primer, probe ratio and concentrations is a must. Primers can compete against recombinase proteins, thus suppressing a reaction. Some examples include a real-time fluorescent duplex RPA for *C. coli* and *C. jejuni* in chicken products and the identification of different MRSA alleles and internal control (Kerting *et al.*, 2014; Kim & Lee, 2016; Piepenburg *et al.*, 2018; Hill-Cawthorne *et al.*, 2014).

TABLE 18.1

Different types of kits for RPA reaction with specific targets, detection system and features

S.No.	Kit	Target	Incubation Temp (°C)	Probe Detection?	Post-amplification Purification?	Detection system	Features	Pathogen	Reference
1	Basic	DNA	37–39	No	Yes	Agarose gel	Fast DNA amplification, hyper-sensitive single molecule detection, multiplexable, 96 reactions	-	Piepenburg *et al.* (2014); Daher *et al.* (2016)
2	Basic RT (reverse transcription)	RNA	40–42	No	Yes	Agarose gel	Fast DNA amplification, hyper-sensitive single molecule detection, multiplexable, 96 reactions	-	Piepenburg *et al.* (2014); Daher *et al.* (2016)
3	Nfo nuclease (lateral-flow detection)	DNA	37–39	Yes	Yes (agarose gel detection)	Lateral flow/ Real time/ agarose gel	End-point detection, multiplexable, 96 reactions	*Salmonella*, red snapper	Piepenburg *et al.* (2014); Daher *et al.* (2016)
4	Exo (exonuclease III real-time detection)	DNA	37–39	Yes	No	Real time	Fast DNA amplification, multiplexable, 96 reactions	*Salmonella*, *Listeria monocytogenes*, *Campylobacter*	Piepenburg *et al.* (2014); Daher *et al.* (2016)
5	Exo RT (exonuclease III real-time detection)	RNA	40–42	Yes	No	Real time	Fast DNA amplification, sensitive, multiplexable, 96 reactions	Influenza A virus	Piepenburg *et al.* (2014); Daher *et al.* (2016)
6	Fpg (fpg nuclease real-time detection)	DNA	37–39	Yes	Yes (only agarose gel detection	Real time, Agarose gel	Fast DNA amplification, sensitive, multiplexable, 96 reactions	-	Piepenburg *et al.* (2014); Daher *et al.* (2016)
7	Liquid basic	DNA	37–42	No	Yes	Agarose gel	Fast DNA amplification, uses flexible reaction volume, flexible reagent component ratio, reagents for at least 100 reactions (dependent on the volume used), multiplexable		www.twistdx.co.uk

(continued)

TABLE 18.1

Different types of kits for RPA reaction with specific targets, detection system and features (Cont.)

S.No.	Kit	Target	Incubation Temp (°C)	Probe Detection?	Post-amplification Purification?	Detection system	Features	Pathogen	Reference
8	Liquid exo	DNA	37–42	Yes	No	Real time	Fast DNA amplification, uses flexible reaction volume, flexible reagent component ratio, reagents for at least 100 reactions (dependent on the volume used), multiplexable		www.twistdx.co.uk
9	AmplifyRP Discovery kit								
9a	AmplifyRP Acceler8 i	DNA	39	Yes	No	Lateral flow	Allows an end-point detection of amplified products using a lateral-flow strip		www.agdia.com
9b	AmplifyRP XRT	DNA	39	Yes	No	Real time	Allows real-time detection of amplified products		www.agdia.com

TABLE 18.2

Various reagents along with concentration required in RPA and specific functions

S.No.	Concentration	Reagents	Functions	References
1	420 nM	Primers of RT-RPA	Guides the amplification event to homologous binding towards the target of nucleic acid interest, providing 3'-OH necessary for the polymerase to extend the strand	www.twistdx.com.uk
2	120 nM	Exo probes RT-RPA	Recombinase has a major role in genetic recombination, DNA repair and replication and is a central component in the related process of recombination DNA repair and homologous genetic recombination that is the ortholog of the UvsX protein	Griffith *et al.* (1985); Bianchi *et al.* (1985)
3	2 U	Reverse transcriptase, transcriptor (Roche, Mannheim, Germany)	The enzyme has RNA-directed DNA polymerase activity, DNA-dependent DNA polymerase activity, unwinding activity	www.twistdx.com.uk
4	20 U	RiboLockRNase inhibitor (Fisher, Schwerte, Germany)	RNase H degrading RNA in RNA-DNA hybrids	www.twistdx.co.uk
5	2 μM	DTT (Roche, Mannheim, Germany)	Enzyme stabilization by exhibiting free sulf-hydryl groups	Fjelstrup *et al.* (2017)
6	14 mM	Mg acetate	Mg acetate if added begins the RPA reaction as it acts as a co-factor for enzyme performance	www.twistdx.co.uk
7	4 X	TwistAmpTM rehydration buffer (TwistDx)	It makes easy amplification by increasing the enzymes' catalytic activity. Tris stabilize and solubilize the DNA in the solution	Piepenburg *et al.* (2006); www.cambio.co.uk/18/applications/lab-reagents/
8	1 μl	Template	The oligonucleotides to which primers attach to make new oligonucleotides	Piepenburg *et al.* (2006); www.cambio.co.uk/18/applications/lab-reagents/

18.4 Major Applications of RPA Technique

18.4.1 Multiple Target Detection

Multiple targets, such as bacteria, parasites, fungi, GMOs, cancer and viruses etc., can be detected through RPA technology. It is used efficiently to amplify both DNA and RNA templates. Amplicon size, size of sequence, type of sample and primer are the factors upon which detection of targets and identification time depends. The development and adaptation of novel and existing isothermal amplification technologies for molecular diagnosis of pathogens has increased in the last decade.

18.4.2 Seed Testing and Other Agricultural Assays

RPA is a robust and adaptive technology for the identification of various pathogens and agricultural testing. The RPA assay successfully detects various pathogens, like bacteria (Piepenburg *et* al., 2018) and viruses in plants (Londoño *et al.*, 2016). RPA also offers a portable, rapid and highly specific isothermal substitute to PCR and is ideally suited to point-of-use molecular assays for the detection of GMOs (Xu *et al.*, 2014).

18.4.3 On-site Microbial Testing

RPA is an excellent technique for monitoring various on-site water resources like rivers and lakes etc. Food safety research and monitoring applications for insects can also be studied using RPA. Its benefits include on-the-spot and field-use diagnostics. It is useful for patients in rural and remote areas where travel over long distances is difficult. It has various characteristics which make it suitable for a variety of microfluidic devices. Various research studies have shown that common digital methods can be added to RPA to make it more advanced (www.twistdx.com.uk).

18.4.4 Disease Detection in Animals

In veterinary medicine, the benefits of RPA are similar to those of human diagnostics. Whether for the identification of diseases in domestic animals or the monitoring of the prevalence of economically important infections in farm animals, RPA can be used to establish a fast, highly sensitive and accurate testing technique. RPA amplifies only a few nucleic acid molecules in three to ten minutes at average temperatures of 37–42°C, although this depends on the target size. It has the advantage that one person can take the sample, plan, run the test and get results in half an hour without advanced training. We can compare this to the normal 24-hour turnaround times for clinical samples that must be submitted for processing to central laboratories for diagnosis, which is time-consuming and requires extra human resources (www.twistdx.com.uk).

18.4.5 Medical Diagnostics

Researchers are being encouraged to use/develop RPA to conduct rapid tests on the most fatal diseases of the world. Currently, the treatment of infectious diseases should be fast, commenced immediately to save lives. Rural/remote areas have patients who have to travel long distances, thereby also making communication very difficult. Where patients have previously needed to submit clinical samples to centrally located PCR laboratories or microbiological cultures over periods of 48 hours or longer, on-the-spot RPA checks have made the process very easy. Recently, an RPA assay has been developed for targeting SARS-CoV-2 (severe acute respiratory syndrome coronavirus-2) for the N gene. Its sensitivity was determined to be 7.74 (95% CI: 2.87–27.39) RNA copies per reaction (Behrmann *et al.*, 2020).

18.5 Comparison with Other Isothermal Techniques

There are various differing parameters for both single and multiplex reactions, such as the mechanism, operating conditions, and advantages and disadvantages. In most techniques, an ssDNA template is created during the initial heating step at 95°C for further amplification. This makes the protocol very complicated and also requires specific equipment for temperature control. There are many significant differences between RPA and other amplification techniques which make RPA a superior technique. Some are listed below.

a) *Temperature*. RPA can work at 20°C but its optimum temperature ranges from 37 to 42°C. It does not require tight temperature control. On the other hand, other techniques like LAMP, PCR etc.

are highly sensitive methods which only work at 30–65°C after initial pre-melting for the detection of bacterial infections (Saharan *et al.*, 2014; Gahlawat *et al.*, 2009).

b) *Storage*. RPA reagents are available in lyophilized form and are stable at ambient temperature for about six months, whereas other techniques require refrigeration.

c) *Primers*. RPA requires only a set of two short primers (forward and reverse) (Higgins *et al.*, 2019). Short primers have the advantage of being compatible with solid-phase amplification, which can potentially be combined with detection, as longer primers may lead to the formation of secondary structures (Lobato & Sullivan, 2018). LAMP and SDA need the most complex primer designs compared to other isothermal techniques.

d) *Speed*. Reaction speed is another advantage of multiplexed RPA as compared to LAMP and other techniques, which require a minimum of 90 minutes. A high degree of flexibility (from 1 to over 16 targets) makes RPA well-suited for multiplexing.

e) *Amplification end product*. The structure of the amplification end product is another important parameter for the choice of isothermal technology. Several detection techniques can be used following amplification to determine the presence or absence of a targeted nucleic acid sequence. Agarose gel electrophoresis is a widely used technique for the visualization of amplification products, but in certain cases it is necessary to purify the amplicons to avoid smeared bands on the gel due to the presence of proteins and the crowding agent in the amplification mix. Therefore, RPA needs purification after amplification so that the substance can be properly visualized/detected. For more clarity colorimetric and fluorescence detection methods may also be used in RPA (Lobato & Sullivan, 2018). Since the molecular methods are highly sensitive and precise, most laboratories prefer these methods for quick and accurate disease diagnostics (Steyer *et al.*, 2016). The key aim of these approaches is to amplify DNA or RNA by various nucleic acid amplifiers. Several techniques for rapid and reliable diagnostics have been developed so far (Malik *et al.*, 2019). A few advanced techniques have been listed in Table 18.3.

18.6 Advantages Over Real-time PCR

Real-time RT-PCR testing is fairly expensive technology. It requires well-equipped laboratories and is not ideal for on-site screening. In other respects, RPA is less tedious than real-time PCR with the use of reverse transcriptase recombinase polymerase amplification (RT-RPA). RPA is much more sensitive and less time-consuming than traditional PCRs. In certain ways, RT-RPA is better than RT-qPCR, as it takes less time and completes in 20–30 minutes, whereas RT-qPCR takes approximately one hour to complete. RT-RPA is more specific and sensitive than real-time PCR. A recombinase polymerase amplification lateral-flow dipstick (RPA-LFD) also works in the field, requiring only a detection chamber and the lateral-flow strips, which are easy to carry, whereas real-time PCR is not operated in the field as it requires well-equipped laboratories. Table 18.4 shows the benefits of RPA over PCR, RT-PCR and qPCR.

An RPA-LFD assay gives better results, i.e., 120 copies/reaction in 30 minutes for *Pasteurella multocida* causing bovine respiratory disease and hemorrhagic septicemia in livestock, as compared to q-PCR, which is less sensitive and more time-consuming (Zhao *et al.*, 2019). RPAs displayed a high degree of sensitivity for the virus of Newcastle disease (NDV) and bronchitis infectious virus (IBV). A total detection time of 20 minutes is required for the performance of an NDV test. Both NDV and IBV are poultry diseases which affect the chicken respiratory tract and cause significant economic losses. To increase the implementation of effective control steps, the rapid identification of these viruses is crucial (Tholoth *et al.*, 2019).

RPA findings of the ASFV p72 gene with LFD revealed that the sensitivity of RPA with a lateral-flow dipstick (RPA-LFD) for ASFV was 150 copies per reaction, giving results within ten minutes at 38°C. ASFV is responsible for the elimination of haemorrhagic fever in domestic pigs in the pig industry. The test, which is highly specific for ASFV, does not react with other swine viruses, including CSFV. RPA-LFD is a new choice for the quick, responsive and accurate identification of ASFV (Miao *et al.*, 2019).

TABLE 18.3

Various diagnostic techniques and their recent modifications

S. No.	Techniques	Principle	Modifications	References
1	NASBA	Useful for RNA detection; uses two primers, one for initial binding of T7 RNA polymerase and the second for binding to the cDNA formed; also utilizes the activity of reverse transcriptase, T7 RNA polymerase and RNase H	Paper-based cell-free systems and synbody-based viral enrichment	Ma *et al.* (2018)
2	Real-time RT-qPCR	Real-time amplification of DNA/RNA using fluorescent reporter	Nanofluidic RT-qPCR, multiplex RT-qPCR, aptamer-based RT-qPCR	Monteiro and Santos (2017); Wongboot *et al.* (2018); Liu *et al.* (2019)
3	LAMP	Isothermal amplification of a targeted sequence in loop-mediated displacement	Real-time RT-LAMP, Paper-LAMP	Lundberg *et al.* (2011)
4	PLA	Amplification of ligated oligonucleotides by connector sequence, bound to antibodies	Amplification of ligated oligonucleotides by connector sequence, bound to antibodies	Assarsson *et al.* (2014)
5	PCR	Amplification of sequence in the presence of Taq polymerase containing stages of annealing and extension per cycle	Multiplex PCR	Liu *et al.* (2019)
6	RPA	Isothermal amplification using a recombinase and a single-stranded DNA-binding protein (SSB) and strand-displacing polymerase	Lateral-flow strip-RPA	Liu *et al.* (2018)

For the detection of Marek's disease in poultry, a real-time RPA assay has also been developed and shows more sensitivity 10^2 copies/reaction in 20 minutes, while PCR requires 60 minutes to finish the test (Zeng *et al.*, 2019). For disease diagnosis in aquaculture, RPA also works better than conventional PCR or RT-qPCR. Soliman *et al.* (2018) developed an RPA-LF assay for the pathogen *Tetracapsuloides bryosalmonae*, responsible for proliferative kidney disease in salmonids, which shows ten times more sensitivity than PCR with a detection time of 25 minutes, while PCR takes one hour.

Moore & Jaykus (2016) developed an RPA process which amplifies and detects nucleic acids in near real-time using a simple computer, based on an RT-RPA study targeted at a recent human norovirus (GII.4 New Orleans) outbreak. This study successfully identified the norovirus. RNA isolated from several outbreak isolates of patients had a 3.40 ± 0.20 log10 copies detection limit (LGCs), comparable to most other recorded amplification methods for the isothermic norovirus. The test also detected noroviruses in directly boiled stools and showed better inhibitor resistance than for a typical RT-qPCR test. The study was unique because nine non-related enteric viruses and bacteria did not replicate genomes. Many tests have detected noroviruses in as little as six minutes and can be completed in less than 30 minutes in the entire detection cycle. The RT-RPA process is the fastest human norovirus amplification tool to date for the rapid point-of-care identification of human outbreaks of norovirus.

18.7 Conclusion

PCR is a revolutionary change in the testing of nucleic acid; however, RPA is a substitute to PCR, which operates at low temperature and performs nucleic acid replication more rapidly. While RPA was

TABLE 18.4

Comparison of RPA with other molecular techniques

S. No.	Host/Organism	Pathogen/Disease	Type of Sample/Nucleic Acid for Test	Techniques Used	Detection Time	Detection Limit/ Sensitivity	References
1	Cattle, buffaloes and bison	*Pasteurella multocida* cause bovine respiratory disease (BRD) and haemorrhagic septicaemia (HS)	Nasal swabs and lung sample DNA	RPA-LFD, qPCR and culture method	30 min.	120 copies/reaction	Zhao *et al.* (2019)
2	Livestock (sheep and cattle)	Brucellosis	Vaginal swabs, aborted fetus tissue samples, milk samples from cattle and sheep DNA	RT-RPA, LFD-RPA combined with SYBR-Green recombinase polymerase amplification (RPA) and PCR, real-time PCR	10–30 min.	4 (RT-RPA) and 6 (LFD-RPA) copies/ reaction	Gumaa *et al.* (2019)
3	Cattle	*Mycoplasma bovis*	Nasal swabs, fresh lung, joint fluid and milk sample DNA	RPA- LFD, qPCR	30 min.	20 copies/reaction	Zhao *et al.* (2018)
4	Cattle	Bovine ephemeral fever virus (BEFV)	Tissue and blood samples from calf DNA/RNA	LFD-RPA and RT-PCR	20 min.	8 copies/reaction	Hou *et al.* (2018)
5	Cattle	Infectious bovine rhinotracheitis virus (IBRV)	Fecal, blood, nasal swab and tissue specimen DNA/RNA	LFD-RPA, SYBR Green I-based real-time PCR	25 min.	5 copies/reaction	Hou *et al.* (2017)
6	Cattle	*Mycobacterium bovis*	Blood sample DNA,	Phage-RPA, PCR	48 h.	10 cells/ml	Swift *et al.* (2016)
7	Cattle	Lumpy skin disease virus (LSDV)	Skin nodule DNA	RPA, qPCR	15 min.	179 copies/reaction	Shalaby *et al.* (2016)
8	Cats	Feline herpesvirus type 1 (FHV-1)	Nasal and ocular conjunctival swab sample DNA	RPA-LFD assay and PCR	20 min.	10^3 copies/reaction	Liu *et al.* (2018)
9	Dogs	Canine distemper virus	Nasal/oropharyngeal swab RNA/DNA	LFS RT-RPA, real-time RT-PCR	20 min.	9.4×10^1 copies/ reaction	Wang *et al.* (2018)

(continued)

TABLE 18.4

Comparison of RPA with other molecular techniques (Cont.)

S. No.	Host/Organism	Pathogen/Disease	Type of Sample/Nucleic Acid for Test	Techniques Used	Detection Time	Detection Limit/ Sensitivity	References
10	Dogs	Canine parvovirus type 2 (CPV-2)	Swab, fecal sample DNA/RNA	qRPA, qPCR	20 min.	10^1 copies/reaction	Geng *et al.* (2017)
11	Dogs	Canine parvovirus type 2 (CPV-2)	Fecal sample DNA/RNA	RPA and conventional PCR	40 min.	10 copies/reaction	Wang *et al.* (2016)
12	Sheep	Peste des petits ruminant virus (PPRV)	Tissue sample RNA	Real-time RT-RPA, LFS RT-RPA	25 min.	100 copies, 150 copies/reaction	Yang *et al.* (2017)
13	Goats	Orf virus	Nasal swabs, tissues sample DNA	RPA- LFD, qPCR	25 min.	80 copies/reaction	Yang *et al.* (2016)
14	Goats	*Mycoplasma capricolum* subsp. *capripneumoniae*	Pleural fluid sample, lung sample, bacterial culture DNA	RPA	15–20 min.	5×10^6 to 5×10^6 copies/reaction	Liljander *et al.* (2015)
15	Pigs	Porcine delta coronavirus (PDCoV)	Intestine specimen, fecal sample RNA	RT-RPA, RT-qPCR	20 min.	100 copies/reaction	Zeng *et al.* (2019)
16	Pigs	African swine fever virus (ASFV)	-	-	10 min.		Miao *et al.* (2019)
17	Pigs, cattle	Foot-and-mouth disease virus (FMDV)	Vesicular fluid, epithelium tissue (LFS RT-PCR) and serum samples (RT-PCR) DNA/RNA	LFS RT-RPA and real-time PCR	20 min.	1.0 × 102 copies/ reaction	Liu *et al.* (2018)
18	Pigs	*Glaesserella parasuis* disease	Synovial fluid sample DNA	RPA-LF, PCR	1 hr.	100 copies	Zhang *et al.* (2018)
19	Poultry	Newcastle disease virus (NDV) and infectious bronchitis virus (IBV)	Oropharyngeal swab DNA	RPA-nucleic acid lateral-flow (NALF) immunoassay and real-time PCR	40 min.	10 copies/reaction	Tholoth *et al.* (2019)
20	Poultry	Marek's disease virus	Tissue sample DNA/RNA	qPCR and conventional PCR	20 min.	10^2 copies/reaction	Zeng *et al.* (2019)

21	Poultry	H9N2 avian influenza virus	Cloacal swabs DNA/RNA	RT-RPA-LFD, RT-PCR	20 min.	1.5 pg copies/reaction	Wang *et al.* (2019)
22	Avians	H7 subtype avian influenza virus (IAV)	Tissue sample RNA	RT-RAA, RT-PCR, PCR	20 min.	10^2 copies/reaction	Wang *et al.* (2019)
23	Fish	*Tetracapsuloides bryosalmonae*	Kidney tissue DNA	RPA-LFD, PCR	25 min.	Ten times more than PCR	Soliman *et al.* (2018)
24	Fish	Cyprinid herpesvirus 2 (CyHV-2)	Tissue sample DNA	RPA-LFD, PCR	50 min.	30%	Wang *et al.* (2018)
25	*Hediste diversicolor*, fish	Abalone herpes-like virus (AbHV)	Brain tissue DNA/RNA	qRPA, qPCR	20 min.	100 copies/reaction	Gao *et al.* (2017)
26	Fish (koi)	Cyprinid herpesvirus 3 (CyHV-3)	Colony, white blood cell DNA	RPA, RT-PCR	20 min.	10 copies/reaction	Prescott *et al.* (2016)

introduced comparatively late as an isothermal amplification method, it is one of the fastest-developing methods. RPA is a promising tool for the identification of pathogens both at the point of treatment and in the field and should be further improved in future years. RPA as a recent technique for isothermal amplification is likely to develop thanks to its various advantages, including quick lead times, portability, trustworthiness, simplicity and sensitivity. With the increasing demand for the simultaneous detection of multiple markers, it can be expected that there will be remarkable uptake of approaches for multiplexed amplification and detection. RPA is completely compliant and truly meets the specifications of assured devices for use at the point of need. RPA technology is maturing for application in the clinic; however, it is still in a transition period towards on-site or field application. With its continued fast development, we foresee that RPA technology will ultimately become a robust mobile and point-of-need application in the future. The biggest problem for RPA kits is that they are only available from one supplier, which can directly influence pricing, and customers have little choice when formulating kits. Often available are custom-built kits, but they are costly and are only produced in low volumes. Another limitation is that the reagents are as yet only available in pellet form and there is limited flexibility of formulation. RPA reagents being available in liquid form would increase the flexibility of kit formulation, potentially facilitating easier optimization of assay conditions.

References

Assarsson, E., Lundberg, M., Holmquist, G., Björkesten, J., Thorsen, S.B., Ekman, D., & Fredriksson, S. (2014). Homogenous 96-plex PEA immunoassay exhibiting high sensitivity, specificity, and excellent scalability. *PloS One*, 9(4), e95192.

Behrmann, O., Bachmann, I., Spiegel, M., Schramm, M., El Wahed, A.A., Dobler, G., & Hufert, F.T. (2020). Rapid detection of SARS-CoV-2 by low volume real-time single tube reverse transcription recombinase polymerase amplification using an exo probe with an internally linked quencher (exo-IQ). *Clinical Chemistry*, 66(8), 1047–1054.

Bianchi, M., Riboli, B., & Magni, G. (1985). *E. coli* recA protein possesses a strand separating activity on short duplex DNAs. *The EMBO Journal*, 4(11), 3025–3030.

Daher, R.K., Stewart, G., Boissinot, M., & Bergeron, M.G. (2016). Recombinase polymerase amplification for diagnostic applications. *Clinical Chemistry*, 62(7), 947–958.

El Wahed, A.A., El-Deeb, A., El-Tholoth, M., El Kader, H.A., Ahmed, A., Hassan, S., & Weidmann, M. (2013). A portable reverse transcription recombinase polymerase amplification assay for rapid detection of foot-and-mouth disease virus. *PloS One*, 8(8), e71642.

El-Tholoth, M., Branavan, M., Naveenathayalan, A., & Balachandran, W. (2019). Recombinase polymerase amplification–nucleic acid lateral flow immunoassays for Newcastle disease virus and infectious bronchitis virus detection. *Molecular Biology Reports*, 46(6), 6391–6397.

Euler, M., Wang, Y., Nentwich, O., Piepenburg, O., Hufert, F.T., & Weidmann, M. (2012). Recombinase polymerase amplification assay for rapid detection of Rift Valley fever virus. *Journal of Clinical Virology*, 54(4), 308–312.

Fjelstrup, S., Andersen, M.B., Thomsen, J., Wang, J., Stougaard, M., Pedersen, F.S., and Knudsen, B.R. (2017). The effects of dithiothreitol on DNA. *Sensors*, 17(6), 1201.

Gahlawat, S.K., Ellis, A.E., & Collet, B. (2009). A sensitive loop-mediated isothermal amplification (LAMP) method for detection of *Renibacterium salmoninarum*, causative agent of bacterial kidney disease in salmonids. *Journal of Fish Diseases*, 32, 491–497.

Gao, F., Jiang, J.Z., Wang, J.Y., and Wei, H.Y. (2017). Real-time isothermal detection of Abalone herpes-like virus and red-spotted grouper nervous necrosis virus using recombinase polymerase amplification. *Journal of Virological Methods*, 251, 92–98.

Geng, Y., Wang, J., Liu, L., Lu, Y., Tan, K., & Chang, Y.Z. (2017). Development of real-time recombinase polymerase amplification assay for rapid and sensitive detection of canine parvovirus 2. *BMC Veterinary Research*, 13(1), 311.

Griffith, J. & Formosa, T. (1985). The uvsX protein of bacteriophage T4 arranges single-stranded and double-stranded DNA into similar helical nucleoprotein filaments. *Journal of Biological Chemistry*, 260(7), 4484–4491.

Gumaa, M.M., Cao, X., Li, Z., Lou, Z., Zhang, N., Zhang, Z., Fu, B., *et al.* (2019). Establishment of a recombinase polymerase amplification (RPA) assay for the detection of Brucella spp. Infection. *Molecular and Cellular Probes*, 47, 101434.

Hakenberg, S., Hügle, M., Weidmann, M., Hufert, F., Dame, G., & Urban, G.A. (2012). A phaseguided passive batch microfluidic mixing chamber for isothermal amplification. *Lab on a Chip*, 12(21), 4576–4580.

Higgins, M., Ravenhall, M., Ward, D., Phelan, J., Ibrahim, A., Forrest, M.S., & Campino, S. (2019). Primed RPA: Primer design for recombinase polymerase amplification assays. *Bioinformatics*, 35(4), 682–684.

Hill-Cawthorne, G.A., Hudson, L.O., Abd El Ghany, M.F., Piepenburg, O., Nair, M., Dodgson, A., & Pain, A. (2014). Recombinations in staphylococcal cassette chromosome mec elements compromise the molecular detection of methicillin resistance in Staphylococcus aureus. *PloS One*, 9(6), e101419.

Hou, P., Wang, H., Zhao, G., He, C., & He, H. (2017). Rapid detection of infectious bovine Rhinotracheitis virus using recombinase polymerase amplification assays. *BMC Veterinary Research*, 13(1), 386.

Hou, P., Zhao, G., Wang, H., He, C., Huan, Y., and He, H. (2018). Development of a recombinase polymerase amplification combined with lateral-flow dipstick assay for detection of bovine ephemeral fever virus. *Molecular and Cellular Probes*, 38, 31–37.

Kersting, S., Rausch, V., Bier, F.F., & von Nickisch-Rosenegk, M. (2014). Rapid detection of *Plasmodium falciparum* with isothermal recombinase polymerase amplification and lateral flow analysis. *Malaria Journal*, 13(1), 99.

Kim, J.Y. & Lee, J.L. (2016). Rapid detection of *Salmonella enterica* serovar enteritidis from eggs and chicken meat by real-time recombinase polymerase amplification in comparison with the two-step real-time PCR. *Journal of Food Safety*, 36(3), 402–411.

Li, J., Macdonald, J., & von Stetten, F. (2018). A comprehensive summary of a decade development of the recombinase polymerase amplification. *Analyst*, 144(1), 31–67.

Liljander, A., Yu, M., O'Brien, E., Heller, M., Nepper, J.F., Weibel, D.B., Jores, J., *et al.* (2015). Field-applicable recombinase polymerase amplification assay for rapid detection of *Mycoplasma capricolum* subsp. *capripneumoniae*. *Journal of Clinical Microbiology*, 53(9), 2810–2815.

Lillis, L., Lehman, D., Singhal, M.C., Cantera, J., Singleton, J., Labarre, P., & Overbaugh, J. (2014). Non-instrumented incubation of a recombinase polymerase amplification assay for the rapid and sensitive detection of proviral HIV-1 DNA. *PloS One*, 9(9), e108189.

Lillis, L., Siverson, J., Lee, A., Cantera, J., Parker, M., Piepenburg, O., Boyle, D.S., *et al.* (2016). Factors influencing recombinase polymerase amplification (RPA) assay outcomes at point of care. *Molecular and Cellular Probes*, 30(2), 74–78.

Liu, L., Wang, J., Zhang, R., Lin, M., Shi, R., Han, Q., Yuan, W., *et al.* (2018). Visual and equipment-free reverse transcription recombinase polymerase amplification method for rapid detection of foot-and-mouth disease virus. *BMC Veterinary Research*, 14(1), 1–8.

Liu, M.Z., Han, X.H., Yao, L.Q., Zhang, W.K., Liu, B.S., & Chen, Z.L. (2019). Development and application of a simple recombinase polymerase amplification assay for rapid point-of-care detection of feline herpesvirus type 1. *Archives of Virology*, 164(1), 195–200.

Lobato, I.M. & O'Sullivan, C.K. (2018). Recombinase polymerase amplification: basics, applications and recent advances. *Trac Trends in Analytical Chemistry*, 98, 19–35.

Londoño, M.A., Harmon, C.L., & Polston, J.E. (2016). Evaluation of recombinase polymerase amplification for detection of begomoviruses by plant diagnostic clinics. *Virology Journal*, 13(1), 1–9.

Lundberg, M., Eriksson, A., Tran, B., Assarsson, E., & Fredriksson, S. (2011). Homogeneous antibody-based proximity extension assays provide sensitive and specific detection of low-abundant proteins in human blood. *Nucleic Acids Research*, 39(15), e102.

Ma, L., Zeng, F., Cong, F., Huang, B., Zhu, Y., & Wu, M. (2018). Development and evaluation of a broadly reactive reverse transcription recombinase polymerase amplification assay for rapid detection of murine norovirus. *BMC Veterinary Research*, 14, 399.

Malik, Y.S., Verma, A.K., Kumar, N., Touil, N., Karthik, K., Tiwari, R., Abdel-Moneim, A.S., *et al.* (2019). Advances in Diagnostic approaches for viral etiologies of diarrhea: from the lab to the field. *Frontiers in Microbiology*, 10, 1957.

Mayboroda, O., Benito, A.G., Del Rio, J.S., Svobodova, M., Julich, S., Tomaso, H., O'Sullivan, C.K., & Katakis, I. (2015). Isothermal solid-phase amplification system for detection of Yersinia pestis. *Analytical and Bioanalytical Chemistry*, 408(3), 671–676.

Miao, F., Zhang, J., Li, N., Chen, T., Wang, L., Zhang, F., Zhou, X., *et al.* (2019). Rapid and sensitive recombinase polymerase amplification combined with lateral flow strip for detecting African swine fever virus. *Frontiers in Microbiology*, 10, 1004.

Monteiro, S. & Santos, R. (2017). Nanofluidic digital PCR for the quantification of Norovirus for water quality assessment. *PloS One*, 12(7), e0179985.

Moore, M.D. & Jaykus, L.A. (2016). Recombinase polymerase amplification: a promising point-of-care detection method for enteric viruses. *Future Virology*, 12(8), doi: 10.2217/fvl-2017-0034.

Piepenburg, O., Williams, C.H., Stemple, D.L., & Armes, N.A. (2006). DNA detection using recombination proteins. *PLoS Biology*, 4(7), e204.

Piepenburg, O., Armes, N.A., & Parker, M.J.D. (2011). U.S. Patent No. 8,071,308. Washington, DC: US Patent and Trademark Office.

Piepenburg, O., Williams, C.H., & Armes, N.A. (2014). Methods for multiplexing recombinase polymerase amplification. Patent US8062850B2.

Piepenburg, O., Williams, C.H., & Armes, N.A. (2018). U.S. Patent No. 9,932,577. Washington, DC: US Patent and Trademark Office.

Prescott, M.A., Reed, A.N., Jin, L., & Pastey, M.K. (2016). Rapid detection of Cyprinid herpesvirus 3 in latently infected koi by recombinase polymerase amplification. *Journal of Aquatic Animal Health*, 28(3), 173–180.

Saharan, P., Dingolia, S., Khatri, P. Duhan, J.S., & Gahlawat, S.K. (2014). Loop-mediated isothermal amplification (LAMP) based detection of bacteria: A review. *African Journal of Biotechnology*, 13(19), 1920–1928.

Shalaby, M.A., El-Deeb, A., El-Tholoth, M., Hoffmann, D., Czerny, C.P., Hufert, F.T., El Wahed, A.A., *et al.* (2016). Recombinase polymerase amplification assay for rapid detection of lumpy skin disease virus. *BMC Veterinary Research*, 12(1), 244.

Sharma, N., Hoshika, S., Hutter, D., Bradley, K.M., & Benner, S.A. (2014). Recombinase-based isothermal amplification of nucleic acids with self-avoiding molecular recognition systems (SAMRS). *ChemBioChem*, 15(15), 2268–2274.

Soliman, H., Kumar, G., & El-Matbouli, M. (2018). Recombinase polymerase amplification assay combined with a lateral flow dipstick for rapid detection of *Tetracapsuloides bryosalmonae*, the causative agent of proliferative kidney disease in salmonids. *Parasites and Vectors*, 11(1), 234.

Steyer, A., Jevšnik, M., Petrovec, M., Pokorn, M., Grosek, Š., Steyer, A.F., & Strle, F. (2016). Narrowing of the diagnostic gap of acute gastroenteritis in children 0–6 years of age using a combination of classical and molecular techniques, delivers challenges in syndromic approach diagnostics. *The Pediatric Infectious Disease Journal*, 35(9), e262.

Swift, B.M., Convery, T.W., & Rees, C.E. (2016). Evidence of *Mycobacterium tuberculosis* complex bacteremia in intradermal skin test positive cattle detected using phage-RPA. *Virulence*, 7(7), 779–788.

Wang, H., Sun, M., Xu, D., Podok, P., Xie, J., Jiang, Y., & Lu, L. (2018). Rapid visual detection of cyprinid herpesvirus 2 by recombinase polymerase amplification combined with a lateral flow dipstick. *Journal of Fish Diseases*, 41(8), 1201–1206.

Wang, J., Liu, L., Li, R., Wang, J., Fu, Q., & Yuan, W. (2016). Rapid and sensitive detection of canine parvovirus type 2 by recombinase polymerase amplification. *Archives of Virology*, 161(4), 1015–1018.

Wang, Z., Yang, P.P., Zhang, Y.H., Tian, K.Y., Bian, C.Z., & Zhao, J. (2019). Development of a reverse transcription recombinase polymerase amplification combined with lateral-flow dipstick assay for avian influenza H9N2 HA gene detection. *Transboundary and Emerging Diseases*, 66(1), 546–551.

Wee, E.J. & Trau, M. (2016). Simple isothermal strategy for multiplexed, rapid, sensitive, and accurate miRNA detection. *ACS Sensors*, 1(6), 670–675.

Wongboot, W., Okada, K., Chantaroj, S., Kamjumphol, W., & Hamada, S. (2018). Simultaneous detection and quantification of 19 diarrhea-related pathogens with a quantitative real-time PCR panel assay. *Journal of Microbiological Methods*, 151, 76–82.

Xia, X., Yu, Y., Weidmann, M., Pan, Y., Yan, S., & Wang, Y. (2014). Rapid detection of shrimp white spot syndrome virus by real time, isothermal recombinase polymerase amplification assay. *PLoS One*, 9(8), e104667.

Xu, C., Li, L., Jin, W., & Wan, Y. (2014). Recombinase polymerase amplification (RPA) of CaMV-35S promoter and nos terminator for rapid detection of genetically modified crops. *International Journal of Molecular Sciences*, 15(10), 18197–18205.

Yang, Y., Qin, X., Song, Y., Zhang, W., Hu, G., Dou, Y., Zhang, Z., *et al.* (2017). Development of real-time and lateral flow strip reverse transcription recombinase polymerase Amplification assays for rapid detection of peste des petits ruminants virus. *Virology Journal*, 14(1), 24.

Yang, Y., Qin, X., Wang, G., Jin, J., Shang, Y., and Zhang, Z. (2016). Development of an isothermal amplification-based assay for rapid visual detection of an Orf virus. *Virology Journal*, 13(1), 46.

Zeng, F., Wu, M., Ma, L., Han, Z., Shi, Y., Zhang, Y., & Liu, S. (2019). Rapid and sensitive real-time recombinase polymerase amplification for detection of Marek's disease virus. *Molecular and Cellular Probes*, 48, 101468.

Zhao, G., He, H., & Wang, H. (2019). Use of a recombinase polymerase amplification commercial kit for rapid visual detection of *Pasteurella multocida*. *BMC Veterinary Research*, 15(1), 154.

Zhao, G., Hou, P., Huan, Y., He, C., Wang, H., & He, H. (2018). Development of a recombinase polymerase amplification combined with a lateral flow dipstick assay for rapid detection of the *Mycoplasma bovis*. *BMC Veterinary Research*, 14(1), 412.

Zheng, W.B., Wu, Y.D., Ma, J.G., Zhu, X.Q., & Zhou, D.H. (2015). Recombinase polymerase amplification and its applications in parasite detection. *Zhongguo ji sheng chong xue yu ji sheng chong bing za zhi (Chinese Journal of Parasitology and Parasitic Diseases)*, 33(5), 382–386.

19

Global Rules, Regulations and Intellectual Property Rights on Diagnostic Methods

Anil Ghanghas,[1] Sarvar Gahlawat,[2] Neer Gahlawat[2] and Asha Poonia[3]
[1] Department of Law, Chaudhary Devi Lal University, Sirsa-125055, Haryana, India
[2] O.P. Jindal Global University, Sonepat-131001, Haryana, India
[3] Department of Zoology, Chaudhary Bansi Lal University, Bhiwani-127021, Haryana, India
Corresponding author: Asha Poonia, *asha.poonia@gmail.com*

19.1 Introduction

Patenting is the most common method used by developers of inventions including diagnostic methods to enjoy exclusive economic rights on their invention, which is generally for a period of 20 years (TRIPS, 1994). It can be interpreted that patents enable patent holders to have a monopoly over the use and exploitation of the patented invention. Patent monopolies and free trade do not go hand in hand and many question whether patent monopolies actually promote economic progress (Machlup and Penrose, 1950; Plomer, 2019).

There are two very different mindsets when it comes to the rationalization of patenting. The first group generally belongs to modern liberal economies such as the USA, which sees patents as incentives to the inventor for his hard work and efforts to make a new unique product. This group believes that patents promote innovation as well as economic growth (Guellec and Potterie, 2007; Daiko *et al.*, 2017). The other group includes the followers of the "social bargain", who believe that if the technical details of all inventions were disclosed from patent applications, all of society would benefit (Scotchmer, 1991). This debate has been going on for ages and both groups have valid reasons for their thinking. If we look exclusively at the health sector, the corporations most benefitted by patents are the large corporations of economically advanced Western countries (UN SG High-Level Panel, 2016).

Presently, all countries have more or less the same rules for patenting. The efforts to have similar global rules for intellectual property rights (IPR) began with the Paris Convention for the Protection of Industrial Property (1883), which was later followed by the Berne Convention for the Protection of Literary and Artistic Works (1886). Both treaties were incorporated into TRIPS (TRIPS, 1994) and IP protection was expanded in the GATT negotiations (Uruguay Round), leading to the formation of the World Trade Organization (WTO). Some recognize TRIPS as one of the most important treaties of the present century as it led to the implementation of minimum standards of intellectual property protection in all member countries of the WTO.

A focus of the present research in bio-science is the development of methods, techniques and products of industrial value, including diagnostic methods for human welfare. Patenting them can lead to successful commercial exploitation of these discoveries around the world by making them available to society at large (Trieste, 2017). Not all novel and non-obvious diagnostic methods make their way to market without patent protection. Many reasons narrow the scope of patentability of diagnostic methods due to controversy among ethics, novelty, non-obviousness, environmental safety, issues relating to expressed sequence tags (ESTs) of partial gene sequences and stem cells, and the need felt in most countries to not restrict medical professionals from carrying out their duties towards patients (Kankanala, 2007; Chandrasekharan and Deegan, 2009; Wu, 2010; Brinckerhoff, 2019). Among diagnostic methods, not all are treated equally by the patent offices and courts of various countries. What makes them unique from other practices of medicine is the evolution of diagnostics based on technology, mostly with the involvement of technicians, where doctors are involved only in the last step to make diagnosis easier, faster and more convenient and accessible. Still, developing such methods requires patent incentives for rapid advancement (Kankanala, 2007; Huys *et al.*, 2011),

In the scenario of the present race against time, the development of diagnostic methods after COVID-19 has heated the debate about the patentability of such techniques. Clear-cut rules may help in the accelerated development and wider availability of testing kits through IP sharing (Tietze *et al.*, 2020). Still, the debate about genetic diagnostic methods and whether they can be regarded as inventions is ongoing. One group renders them eligible for patent protection, while the other regards them as mere discoveries or principles of nature, or as against ethics, and advocates their exclusion from patentability (Chandrasekharan and Deegan, 2009).

It is well established that patent eligibility of diagnostic methods is different in different countries (Huys *et al.*, 2011). This leads to confusion among researchers and pharmaceutical companies who want to patent diagnostic methods. It also delays the process of development and the availability of important technologies. The IPR question is just one undervalued challenge among various others in the present scenario. Governments worldwide are facing shortages of necessary medical infrastructure, equipment and diagnostic kits for COVID-19, a cure for which is yet to be found. This has made these medical resources essential commodities whose supply is urgently required for the greater good. However, the lack of a proper IPR law system might hinder the process as manufacturing firms, especially those that were competitors before COVID-19, may not show much zeal in the development and mass manufacturing of these essential commodities.

Advances in technology also pose new and dynamic challenges to patentees and patent offices. Hence, uniform guidelines and consistent practices are the need of the hour while examining patent applications for diagnostic methods to achieve uniformity and consistency (Office of the Controller General of Patents, Designs and Trade Marks, 2013).

The present chapter focuses on the need for uniform guidelines in the patenting of diagnostic methods and calls for consistent global rules, regulations and IPR on diagnostic methods with a focus on and examples from India, the USA and Europe.

Before we proceed, it is important to know the definition of a patent. Although it has been defined by various agencies using different words (including the USPTO, Wikipedia and IP India), the gist remains the same.

> A patent is granted by a sovereign authority (usually a patent office) of a given country, conferring on its owner the exclusive right over the exploitation of the invention for a limited period of time in return for disclosing the invention to the public. Thus, in general, the patent owner (patentee) can prevent others from making, using, offering for sale, selling or importing for those purposes the patented invention without the patentee's permission. This exclusive right is given for a limited period of time, generally for 20 years from the filing date, as long as annual maintenance fees are paid, and has no effect beyond the territory of the country in which the patent was granted. In some countries, and in the case of pharmaceutical and agro-chemical inventions, this period can be extended for an additional five years, by acquiring a Supplementary Protection Certificate.
>
> (Trieste, 2017)

As almost every country addresses issues of novelty, non-obviousness and usefulness in considering patents, it is useful to discuss them in detail here.

Novelty means that the invention is new and has never appeared before in any print media or on digital platforms, television or in a seminar/conference. If the invention has been discussed anywhere before the filling of the patent application, it ceases to be novel in the global context. Thus, academicians are advised that if they invent something, they must go for the patent first, before publishing a paper on it. Use of the invention before its filing date may also destroy the novelty. Not much detailed information about patent documents is published; hence, it is critical beforehand to extensively search the literature and patent libraries to ascertain novelty for a claim. Another misconception is that a claim must be based on a large breakthrough to have novelty. In fact, an invention may be large or small when it comes to IPR. All useful modifications which have commercial value to arts, processes, products, reactants, catalysts, processes or conditions may be patented if they are novel (Saha, 2020).

Inventiveness/non-obviousness means that the claim should be such that if a skilled person from the specific specialization were to look at the claim, the technology would not be an obvious thing to him/her. Even a simple invention can be patented if it is new and improves drastically upon the existing knowledge. Moreover, unpublished patents cannot be taken into account while ascertaining the novelty of a claim. Presently, with such a magnitude of increase in technology, it is becoming difficult to establish inventiveness as it also depends on "the interpretative skills of the inventor" (Saha, 2020).

Usefulness means the claim must have a utility and a commercial value. A patent is not granted to any claim if it does not have any function/utility, however novel it may be. While a filing patent application, the uses of the claim have to be mentioned, whether it is for a product or process (Saha, 2020).

19.2 Patent Law in India

Before 2002, India did not grant patents for "any living organisms, biological materials/materials having replicating properties or substances derived from such materials and any processes for the production of living substances/entities including nucleic acids" (Article 27(3), Section 5, Part II, TRIPS, 1994). Diagnostic methods were excluded from patentability by the Indian Patents Act (Section 3(i)) along with "Medicinal methods, Surgical methods, Curative methods, Prophylactic methods, any other method of treatment of animal to render them free of disease or to increase their economic value or that of their products and any diagnosis practiced on the human or animal body…", among with various others. If diagnostic methods were used on living organisms, they were not patentable. However, if the diagnostic method was applied outside a living body such as on a dead body or any tissue/fluid taken from a living organism, it was patentable (Patent Amendment Act, 2005). Patents were awarded for surgical, therapeutic or diagnostic instruments/apparatus and fragments/ESTs if they satisfied the conditions of being useful and having commercial value along with other conditions.

Presently, India is a signatory to TRIPS (1994), the Budapest Treaty (1977), the Patent Cooperation Treaty (1998), the Paris Convention (1998) and the WTO Agreement (1995), among others. The landmark judgment in the case of *Dimminaco AG v Controller of Patents and Designs* and pressure to enforce TRIPS guidelines from the WTO allowed patent grants to processes containing living microorganisms for the first time. The Patents Act 1970 was amended by the Patents (Amendment) Act 2002 and later by the Patents (Amendment) Acts 2005 and 2006 (*Dimminaco AG v Controller of Patents and Designs*, 2002) to follow TRIPS, which allowed the patenting of microorganisms and pharmaceutical products, among others. India also has an Appellate Board for speeding up legal proceedings. This does not mean, however, that the present Indian Patent Act offers a very easy procedure for patenting diagnostic methods.

As per the Manual, any method which diagnoses a medical disorder/disease would not be patentable, whether it was performed by a medical professional or a machine (Office of the Controller General of Patents, Designs and Trademarks, 2005). Though the patent law of India is somewhat similar to EPO guidelines on the patenting of diagnostic methods, it does not have much legislative history and has not been interpreted fully by case law. Its exact scope is not clearly defined. To obtain a patent in India, the claim must fulfill the conditions of novelty, non-obviousness, usefulness and commercial value.

The Manual provides that "a method is considered to be a diagnostic method if it identifies the presence of a disorder in a person or animal suffering from a medical disorder" (Office of the Controller General of Patents, Designs and Trademarks, 2005). Presently, the Indian Patents Act gives a list of certain things which are not considered novel or inventions and hence are not patentable, which includes the following:

> (a) an invention which is frivolous or which claims anything obviously contrary to well established natural laws; (b) an invention the primary or intended use or commercial exploitation of which could be contrary to public order or morality or which causes serious prejudice to human, animal or plant life or health or to the environment; (c) the mere discovery of a scientific principle or the formulation of an abstract theory or discovery of any living thing or non-living substance occurring in nature; (d) the mere discovery of a new form of a known substance which does not result in the enhancement of the known efficacy of that substance or the mere discovery of any new property or new use for a known substance or of the mere use of a known process, machine or apparatus unless such known process results in a new product or employs at least one new reactant; (e) a substance obtained by a mere admixture resulting only in the aggregation of the properties of the components thereof or a process for producing such substance; (f) the mere arrangement or re-arrangement or duplication of known devices each functioning independently of one another in a known way; (g) Omitted by the Patents (Amendment) Act 2002: (h) a method of agriculture or horticulture; (i) any process for the medicinal, surgical, curative, prophylactic diagnostic, therapeutic or other treatment of human beings or any process for a similar treatment of animals to render them free of disease or to increase their economic value or that of their products; (j) plants and animals in whole or any part thereof other than microorganisms but including seeds, varieties and species and essentially biological processes for production or propagation of plants and animals; (k) a mathematical or business method or a computer programme per se or algorithms; (l) a literary, dramatic, musical or artistic work or any other aesthetic creation whatsoever including cinematographic works and television productions; (m) a mere scheme or rule or method of performing a mental act or method of playing a game; (n) a presentation of information; (o) topography of integrated circuits; (p) an invention which in effect is traditional knowledge or which is an aggregation or duplication of known properties of traditionally known component or components.

Hence, for the granting of a patent, first the patent seeker has to prove that their claim has novelty and does not in any way come under the above-mentioned conditions.

As most diagnostic methods involve the application of genetic resources/biotechnology in one way or another, they also come under the purview of the Biological Diversity Act, 2002. This provides a mechanism to access genetic resources and benefits which arise from them. Section 6 of the Biological Diversity Act is very important, making it compulsory to first seek approval from the National Biodiversity Authority (NBA) if Indian biological resources are being used and to disclose their source and geographical origin during any patent claim so that benefits may be shared equitably. No patent can be claimed on Indian traditional knowledge, as per Section 3(p) of Biological Diversity Act.

A patent for a diagnostic procedure is given after the fulfillment of a few other requirements, which include the inventive step and fulfilling Section 6 of the Biological Diversity Act 2002, among others (*Raj Praksh v Mangatram Chowdhury*, 1978; Biological Diversity Act, 2002). The procedure of obtaining a patent is described through the flowchart in Figure 19.1.

The judiciary has also made it clear that a claimed invention should enable the industry concerned to begin its production/use without more research, and that it should not be unnecessarily difficult to follow the instructions at the filling date itself. If the diagnostic process includes any polynucleotides/polypeptide sequences, its analogues or variants may be infinite. If such a case arises, only those variants having the specific activity with one another as described in the specification are included in the patent. If such sequences/antibodies hybridize with a specifically identified probe/target protein, then the claim will be

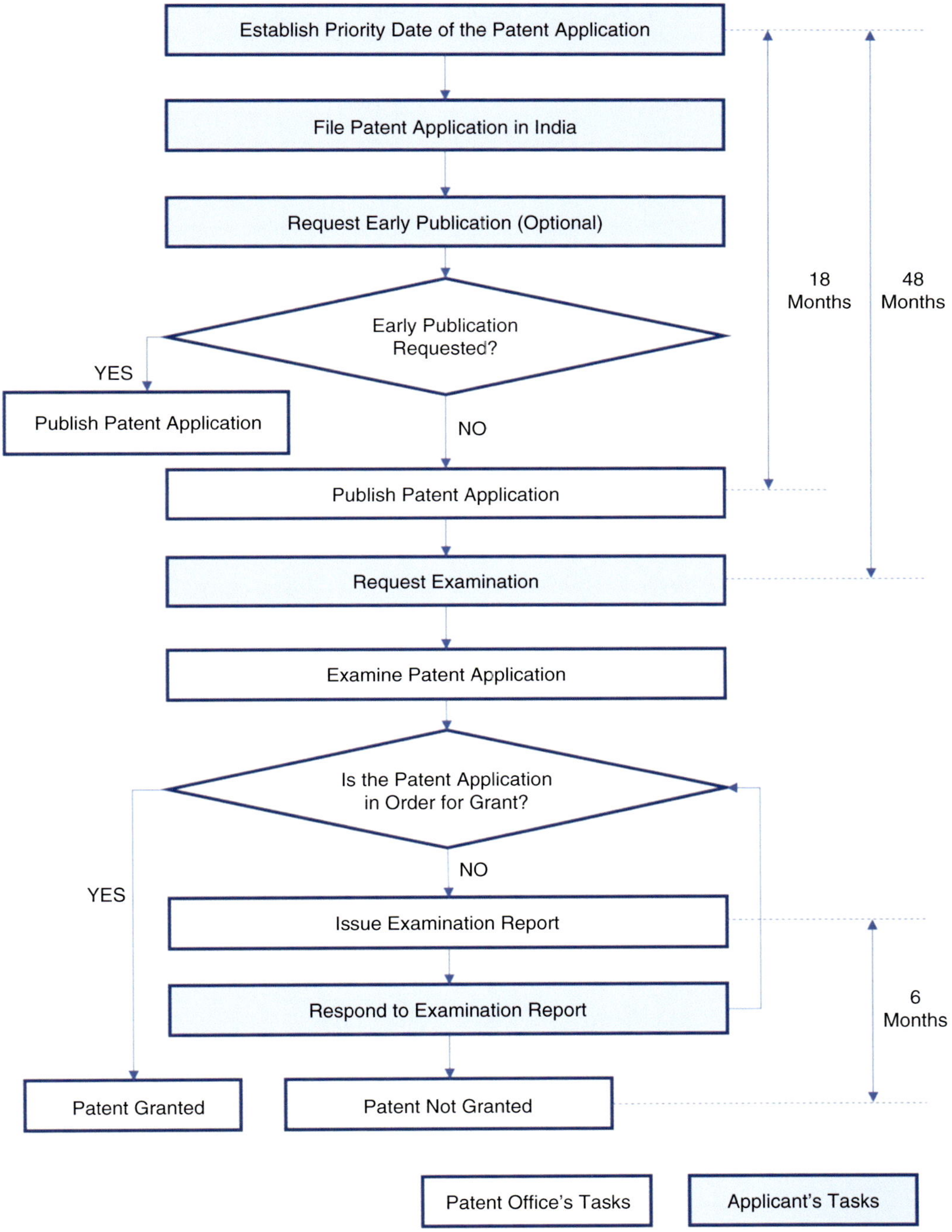

FIGURE 19.1 Flowchart showing timeline and patent grant procedure in India.
Adapted from www.invntree.com/blogs/indian-patenting-process-timeline#more-468

invalid if hybridization conditions are not specified and the role for the target protein has not been identified and proved in the specific disease.

When India amended the Patents Act in 2005 according to the TRIPS agreement, there were views that it would adversely affect India's generic pharmaceutical producers. The reasons for this were two key changes in the law: first, an increase in the patent term from 5 years to 20 years; and, second, the introduction of product patents, replacing the process patent regime. Various countries faced a dilemma over these, as their non-inclusion leads to negativity towards research and development by pharmaceutical companies, making the market anti-competitive and anti-innovative. However, an analysis of the Indian pharmaceutical industry showed that economic activities have almost remained unaffected. Even the profit rates of the Indian pharmaceutical industry were higher than for other manufacturing industry sectors of India (Dhar and Joseph, 2019).

TRIPS has also led to the departure of Indian pharmaceutical companies from their "conventional business model—exclusively #1 producing generic drugs #2 utilizing reverse engineering #3 technology" (Mitsumori, 2018). These companies have increased their investment in "Research and Development (R&D) to develop value-added generic drugs and/or new chemical entities since the mid-1990s to avoid the negative impacts of patent introduction on business performance by developing branded generic drugs #4 and brand-name drugs #5, in addition to the conventional simple generic drugs" (Mitsumori, 2018).

India dealt with these by making use of the liberty of "elbow room" by "bringing a law in a manner conducive to social and economic welfare and to a balance of rights and obligations", offered by Article 1 of TRIPS, which gives a choice to the member country for determination of the appropriate method for implementation of the provisions of this agreement (*Novartis AG v Union of India*, 2007). The Patents Act Section 3(d) states the insufficiency of a "mere discovery of a new form of a known substance which does not result in the enhancement of the known efficacy of that substance or the mere discovery of any new property or new use for a known substance or of the mere use of a known process, machine or apparatus unless such known process results in a new product or following: employs at least one new reactant". This has been explained as follows by the Patents Act: "salts, esters, ethers, polymorphs, metabolites, pure form, particle size, isomers, mixtures of isomers, complexes, combinations and other derivatives of known substance shall be considered to be the same substance, unless they differ significantly in properties with regard to efficacy". These are two very meaningful phrases when talking about diagnostic methods/procedures, as most have a key component in one form or another. This exclusion is very important to ensure that a patent can be granted only if the claim provides "enhanced efficiency" over an existing product and to avoid the "ever-greening" of patents (Technical Expert Group on Patent Law Issues, 2006). Examples of the use of these provisions can be seen in many cases, such as *Novartis AG v Union of India*. This first case to be discussed concerns when Novartis filed an appeal to Intellectual Property Appellate Board (IPAB) against the ruling of the Patent Office for a beta crystalline form of imatinib mesylate as an anti-cancer drug (*Novartis AG v Union of India*, 2007). However, the Board rejected its appeal, citing "the objective of amended section 3(d) of the Act is nothing but a requirement of higher standard of inventive step in the law particularly for the drug/pharmaceutical substances" (*Novartis AG v Union of India*, 2013). It added that the claim lacked novelty and non-obviousness to a person skilled in the art. Later, the Supreme Court also denied the patent on the same grounds. The honorable Court also clarified that Section 3(d) of the Act "clearly sets up a second tier of qualifying standards for chemical substances/pharmaceutical products in order to leave the door open for true and genuine inventions but, at the same time, to check any attempt at repetitive patenting or extension of the patent term on spurious grounds" (*Novartis AG v Union of India*, 2013).

Another important feature of Indian patent law is its adoption of compulsory licensing . Compulsory licensing is generally invoked if the patent monopoly is against the interests of the general public and is allowed only after three years of the grant of the patent. The term of three years can be neglected in cases of national or extreme emergency. Section 84 of the Patents Act clarifies the grounds of compulsory licensing, outlining under which circumstances it may be invoked:

> (a) that the reasonable requirements of the public with respect to the patented invention have not been satisfied, or (b) that the patented invention is not available to the public at a

> reasonably affordable price, or (c) that the patented invention is not worked in the territory of India.
>
> (Section 84 of the Patents Act 1970)

The only example of invocation of compulsory licensing post-TRIPS is the case of sorafenib tosylate, an anti-cancer drug which was available by the brand name Nexavar, manufactured and sold by the Bayer Corporation. Bayer charged a very high price for the drug (Rs. 2,800,000 for a month's supply), yet still it was not supplied to India in the demanded quantity. Natco Pharma Ltd. applied for licensing to produce the drug domestically and made assurances that it could produce the medicine at a much lower price (Rs. 8,000 for a month's supply). The court ruled in favor of Natco Pharma's application on the condition that it would pay Bayer 6% of the drug's net sales as a royalty (*Natco Pharma Ltd. v Bayer Corporation*, 1970).

In the last few years, India has seen much progress towards strengthening its IPR system. The first step towards this was the "National Intellectual Property Rights policy" and the "Cell for IPR Promotion and Management (CIPAM)" (National IPR Policy, 2020; CIPAM, 2020). The priorities for India are to clear patent and trademark applications and to encourage start-ups to seek protection of their IP and to file patent applications. For this, India has undertaken a large-scale digitization in the process, recruiting a large number of examiners and facilitators, which has led to massive increases in the examination as well as granting of patents.

The judiciary has also started listening more on IPR, and has begun to grant interim injunctions (which were very rare earlier in matters of IPR), which is another positive change. A recent example of this is *Sterlite Technologies v ZTT India Private* (2019). Although recent efforts have given wings to IPR in India, diagnostic methods and their development have not enjoyed changes on this scale due to Section 3 of the Indian Patents Act, which has made inventions related to derivatives of a pharmaceutical drug, stem cells, diagnostic methods and kits, and isolated DNA sequences a non-patentable matter, which has led to more examination and scrutiny in these matters (Narula, 2019). Multinational companies still are expecting better protection of their IP in India, as shown by a 2018 Special Report by the USTR (USTR Special 301 Report, 2018).

Patents for diagnostic methods have also been obtained by minutely changing a few words or phrases in patent applications to avoid legal vocabulary in many cases; for example, Patent No. 278579 was granted after the addition of "wherein the assay is not a method of diagnosis of an ailment associated with a human being and/or animal"; Patent No. 298259 was granted after an explanation: "a method of determining a value indicative of … viral infection in an untreated whole blood sample"; Patent No. 299791, after deletion of "by a method as claimed in claim 1"; Patent No. 285429 after adding that it is "an in vitro method for analyzing a sample for the presence of *Bacillus anthracis*"; Patent No. 298524 after deletion of the word "diagnostic" and the phrase "providing a sample of a bodily fluid from said subject suffering from a primary non-infectious disease" etc. However, this is not successful in every case. There are also various examples of diagnostic methods whose claims were rejected due to ambiguous interpretation of the Patents Act; for example, "a method of diagnosing liver fibrosis in a human subject, obtaining a blood sample from a human subject suspected of having liver fibrosis…"; "relating to biomarkers for COPD diagnosis to determine course of treatment"; "relating to determining the correlation between HBP levels and prediction of severe sepsis"; "relating to a method of detecting the presence or absence of a Chikungunya virus (CHIK) strain in a biological sample" etc. (Malhotra and Lakshmikumaran, 2018).

It may be concluded that the Patents Act needs to be interpreted by courts so that the ambiguity and discrepancy associated with it may be reduced. As the world is now more connected than ever and with such a fast pace of development in technology having led to a boom in research and innovation in biotechnology and medical fields, it is becoming more important for India to keep pace with rapidly changing IPR regulations throughout the globe. It should, however, be done with proper acknowledgement of the public health and social and economic conditions of the country. Presently there is a need to balance the greater good of the population by making all knowledge public and to protect the interests of pharma companies to continue more research and innovation in this field (Malhotra and Lakshmikumaran, 2018).

19.3 Patent Law in the USA

In general, the United States Patent and Trademark Office (USPTO) is responsible for the granting and issuing of patents as well as for making information regarding patents public. In US patent law, 35 USC y101 lists the general requirements for patentability, which state that "any new and useful process, machine, manufacture or composition of matter, or any new and useful improvement thereof is patentable subject to the conditions and requirements of this title." As diagnostic methods are a process, they are patentable if they satisfy all other patentability requirements.

The conditions of obtaining patents are described below, as per 35 USC y101.

1. 35 USC 102. Conditions for patentability; novelty. "A person shall be entitled to a patent unless: (1) the claimed invention was patented, described in a printed publication, or in public use, on sale, or otherwise available to the public before the effective filing date of the claimed invention; or (2) the claimed invention was described in a patent issued under section 151, or in an application for patent published or deemed published under section 122(b), in which the patent or application, as the case may be, names another inventor and was effectively filed before the effective filing date of the claimed invention."

2. 35 USC 103. Conditions for patentability; non-obvious subject matter.

> A patent for a claimed invention may not be obtained, notwithstanding that the claimed invention is not identically disclosed as set forth in section 102, if the differences between the claimed invention and the prior art are such that the claimed invention as a whole would have been obvious before the effective filing date of the claimed invention to a person having ordinary skill in the art to which the claimed invention pertains. Patentability shall not be negated by the manner in which the invention was made.

The USA has a Patent Trial and Appeal Board (PTAB) with the following functions.

> (1) on written appeal of an applicant, review adverse decisions of examiners upon applications for patents pursuant to section 134(a); (2) review appeals of reexaminations pursuant to section 134(b); (3) conduct derivation proceedings pursuant to section 135; and (4) conduct inter partes reviews and post-grant reviews pursuant to chapters 31 and 32. (c) 3-Member Panels. Each appeal, derivation proceeding, post-grant review, and inter partes review shall be heard by at least 3 members of the Patent Trial and Appeal Board, who shall be designated by the Director. Only the Patent Trial and Appeal Board may grant rehearings.

If a patent claim involves a method of manufacturing or any product which uses recombinant DNA technology for manufacturing, permission for the commercial marketing/use of the product is given after a regulatory review period (35 U.S.C. 156).

Case law establishes exceptions to patentability in the USA, which include products and laws of nature/natural phenomena/abstract ideas/basic human knowledge/thought (*Diamond v Chakrabarty*, 1980).

Section 287(c) was incorporated by the US Congress through an amendment after a hue and cry from medical professionals outraged due to Pallin's case (*Pallin v Singer*, 1995; the Omnibus Consolidated Appropriations Act, 1997). Pallin had patented a method of surgical incision to the eye which allowed it to self-heal without sutures during cataract surgery. The Court held this patent invalid as there was no novelty/non obviousness in it (*Pallin v Singer*, 1996).

There is no difference between diagnostic methods and other methods of medical treatment in the USA concerning their patentability or enforceability. However, the law treats diagnostic methods differently from other medical methods depending upon the direct involvement of doctors/medical practitioners in them. As most of the steps of diagnostic methods are performed by technicians with the involvement of doctors in the deduction step, it is comparatively easy to get a patent for such methods. The US Court of Appeals of the Federal Circuit (CAFC) in *re Bilski* ruled that a process is patentable if "it is tied to a particular machine or apparatus" or "it transforms a particular article into a different state or thing" (*re Bilski*, 2008). In *Prometheus Laboratories Inc. v Mayo Collaborative Services*, a method claim was sought in which the patient was first administered with a drug and then his metabolite rate was checked to adjust future drug doses. The CAFC declared that these steps were a "method of treatment" and were transformative in nature (Huys *et al.*, 2011). Doctors are protected from patent enforcement by US patent law but technicians, institutes or companies and other such persons/parties are not who may be involved at any step of a patented diagnostic method. Under US law these people/companies/institutions can be made liable for infringement. It can be concluded that patent law in the USA balances patent incentives which are necessary for the promotion of diagnostic technology with the right of doctors to provide adequate medical care without worrying about patents (Kankanala, 2007).

Under the US Patent Act, medical treatment methods can be patented, but Section 287(c) (1) is another section which abrogates the remedy for the infringement when it states that patents cannot be granted against medical professionals for carrying out any medical/surgical procedure which is related to the treatment of any disease of humans (35 USC 287(c)(1), 2003). This exemption is only applicable to licensed medical practitioners and does not include "machine, manufacture, or composition of matter" (35 USC 287(c)(1), 2003).

The method of getting a patent in the USA is described with the help of the flowchart in Figure 19.2, which was made by the USPTO.

More clarification on the subject was brought out by in *AMP v USPTO*, whereby the Court applied the machine-or-transformation test for the first time (*re Bilski*, 2008) for a claim on a genetic diagnostic method (*Association of Molecular Pathology v U.S. Patent and Trademark Office*, 2010). The honorable Court wanted to assess whether the method claim was only an application of a fundamental principle which is not patentable, or if the method was of a transformative character (which is patentable). The Court ordered that analyzing and comparing gene sequences is not a transformative method and hence cannot be patented (Huys *et al.*, 2011).

The Court was of the opinion that DNA isolation and sequencing are common procedures, while the invention was basically the mathematical algorithm in this case, which was not patentable (Huys *et al.*, 2011). This decision again stands in line with the famous breast cancer (BRCA) genes case (Kesselheim and Mello, 2010).

Another case where a patent was awarded for a diagnostic method after re-appeal was *re Lee*, Appeal 2017-011014 (January 14, 2019). Here the claim was for a diagnostic method to indicate that an asymptomatic person may be diagnosed for risk of colorectal cancer if all three M-dist values of SEQ ID NO: 1, 21 and 23 were found to be greater than the ninety-fifth percentile of the database's values taken from control subjects (Brinckerhoff, 2019). Here the Court said that although the claims were directed to "a law of nature", the steps included were "routine in the art". The PTAB said that the claimed steps, as an ordered combination, were not routine but "something more", for which they may be considered inventive.

Presently, for a claim for a diagnostic method to be successful, first it is determined whether it is directed to "natural law". If so, then the second step is to determine if the "patent claim is sufficient enough to be more than natural law". This step leads to the invalidation of the patent claim for a diagnostic method which contains laboratory or analytic techniques which may be used for the diagnosis of any natural physical phenomenon, even if the diagnosis carried out by them is novel. The success of these claims depends upon their innovative methods/practical applications. During the last few years, US courts have been paying a decent amount of attention to medical diagnostic methods.

One very famous case regarding medical diagnostic methods is the Athena case (*Athena Diagnostics Inc. v Mayo Collaborative Services*, 2019). The case received eight separate court opinions, of which four were concurring while four were dissenting regarding the dismissal of U.S. Patent No. 7,267,820 (the "820 Patent"), highlighting the "uncertainties and difficulties faced by courts when deciding what constitutes patent-eligible subject matter in the area of medical diagnostic methods" (Bluni and Massengill, 2019). Athena had received this patent to diagnose patients suffering from myasthenia gravis (MG). Athena submitted that MG patients produce autoantibodies which attach to a membrane protein (MuSK), which is used to diagnose MG in the said patent. Mayo asked the court to invalidate the patent, citing that the diagnostic method patented was a "law of nature". The Court used its pre-established routine from *Alice Corp. v CLS Bank Int'l* and *Mayo Collaborative Services v Prometheus Laboratories* to determine "(1) whether the claims are indeed directed to a law of nature, and if so, (2) whether the limitations of the

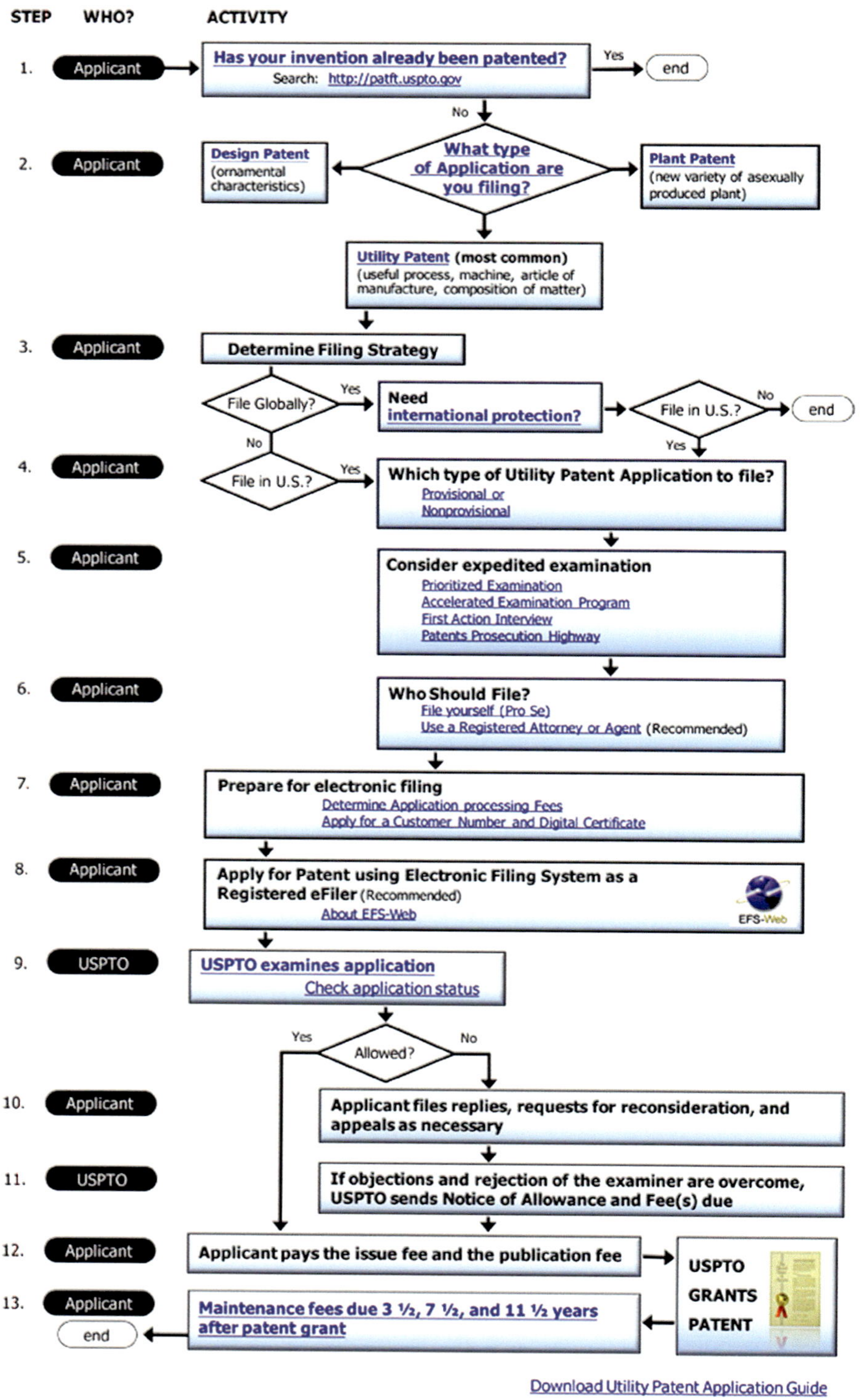

FIGURE 19.2 Flowchart showing patent grant procedure in the United States of America. Retrieved from www.uspto.gov/patents-getting-started/patent-basics/types-patent-applications/utility-patent/process-obtaining

claim apart from the law of nature, considered individually and as an ordered combination, transform the nature of the claim into a patent-eligible application as amounting to something significantly more than a patent of the natural law itself" (Bluni and Massengill, 2019).

The Court found it to be a "law of nature" and disqualified Athena from the patent. Court held that the patent only discovered the link between MuSK autoantibodies and MG. After losing at the appellate level, Athena petitioned the Federal Court to a full court of judges, but lost again.

It may be concluded that presently US courts are following a two-step process commonly called the Alice test (*Alice Corp. v CLS Bank International*, 2014) to analyze the patentability of any claim. In the first step, the claim is analyzed for a judicial exception. If the claim fails, in the second step each claim element is analyzed individually as well as in combination with other elements, leading to a concrete determination of whether the claim has added something "significantly more" than the ineligible concept. Some, however, do not agree with the excessive use of the Alice test by US courts in last few years as it may lead to a decline in research into diagnostic methods and personalized medicines (Stoll, 2019).

In view of the above, the USPTO published revised guidelines to improve consistency in the examination of patent claims for examiners (USPTO Guidelines, 2019). The guidelines provide more clarity on the second step of the Alice test.

19.4 Patent Law in Europe

In Europe, the European Patent Organisation (EPO) is the main and most powerful organization when it comes to IPR. The EPO was established in 1973 under the European Patent Convention (EPC). The EPO is responsible for the granting of European patents, which are potentially enforced in all the member countries of the EPC, unlike national patents (Article 4 EPC). While the European Patent Organisation is not a representative of European Union (EU) and is presented as a functionalist political organization, it is also a legal institution which determines patent policy and the patent laws of Europe and has the supreme authority to interpret the European Patent Convention (EPC). Practically, the EPO exercises similar functions to the EU while being insulated from national legislature control and the EU itself on IPR (Plomer, 2019). The EPC very clearly states that the Treaty creates "a system of law, common to the Contracting States, for the grant of patents for invention" (Article 1 EPC).

In Europe, the process of obtaining a patent is fairly complex. The patent application may be filed in a national patent office, or for a European patent at the EPO. EPC Article 52, Paragraph 1 holds that "patents can be granted for any inventions which are new/have inventive step and have industrial application" (Article 52, Convention on the Grant of European Patents, 2000). Paragraph 4 puts an exception on Paragraph 1 for methods for treatments of humans/animals by surgery/therapy/diagnosis to be not included as inventions even if they fulfill Paragraph 1 of Article 52, EPC (35 USC 287(c)(1), 2003). The EPC excludes these from patentability due to socio-ethical considerations. Article 53(c) of the EPC clarifies that diagnostic methods on humans are not patentable. However, those which are not directly carried out on humans may be patented. The EPC has not given any clear definition of invention but certain courts/legislators have clarified the issue (*Iogen Inc. v Medeva Plc.*, 1997). The EPC has specified that invention must have technical features, should be related to a technical field and should be concerned with a technical problem. "Technicality" is a very important aspect in qualification for a patent in Europe. EPC Articles 52(2) and 52(3) contain a list of exclusions, which include discoveries/scientific theories/methods to perform mental acts which are not regarded as inventions as their nature is abstract or non-technical in nature. These provisions, however, are not applicable to products. The Board of Appeals has also not been very clear itself and has offered conflicting opinions on the patentability of diagnostic methods, such as in *R v CYGNUS/Diagnostic method* and *Bruker/non-invasive measurement* among various others, so the enlarged Board of Appeals listened to these cases. The enlarged Board later provided clarification on the laws relating to the scope of the exclusion from patentability.

The enlarged Board of Appeal has defined diagnostic methods for the human body as containing the following four steps:

> (1) the examination phase involving the collection of data, (2) the comparison of these data with standard values, (3) the finding of any significant deviation, that is, a symptom, during the comparison and (4) the attribution of the deviation to a particular clinical picture, that is, the deductive medical or veterinary decision phase.

These steps must be incorporated for the exclusion from patentability of a diagnostic method. *In vitro* diagnostic methods, however, are patentable.

The enlarged Board of the EPO has given highly relevant findings on the matter of patentability of diagnostic methods. The Board gave a narrow definition of a diagnostic method when it clarified it as a method for "the determination of the nature of a medicinal condition intended to identify a pathology", which is not in the purview of industrial application as it is related to socio-ethical issues in general and public health in particular, and may affect the medical/veterinary professionals by patenting. However, a medical condition diagnosed with the help of a diagnostic tool is patentable. The Board explained that the criterion "practiced on the human body" is considered only while talking about the technical method steps. The last step, whereby, using all the data, deduction of the medical condition is carried out, is a purely intellectual step and is non-technical, and claims for this step are a mental act and hence are not patentable as per Article 52(2) EPC. If one wants to patent such a method, then it must first include technical steps which are not practiced on the human body. The Board also clarified that diagnostic methods which make use of *in vitro* techniques which are performed in the laboratory and not on the human body, including genetic diagnostic methods (DNA sequencing/PCR/microarrays), are of a purely technical nature and hence are patentable.

The above reason led to the patent of BRCA1 by the EPO in the T80/05, T666/08 and T1213/05 cases, for the diagnosis of breast and ovarian cancer in females. In Europe, many other claims relating to genes and genetic diagnostic methods have been patented with a narrow scope (Matthijs, 2006). The Board elaborated that it has a narrow interpretation of the diagnostic methods exclusion as Article 52 does not make reference to particular steps of diagnostic methods and it is very tough for doctors to determine to which steps of diagnostic methods the exclusion is applied. Moreover, diagnosis involves technology which also limits the role of doctors in diagnosis. Furthermore, diagnostic tool companies need patent incentives. It was further clarified by the Board that the definition of a diagnostic method should be based on essential/non-essential steps involved, and should not be defined by involvement/non-involvement of doctors/technical staff/patients. The enlarged Board added that technicality may be involved in the practice of a step of a diagnostic method on a human or animal body.

It may be concluded from the observations of the diagnostic methods enlarged Board that

> a diagnostic method practiced on the human or animal body containing the feature pertaining to the diagnosis for curative purposes as a purely intellectual exercise representing the deductive medical or veterinary decision phase as well as the features relating to the preceding steps which are constitutive for making the diagnosis and the specific interactions with the human or animal body which occur when carrying those out among said preceding steps which are of a technical nature are excluded from patentability under Article 52(4) of EPC.

Max Weber (1978) has noted that "the fundamental building block of every successful capitalist market is a secure predictability interest". A few scholars argue that it is essential "to promote economic growth and encourage investment through the adoption of predictable laws governing the marketplace and a legal regime that protects capital formation and ensures property rights" (Hirschl, 2007). Plomer has said the same about the EPO, also stating that UPC are also on the same line, with an existence parasitic on the EPO. The UPC acts as an integrated court with unitary effect (EUPUE) with the help of EPO (Regulation (EU) No. 1257/2012 of the European Parliament). The UPC has exclusive jurisdiction over the EU.

The general outline of obtaining a patent is given in Figure 19.3 with the help of a flowchart.

Once the patent is granted by the EPO, it is enforced with the same legal effect in national courts in accordance with national laws (Article 2, EPC).

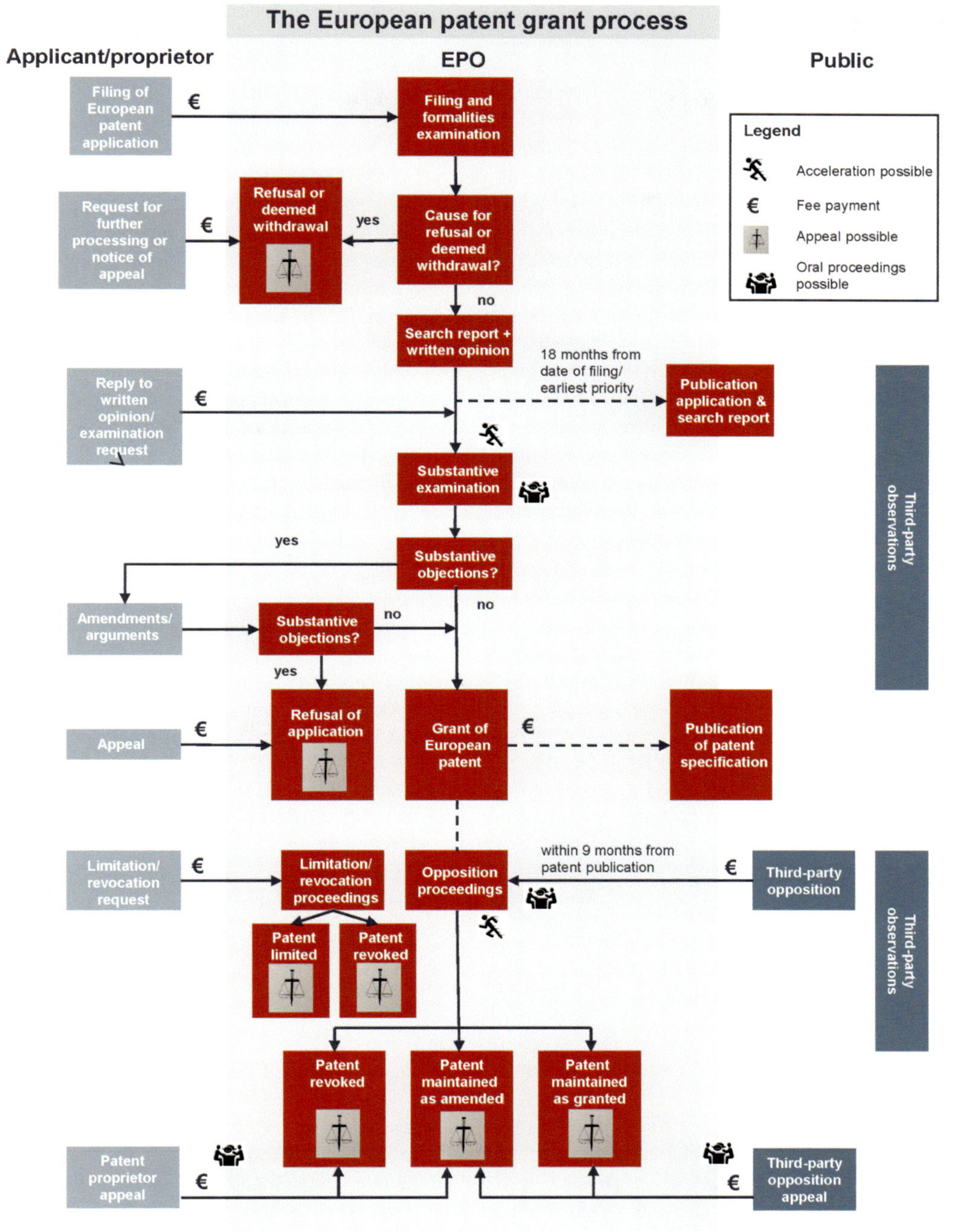

Schematic overview of the main procedural steps in the EP direct proceedings. For a complete guide to every stage of the grant procedure, please consult the Guidelines for Examination in the EPO.

FIGURE 19.3 Flowchart showing patent grant procedure in Europe.
Retrieved from www.epo.org/applying/european/Guide-for-applicants/html/e/ga_ai.html

In view of this, the European patent is also called "a bundle of patents". After granting of the patent, the applicant may designate the countries of their choice in which they wish to enforce the patent, which are generally four or five countries. The applicant will now bring proceedings in the courts of these countries only, according to their national laws. The EPC may challenge the validity of any patent at the

EPO. There are several divisions in the EPO. It also includes an internal appeals procedure which may be against patents by the examining division. It may also lead to invalidation of previously granted patents for lack of any of the conditions for patentability, such as novelty/inventive step/industrial application. Part V of the EPC details the opposition procedure. Another very important decision-making body of the EPO is the Technical Board of Appeal, whose details may be obtained from the EPO's official website where the details are given in "case law". Member states' national courts do not have a legal obligation to follow the case law of the EPO, but as they have agreed to the uniform legal structure of the EPO, they try to follow the EPO's interpretation of case law (Plomer, 2019). Hence, the EPO is the main decision-making body with authority and discretion on the interpretation of EPC guidelines on all matters related to IPR. Due to different opinions while interpreting EPC rules and guidelines, different national courts may sometimes have different opinions over the same patent (Graham and Zeebroeck, 2014). This is one of the main reasons for the creation of a Unified Patent Court (UPC) by the EU, which is a single, central court for the post-grant enforcement of patents (Ullrich, 2002).

It is very clear from the above that while considering diagnostic methods, the guidelines laid by the enlarged Board of Appeals are followed in Europe. As diagnosis in general or diagnostic methods involve technology generally in the form of a tool or methods whose intermediate steps are patentable, it can be concluded that Europe ensures the availability of patent incentives to pharmaceutical companies and researchers to promote research and development of diagnostic methods while their scope of exclusion is narrow. European patent law also protects medical professionals by excluding diagnostic methods which involve all the four steps mentioned earlier.

19.5 Analysis and Conclusion

Presently, not much attention is being given to IPR among public laws, as observed in the international conference "Courts, Power and Public Law". The conference included many presentations on constitutional and international courts, commercial tribunals and the World Trade Organization (WTO), but just one panel addressed the topic of intellectual property and specialist patent courts.

There are two schools of thought while talking about patenting in medical methods. One believes that IPR rights have a negative effect on the diffusion of knowledge, referring to them as "neo-colonism" (Boyle, 2008; Drahos, 2010; Heller, 1998; Maskus and Reichman, 2004; Stiglitz, 1999; Plomer, 2015) and suggesting that they have erected barriers against fundamental human rights. One example of this school of thought was the suit against the Mandela government by 39 pharmaceutical companies to oblige TRIPS in South Africa against the import of generic, lifesaving, essential medicines during the AIDS crisis, when 8 million lives were at stake (Médecins Sans Frontières, 2001). This situation may arise amid the COVID-19 outbreak in the present scenario.

A UN panel has also reported that patent monopolies lead to higher costs of drugs and other essential lifesaving commodities and prevent their access, especially in developing countries (UN SG High Level Panel, 2016). Another important point raised concerns the controversial decisions in similar cases as discussed earlier in this chapter.

Another school of thought strongly believes that "IPR rights are very important in the face of changing trade environment which is characterized by … global competition, high innovation risks, short product cycle, need for rapid changes in technology, high investments in research and development (R&D), production and marketing and need for highly skilled human resources" (Saha, 2020). It insists that drugs and pharmaceuticals require large funding to complete research and development (R&D), citing that the introduction of new drug may cost from $300 million to $600 million (Saha, 2020).

While both the arguments are valid, it cannot be overlooked that the "free flow of information saves life" in every area (Page, 2020). If China had told the world about the new coronavirus in time, i.e., December 2019 itself, when Dr Li Wenling first raised the alarm (BBC News, 2020), the world may have been a little different today (Johnson and Bailey, 2020). It can also be deducted that if a low standard is maintained while granting patents, which are costly to challenge and are able to distress markets, it will lead to "ever-greening" by pharmaceutical corporations, leading to detrimental consequences. It is necessary to have checks on this (Breyer, 1998).

A special body of judges as appointed by the EPO in a CJEU which specializes in patent laws is a great step, as this is a very technical field, the most important part of the law being determining whether the claim is really an invention or contains an "innovative step". This requires a "high level of technical knowledge in highly specialized field", as judges normally lack such specialization (WIPO, 2018).

Patent law throughout the world faces challenges while trying to balance the patent incentives for researchers and pharmaceutical companies for rapid development and research in the field of medical technology against the protection of the interests of medical professionals. Different countries try to achieve this objective using different methods, the USA by "limiting enforceability of diagnostic methods against medical practitioners" and Europe by "construing the scope of diagnostic methods excluded from patentability narrowly". India, however, provides incentives to researchers and pharmaceutical companies by "allowing *in vitro* diagnostic methods and intermediate steps in a diagnostic method to be patentable but the scope and extent of excluded methods is not clear" (Huys *et al.*, 2011). This chapter finally concludes that uniform diagnostic method patent models are the need of the hour to stop unnecessary chaos especially in the present scenario of a novel coronavirus (Johnson and Bailey, 2020; Tietze *et al.*, 2020).

References

Alice Corp. v CLS Bank International, 573 U.S. 208 (2014).

Association of Molecular Pathology v U.S. Patent and Trademark Office, USDC SDNY 09 Civ. 4515 (2010).

Athena Diagnostics Inc. v Mayo Collaborative Services LLC, No. 17-2508 (Fed. Cir. 2019) (2019).

BBC News (2020) Li Wenliang: Coronavirus Kills Chinese Whistleblower Doctor, BBC News (March 7), retrieved from www.bbc.com/news/world-asia-china-51403795 on April 4, 2020.

Bluni S, Massengill B (2019) Understanding Medical Diagnostic Method Patent Eligibility, Med Device Online (July 31), retrieved from www.meddeviceonline.com/doc/understanding-medical-diagnostic-method-patent-eligibility-0002 on April 15, 2020.

Boyle J (2008) *The Public Domain: Enclosing the Commons of the Mind*. Yale University Press.

Breyer S (1998) The Interdependence of Science and Law. *Judicature* 82: 25.

Brinckerhoff CC (2019) A Patent-Eligible Diagnostic Method Claim, Pharma Patents (October 1), retrieved from www.foley.com/en/insights/publications/2019/10/a-patent-eligible-diagnostic-method-claim on April 23, 2020.

Bruker/non-invasive measurement, Technical Board of Appeal 3.4.1, E.P.O.R. 357 (1988).

Chandrasekharan S, Cook-Deegan R (2009) Gene Patents and Personalized Medicine – What Lies Ahead? *Genome Medicine* 1: 92.

Daiko T, Dernis H, Dosso M, *et al.* (2017) *World Corporate Top R&D Investors: Industrial Property Strategies in the Digital Economy*. A JRC and OECD Common Report, Publications Office of the European Union.Dhar B, Joseph RK (2019) The Challenges, Opportunities and Performance of the Indian Pharmaceutical Industry Post-TRIPS. In Liu KC, Racherla U (eds) *Innovation, Economic Development, and Intellectual Property in India and China*. ARCIALA Series on Intellectual Assets and Law in Asia. Springer, pp. 299–323.

Diagnostic Methods, Enlarged Board of Appeal, G1/04 (2006).

Diamond v Chakrabarty, 447 US 303 (1980).

Dimminaco AG v Controller of Patents and Designs, I.P.L.R. July 255, Kolkata High Court (2002).

Drahos P (2010) *The Global Governance of Knowledge: Patent Offices and their Clients*. Cambridge University Press.

Graham SJH, Zeebroeck N (2014) Comparing Patent Litigation across Europe: A First Look. *Stanford Technology Law Review* 17: 655.

Guellec D, de la Potterie BVP (2007) *The Economics of the European Patent System: IP Policy for Innovation and Competition*. Oxford University Press.

Heller MA (1998) The Tragedy of the Anticommons: Property in the Transition from Marx to Markets. *Harvard Law Review* 111: 621–688.

Hirschl R (2007) *Towards Juristocracy: The Origins and Consequences of the New Constitutionalism*. Harvard University Press.

Huys I, Van Overwalle G, Matthijs G (2011) Gene and Genetic Diagnostic Method Patent Claims: A Comparison under Current European and US Patent law. *European Journal of Human Genetics* 19: 1104–1107.
ICON-S (2017) Conference on "Courts, Power, Public Law", Copenhagen, July 5–7, 2017.
Iogen Inc. v. Medeva Plc, Hepatitis-B-virus, R.P.C. 1 (41–42) (1997).Johnson EE, Bailey TC (2020) Urgent Legal Lessons from a Very Fast Problem: COVID-19. *Stanford Law Review Online*.
Kankanala KC (2007) "Diagnostic Method" Patent Model: Patent Incentives and Socio-Ethical Concerns. *Journal of Intellectual Property Rights* 12: 104–110.
Kesselheim AS, Mello MM (2010) Gene Patenting: Is the Pendulum Swinging Back? *New England Journal of Medicine* 362: 1855–1858.
Machlup F, Penrose E (1950) The Patent Controversy in the Nineteenth Century. *The Journal of Economic History* 10: 1–29.
Malhotra D, Lakshmikumaran M (2018) Scope of Section 3(i): An Analysis on Diagnostic Methods of Treatment (November 21), retrieved from www.lakshmisri.com/insights/articles/scope-of-section-3-i-an-analysis-on-diagnostic-methods-of-treatment/# on April 30, 2020.
Maskus KE, Reichman JH (2004) The Globalization of Private Knowledge Goods and the Privatization of Global Public Goods. *Journal of International Economic Law* 7: 279.
Matthijs G (2006) The European Opposition against the BRCA Gene Patents. *Familial Cancer* 5: 95–102.
Mayo v. Prometheus, 566 U.S. 66 (2012).
Médecins Sans Frontières (2001) 39 Drug Companies vs South Africa: People Die for Affordable Drugs as Inhumane Industry Ignores Reality. Press release, March 5, 2001.
Mitsumori Y (2018) *The Indian Pharmaceutical Industry: Impact of Changes in the IPR Regime*. Springer.
National IPR Policy (2020) National IPR Policy, Department for Promotion of Industry and Internal Trade, retrieved from www.dipp.gov.in as retrieved from https://dipp.gov.in/policies-rules-and-acts/policies/national-ipr-policy on April 24, 2020.
Narula R (2019) India: Challenges Faced in the Protection and Enforcement of Patent Rights, Managing IP (September 18), retrieved from www.managingip.com/article/b1kbm12wlgsgt6/india-challenges-faced-in-the-protection-and-enforcement-of-patent-rights on April 24, 2020.
Natco Pharma Ltd. v Bayer Corporation, Application for Compulsory Licence Under Section 84(1) of the Patents Act, 1970 in respect of Patent No. 215758.
Novartis AG v Union of India, High Court of Madras (2007).
Novartis AG v Union of India, The Supreme Court of India (2013).
Office of the Controller General of Patents, Designs and Trademarks (2005) Manual of Patent Practice and Procedure, retrieved from www.ipindia.nic.in/writereaddata/Portal/Images/pdf/Manual_for_Patent_Office_Practice_and_Procedure_.pdf on March 22, 2020.
Office of the Controller General of Patents, Designs and Trademarks (2011) Manual of Patent Practice and Procedure, retrieved from https://ipindia.gov.in/writereaddata/Portal/IPOGuidelinesManuals/1_28_1_manual-of-patent-office-practice_and-procedure.pdf on February 12, 2021.
Office of the Controller General of Patents, Designs and Trademarks (2019) Guidelines for Examination of Biotechnology Applications for Patent, retrieved from www.ipindia.nic.in/writereaddata/Portal/IPOGuidelinesManuals/1_38_1_4-biotech-guidelines.pdf on April 12, 2020.
Page J (2020) China's Early Missteps Fed Epidemic: As Doctors Raised Alarms, Officials Dragged their Feet to Take Action against the Coronavirus, *Wall Street Journal* (March 7), A1.
Pallin v Singer, 1995 WL 608365 (D Vt, 1995) (1995).
Pallin v Singer, 1996 WL 274407 (D Vt, 1996) (1996).
Plomer A (2015) *Patents, Human Rights and Access to Science*. Edward Elgar.
Plomer A (2019) The EPO as Patent Law-maker in Europe. *European Law Journal* 25(1): 57–74.
Prometheus Laboratories, Inc. v Mayo Collaborative Services, No. 2008–1403 (Fed. Cir. 2009) (2009).
R v CYGNUS/Diagnostic method, Technical Board of Appeal 3.4.1, E P O R 280 (2002).
Raj Praksh v Mangatram Chowdhury, AIR (1978).
re Bilski, 545 F.3d at 961-2 (Fed. Cir. 2008) (2008).
Saha R (2020) Management of Intellectual Property Rights in India, retrieved from www.pfc.org.in/workshop/workshop.pdf on March 15, 2020.
Scotchmer S (1991) Standing on the Shoulders of Giants: Cumulative Research and the Patent Law. *Journal of Economic Perspectives* 5(1): 29–41.

Sterlite Technologies v ZTT India Private, CS [COMM] 314/2019, IA No. 8386/2019, IA No. 8389/2019 & IA No. 8390/2019 (2019).

Stiglitz JE (1999) Knowledge as a Global Public Good. In Kaul I, Grunberg I, Stern M (eds) *Global Public Goods: International Cooperation in the 21st Century*. Oxford University Press, pp. 308–326.

Stoll R (2019) What Happens to Diagnostic Method Patents After *Athena*?, IP Watchdog (March 6), retrieved from www.ipwatchdog.com/2019/03/06/diagnostic-method-patents-athena/id=107058/ on April 25, 2020.

Technical Expert Group on Patent Law Issues (2006), Report of the Technical Expert Group on Patent Law Issues, retrieved from www.ipindia.nic.in/writereaddata/images/pdf/report-of-technical-expert-group.pdf on April 30, 2020.

Tietze PF, Vimalnath P, Aristodemou L, Molloy J (2020) Crisis-Critical Intellectual Property: Findings from the COVID-19 Pandemic. arXiv:2004.03715 2020. https://doi.org/10.17863/CAM.51142.

TRIPS (1994), Trade Related Agreement on Intellectual Property Rights, retrieved from www.wto.org/english/docs_e/legal_e/27-trips_01_e.htm on April 30, 2020.

Ullrich H (2002) Patent Protection in Europe: Integrating Europe into the Community or the Community into Europe? *European Law Journal* 4: 433–491.

UN SG High Level Panel (2016) United Nations Secretary-General's High-Level Panel on Access to Medicines Report, retrieved from www.unsgaccessmeds.org/final-report on April 30, 2020.

USPTO (n.d.) Patent Process Overview, retrieved from www.uspto.gov/patents/basics/patent-process-overview on March 23, 2020.

USPTO (2019), USPTO Guidelines, retrieved from www.uspto.gov/patent/laws-and-regulations/examination-policy/subject-matter-eligibility on March 23, 2020.

USTR (2018), USTR Special 301 Report, retrieved from https://ustr.gov/sites/default/files/files/Press/Reports/2018%20Special%20301.pdf on April 24, 2020.

Weber M (1978) *Economy and Society: An Outline of Interpretive Sociology*. Berkeley, CA: University of California Press.

WIPO (2018) World Intellectual Property Indicators 2018, retrieved from www.wipo.int/publications/en/details.jsp?id=4369 on February 13, 2021.Wu G (2010) Patenting Biotech beyond the Central doçgma. *Nature Biotechnology* 28: 230–233.

Index